ANDROGENS IN HEALTH AND DISEASE

CONTEMPORARY ENDOCRINOLOGY

P. Michael Conn, SERIES EDITOR

Androgens in Health and Disease, edited by
CARRIE J. BAGATELL AND WILLIAM J. BREMNER,
2003

*Endocrine Replacement Therapy in Clinical
Practice,* edited by A. WAYNE MEIKLE, 2003

Early Diagnosis of Endocrine Diseases, edited
by ROBERT S. BAR, 2003

Type I Diabetes: Etiology and Treatment, edited
by MARK A. SPERLING, 2003

Handbook of Diagnostic Endocrinology, edited
by JANET E. HALL AND LYNNETTE K. NIEMAN,
2003

*Pediatric Endocrinology: A Practical Clinical
Guide,* edited by SALLY RADOVICK
AND MARGARET H. MACGILLIVRAY, 2003

Diseases of the Thyroid, Second Edition, edited
by LEWIS E. BRAVERMAN, 2003

*Developmental Endocrinology: From Research
to Clinical Practice,* edited by ERICA A.
EUGSTER AND ORA HIRSCH PESCOVITZ, 2002

*Osteoporosis: Pathophysiology and Clinical
Management,* edited by ERIC S. ORWOLL
AND MICHAEL BLIZIOTES, 2002

Challenging Cases in Endocrinology, edited by
MARK E. MOLITCH, 2002

*Selective Estrogen Receptor Modulators:
Research and Clinical Applications,* edited
by ANDREA MANNI AND MICHAEL F.
VERDERAME, 2002

Transgenics in Endocrinology, edited by
MARTIN MATZUK, CHESTER W. BROWN,
AND T. RAJENDRA KUMAR, 2001

*Assisted Fertilization and Nuclear Transfer in
Mammals,* edited by DON P. WOLF
AND MARY ZELINSKI-WOOTEN, 2001

Adrenal Disorders, edited by ANDREW N. MARGIORIS
AND GEORGE P. CHROUSOS, 2001

Endocrine Oncology, edited by STEPHEN P. ETHIER,
2000

*Endocrinology of the Lung: Development
and Surfactant Synthesis,* edited by
CAROLE R. MENDELSON, 2000

Sports Endocrinology, edited by MICHELLE P.
WARREN AND NAAMA W. CONSTANTINI, 2000

Gene Engineering in Endocrinology, edited by
MARGARET A. SHUPNIK, 2000

Endocrinology of Aging, edited by JOHN E.
MORLEY AND LUCRETIA VAN DEN BERG, 2000

*Human Growth Hormone: Research
and Clinical Practice,* edited by
ROY G. SMITH AND MICHAEL O. THORNER,
2000

Hormones and the Heart in Health and Disease,
edited by LEONARD SHARE, 1999

Menopause: Endocrinology and Management,
edited by DAVID B. SEIFER
AND ELIZABETH A. KENNARD, 1999

*The IGF System: Molecular Biology,
Physiology, and Clinical Applications,*
edited by RON G. ROSENFELD
AND CHARLES T. ROBERTS, JR., 1999

*Neurosteroids: A New Regulatory Function
in the Nervous System,* edited by
ETIENNE-EMILE BAULIEU, MICHAEL SCHUMACHER,
AND PAUL ROBEL, 1999

Autoimmune Endocrinopathies, edited by
ROBERT VOLPÉ, 1999

Hormone Resistance Syndromes, edited by
J. LARRY JAMESON, 1999

Hormone Replacement Therapy, edited by
A. WAYNE MEIKLE, 1999

Insulin Resistance: The Metabolic Syndrome X,
edited by GERALD M. REAVEN AND AMI LAWS,
1999

Endocrinology of Breast Cancer, edited by
ANDREA MANNI, 1999

Molecular and Cellular Pediatric Endocrinology,
edited by STUART HANDWERGER, 1999

Gastrointestinal Endocrinology, edited by
GEORGE H. GREELEY, JR., 1999

The Endocrinology of Pregnancy, edited by
FULLER W. BAZER, 1998

Clinical Management of Diabetic Neuropathy,
edited by ARISTIDIS VEVES, 1998

G Proteins, Receptors, and Disease, edited by
ALLEN M. SPIEGEL, 1998

Natriuretic Peptides in Health and Disease,
edited by WILLIS K. SAMSON
AND ELLIS R. LEVIN, 1997

Endocrinology of Critical Disease, edited by
K. PATRICK OBER, 1997

*Diseases of the Pituitary: Diagnosis and
Treatment,* edited by
MARGARET E. WIERMAN, 1997

Endocrinology of the Vasculature, edited by
JAMES R. SOWERS, 1996

ANDROGENS

IN HEALTH

AND DISEASE

Edited by

CARRIE J. BAGATELL, MD

Clinical Assistant Professor
Department of Medicine
University of Washington School of Medicine
Seattle, WA

and

WILLIAM J. BREMNER, MD, PhD

The Robert G. Petersdorf Professor and Chairman
Department of Medicine
University of Washington School of Medicine
Seattle, WA

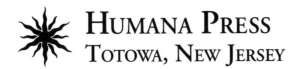

HUMANA PRESS
TOTOWA, NEW JERSEY

BS

The content and opinions expressed in this book are the sole work of the authors and editors, who have warranted due diligence in the creation and issuance of their work. The publisher, editors, and authors are not responsible for errors or omissions or for any consequences arising from the information or opinions presented in this book and make no warranty, express or implied, with respect to its contents.

Due diligence has been taken by the publishers, editors, and authors of this book to assure the accuracy of the information published and to describe generally accepted practices. The contributors herein have carefully checked to ensure that the drug selections and dosages set forth in this text are accurate and in accord with the standards accepted at the time of publication. Notwithstanding, since new research, changes in government regulations, and knowledge from clinical experience relating to drug therapy and drug reactions constantly occur, the reader is advised to check the product information provided by the manufacturer of each drug for any change in dosages or for additional warnings and contraindications. This is of utmost importance when the recommended drug herein is a new or infrequently used drug. It is the responsibility of the treating physician to determine dosages and treatment strategies for individual patients. Further, it is the responsibility of the health care provider to ascertain the Food and Drug Administration status of each drug or device used in their clinical practice. The publishers, editors, and authors are not responsible for errors or omissions or for any consequences from the application of the information presented in this book and make no warranty, express or implied, with respect to the contents in this publication.

This publication is printed on acid-free paper. ∞

ANSI Z39.48-1984 (American National Standards Institute) Permanence of Paper for Printed Library Materials.

Cover design by Patricia F. Cleary.
Production Editor: Jessica Jannicelli.

For additional copies, pricing for bulk purchases, and/or information about other Humana titles, contact Humana at the above address or at any of the following numbers: Tel: 973-256-1699; Fax: 973-256-8341; E-mail: humana@humanapr.com or visit our website at http://humanapress.com

Photocopy Authorization Policy:
Authorization to photocopy items for internal or personal use, or the internal or personal use of specific clients, is granted by Humana Press Inc., provided that the base fee of US $20.00 per copy is paid directly to the Copyright Clearance Center at 222 Rosewood Drive, Danvers, MA 01923. For those organizations that have been granted a photocopy license from the CCC, a separate system of payment has been arranged and is acceptable to Humana Press Inc. The fee code for users of the Transactional Reporting Service is: [1-58829-029-8/03 $20.00].

Printed in the United States of America. 10 9 8 7 6 5 4 3 2 1

Library of Congress Cataloging-in-Publication Data

Androgens in health and disease / edited by Carrie Bagatell and William J. Bremner.
      p. ; cm.
   Includes bibliographical references and index.
   ISBN 1-58829-029-8 (alk. paper) eISBN 1-59259-388-7
    1. Androgens--Physiological effect. 2. Androgens--Therapeutic use. I. Bagatell, Carrie,
MD. II. Bremner, William J.
   [DNLM: 1. Androgens--physiology. 2. Androgens--therapeutic use. 3. Gonadal
Disorders--drug therapy. WJ 875 A5746 2003]
   QP572.A5.A538 2003
   612.6'1--dc21

                                                                                2003043012

8/27/04

PREFACE

The products of the testes have been recognized as essential to the development and maintenance of male physique and virility since ancient times. However, only in the past few decades has the entire spectrum of influence and action of testosterone, its metabolites, and its analogs begun to be fully investigated and appreciated. As we understand more about how androgens act and how they influence a myriad of physiological functions, we are able to use androgens in a wider variety of clinical settings. Unfortunately, use is frequently accompanied by abuse; over the last 20 years, abuse of anabolic agents has become widespread in some communities of athletes, sometimes with untoward consequences.

In *Androgens in Health and Disease,* we have brought together reviews of our latest understanding of andrology in both basic science and clinical medicine. In the first section of the book, the biology of androgens, androgen metabolites, and androgen receptors is presented from several different perspectives. We hope that clinicians as well as basic scientists will find this section useful. The next two sections explore the roles of androgens in development and in the modulation of a wide variety of physiologic systems. Although the lay public tends to view androgens primarily as agents of virility and muscularity, androgens actually regulate nearly every physiologic system in some way, as these chapters demonstrate.

In the last two sections of the book, several newer uses of androgens are presented. Most endocrinologists and urologists, as well as some practitioners with broader scopes of practice, are familiar with the use of androgens in delayed puberty and in young men with acquired hypogonadism. However, fewer clinicians are aware that testosterone can be a useful adjunct to the treatment of many other disease states, particularly those in which catabolism and loss of muscle mass occur. In addition, it is becoming increasingly apparent that many older men experience "andropause," analogous but certainly not identical to menopause. Although not appropriate for all older men, androgens may improve physical function and enhance the quality of life for many individuals. As with hormone replacement, the development of hormonal male contraception lags far behind that which is available for women. However, several recent studies have demonstrated the potential utility of androgens, often combined with other hormonal agents, in suppressing spermatogenesis consistently and reversibly. These potential indications are much more prevalent than is "classical" hypogonadism, and thus the potential future uses of androgens as therapeutic agents are extensive.

The last section of the book presents recent developments in the role of androgens in regulating female physiology. Excessive androgens, either in the serum or at the tissue level, can cause a wide range of symptoms and physical findings in women, and hyperandrogenism may also be associated with an increased risk of cardiovascular disease. Conversely, androgen deficiency in women is not often recognized, but it too may impact the physical and emotional well-being of women, particularly after menopause.

We hope *Androgens in Health and Disease* will serve as a valuable resource to researchers and clinicians alike and will broaden the reader's concept of how and why androgens exert their effects. We are grateful to all of the authors for contributing their time and expertise to this endeavor. We offer sincere thanks to Ms. Tetana Oguara for her expert and enthusiastic support in coordinating and compiling the manuscripts.

Carrie Bagatell, MD
William J. Bremner, MD, PhD

CONTENTS

Preface .... *v*

Contributors .... *ix*

I   GENERAL ANDROLOGY

1   Testosterone Synthesis, Transport, and Metabolism
Stephen J. Winters and Barbara J. Clark *3*

2   Androgen Action
Terry R. Brown *23*

3   Hypogonadism in Men: *An Overview*
Stephen R. Plymate *45*

4   Dihydrotestosterone and 5α-Reductase: *Normal Physiology
and Inhibition*
Paul R. Sutton, John K. Amory, and Richard V. Clark *77*

5   Estrogen Action in Males: *Insights Through Mutations
in Aromatase and Estrogen-Receptor Genes*
Jonathan Lindzey and Kenneth S. Korach *89*

6   Alterations of Androgen Action Caused by Mutation
of the Human Androgen Receptor
Michael J. McPhaul *103*

7   Androgen Excess Disorders in Women
Richard S. Legro *123*

8   Androgen Pharmacology and Delivery Systems
Christina Wang and Ronald S. Swerdloff *141*

II   ANDROGEN EFFECTS ON PHYSIOLOGIC SYSTEMS

9   Androgen Signaling in Prostatic Neoplasia and Hyperplasia
*Marco Marcelli, Dolores J. Lamb, Nancy L. Weigel,
and Glenn R. Cunningham* *157*

10   Androgens and Coronary Artery Disease
Frederick C. W. Wu and Arnold von Eckardstein *191*

11   Androgens and Bone
Anne M. Kenny and Lawrence G. Raisz *221*

12   Androgens and the Hematopoietic System
Shehzad Basaria and Adrian S. Dobs *233*

13   Androgens and Body Composition
     Laurence Katznelson *243*

14   Androgens and Sexual Function in Men and Women
     John Bancroft...*259*

15   Androgens and Cognition
     Monique M. Cherrier and Suzanne Craft *291*

III APPLIED ANDROLOGY

16   Androgen Treatment of the Hypogonadal Male
     Alvin M. Matsumoto *313*

17   Androgens and Puberty
     Erick J. Richmond and Alan D. Rogol *335*

18   Androgens in Older Men
     J. Lisa Tenover *347*

19   Rationale for Treating Hypoandrogenism in Women
     Susan R. Davis *365*

20   Androgens as Anabolic Agents
     Shalender Bhasin, Linda J. Woodhouse,
     and Thomas W. Storer *381*

21   Androgens and Male Contraception
     John K. Amory *405*

22   Androgens in Primary Care
     Bradley D. Anawalt *419*

Index *439*

CONTRIBUTORS

JOHN K. AMORY, MD, *Department of Medicine, University of Washington School of Medicine, Seattle, WA*

BRADLEY D. ANAWALT, MD, *Department of Medicine, VA Puget Sound Health Care System, Seattle, WA*

CARRIE J. BAGATELL, MD, *Department of Medicine, University of Washington School of Medicine, Seattle, WA*

JOHN BANCROFT, MD, *The Kinsey Institute for Research in Sex, Gender, and Reproduction, Indiana University, Bloomington, IN*

SHEHZAD BASARIA, MD, *Division of Endocrinology, Department of Medicine, Johns Hopkins University School of Medicine, Baltimore, MD*

SHALENDER BHASIN, MD, *Division of Endocrinology, Metabolism, and Molecular Medicine, Department of Internal Medicine, Charles R. Drew University of Medicine and Science, Los Angeles, CA*

WILLIAM J. BREMNER, MD, PhD, *Department of Medicine, University of Washington School of Medicine, Seattle, WA*

TERRY R. BROWN, PhD, *Department of Biochemistry and Molecular Biology, Johns Hopkins University Bloomberg School of Public Health, Baltimore, MD*

MONIQUE M. CHERRIER, PhD, *Department of Psychiatry and Behavioral Sciences, University of Washington School of Medicine, Seattle, WA*

BARBARA J. CLARK, PhD, *Department of Biochemistry and Molecular Biology, University of Louisville, Louisville, KY*

RICHARD V. CLARK, MD, PhD, *GlaxoSmithKline, Research Triangle Park, NC*

SUZANNE CRAFT, PhD, *Department of Psychiatry and Behavioral Sciences, University of Washington School of Medicine; and VA Puget Sound Health Care System, Seattle, WA*

GLENN R. CUNNINGHAM, MD, *Departments of Medicine and Molecular and Cellular Biology, Baylor College of Medicine, Houston, TX*

SUSAN R. DAVIS, PhD, MBBS, FRACP, *The Jean Hailes Foundation, Clayton, Australia*

ADRIAN S. DOBS, MD, MHS, *Division of Endocrinology, Department of Medicine, Johns Hopkins University School of Medicine, Baltimore, MD*

LAURENCE KATZNELSON, MD, *Neuuroendocrine Unit, Massachusetts General Hospital, Boston, MA*

ANNE M. KENNY, MD, *Center on Aging, University of Connecticut Health Center, Farmington, CT*

KENNETH S. KORACH, PhD, *Laboratory of Reproductive and Developmental Toxicology, National Institute of Environmental Health Sciences, Research Triangle Park, NC*

DOLORES J. LAMB, PhD, *Departments of Molecular and Cellular Biology and Urology, Baylor College of Medicine, Houston, TX*

RICHARD S. LEGRO, MD, *Department of Obstetrics and Gynecology, Penn State College of Medicine, Hershey Medical Center, Hershey, PA*

JONATHAN LINDZEY, PhD, *Department of Biology, University of South Florida, Tampa, FL*

MARCO MARCELLI, MD, *Department of Medicine and Molecular and Cellular Biology, Baylor College of Medicine, Houston, TX*

ALVIN M. MATSUMOTO, MD, *Department of Medicine, University of Washington, and Geriatric Research, Education and Clinical Center, VA Puget Sound Health Care System, Seattle, WA*

MICHAEL J. MCPHAUL, MD, *Division of Endocrinology and Metabolism, UT Southwestern Medical Center, Dallas, TX*

STEPHEN R. PLYMATE, MD, *Division of Gerentology and Geriatric Medicine, University of Washington School of Medicine, Seattle, WA*

LAWRENCE G. RAISZ, MD, *Lowell P. Weicker General Clinical Research Center, University of Connecticut Health Center, Farmington, CT*

ERICK J. RICHMOND, MD, *Pediatric Endocrinology, University of Virginia, Charlottesville, VA*

ALAN D. ROGOL, MD, PhD, *Pediatric Endocrinology, University of Virginia, Charlottesville, VA*

THOMAS W. STORER, PhD, *Division of Endocrinology, Metabolism, and Molecular Medicine, Department of Internal Medicine, Charles R. Drew University of Medicine and Science, Los Angeles, CA*

PAUL R. SUTTON, MD, PhD, *Department of Medicine, University of Washington School of Medicine, Seattle, WA*

RONALD S. SWERDLOFF, MD, *Division of Endocrinology, Department of Medicine, Harbor-UCLA Medical Center, Torrance, CA*

J. LISA TENOVER, MD, PhD, *Division of Geriatric Medicine and Gerontology, Department of Medicine, Emory University, Atlanta, GA*

ARNOLD VON ECKARDSTEIN, MD, *Institute of Clinical Chemistry, University of Zurich and University Hospital of Zurich, Zurich, Switzerland*

CHRISTINA WANG, MD, *Division of Endocrinology, Department of Medicine, Harbor-UCLA Medical Center, Torrance, CA*

NANCY L. WEIGEL, PhD, *Department of Molecular and Cellular Biology, Baylor College of Medicine, Houston, TX*

STEPHEN J. WINTERS, MD, *Division of Endocrinology and Metabolism, University of Louisville, Louisville, KY*

LINDA J. WOODHOUSE, PhD, *Division of Endocrinology, Metabolism, and Molecular Medicine, Department of Internal Medicine, Charles R. Drew University of Medicine and Science, Los Angeles, CA*

FREDERICK C. W. WU, MD, *Department of Endocrinology, Manchester Royal Infirmary, University of Manchester, Manchester, UK*

I GENERAL ANDROLOGY

1

Testosterone Synthesis, Transport, and Metabolism

Stephen J. Winters, MD
and Barbara J. Clark, PhD

Contents

Introduction
Testosterone Biosynthetic Pathway
LH Regulation of Testosterone Synthesis
Other Factors That Influence Testosterone Synthesis
The Hypothalamus–Pituitary and Testosterone Secretion
Circulating Testosterone Concentrations
SHBG and Testosterone Transport
Testosterone Metabolism
Summary
References

INTRODUCTION

Testosterone, the major androgen in men, is necessary for fetal male sexual differentiation, pubertal development, the maintenance of adult secondary sex characteristics, and spermatogenesis, and functions in many other tissues, including muscle and bone, and in the immune system. The testes are the source of more than 95% of the circulating testosterone in men, although the adrenal cortex produces large amounts of the testosterone precursor steroids dehydroepiandrosterone (DHEA) and androstenedione.

The site of testosterone production in the testis is the Leydig cell *(1)*. These cells are irregularly ovoid and constitute about 5% of the volume of the testis. Leydig cells are found in aggregates in the space between the seminiferous tubules and are connected by gap junctions. The intertubular space also contains blood vessels and lymphatics by which Leydig cells receive signals and into which they secrete their products. Leydig cell cytoplasm is rich in smooth endoplasmic reticulum and in mitochondria. Lipid inclusions are found in the Leydig cells of certain species but are uncommon in human Leydig cells. Rod-shaped structures of up to 20 µm in length, known as crystals of Reinke, are found in human Leydig cells but are of uncertain significance. There is a triphasic pattern of human Leydig cell function. Leydig cells in the fetal testis are thought to develop from mesenchymal precursors into cells that express LH/hCG (luteinizing hormone/human

From: *Contemporary Endocrinology: Androgens in Health and Disease*
Edited by: C. Bagatell and W. J. Bremner © Humana Press Inc., Totowa, NJ

chorionic gonadotropin) receptors and steroidogenic enzymes. Testosterone production peaks toward the end of the first trimester of fetal life and then declines to about 10% of peak values for the remainder of gestation. This temporal pattern is readily superimposed upon the levels of hCG in maternal blood. Following birth, there is a second peak in testosterone secretion that lasts up to 4–6 mo and results from transient activation of gonadotropin-releasing hormone (GnRH) production. Then, there is sharp decline in testosterone production that is associated with a considerable loss of mature Leydig cells. GnRH secretion increases markedly at puberty, at which time Leydig cell differentiation and testosterone production parallel activation of the spermatogenesis process *(2)*.

TESTOSTERONE BIOSYNTHETIC PATHWAY

All mammalian steroid hormones are synthesized from cholesterol by sequential cytochrome P450- and dehydrogenase-dependent enzymatic reactions. Testosterone is a C19 3-keto, 17β-hydroxy Δ4 steroid. Figure 1 illustrates the biosynthetic pathway for testosterone synthesis in Leydig cells. The cyclopentanophenanthrene ring structure of the cholesterol nucleus is retained, and the distinct biological function of the end-product steroid hormone is the result of the stereo-specific modifications of the ring carbons. The first reaction, the conversion of cholesterol to pregnenolone, occurs within mitochondria and is catalyzed by the cytochrome P450 side-chain cleavage enzyme, P450scc *(3,4)*. P450scc is encoded by the CYP11A gene located in the q23-q24 region of chromosome 15 *(5,6)*. P450scc is translated with an amino-terminal signal sequence that targets the protein to the mitochondria, where it is localized in the inner membrane *(7)*. The enzyme is part of an electron-transport complex that includes adrenodoxin reductase and adrenodoxin, an FAD-containing flavoprotein and iron–sulfur protein, respectively, that are required to transfer reducing equivalents from NADPH to P450scc for the mixed-function oxidase reactions *(8)*. P450scc catalyzes two sequential hydroxylations of the cholesterol side chain at C22 and C20, producing 22R-hydroxycholesterol and 20,22-dihydroxycholesterol intermediates *(9,10)*. Subsequent cleavage of the bond between C20 and C22 by P450scc produces pregnenolone and releases isocaproaldehyde.

Pregnenolone diffuses out of the mitochondria and can be converted to testosterone by two alternative routes referred to as the Δ^4 pathway or the Δ^5 pathway, based on whether the steroid intermediates are 3-keto, Δ^4 steroids (Δ^4) or 3-hydroxy, Δ^5 steroids (Δ^5). In the Δ^4 pathway, which predominates in rodents, pregnenolone is metabolized to progesterone by 3β-hydroxysteroid dehydrogenase/Δ^5-Δ^4 isomerase (3βHSD) that catalyzes both the oxidation of the 3β-hydroxyl group to a 3-keto group and the isomerization of the double bond between C5 and C6 to a double bond between C4 and C5 position in an NAD+/–dependent reaction *(11)*. 3βHSD is a member of a family of short-chain dehydrogenases (SDR) of which the type II human enzyme, 3βHSD-II, is the gonad-specific form encoded by the HSD3B2 gene on chromosome 1p13 *(12–15)*. Progesterone is then hydroxylated at C17 to form 17α-hydroxyprogesterone, followed by cleavage of the bond between C17 and C20 to produce androstenedione. Both reactions are catalyzed by cytochrome P450 17α-hydroxylase/C17,20 lyase, an enzyme encoded by the CYP17 gene on chromosome 10q24.3 *(16,17)*. CYP17 is a microsomal enzyme that utilizes a ubiquitous flavoprotein, NADPH–cytochrome P450 reductase, to transfer reducing equivalents from NADPH to the enzyme. Finally, the C17 keto group of androstenedione is reduced to a hydroxyl group to produce testosterone. This reaction

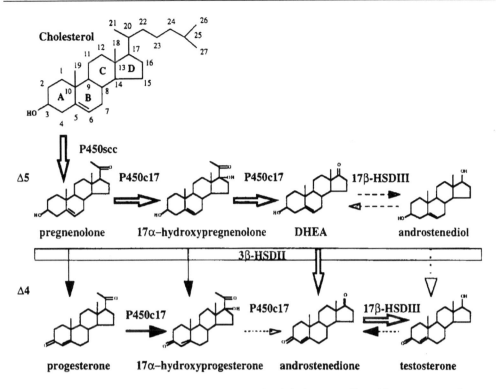

Fig. 1. Biosynthetic pathway for testosterone synthesis in humans. Steroid structures and names are shown. The open arrows indicate the major route of steroidogenesis in human Leydig cells. The enzymes are shown with corresponding reactions (arrows). The box indicates the reactions catalyzed by 3βHSD and schematically separates the Δ5 from the Δ4 pathway.

is catalyzed by 17β-hydroxysteroid dehydrogenase (17βHSD), and the reaction can be reversible in vitro. Activity in vivo is typically unidirectional, however, and depends on the isoform and cofactor requirement *(18,19)*. Several isoforms of 17βHSD have been identified that have different tissue, substrate, and cofactor preferences. The type III "reductive" enzyme (17βHSD-III) is expressed specifically in the testis and converts androstenedione to testosterone in a NADPH-dependent reaction *(20,21)*. The 17βHSD enzymes are also members of the SDR family, and 17βHSD-III is encoded by the HSD17B3 gene located on chromosome 9q22 *(19,21)*. Mutations in the HSD17B3 gene are the basis for male pseudohermaphroditism *(20,22)*.

In the Δ⁵ pathway, the initial reactions are catalyzed by P450c17; C17 hydroxylation of pregnenolone to form 17α-hydroxypregnenolone, and cleavage of the bond between C17 and C20 of 17α-hydroxypregnenolone to produce DHEA, a 3-hydroxy Δ⁵-steroid. Oxidation of the 3β-hydroxy group and isomerization of the double bond between C5 and C6 of DHEA by 3βHSD forms androstenedione that is subsequently bioconverted to testosterone by 17βHSD. Early experiments in which human testicular tissue was incubated with radiolabeled steroids revealed that the C17,20 lyase activity was more efficient with 17α-hydroxypregnenolone as a substrate than with 17α-hydroxypro- gesterone *(23)*. Subsequent cloning and in vitro expression of the human P450c17 cDNA demonstrated that the 17α-hydroxylase activity of P450C17 is equally efficient with pregnenolone or progesterone and confirmed that 17α-hydroxypregnenolone is the preferred substrate for the C17,20 lyase activity of human P450c17, with virtually undetectable metabolism of 17α-hydroxyprogesterone *(24,25)*. For this reason, the Δ^5 pathway is the predominant pathway for testosterone biosynthesis in the human testis.

LH REGULATION OF TESTOSTERONE SYNTHESIS

Luteinizing hormone (LH) activates testosterone synthesis in Leydig cells through a G-protein-associated seven-transmembrane receptor with an uncommonly long extracellular domain *(26)*. As shown in Fig. 2, LH binding initiates a signaling cascade by activating G_s, a small GTPase protein, that stimulates adenylate cyclase activity to increase levels of intracellular cAMP and activate cAMP-dependent protein kinase A (PKA). cAMP-dependent PKA activates two temporally distinct responses that stimulate testosterone synthesis. The acute response, which occurs within minutes of hormonal stimulation, is defined as the stimulated increase in cholesterol transport into the mitochondria. The chronic response, which requires several hours, involves transcriptional activation of the genes encoding the steroidogenic enzymes of the testosterone biosynthetic pathway *(27,28)*.

Acute Regulation

Cholesterol for steroidogenesis is acquired by receptor-mediated endocytosis of circulating low-density lipoprotein (LDL) or cholesterol ester uptake from circulating high-density lipoprotein (HDL) or is synthesized *de novo* from acetyl-CoA. The source of cholesterol in adrenal and gonadal cells appears to be species dependent. Humans have higher circulating levels of LDL compared to HDL, and LDL appears to be the preferred cholesterol source for adrenal and gonadal steroidogenesis under physiological conditions. However, patients with hypercholesterolemia that is a result of decreased cellular uptake of LDL because of mutant LDL receptors, have normal circulating adrenal or gonadal steroid levels. Nor are plasma steroid levels altered when cholesterol synthesis is decreased in these patients by treatment with the statin family of drugs to inhibit 3-hydroxy 3-methylglutaryl-coenzyme A (HMG-CoA) reductase activity, the rate-limiting and regulated step in cholesterol biosynthesis *(29,30)*. These data indicate that the cholesterol supply for steroid hormone biosynthesis is maintained by compensatory mechanisms. Studies in rodents, in which HDL is the major lipoprotein, have established that that scavenger receptor type B, class I (SR-BI) binds HDL, and cholesterol ester uptake occurs without endocytosis and catabolism of the lipoprotein *(31)*. SR-BI is highly expressed in steroidogenic cells and its expression is increased by gonadotropin stimulation and it is positively correlated with increased adrenal steroid production *(32,33)*. The cholesterol derived from HDL can be used directly for cortisol production as determined by radiolabeling studies in cell culture systems. Thus, HDL is the preferred lipoprotein to supply steroidogenic cholesterol in rodents. The human homolog of SR-BI, CLA-1, has been localized to human adrenal, ovary, and testis, and expression in the adrenal cortex is ACTH regulated *(34)*. CLA-1, in cultured human adrenocortical cells, is functional in cholesterol uptake from HDL, but when compared to LDL receptor-mediated endocytosis, HDL is much less efficient *(34,35)*. Nevertheless, HDL uptake appears to be sufficient to maintain steroidogenesis in the absence of LDL or *de novo* synthesis.

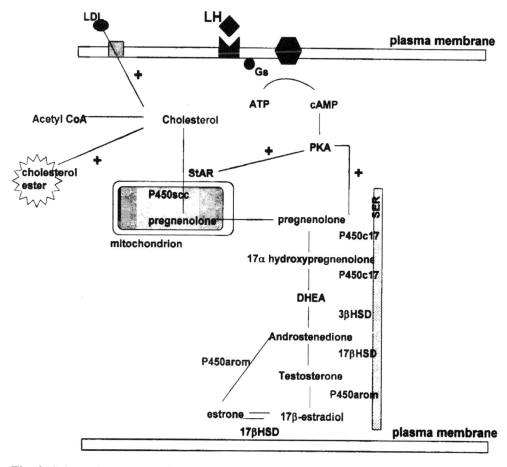

Fig. 2. Schematic representation of the the mechanisms by which LH regulates testosterone biosynthesis. LH activates the cAMP–PKA signaling pathway that, in turn, promotes (+) cholesterol mobilization and StAR synthesis and thereby cholesterol transport to acutely increase steroid secretion. Chronic stimulation is indicated (+) as transcriptional regulation of the steroidogenic cytochrome P450 enzymes P450Scc and P457c17 and the dehydrogenase enzymes 3βHSD and 17βHSD. Gs, stimulatory guanine–nucleotide triphosphate-binding protein; AC, adenylate cyclase; SER, smooth endoplasmic reticulum.

Although the supply of cholesterol for steroidogenesis can be maintained by multiple mechanisms, the rate-limiting step in steroid production is substrate delivery to the P450scc complex (i.e., the transport of cholesterol into the mitochondria). This mitochondrial transport of cholesterol is now established to be regulated by the steroidogenic acute regulatory (StAR) protein *(27).* StAR's critical role in hormone-dependent steroid production in the adrenal and gonads is most clearly demonstrated by the clinical disorder lipoid congenital adrenal hyperplasia (LCAH) in which both adrenal and gonadal steroidogenesis is markedly impaired or absent because of the inability of steroidogenic cells to deliver cholesterol to P450scc. Mutations in the StAR gene, which lead to the production of nonfunctional proteins, have been identified as the underlying basis for LCAH *(36).* StAR is a nuclear-encoded mitochondrial protein encoded on chromosome 8p11.2 *(37,38).* Stimulation of StAR synthesis in Leydig cells by LH acutely increases steroid production (within 30 min in MA-10 mouse Leydig tumor cells) *(39)*. StAR appears to function at the mitochondrial outer membrane, but the mechanism of action for cholesterol transport is not yet known *(40,41)*.

Long-Term Regulation

The mechanism by which LH stimulates testosterone synthesis also involves increased expression of the steroidogenic enzymes P450scc, P450c17, 3βHSD and 17βHSD *(27)*. These enzymes are increased by transcriptional and posttranscriptional mechanisms, but the best characterized response to LH so far is the cAMP-dependent transcriptional activation of P450scc and P450c17. Perhaps the most striking observation from this research is the apparent lack of coordination for regulation of these two genes; both are responsive to cAMP, but distinct promoter elements and transcription factors are required for gene activation *(42)*.

OTHER FACTORS THAT INFLUENCE TESTOSTERONE SYNTHESIS

The concept that testosterone biosynthesis and secretion are under LH control is well established and is underscored by the prepubertal levels of circulating testosterone in men with the complete form of congenital hypogonadotropic hypogonadism *(43)*. The phenotype in these men is that of a normal male presumably because placental hCG stimulates testosterone synthesis in the human male fetus. In support of this view, inactivating mutations of the LH receptor produce XY infants with Leydig cell agenesis and female external genitalia *(44)*. On the other hand, in mice expressing a functionless LH receptor, males are phenotypically normal yet are hypogonadal as adults, implying that other factors activate testicular steroidogensis in fetal rodents but play a lesser role in adulthood *(45)*. One candidate activator of fetal testosterone biosynthesis is pituitary adenylate cyclase-activating polypeptide (PACAP) *(46)*.

Early studies with purified follicle-stimulating hormone (FSH) preparations suggested that FSH enhanced Leydig cell responsiveness to LH. From studies using recombinant gonadotropins (which do not contain other hormones), however, recombinant human (rh)-FSH is now known *(47)* to have a negligible effect on testosterone production in vitro (1 : 100,000 the potency of LH). Moreover, neither treating GnRH-primed juvenile monkeys with rh-FSH *(48)* nor adding rh-FSH to rh-LH treated gonadotropin-deficient men *(49)* increased circulating testosterone levels further. Thus, FSH appears to have little or no direct effect on testosterone production.

Many studies have proposed that prolactin (PRL) affects testosterone production, but the function of PRL in males remains controversial. PRL receptors are found on Leydig cells *(50)*, and PRL may increase LH-stimulated testosterone production by increasing LH binding *(51)*. However, PRL has a dose-dependent biphasic effect on Leydig cell steroidogenesis *(52)*, and PRL knockout mice have normal circulating levels of testosterone and are fertile *(53)*. Men with prolactin-producing pituitary microadenomas have low plasma testosterone levels primarily because pulsatile LH secretion is suppressed *(54)*.

Growth hormone (GH) has been proposed to stimulate testosterone biosynthesis directly, or via testicular insulin-like growth factor-1 (IGF-1) and IGF-1 receptors on Leydig cells *(55)*. In rodents, testicular IGF-1 is upregulated by gonadotropins and may play a role in the differentiation of immature into adult Leydig cells *(56)*. In IGF-1-deficient mice, testosterone levels are 18% of normal, although this may be the result of gonadotropin deficiency *(57)*. The testes are smaller than normal in men with childhood-onset GH deficiency; however, circulating testosterone levels are generally normal *(58)*. In adult men with isolated GH deficiency as a result of hypothalamic–pituitary disease, plasma testosterone levels increased slightly following 6–12 mo of human GH (hGH) therapy, and the testosterone response to hCG stimulation was increased by 20% *(59)*. Thus, GH may play a minor role in testosterone production. There is a direct stimulatory effect of T3 on the production of testosterone and estradiol by Leydig cells, in part, by increasing StAR expression *(60)*.

Paracrine factors produced by Sertoli cells, germ cells, peritubular cells, and macrophages may also regulate Leydig cell function. As noted earlier, PACAP or vasoactive intestinal polypeptide (VIP), which, like LH, activate cAMP-dependent PKA and may stimulate fetal Leydig cells *(46)*. On the other hand, anti-Mullerian hormone may function as a negative modulator of Leydig cell differentiation and function. Corticotropin-releasing hormone (CRH) is secreted by Leydig cells and acts through high-affinity receptors on Leydig cell membranes to negatively regulate LH action by inhibiting gonadotropin-induced cAMP generation and thereby decrease androgen production *(61)*. CRH also increases interleukin-1 (IL-1) in Sertoi cells, and IL-1 inhibits Leydig cell steroidogenesis in vitro *(62)*. In this way, testicular CRH may play a role in the decline in testosterone production with stress and inflammation. Arginine vasopressin (AVP) is present in the testis, receptors for AVP are present in Leydig cells, and AVP inhibits testosterone synthesis in vitro, but the significance of these findings is unknown. Rat and mouse Leydig cells also express receptors for atrial natriuetic peptide. In vitro experiments have shown that inhibin and activin may also influence LH-stimulated steroidogenesis in immature Leydig cells *(63)*. Testicular macrophages produce a lipophilic factor that stimulates testosterone synthesis that may be 25OH-cholesterol *(64)*.

The Leydig cell not only produces testosterone and estradiol but also is a target for the actions of these steroid hormones. Both androgen receptors and estrogen receptor-α (ER-α) are found in Leydig cells *(65)* and may mediate autocrine genomic effects of these hormones. For example, testosterone suppresses P450c17 activity as well as the cAMP-activated transcription of P450c17 *(66)*, and estradiol decreases testosterone production by decreasing the LH receptor concentration and reducing the mRNA for P450C17. Based on experiments in rats treated with the Leydig cell toxin ethane dimethane sulfonate (EDS), estradiol also impairs Leydig cell development *(67)*. Nongenomic mechanisms of steroid action may also occur because the high interstitial fluid concentrations of estradiol and testosterone would allow for membrane signaling. Corticosterone has been shown to reduce LH-stimulated cAMP production and 17βHSD activity in rat Leydig cells *(68)* and may contribute to testosterone deficiency in stress. The gene for P450C17 is also regulated in rat Leydig cells by the orphan nuclear receptor steroidogenic factor-1 (SF-1).

THE HYPOTHALAMUS-PITUITARY
AND TESTOSTERONE SECRETION

The proximate regulator of testosterone synthesis and secretion is GnRH, which is produced in neurons located diffusely throughout the anterior hypothalamus in primates *(69)*. Fundamental experiments in rams revealed that GnRH is released in bursts into hypothalamic portal blood and that each burst of GnRH is associated with an LH secretory pulse *(70)*. GnRH activates a cell surface G-protein-coupled receptor on gonadotrophs following which G proteins hydrolyze membrane phosphoinositides to produce inositol phosphates (Ips) including inositol triphosphate ($I_{1,4,5}$) P3. IP3 mobilizes calcium from intracellular stores and causes extracellular calcium to enter gonadotrophs. The rise in intracellular free calcium results in the fusion of hormone-containing vesicles to the cell membrane with hormone release into pituitary capillaries.

GnRH also increases LH and FSH secretion by upregulating the levels of the mRNAs for the α-subunit, LH-β and FSH-β genes *(71)*. LH-β and FSH-β subunit gene expression are dependent on pulsatile GnRH, whereas either pulsatile or continuous GnRH increase α-subunit mRNA levels *(72,73)*. When administered as pulses, but not continuously, GnRH also increases GnRH-receptor gene expression *(74)*. In addition, gonadotropin glycosylation is increased by GnRH, and this modification influences circulating half-life and receptor-binding activity.

The importance of the LH pulse to normal testicular function is less clear. Although Leydig cells respond to pulses of LH with bursts of testosterone secretion, continuous infusion of LH (into rams rendered gonadotropin deficient by GnRH immunization) also stimulated testosterone secretion and had little effect on the subsequent response to LH *(75)*. Likewise, treatment of men with hCG (with a much longer circulating half-life than LH and therefore little pulsatile variation) also effectively increases testosterone secretion. The action of hCG in gonadotropin-deficient men is biphasic with peaks at 4 h and 72 h *(76)*, which may represent an acute steroidogenic response followed by upregulation of the genes for the steroidogenic enzymes. Very large doses of LH/hCG desensitize rat Leydig cells and downregulate LH receptors *(77)* by decreasing receptor mRNA levels *(78)*. This effect may be applicable to men treated with hCG and to men with hCG-producing tumors among whom testosterone levels are generally not elevated.

Testosterone regulates is own production by negative feedback inhibition of LH secretion. Otherwise, unchecked LH drive would stimulate testosterone production maximally, and undesirable side effects would occur. Testosterone exerts negative feedback effects by suppressing LH secretion within a few hours *(79)* and by downregulating gonadotropin subunit gene expression *(80)*. Most of the testosterone feedback inhibition of LH in men appears to be via GnRH. For example, testosterone and dihydrotestosterone (DHT) decrease LH (and presumably GnRH) pulse frequency in adult men *(79,81)*, and LH pulse frequency is increased in patients with androgen insensitivity *(82)*. Moreover, testosterone inhibition of LH secretion is less effective in men with congenital gonadotropin deficiency treated with pulsatile GnRH than in normal men (in whom testosterone can reduce GnRH production) *(83)*. Experiments in the nonhuman adult male primate rendered gonadotropin deficient by a hypothalamic lesion and reactivated with pulses of GnRH further demonstrate the importance of the GnRH pulse generator in the testosterone control of LH secretion. In that model, removal of the testes produced little change in circulating LH levels until the frequency of the applied GnRH pulses was increased *(84)*. Furthermore, testosterone fails to suppress GnRH-stimulated LH secretion or α-subunit mRNA levels in GnRH-stimulated primate pituitary cell cultures, although these effects are demonstrable using pituitary cell cultures from adult male rats *(85)*.

Estradiol is also an important feedback regulator of LH and, thereby, testosterone secretion in men. In fact, much of feedback inhibition of LH secretion by testosterone can be accounted for by its bioconversion to estradiol *(79,86)*. Recent findings in men with mutations of ER-α *(87)* or the aromatase gene *(88)* reveal that LH levels are increased even though testosterone levels are elevated. The importance of estradiol in the testicular control of LH secretion was predicted some years ago with the findings that the antiestrogen clomiphene *(89)* and the aromatase inhibitor testolactone *(90)* increased LH secretion in men. Furthermore, LH pulse frequency accelerated during clomiphene treatment, indicating that a portion of the estradiol effect is on the GnRH pulse generator *(91)*. Aromatase is expressed in the hypothalamus, and estradiol produced in the brain from testosterone may suppress GnRH secretion by a genomic or transmembrane effects. The importance of central nervous system (CNS) production of estradiol is evident in rams in which intracerebral ventricular (icv) infusion of the aromatase inhibitor fadrozole increased LH pulse frequency with no effect on plasma estradiol concentrations *(92)*. Estradiol also reduces LH pulse amplitude in men *(79)* and suppresses GnRH-stimulated LH secretion in primate pituitary cells *(85)*, indicating a pituitary site of action.

Follicle-stimulating hormone secretion is also suppressed following testosterone and estradiol administration *(86,93)* because FSH production, like LH, production is GnRH dependent. In addition, FSH is negatively regulated at the level of the gonadotroph by testicular inhibin-B *(94)*. A schematic of the interrelationship between gonadotropin and testosterone secretion is shown in Fig. 3.

CIRCULATING TESTOSTERONE CONCENTRATIONS

The usual normal range for testosterone levels in serum samples drawn in the morning from adult men is 3–10 ng/mL (10–40 n*M*), whereas following bilateral orchidectomy, the level of testosterone declines to less than 0.3 ng/mL. The blood production rate of testosterone in normal adult men is estimated to range from 5000 to 7500 µg/24 h *(95)*. The testosterone content of the adult human testis is only about 50 µg (1 µg/g testis), indicating that nearly all of the synthesized testosterone is released into the circulation. Steroid hormones are presumed to diffuse freely and rapidly across cell membranes. As such, following its synthesis, testosterone exits the Leydig cell to enter the testicular interstitial compartment and diffuse across the capillary endothelium into the circulation to produce a secretory pulse. Interestingly, the LH receptor is found in testicular vascular endothelium *(96)*, where it could have a vasoactive function and facilitate diffusion.

In many species, including rams, dogs, and nonhuman primates, frequent blood sampling reveals a tight coupling between LH pulses and testosterone secretory episodes with a lag of about 30 min. In men, however, episodes of testosterone secretion are more difficult to identify by visual inspection in plasma concentration profiles *(97)*, although, as shown in Fig. 4, hourly testosterone secretory episodes are readily apparent in sequential samples of spermatic vein blood *(98)*. The inability to readily identify testosterone secretory episodes in human peripheral blood samples may relate in part to a rapid pulse frequency, because slowing the GnRH pulse generator, as with fluoxymesterone *(99)*, unmasked the circulating testosterone response to LH. However, even under those conditions, testosterone secretory episodes were delayed and prolonged and of relatively low magnitude. Thus, other factors, such as Leydig cell responsiveness to LH and testosterone clearance, appear to contribute to the configuration of the testosterone pulse in men.

Frequent sampling of human spermatic vein blood revealed that the testis secretes pulses of the testosterone precursor steroids, including pregnenolone, 17-hydroxypregnenolone, DHEA, progesterone, 17α-hydroxyprogesterone, and androstenedione

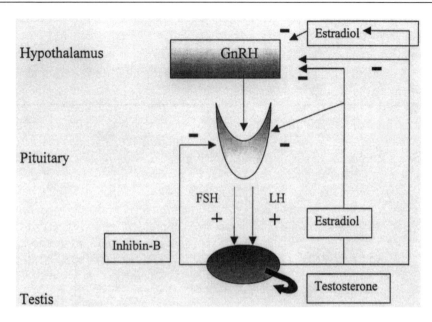

Fig. 3. A schematic of the hypothalamic–pituitary–testicular axis showing the interrelationship between GnRH, LH, FSH, testosterone, estradiol, and inhibin-B.

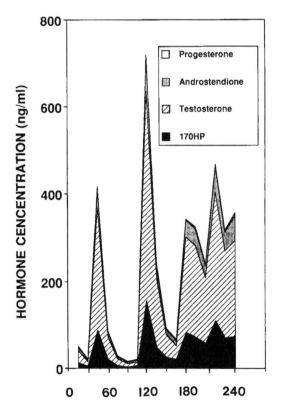

Fig. 4. Secretion into spermatic vein blood of testosterone, 17α-hydroxyprogesterone, androstenedione, and progesterone. Blood samples were drawn every 15 min for 4 h in a man with varicocele-associated infertility undergoing spermatic venography.

together with testosterone, as shown in Fig. 4. Moreover, the relative concentration of these steroids in spermatic vein blood was proportional to their intratesticular concentration *(100)*. One idea is that these precursor steroids are secreted as unnecessary byproducts in the transformation of pregnenolone to testosterone, because none is known to have a physiological function in males.

There is also a diurnal variation in circulating testosterone levels in adult men, with highest levels in the early morning, followed by a progressive fall throughout the day, to nadir levels in the evening and during the first few hours of sleep *(101)*. Peak and nadir values differ by approx 15%, although more pronounced differences are sometimes observed *(102)*. Although a rise in LH precedes the nocturnal rise in testosterone levels in pubertal boys *(103)*, there is no clear diurnal rhythm for LH in most adult men *(104)*, implying that the nocturnal increase in testosterone is only partly LH controlled. Fragmented sleep disrupts the diurnal testosterone rhythm *(105)*, but the link between sleep and testosterone secretion is thus far unknown. Moreover, this rhythm is blunted with aging *(106)* and in men with testicular failure *(107)*.

SHBG AND TESTOSTERONE TRANSPORT

After its release from the testis, testosterone is bound by plasma proteins in the circulation. About 45% of the plasma testosterone in adult men is bound with high affinity to sex hormone-binding globulin (SHBG), 50% is loosely bound to albumin, 1–2% to cortisol-binding globulin, and less than 4% is free (not protein bound) *(108)*. SHBG is a carbohydrate-rich β-globulin produced by the liver. SHBG is a 100,000-kDa dimer, with protomers of 48–52 kDa that convert to a single 39-kDa species after deglycosylation *(109)*. Androgen-binding protein (ABP) is a product of the SHBG gene in testicular Sertoli cells. Expression utilizes a 5' alternative exon to produce a protein with an identical AA sequence but variant glycosylation.

Sex hormone-binding globulin binds testosterone and other steroids and prolongs their metabolic clearance; however, the function of SHBG remains controversial *(110)*. The general view, however, is that SHBG-bound testosterone is not biologically active. SHBG reduces cellular uptake of testosterone in vitro *(111)* as well as testosterone bioactivity *(112)*, implying that SHBG regulates testosterone availability to target cells. SHBG is seemingly absent in rats, mice, and pigs, although there is an SHBG in fetal rats, suggesting that the role of SHBG could be species-specific. ABP is thought to maintain a high level of testosterone in the extracellular space of the male reproductive tract for androgen-dependent sperm maturation. The finding of membrane binding sites for SHBG in the testis, prostate, and other tissues *(113)* and for ABP in the caput epididymis *(114)* and germ cells *(115)* suggest, however, that ligand activation of these binding proteins could directly influence androgen action.

The SHBG levels decrease from infancy to puberty in both sexes *(116,117)* and are lower in adult men than in women. SHBG levels rise as men grow older *(118)*. SHBG levels are reduced in obesity *(119)*, especially with abdominal obesity *(120)*. A high-fat diet decreased SHBG in normal men, whereas a weight-reducing high-protein diet increased SHBG levels *(121)*. Metabolic effects on SHBG are partly mediated by insulin, because insulin levels are increased with visceral obesity *(122)* and with a high-fat diet, and insulin decreases SHBG mRNA *(123)*. Moreover, lowering insulin levels using diazoxide increased plasma SHBG levels *(124)*. However, imperfect correlations

Table 1
Factors Known to Influence
Circulating SHBG Concentrations

Increase	*Decrease*
Estrogens	Insulin
Thyroxine	GH
	Glucocorticoids
	Androgens
	Progestins

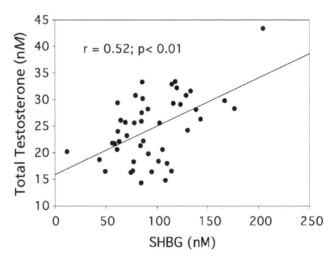

Fig. 5. Relationship between the levels of SHBG and total testosterone in serum in 46 normal young adult men.

between insulin levels and SHBG suggest that other factors related to insulin resistance, including GH and insulin-like growth factors and their binding proteins, or glucorticoids, may contribute to low SHBG as well. Table 1 lists the hormonal factors that are known to influence SHBG concentrations. A low level of SHBG is a marker for visceral obesity, insulin resistance, and hyperinsulinemia and is associated with increased risk for developing diabetes and cardiovascular disease.

Because of its function to bind testosterone with high affinity, the level of SHBG in plasma is a strong predictor of the total testosterone concentration among normal men (*see* Fig. 5). As such, the factors that increase or decrease SHBG levels similarly influence the total testosterone concentration. For example, both SHBG and total testosterone levels tend to be low in obese men *(120)* and increased in men with hyperthyroidism *(118)*.

Because the portion of circulating testosterone that is not bound to SHBG is thought to represent the biologically active fraction, many methods for determining non-SHBG-bound or free testosterone have been developed. Of these methods, there is a high positive correlation between the level of free-testosterone by equilibrium dialysis, non-SHBG testosterone (bioavailable testosterone), and the free-testosterone level calculated from the levels of total testosterone and SHBG *(125)*. These assays are important

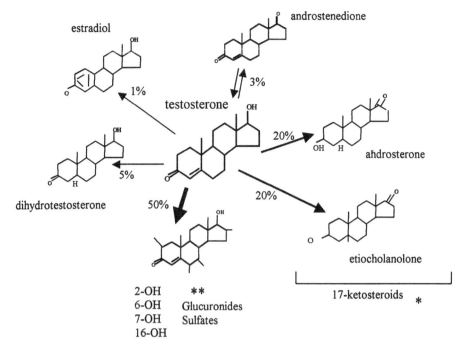

Fig. 6. Pathways for testosterone metabolism. Products have reduced affinityf or the androgen receptor, and because they are hydrophilic, they are excreted in the urine and bile. *Formation of 17-ketosteroids involves oxidation of C17 hydroxyl and reduction of 3-keto groups. **Excreted species are a mixture of polyhydroxyls, and glucuronides and sulfates.

tools in clinical research on the actions of androgens in men and are sometimes needed to establish a correct patient diagnosis. As an example of the former use, non-SHBG-bound testosterone levels in older men were found to be more strongly related to bone mineral density and to muscle strength than were total testosterone concentrations *(126)*.

TESTOSTERONE METABOLISM

As shown in Fig. 6, testosterone is metabolized to two important biologically active products, dihydrotesterone (DHT) and estradiol. The major route of metabolism of testosterone, however, is to monohydroxylated products that are hydrophilic and are excreted in the urine and bile. The metabolism of testosterone is tissue-specific and implies a unique biological role for many of the products in their tissue of origin. This general process has been termed "intracrinology" *(127)*.

Testosterone is converted to DHT by the enzyme steroid 5α-reductase through reduction of a double bond in the A ring. Steroid 5α-reductase is encoded by two genes that have been designated as type-1 and type-2 *(128)*. The genes encoding these isoenzymes have been assigned by *in situ* hybridization to chromosomes 5p15 and 2p23, respectively. The type-1 enzyme has a relatively broad pH optimum from 6.0 to 8.5, whereas the type-2 enzyme has a narrow pH optimum with maximum activity at pH 5.0. These enzymes also reduce other substrates with the Δ4-5, 3-keto structure including progesterone, 17α-hydroxyprogesterone, androstenedione, and cortisol. Expression of the isozymes is hormonally regulated. mRNA expression in (rat) prostate is upregulated by

Table 2
Tissue Distribution of Steroid 5α-Reductase Isozymes in Man

Tissue	Type 1	Type 2
Prostate, epididymis, seminal vesicle, genital skin	–	++
Liver	+	+
Nongenital skin	++	–
Testis, ovary, adrenal, brain, kidney	–	–

Source: ref. *129*.

its product, DHT. In human genital skin fibroblasts, activity is increased by androgens, transforming growth factor (TGF)-β, and activin *(129)*. Isozyme expression is also species- and tissue-specific *(130)*. The major sites of distribution in human tissues are summarized in Table 2.

Dihydrotestosterone is inactivated by conversion to 3α- and 3β-androstanediol (adiol) by 3αHSD and 3βHSD, respectively. High levels of 3αHSD mRNA are found in the prostate, liver, small intestine, colon, lung, and kidney *(131)*, suggesting that this reversible interconversion between a very active androgen (DHT) and an inactive metabolite (adiol) may influence androgen effects on target tissues.

Testosterone is converted to estradiol by aromatase P450, the product of the CYP19 gene *(132)* localized to chromosome 15q21.1. This microsomal enzyme oxidizes the C19 angular methyl group to produce a phenolic A ring and utilizes NAPDH–cytochrome P450 reductase to transfer the reducing equivalents, as described earlier for P450c17 (*see* Fig. 1). Aromatase is expressed in the Leydig cells of the adult testis, where it is upregulated by LH/hCG *(133)*. This regulation accounts for the high level of estradiol relative to testosterone in the plasma of men with primary testicular failure, or with hCG-producing neoplasms. Sertoli cell cultures from immature primates produce estradiol under the control of FSH.

Studies using radiolabeled androstenedione indicate that the testes of normal men produce only about 15% of the circulating estrogens *(134)*. Instead, most estrogen in men is from aromatase in adipose and skin stromal cells, with a lesser contribution from aortic smooth muscle cells, kidney, skeletal cells, and the brain. The promoter sequences of the P450 aromatase genes are tissue-specific because of differential splicing, but the translated protein appears to be the same in all tissues. Thus, glucocorticoids and serum growth factors (e.g., IL-6 and leukemia inhibitory factor) stimulate androgen bioconversion to estrogen in human adipose stromal cells but not in testis. Aromatase in adipose tissue leads to increased bioconversion of androgens to estrogens with obesity *(135)* and, perhaps, with aging.

Awareness of the importance of estradiol in men has increased substantially with the description of an adult man with an inactivating mutation of ER-α and of men with mutations of the CYP19 aromatase gene *(136)*. Striking findings in these men include high levels of LH and testosterone, delayed epiphyseal closure and osteopenia, as well as hyperinsulinemia in the ER-α-deficient man. Estrogen synthesis in target tissues may play an important role in the function of these tissues. For example, testosterone converted to estradiol in the brain is thought to mediate masculinization behavior, at least in rats *(137)*, and it is important in the testicular feedback inhibition of GnRH. Both ER-α and ER-β are expressed in the testis. ER-α is found in testicular Leydig cells and ER-β is present in seminiferous tubules. Studies of the ER-α knockout mouse indicate that estrogens regulate the efferent ductules of the testis, whereas male mice deficient in aromatase, although fertile in young adulthood, progressively develop infertility *(138)*. Therefore, conversion of testosterone to estrogens is essential for male fertility.

The reversible interconversion between testosterone and the inactive 17-ketosteroid, androstenedione, is catalyzed by the 17βHSDs. These enzymes also catalyze the interconversion between the biologically active estrogen, estradiol, and the relatively inactive estrogen, estrone. Several distinct 17βHSD isoenzymes have been characterized with unique tissue distribution patterns that imply a specific function, and at least seven 17βHSDs have already been identified in humans. 17βHSD-I is a reductase found in Leydig cells, where it is essential for testosterone biosynthesis, as described earlier. 17βHSD-II is a dehydrogenase that is widely expressed in tissues, including the prostate, liver, and kidney and in the breast and uterus in females. 17βHSD types I, III, IV, and V are found in the brain *(139)*.

The major route of metabolism of testosterone is by a family of hepatic microsomal CYP P450 enzymes (P450 3A isoforms) that produce monohydroxylated products at the 2, 6, 7, and 16 positions. Oxidation of the D ring produces the 17-ketosteroids androsterone (3α-hydroxy-5α-androstane-17-one) and etiocholanolone (3α-hydroxy-5β-androstane-17-one). These products are excreted in the urine and bile. Although these hydroxylations occur primarily in the liver, activity is also found in other tissues, including the kidney, adipose, brain, and prostate. The finding that the formation of hydroxylated steroids is under developmental and hormonal control and is influenced by drugs and by environmental factors raises the possibility that metabolism influences the action of testosterone in certain target cells. Moreover, the hydroxylated products of testosterone may themselves have a biological function and could play a role in disease processes.

Testosterone and its hydroxylated metabolites are also conjugated at the 3 or 17 position by glucuronyltransferases and sulfotransferases to produce water-soluble conjugates that are readily excreted in the urine and bile. Finally, a small fraction (2%) of the circulating testosterone is excreted unchanged in the urine.

SUMMARY

Molecular methods have exponentially increased our understanding of how testosterone is synthesized and secreted by Leydig cells. Yet, these mechanisms remain far from clear. Stimulation of StAR synthesis by LH acutely increases steroid production, but how cholesterol is transported from lipid droplets to P450scc in the inner mitochondrial membrane is not yet known. The importance of pulses of LH to this process also remains uncertain. Local control mechanisms are complex. Leydig cells synthesize many proteins that are not steroidogenic enzymes, most of which have not been identified or sequenced, and their physiological actions remain to be established. Finally, the function of SHBG remains controversial, and our understanding of the tissue-specific metabolism of testosterone is rudimentary. However, there is a wealth of information that provides a basis for understanding testosterone deficiency and justifies androgen-replacement therapies.

REFERENCES

1. Payne AH, Hardy MP, Russell LD (eds). The Leydig Cell, Cahce River Press, St. Louis, MO, 1996.
2. Prince FP. The triphasic nature of Leydig cell development in humans, and comments on nomenclature. J Endocrinology 2001;168:213–216.
3. Karaboyas G, Koritz S. Identity of the site of action of cAMP and ACTH in corticosteroidogenesis in rat adrenal and beef adrenal cortex slices. Biochemistry 1965;4:462–468.
4. Stone D, Hechter O. Studies on ACTH action in perfused bovine adrenals: site of action of ACTH in corticosteroidogenesis. Arch Biochem Biophys 1954;51:457–469.
5. Chung BC, Matteson KJ, Voutilainen R, et al. Human cholesterol side-chain cleavage enzyme, P450scc: cDNA cloning, assignment of the gene to chromosome 15, and expression in the placenta. Proc Natl Acad Sci USA 1986;83:8962–8966.
6. Durocher F, Morissette J, Simard J. Genetic linkage mapping of the CYP11A1 gene encoding the cholesterol side-chain cleavage P450scc close to the CYP1A1 gene and D15S204 in the chromosome 15q22.33-q23 region. Pharmacogenetics 1998;8:49–53.
7. Matocha M F, Waterman MR. Synthesis and processing of mitochondrial steroid hydroxylases. In vivo maturation of the precursor forms of cytochrome P-450scc, cytochrome P-450 (11) beta, and adrenodoxin. J Biol Chem 1985;260:12,259–12,265.
8. Hanukoglu I. Steroidogenic enzymes: structure, function, and role in regulation of steroid hormone biosynthesis. J Steroid Biochem Mol Biol 1992;43:779–804.
9. Burstein S, Middleditch BS. Enzymatic formation of ($20R$, $22R$)-20,22-dihdroxycholesterol from cholesterol and a mixture of 16O2 and 18O2: random incorporation of oxygen atoms. Biochem Biophys Res Commun 1974;61:692–697.
10. Hume R, Boyd GS. Cholesterol metabolism and steroid-hormone production. Biochem Soc Trans 1978;6:893–898.
11. Thomas JL, Frieden C, Nash WE, Strickler RC. An NADH-induced conformational change that mediates the sequential 3 beta-hydroxysteroid dehydrogenase/isomerase activities is supported by affinity labeling and the time-dependent activation of isomerase. J Biol Chem 1995;270:21,003–21,008.
12. Lachance Y, Luu-The, V, Verreault H, et al. Structure of the human type II 3 beta-hydroxysteroid dehydrogenase/delta 5-delta 4 isomerase (3 beta-HSD) gene: adrenal and gonadal specificity. DNA Cell Biol 1991;10:701–711.
13. Jornvall H, Persson B, Krook M, et al. Short-chain dehydrogenases/reductases (SDR). Biochemistry 1995;34:6003–6013.
14. Penning TM. Molecular endocrinology of hydroxysteroid dehydrogenases. Endocr Rev 1997;18:281–305.
15. Rheaume E, Lachance Y, Zhao HF, et al. Structure and expression of a new complementary DNA encoding the almost exclusive 3 beta-hydroxysteroid dehydrogenase/delta 5-delta 4-isomerase in human adrenals and gonads. Mol Endocrinol 1991;5:1147–1157.
16. Sparkes RS, Klisak I, Miller WL. Regional mapping of genes encoding human steroidogenic enzymes: P450scc to 15q23-q24, adrenodoxin to 11q22; adrenodoxin reductase to 17q24-q25; and P450c17 to 10q24-q25. DNA Cell Biol 1991;10:359–365.
17. Zuber MX, Simpson ER, Waterman MR. Expression of bovine 17 alpha-hydroxylase cytochrome P-450 cDNA in nonsteroidogenic (COS 1) cells. Science 1986;234:1258–1261.
18. Luu-The V, Zhang Y, Poirier D, Labrie F. Characteristics of human types 1, 2 and 3 17 beta-hydroxysteroid dehydrogenase activities: oxidation/reduction and inhibition. J Steroid Biochem Mol Biol 1995;55:581–587.
19. Peltoketo H, Luu-The V, Simard J, Adamski J. 17beta-hydroxysteroid dehydrogenase (HSD)/17-ketosteroid reductase (KSR) family; nomenclature and main characteristics of the 17HSD/KSR enzymes. J Mol Endocrinol 1999;23:1–11.
20. Andersson S, Geissler WM, Wu L, et al. Molecular genetics and pathophysiology of 17 beta-hydroxysteroid dehydrogenase 3 deficiency. J Clin Endocrinol Metab 1996;81:130–136.
21. Geissler WM, Davis DL, Wu L, et al. Male pseudohermaphroditism caused by mutations of testicular 17 beta-hydroxysteroid dehydrogenase 3. Nat Genet 1994;7:34–39.
22. Saez JM, Morera AM, De Peretti E, et al. Further in vivo studies in male pseudohermaphroditism with gynecomastia due to a testicular 17-ketosteroid reductase defect (compared to a case of testicular feminization). J Clin Endocrinol Metab 1972;34:598–600.
23. Yanaihara T, Troen P. Studies of the human testis. I. Biosynthetic pathways for androgen formation in human testicular tissue in vitro. J Clin Endocrinol Metab 1972;34:783–792.

24. Conley AJ, Bird IM. The role of cytochrome P450 17 alpha-hydroxylase and 3 beta-hydroxysteroid dehydrogenase in the integration of gonadal and adrenal steroidogenesis via the delta 5 and delta 4 pathways of steroidogenesis in mammals. Biol Reprod 1997;56:789–799.

25. Fevold HR, Lorence MC, McCarthy JL, et al. Rat P450(17 alpha) from testis: characterization of a full-length cDNA encoding a unique steroid hydroxylase capable of catalyzing both delta 4- and delta 5-steroid-17,20-lyase reactions. Mol Endocrinol 1989;3:968–975.

26. Dufau ML. The luteinizing hormone receptor. Annu Rev Physiol 1998;60:461–496.

27. Parker KL, Schimmer BP. Transcriptional regulation of the genes encoding the cytochrome P-450 steroid hydroxylases. Vitam Horm 1995;51:339–370.

28. Stocco DM, Clark BJ. Regulation of the acute production of steroids in steroidogenic cells. Endocr Rev 1996;17:221–244.

29. Dobs AS, Schrott H, Davidson MH, et al. Effects of high-dose simvastatin on adrenal and gonadal steroidogenesis in men with hypercholesterolemia. Metabolism 2000;49:1234–1238.

30. Travia D, Tosi F, Negri C, et al. Sustained therapy with 3-hydroxy-3-methylglutaryl-coenzyme-A reductase inhibitors does not impair steroidogenesis by adrenals and gonads. J Clin Endocrinol Metab 1995;80:836–840.

31. Krieger M. Charting the fate of the "good cholesterol": identification and characterization of the high-density lipoprotein receptor SR-BI. Annu Rev Biochem 1999;68:523–558.

32. Cao G, Zhao L, Stangl H, et al. Developmental and hormonal regulation of murine scavenger receptor, class B, type 1. Mol Endocrinol 1999;13:1460–1473.

33. Rigotti A, Edelman ER, Seifert P, et al. Regulation by adrenocorticotropic hormone of the in vivo expression of scavenger receptor class B type I (SR-BI), a high density lipoprotein receptor, in steroidogenic cells of the murine adrenal gland. J Biol Chem 1996;271:33,545–33,549.

34. Liu J, Heikkila P, Meng QH, et al. Expression of low and high density lipoprotein receptor genes in human adrenals. Eur J Endocrinol 2000;142:677–682.

35. Martin G, Pilon A, Albert C, et al. Comparison of expression and regulation of the high-density lipoprotein receptor SR-BI and the low-density lipoprotein receptor in human adrenocortical carcinoma NCI-H295 cells. Eur J Biochem 1999;261:481–491.

36. Lin D, Sugawara T, Strauss JF 3rd, et al. Role of steroidogenic acute regulatory protein in adrenal and gonadal steroidogenesis. Science 1995;267:1828–1831.

37. Clark BJ, Wells J, King SR, Stocco DM. The purification, cloning, and expression of a novel luteinizing hormone-induced mitochondrial protein in MA-10 mouse Leydig tumor cells. Characterization of the steroidogenic acute regulatory protein (StAR). J Biol Chem 1994;269:28,314–28,322.

38. Sugawara T, Holt JA, Driscoll D, et al. Human steroidogenic acute regulatory protein: functional activity in COS-1 cells, tissue-specific expression, and mapping of the structural gene to 8p11.2 and a pseudogene to chromosome 13. Proc Natl Acad Sci USA 1995;92:4778–4782.

39. Clark BJ, Combs R, Hales KH, et al. Inhibition of transcription affects synthesis of steroidogenic acute regulatory protein and steroidogenesis in MA-10 mouse Leydig tumor cells. Endocrinology 1997;138:4893–4901.

40. Miller WL, Strauss JF 3rd. Molecular pathology and mechanism of action of the steroidogenic acute regulatory protein, StAR. J Steroid Biochem Mol Biol 1999;69:131–141.

41. Stocco, DM. Steroidogenic acute regulatory protein. Vitam Horm 1999;55:399–441.

42. Kagawa N, Bischof LJ, Cheng PY, et al. Biochemical diversity of peptide-hormone-dependent regulation of steroidogenic P450s. Drug Metab Rev 1999;31:333–342.

43. Waldstreicher J, Seminara SB, Jameson JL, et al. The genetic and clinical heterogeneity of gonadotropin-releasing hormone deficiency in the human. J Clin Endocrinol Metab 1996:81:4388–4395.

44. Themmen APN, Huhtaniemi IT. Mutations of gonadotropins and gonadotropin receptors: elucidating the physiology and pathophysiology of pituitary-gonadal function. Endocr Rev 2000;21:551–583.

45. Zhang FP, Poutanen M, Wilbertz J, et al. Normal prenatal but arrested postnatal sexual development of luteinizing hormone receptor knockout (LuRKO) mice. Mol Endocrinol 2001;15:172–183.

46. El-Gehani F, Tena-Sempere M, Huhtaniemi I. Evidence that pituitary adenylate cyclase-activating polypeptide is a potent regulator of fetal rat testicular steroidogenesis. Biol Reprod 2000;63:1482–1489.

47. Mannaerts B, de Leeuw R, Geelen J, et al. Comparative in vitro and in vivo studies on the biological characteristics of recombinant human follicle-stimulating hormone. Endocrinology 1991;129:2623–2630.

48. Majumdar SS, Winters SJ, Plant TM. A study of the relative roles of follicle-stimulating hormone and luteinizing hormone in the regulation of testicular inhibin secretion in the rhesus monkey (*Macaca mulatta*). Endocrinology 1997;138:1363–1373.

49. Young J, Couzinet B, Chanson P, et al. Effects of human recombinant luteinizing hormone and follicle-stimulating hormone in patients with acquired hypogonadotropic hypogonadism: study of Sertoli and Leydig cell secretions and interactions. J Clin Endocrinol Metab 2000;85:3239–3244.

50. Manna PR, El-Hefnawy T, Kero J, et al. Biphasic action of prolactin in the regulation of murine Leydig tumor cell functions. Endocrinology 2001;142:308–318.

51. Bex FJ, Bartke A. Testicular LH binding in the hamster: modification by photoperiod and prolactin. Endocrinology 1977;100:1223–1226.

52. Weiss-Messer E, Ber R, Barkey RJ. Prolactin and MA-10 Leydig cell steroidogenesis: biphasic effects of prolactin and signal transduction. Endocrinology 1996;137:5509–5518.

53. Steger RW, Chandrashekar V, Zhao W, et al. Neuroendocrine and reproductive functions in male mice with targeted disruption of the prolactin gene. Endocrinology 1998;13:3691–3695.

54. Winters SJ, Troen P. Altered pulsatile secretion of luteinizing hormone in hypogonadal men with hyperprolactinemia. Clin Endocrinol 1984;21:257–263.

55. Bartke A. Effects of growth hormone on male reproductive function. J Androl 2000;21:181–188.

56. Benton L, Shan LX, Hardy MP. Differentiation of adult Leydig cells. J Steroid Biochem Mol Biol 1995;53:61–68.

57. Baker J, Liu JP, Robertson EJ, et al. Role of insulin-like growth factors in embryonic and postnatal growth. Cell 1993;75:73–82.

58. Juul A, Andersson AM, Pedersen SA, et al. Effects of growth hormone replacement therapy on IGF-related parameters and on the pituitary-gonadal axis in GH-deficient men. Horm Res 1998;49:269–278.

59. Carani C, Granata AR, De Rosa M, et al. The effect of chronic treatment with GH on gonadal function in men with isolated GH deficiency. Eur J Endocrinol 1999;140:224–230.

60. Manna PR, Tena-Sempere M, Huhtaniemi IT. Molecular mechanisms of thyroid hormone-stimulated steroidogenesis in mouse leydig tumor cells. Involvement of the steroidogenic acute regulatory (StAR) protein. J Biol Chem 1999;274:5909–5918.

61. Dufau ML, Tinajero JC, Fabbri A. Corticotropin-releasing factor: an antireproductive hormone of the testis. FASEB 1993;7:299–307.

62. Calkins JH, Sigel MM, Nankin HR, et al. Interleukin-1 inhibits Leydig cell steroidogenesis in primary culture. Endocrinology 1988;123:1605–1610.

63. Lejeune H, Chuzel F, Sanchez P, et al. Stimulating effect of both human recombinant inhibin A and activin A on immature porcine Leydig cell functions in vitro. Endocrinology 1997;138:4783–4791.

64. Nes WD, Lukyanenko YO, Jia ZH, et al. Identification of the lipophilic factor produced by macrophages that stimulates steroidogenesis. Endocrinology 2000;141:953–958.

65. Pelletier G, Labrie C, Labrie F. Localization of oestrogen receptor alpha, oestrogen receptor beta and androgen receptors in the rat reproductive organs. J Endocrinol 2000;165:359–370.

66. Burgos-Trinidad M, Youngblood GL, Maroto MR, et al. Repression of cAMP-induced expression of the mouse P450 17 alpha-hydroxylase/C17-20 lyase gene (Cyp17) by androgens. Mol Endocrinol 1997;11:87–96.

67. Abney TO. The potential roles of estrogens in regulating Leydig cell development and function: a review. Steroids 1999;64:610–617.

68. Sankar BR, Maran RR, Sivakumar R, et al. Chronic administration of corticosterone impairs LH signal transduction and steroidogenesis in rat Leydig cells. J Steroid Biochem Mol Biol 2000;72:155–162.

69. Goldsmith PC, Thind KK, Song T, et al. Location of the neuroendocrine gonadotropin-releasing hormone neurons in the monkey hypothalamus by retrograde tracing and immunostaining. J Neuroendocrinol 1990;2:157–168.

70. Caraty A, Locatelli A. Effect of time after castration on secretion of LHRH and LH in the ram. J Reprod Fertil 1988;82:263–269.

71. Shupnik MA. Gonadotropin gene modulation by steroids and gonadotropin-releasing hormone. Biol Reprod 1996;54:279–286.

72. Marshall JC, Dalkin AC, Haisenleder DJ, et al. Gonadotropin-releasing hormone pulses: regulators of gonadotropin synthesis and ovulatory cycles. Recent Prog Horm Res 1991;47:155–187.

73. Chedrese PJ, Kay TW, Jameson JL. Gonadotropin-releasing hormone stimulates glycoprotein hormone alpha-subunit messenger ribonucleic acid (mRNA) levels in alpha T3 cells by increasing transcription and mRNA stability. Endocrinology 1994;134:2475–2481.

74. Kaiser UB, Jakubowiak A, Steinberger A, Chin WW. Regulation of rat pituitary gonadotropin-releasing hormone receptor mRNA levels in vivo and in vitro. Endocrinology 1993;133:931–934.

75. Chase DJ, Schanbacher BD, Lunstra DD. Effects of pulsatile and continuous luteinizing hormone (LH) infusions on testosterone responses to LH in rams actively immunized against gonadotropin-releasing hormone. Endocrinology 1988;123:816–826.

76. Saez JM, Forest MG. Kinetics of human chorionic gonadotropin-induced steroidogenic response of the human testis. I. Plasma testosterone: Implications for human chorionic gonadotropin stimulation test. J Clin Endocrinol Metab 1979;49:278–283.

77. Hsueh AJ, Dufau ML, Catt KJ. Gonadotropin-induced regulation of luteinizing hormone receptors and desensitization of testicular 3':5'-cyclic AMP and testosterone responses. Proc Natl Acad Sci USA 1977;74:592–595.

78. Chuzel F, Schteingart H, Vigier M, et al. Transcription and post-transcriptional regulation of luteotropin/chorionic gonadotropin receptor by the agonist in Leydig cells. Eur J Biochem 1995;229:316–325.

79. Santen RJ. Is aromatization of testosterone estradiol required for inhibition of luteinizing hormone secretion in men? J Clin Invest 1975;56:1555–1563.

80. Winters SJ, Ishizaka K, Kitahara S, et al. Effects of testosterone on gonadotropin subunit messenger RNAs in the presence or absence of GnRH. Endocrinology 1992;130:726–735.

81. Winters S, Sherins RJ, Troen P. The gonadotropin suppressive activity of androgen is increased in elderly men. Metabolism 1984;33:1052–1059.

82. Boyar RM, Moore RJ, Rosner W, et al. Studies of gonadotropin–gonadal dynamics in patients with androgen insensitivity. J Clin Endocrinol Metab 1978;47:1116–1122.

83. Finkelstein JS, Whitcomb RW, O'Dea LS, et al. Sex steroid control of gonadotropin secretion in the human male. I. Effects of testosterone administration in normal and gonadotropin-releasing hormone-deficient men. J Clin Endocrinol Metab 1991;73:609–620.

84. Plant TM, Dubey AK. Evidence from the rhesus monkey (*Macaca mulatta*) for the view that negative feedback control of luteinizing hormone secretion by the testis is mediated by a deceleration of hypothalamic gonadotropin-releasing hormone pulse frequency. Endocrinology 1984;115:2145–2153.

85. Kawakami S, Winters SJ. Regulation of luteinizing hormone secretion and subunit messenger ribonucleic acid expression by gonadal steroids in perifused pituitary cells from male monkeys and rats. Endocrinology 1999;140:3587–3593.

86. Sherins RJ, Loriaux DL. Studies on the role of sex steroids in the feedback control of luteinizing hormone in normal men. J Clin Endocrinol Metab 1973;36:886–893.

87. Smith EP, Boyd J, Frank GR, et al. Estrogen resistance caused by a mutation in the estrogen-receptor gene in a man. N Engl J Med 1994;331:1056–1061.

88. Morishima A, Grumbach MM, Simpson ER, et al. Aromatase deficiency in male and female siblings caused by a novel mutation and the physiological role of estrogens. J Clin Endocrinol Metab 1995;80:3689–3698.

89. Naftolin F, Judd HL, Yen SSC. Pulsatile patterns of gonadotropins and testosterone in man: the effects of clomiphene with and without testosterone. J Clin Endocrinol Metab 1973;36:285–288.

90. Marynick SP, Loriaux DL, Sherins RJ, et al. Evidence that testosterone can suppress pituitary gonadotropin secretion independently of peripheral aromatization. J Clin Endocrinol Metab 1979; 49:396–398.

91. Winters SJ, Troen P. Evidence for a role of endogenous estrogen in the hypothalamic control of gonadotropin secretion in men. J Clin Endocrinol Metab 1985;61:842–845.

92. Sharma TP, Blache D, Blackberry MA, Martin GB. Role of peripheral and central aromatization in the control of gonadotrophin secretion in the male sheep. Reprod Fertil Dev 1999;11:293–302.

93. Finkelstein JS, O'Dea LS, Whitcomb RW, et al. Sex steroid control of gonadotropin secretion in the human male. II. Effects of estradiol administration in normal and gonadotropin-releasing hormone-deficient men. J Clin Endocrinol Metab 1991;73:621–628.

94. Burger HG, Robertson DM. Inhibin in the male—progress at last. [editorial] Endocrinology 1997;138: 1361–1362.

95. Vierhaper H, Nowotny P, Waldhausal W. Production rats of testosterone in patients with Cushing's syndrome. Metabolism 2000;49:229–231.

96. Ghinea N, Mai TV, Groyer-Picard MT, Milgrom E. How protein hormones reach their target cells. receptor mediated transcytosis of hCG through endothelial cells. J Cell Biol 1994;125:87–97.

97. Veldhuis JD, King JC, Urban RJ, et al. Operating characteristics of the male hypothalamo–pituitary–gonadal axis: pulsatile release of testosterone and follicle-stimulating hormone and their temporal coupling with luteinizing hormone. J Clin Endocrinol Metab 1987;65:929–941.

98. Winters SJ, Troen P. Testosterone and estradiol are co-secreted episodically by the human testis. J. Clin Invest 1986;78:870–874.

99. Vigersky RA, Easley RB, Loriaux DL. Effect of fluoxymesterone on the pituitary–gonadal axis: the role of testosterone–estradiol-binding globulin. J Clin Endocrinol Metab 1976;43:1–9.

100. Winters SJ, Troen P, Takahashi J. Secretion of testosterone and its delta-4 precursor steroids into spermatic vein blood in men with varicocele-associated infertility. J Clin Endocrinol Metab 1999;84:997–1001.

101. Resko JA, Eik-Nes KB. Diurnal testosterone levels in peripheral plasma of human male subjects. J Clin Enodcrinol Metab 1966;26:573–576.

102. Spratt DI, O'dea LSL, Schoenfeld D, et al. Neuroendocrine-gonadal axis in men: frequent sampling of LH, FSH, and testosterone. Am J Physiol 1988;254:E658–E666.

103. Boyar RM, Rosenfeld RS, Kapen S, et al. Human puberty. Simultaneous augmented secretion of luteinizing hormone and testosterone during sleep. J Clin Invest 1974;54:609–618.

104. Tenover JS, Matsumoto AM, Clifton DK, Bremner WJ. Age-related alterations in the circadian rhythms of pulsatile luteinizing hormone and testosterone secretion in adult men. J Gerontol 1988;43:163–169.

105. Luboshitzky R, Zabari Z, Shen-Orr Z, et al. Disruption of the nocturnal testosterone rhythm by sleep fragmentation in normal men. J Clin Endocrinol Metab 2001;86:1134–1139.

106. Bremner WJ, Vitiello MV, Prinz PN. Loss of circadian rhythmicity in blood testosterone levels with aging in normal men. J Clin Endocrinol Metab 1983;56:1278–1281.

107. Winters SJ. Diurnal rhythm of testosterone and luteinizing hormone in hypogonadal men. J Androl 1991;12:185–190.

108. Dunn JF, Nisula BC, Rodbard D. Transport of steroid hormones: binding of 21 endogenous steroids to both testosterone-binding globulin and corticosteroid-binding globulin in human plasma. J Clin Endocrinol Metab 1981;53:58–68.

109. Joseph DR. Structure, function, and regulation of androgen-binding protein/sex hormone-binding globulin. Vitam Horm 1994;49:197–280

110. Hammond GL. Potential functions of plasma steroid-binding proteins. Trends Endocrinol Metab 1995;6:298–304.

111. Damassa DA, Lin TM, Sonnenschein C, Soto AM. Biological effects of sex hormone-binding globulin on androgen-induced proliferation and androgen metabolism in LNCaP prostate cells. Endocrinology 1991;129:75–84.

112. Raivio T, Palvimo JJ, Dunkel L, et al. Novel assay for determination of androgen bioactivity in human serum. J Clin Endocrinol Metab 2001;86:1539–1544.

113. Hryb DJ, Khan MS, Romas NA, Rosner W. Solubilization of partial characterization of the sex hormone-binding globulin receptor from human prostate. J Biol Chem 1989;264:5378–5383.

114. Hermo L, Barin K, Oko R. Androgen-binding protein secretion and endocytosis by principal cells in the adult rat epididymis and during postnatal development. J Androl 1998;19:527–541.

115. Gerard A, en Nya A, Egloff M, et al. Endocytosis of human sex-steroid-binding protein in monkey germ cells. Ann NY Acad Sci 1992;637:258–276.

116. Bartsch W, Horst HJ, Derwahl DM. Interrelationships between sex hormone-binding globulin and 17 beta-estradiol, testosterone, 5 alpha-dihydrotestosterone, thyroxine, and triiodothyronine in prepubertal and pubertal girls. J Clin Endocrinol Metab 1980;50:1053–1056.

117. Belgorosky A, Rivarola MA. Progressive decrease in serum sex hormone-binding globulin from infancy to late prepuberty in boys. J Clin Endocrinol Metab 1986;63:510–512.

118. Anderson DC. Sex-hormone-binding globulin. Clin Endocrinol 1980;3:69–96.

119. Glass AR, Swerdloff RS, Bray GA, et al. Low serum testosterone and sex hormone binding-globulin in massively obese men. J Clin Endocrinol Metab 1977;45:1211–1219.

120. Longcope C, Feldman HA, McKinlay JB, Araujo AB. Diet and sex hormone-binding globulin. J Clin Endocrinol Metab 2000;85:293–296.

121. Vermeulen A, Kaufman JM, Giagulli VA. Influence of some biological indexes on sex hormone-binding globulin and androgen levels in aging or obese males. J Clin Endocrinol Metab 1996;81:1821–1826.

122. Pugeat M, Crave JC, Elmidani M, et al. Pathophysiology of sex hormone binding globulin (SHBG): relation to insulin. J Steroid Biochem Mol Biol 1991;40:841–849.

123. Plymate SR, Jones RE, Matej LA, Friedl KE. Regulation of sex hormone binding globulin (SHBG) production in Hep G2 cells by insulin. Steroids 1988;52:339–340.

2   Androgen Action

Terry R. Brown, PhD

Contents

Introduction
Androgens and Antiandrogens
Sex Hormone-Binding Globulin
Andtrogen Methbolism
Steroid 5α-Reductase Enzyme
Androgen Receptor
Androgen Receptor and Human Pathology
Summary
References

INTRODUCTION

Androgen action in human male subjects is predominantly the result of the biological activities of testosterone and 5α-dihydrotestosterone (DHT) (*see* Fig. 1). Although the former steroid is the predominant androgen present in the peripheral circulation at a 10-fold to 12-fold greater concentration, the local tissue concentration of DHT may be greater, as is its biological potency. Testosterone is synthesized within Leydig cells and secreted by the testes, whereas DHT is formed primarily as a metabolic product in peripheral tissues expressing steroid 5α-reductase activity. The equilibrium kinetic properties of lipophilic steroids suggest that testosterone can enter cells by passive diffusion across the cell membrane. However, only 1–2% of the testosterone present in the blood is free to diffuse into tissues, because the vast majority of the steroid is bound to sex hormone-binding globulin (SHBG; 40–50%) and to albumin (50–60%). Normal physiologic levels of circulating testosterone are necessary for adequate androgen biologic activity; however, some actions of androgens within tissues require the local conversion of testosterone to its more biologically active metabolite, DHT. A single molecular form of the androgen receptor (AR) exists within androgen target cells. The inactive cytoplasmic AR is a member of a large macromolecular chaperone complex, which dissociates upon the binding of testosterone or DHT to its receptor. The binding of steroid produces a conformational (or allosteric) change to an activated receptor complex that translocates into the nucleus and binds with high affinity as homodimers

From: *Contemporary Endocrinology: Androgens in Health and Disease*
Edited by: C. Bagatell and W. J. Bremner © Humana Press Inc., Totowa, NJ

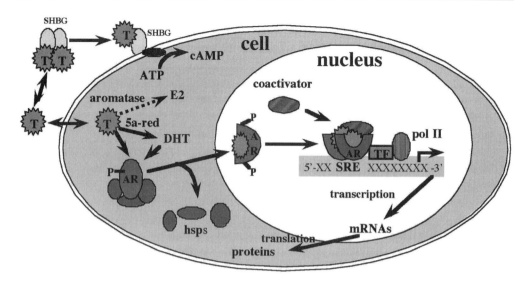

Fig. 1. Mechanism for androgen action in target organs. Testosterone (T) circulates in the blood predominantly bound to carrier proteins, such as the dimers formed by sex hormone-binding globulin (SHBG). SHBG–T or SHBG–DHT complexes can bind to receptors on the cell surface and activate the cyclic AMP-dependent protein kinase A pathways. Alternatively, free T enters cells by passive diffusion. Within the target cell, T may act by itself or be converted to its active metabolites, dihydrotestosterone (DHT) by steroid 5α-reductase or estradiol (E$_2$) by the aromatase pathway. E$_2$ acts through the estrogen receptor pathway (not shown). The cytoplasmic androgen receptor (AR) is a phosphoprotein (P) that forms a large macromolecular complex with various chaperone molecules, including heat shock proteins (hsps). Upon binding of androgen, T, or DHT, the receptor undergoes a conformational change and hsps are released. The AR complex undergoes further phosphorylation and acquires increased avidity for binding to DNA. The activated AR–T/DHT steroid complexes bind as dimers to specific steroid response elements (SREs) defined by DNA nucleotide sequences in regulatory regions of androgen-responsive genes. The chromatin-bound receptors are complexed with other nuclear proteins that function as coactivators (or corepressors) of gene transcription that may act to modify the chromatin structure (histone acetylation/deacetylation) and/or interact with the transcriptional initiation complex composed of various transcription factors (TFs) and RNA polymerase II (pol II). This complex acts to facilitate or repress transcription of specific mRNAs, which are subsequently translated into cellular/secretory proteins.

to specific binding sites on nuclear chromatin adjoining androgen-responsive genes. ARs function as transcription factors and form larger complexes via interactions with additional nuclear proteins that serve as transcriptional coactivators or adaptors, some of which possess intrinsic kinase, methyltransferase, or histone acetyltransferase activities. These multifactorial transcriptional complexes activate (or repress) androgen-regulated gene transcription by RNA polymerase, which alters the levels of specific mRNAs. The translation of mRNAs on cytoplasmic ribosomes directs the synthesis of proteins responsible for androgen-induced changes in cell function, growth, or differentiation.

It is important to remember that testosterone also serves as a precursor for estrogen biosynthesis. Therefore, estrogenic actions can occur in men following aromatization of testosterone to estradiol and binding of the latter steroid to nuclear estrogen receptors.

Hence, the local tissue metabolism and concentration of testosterone, DHT, or estradiol will determine the specific hormonal responses that are observed.

This chapter will address the biochemical events and molecular biology of androgen action, with a particular emphasis on the molecular mechanisms of androgen action at the cellular level. The androgen receptor is the key intracellular molecule involved in mediating androgen action and much of this chapter describes the multiple dimensions of its molecular structure and biologic function. Various human pathologic conditions associated with abnormal androgen action are discussed briefly, with emphasis on how studies of these conditions have increased our overall understanding of androgen action.

ANDROGENS AND ANTIANDROGENS

Androgens are steroid hormones that induce the differentiation and maturation of the male reproductive organs, the development of male secondary sex characteristics, and the behavioral manifestations consistent with the male role in reproduction *(1)*. The two most important endogenous steroid hormones of the adult male that manifest both androgenic and anabolic activities are testosterone and DHT. Synthetic analogs of testosterone, such as nandrolone decanoate, oxandrolone, and stanozolol, produce primarily anabolic actions on muscle and skeleton and are often substances abused by bodybuilders and athletes. Antiandrogens are synthetic compounds that compete with androgens for binding to AR, but do not generate androgenic effects *(2)*. These compounds are used primarily in the treatment of prostate cancer and include cyproterone acetate, flutamide, and bicalutamide. Although cyproterone acetate acts as an inhibitor of androgen action, it is also a strong progestin with central antigonadotropic effects and is a weak glucocorticoid. Flutamide and bicalutamide are pure antiandrogens with no inherent glucocorticoid, progestational, androgenic, or estrogenic activities. Bicalutamide has an affinity for AR approximately fourfold greater than hydroxyflutamide, the active metabolite of flutamide. Bicalutamide also has a significantly longer half-life that is compatible with single daily administration.

SEX HORMONE-BINDING GLOBULIN

Sex hormone-binding globulin (SHBG) is synthesized in the liver and forms a homodimer that is glycosylated and secreted into the blood as a 95-kDa β-globulin *(3)*. Several different isoforms of SHBG, represented by differential posttranslational glycosylation, normally appear in blood and a variant allele of the gene is present in a subpopulation of individuals. Each of the protein subunits is capable of binding a molecule of steroid near its dimeric interface *(4)*. SHBG binds testosterone, DHT, and, more weakly, estradiol *(5)*. Under physiologic conditions, about 40–50% of testosterone is bound with higher affinity to SHBG. Some evidence suggests that the actual in vivo bioavailable testosterone includes both the free steroid as well as the lower-affinity, readily dissociable albumin-bound steroid, or about half of the total testosterone *(6)*. The level of SHBG in blood is increased by estrogens, but decreased by androgens. The suppression of SHBG levels following exogenous administration of testosterone has been employed clinically as an index of human androgen sensitivity in cases of suspected androgen-insensitivity syndrome resulting from mutations in the AR gene. Recent studies have also demonstrated that SHBG–steroid complexes may be biologically active via their binding to cell surface SHBG receptors that evoke an increase in intracellular cAMP levels *(7)*. Androgen-binding protein (ABP) is a product of the same gene that is expressed in testicular Sertoli cells and secreted into the seminiferous tubules, where it binds a significant proportion of the testosterone and/ or DHT present in the intratubular fluid of the testes and epididymides. This may explain, in part, the apparent requirement for high intratesticular levels of testosterone in the maintenance of spermatogenesis.

ANDROGEN METABOLISM

Testosterone is, itself, an active steroid with both androgenic actions to promote spermatogenesis in the testes and anabolic actions to increase tissue mass in muscle. In sexual tissues, such as the skin and prostate, testosterone is irreversibly converted primarily to the active metabolite DHT *(8)*. DHT can be further reduced to 5α-androstane-3α-, 17β-diol (3α-diol) and subsequently conjugated with glucuronide to form 3α-diol glucuronide *(9)*. These latter reactions are reversible such that 3α-diol, or its glucuronide, can be converted back to DHT. Most of the DHT, 3α-diol, and their glucuronides that appear in blood are derived from extrasplanchnic metabolism. Inactivation of testosterone occurs primarily in the liver and involves the formation of 17-ketosteroids via oxidation of the 17-OH group, reduction of the A ring, and reduction of the 3-keto group with the formation of polar metabolites that include diols, triols, and their conjugates *(10)*. Testosterone and its synthetic precursor androstenedione can be aromatized to estradiol and estrone, respectively, by the cytochrome P450 aromatase enzyme, designated CYP19 *(11)*. The enzyme complex catalyzes a multistep reaction leading to removal of the methyl group as formic acid and the rearrangement of the steroid A ring to an aromatic structure. This reaction requires NADPH as a cofactor for NADPH–cytochrome P450 reductase to enable the transfer of reducing equivalents to the enzyme, with 3 mol of oxygen being consumed in the sequence of hydroxylation reactions. Approximately 60–70 µg of estradiol are formed each day in normal men, primarily within adipose tissue, and this serves to further diversify the biological actions derived from androgens at the individual tissue level.

STEROID 5α-REDUCTASE ENZYME

The conversion of testosterone to a variety of 5α- and 5β-reduced metabolites was known prior to the discovery that the 5α-reduced metabolite DHT was the principal intracellular androgen concentrated within the nuclei of many androgen-responsive target tissues, such as the prostate *(8)*. DHT proved to be twice as potent as testosterone in bioassays. Its physiologic importance was confirmed in human subjects with abnormal male sex differentiation and decreased serum concentrations of DHT resulting from genetic deficiency of steroid 5α-reductase enzyme activity *(12)*. Russell and Wilson *(8)* discovered that steroid 5α-reductase was present as two isoforms encoded by different genes, each containing 5 exons and having 50% identity of their nucleotide sequences. The 28- to 29-kDa enzyme proteins are localized to the endoplasmic reticulum and nuclear membranes, bind testosterone as a substrate, and require NADPH as a cofactor. The human type 1 isoform is present at low levels in the prostate but is the predominant isozyme expressed in the skin and liver. It is encoded by a gene on the short arm of chromosome 5, has an optimal activity across a broad pH range from 6.5 to 8.0, has a high K_m (1–5 µM) for testosterone, and is relatively insensitive (K_i = 300–500 nM) to the

4-azasteroid inhibitor finasteride. The type 2 isozyme is encoded by its gene on the short arm of chromosome 2, has an acidic pH (5.0) optimum, and a low K_m (0.1–1.0 μM) for testosterone and is sensitive to inhibition by finasteride ($K_i = 3–5$ nM). As discussed in a later chapter, molecular defects in the type 2 isozyme are responsible for the reduced serum and tissue DHT concentrations and inadequate virilization of the urogenital sinus and external genitalia observed in some infants with male pseudohermaphroditism because of steroid 5α-reductase enzyme deficiency.

ANDROGEN RECEPTOR

The AR is a member of the larger superfamily of nuclear ligand-dependent transcription factors that includes all of the steroid receptors among its members [13]. Thus, the AR gene and protein share homology and conservation of structure and function with the other steroid receptors [14] (see Fig. 2). The human AR gene locus resides on the X chromosome between q11 and q12 and is estimated to span a region of approx 90 kb [15,16]. The gene encodes eight exons and transcription is initiated from one of two sites within a 13-bp region of a single promoter that lacks a TATA or a CCAAT box [17]. The AR promoter contains a GC box near the initiation site and an adjacent upstream homopurine/homopyrimidine stretch. Transcription from the initiation site at +13, but not +1, is dependent on binding of Sp1 to the GC box. The purine/pyrimidine region can bind Sp1 in its normal double-stranded B-DNA conformation, but a novel single-strand binding protein may also be involved [18]. Relative to the rather large size of the AR gene, the predominant mRNA transcript is 10.6 kb, with a minor 8.5-kb transcript also detected in various tissues. The 10.6-kb transcript includes a 1.1-kb 5' untranslated region (UTR), the 2.7-kb open reading frame (ORF) and a relatively long 3' UTR of 6.8 kb, whereas the shorter, alternative 8.5-kb mRNA transcript arises from differential splicing in the 3' UTR. Recently, unique androgen-responsive regulatory regions within exons 4 and 5 have been postulated to mediate upregulation of AR mRNA transcription that occurs in several cell types in response to androgen [19]. A portion of the 5' UTR of AR mRNA is capable of forming a stem-loop secondary structure that has been suggested to play a role in the induction of AR translation [20].

Variations in the coding region of the cDNA clones for the human AR arise as a result of polymorphisms in two stretches of the nucleotide sequence that encode amino acid polymeric repeats for glutamine and glycine within the amino terminus of the approx 110-kDa protein. Hence, the number of amino acids reported in the literature for AR vary between 910 and 919. All numeric references to amino acid residues in this chapter are derived from the original AR cDNA cloned by Lubahn et al. [21] and have been adopted as the international reference standard for the Human Androgen Receptor Mutation Database maintained at McGill University [22].

Posttranslational modification of AR occurs via phosphorylation on several serine residues and results in a shift in the apparent molecular weight (MW) to 112–114 kDa [23,24]. The translation of an 87-kDa (AR-A) minor isoform of the receptor has been reported to occur from an alternative initiation methionine codon at position 189, but this isoform generally represents less than 20% of the total AR protein expressed in tissues [26]. Interestingly, cell transfection studies showed that transcriptional activation by the amino truncated AR-A isoform could not be distinguished from the full-length AR-B isoform. More recent studies, however, suggest that the entire amino terminus plays a

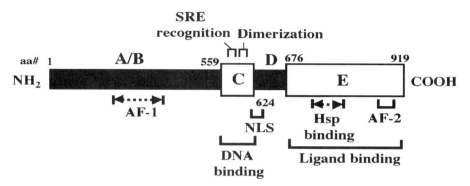

Fig. 2. Structural and functional domains of the human androgen receptor. The human AR is a 919-amino-acid protein with homology of structure and function with other members of the nuclear steroid-receptor family. Five representative structural and functional domains indicated by the letters A–E are conserved within these receptor proteins. The amino-terminal A/B region is characterized by significant divergence of amino acid sequence and number among the various receptors presenting differences in epitope recognition and in properties related to transcriptional activation. A strong transcriptional activating function (AF-1) resides within the A/B domain of AR. The central C region contains the two zinc fingers required for DNA binding, with the first zinc finger containing the "P-box" for specific recognition of steroid response elements (SREs) on DNA and the second zinc finger containing the "D box" that promotes receptor dimerization. A nuclear localization signal (NLS) sequence resides in the region linking the DNA-binding and hinge (D) domains. The hinge region provides conformational flexibility within the molecule between the DNA-binding and ligand-binding (E) domains. The E domain also contains putative sites for binding of chaperones, such as the heat shock proteins (hsps), and a second, ligand-dependent activating function (AF-2) where coactivators may bind to AR.

critical role in the conformation and stability of the ligand-bound receptor. Like other nuclear steroid receptors and as discussed in the forthcoming subsections, the AR shares a molecular architecture that includes a poorly conserved amino-terminal transactivation domain, a highly conserved DNA-binding domain, a connecting hinge region, and a discrete ligand-binding domain (*see* Fig. 2).

Amino-Terminal Transactivation Domain

The amino terminus is the least conserved region and varies significantly in length among members of the steroid-receptor superfamily. The relatively long amino terminus of the AR includes 538 amino acids and is entirely encoded by the first exon of the AR gene *(26)*. Assays of transcriptional activity that examined the effects of deleting different portions of the AR cDNA, initially ascribed a transcriptional activation domain to the amino terminus of AR *(14)*. However, only recently have more detailed structural analyses revealed additional significant biological functions of this region. The entire amino-terminal domain is required for full activity of the receptor *(27,28)*. More specifically, a core region was defined between amino acids 101 and 360, termed tau-1, that contributes 50% of the activity. However, in the absence of the carboxyl-terminal ligand-binding domain, a different region, termed tau-5 (residues 370–494), can also mediate activation. A functional interaction occurs between the amino-terminal domain, which contains the so-called activation function (AF)-1, and the carboxy-terminal ligand-binding domain, which contains a second activation domain referred to as AF-2. Within the amino terminus of AR, the subregions encompassing amino acid residues 14–36 and 371–494 were subsequently implicated in these interactions with the ligand-binding domain. Most recently, the FXXLF motif represented by the amino acid sequence FQNLF (aa 23–27) and the WXXLF motif represented by the amino acid sequence WHTLF (aa 433–437) have been identified as the specific regions within the amino terminus of AR that interact with other regions within the carboxy-terminal ligand-binding domain *(29)*. The increased stability of the AR that is observed when it is bound to androgen has been attributed to the intramolecular interactions that occur between the amino- and carboxy-terminal regions of AR. Moreover, the conformational change imposed by such intramolecular interaction may interfere with the recruitment and interaction of the commonly recognized LXXLL motifs that reside within most nuclear coactivators and their recognition by the AF-2 domain found in most steroid receptors, including AR (discussed in more detail under the headings Ligand-Binding Domain and Coactivators). Recent reports have inferred that AR interaction with nuclear coactivators relies less upon the AF-2 domain and more on the AF-1 domain for enhanced transcriptional activity *(29–31)*. Furthermore, the AF-1 domain to which coactivators binds appears to be distinct from the region involved in the amino- and carboxy-terminal interaction within the AR protein.

A unique, polymorphic polyglutamine stretch encoded by (CAG)nCAA and polymorphic polyglycine sequence encoded by (GGN)n, are present in the human AR amino terminus, in addition to polyalanine and polyproline amino acid repeats *(21)*. Within the normal population, the number of glutamine repeats varies from 9–33 residues and the glycine stretch ranges between 16 and 27 residues *(32,33)*. The polymorphic nature of these amino acid repeats accounts for natural variations in the length of the cDNAs that were cloned for the human AR and in the assignment of amino acid numbers encoded within the protein. Acidic polyproline and polyglutamine sequence motifs are generally believed to confer a transcriptional activation function when present in various proteins. Indeed, fewer numbers of glutamine residues in this region of AR are associated with higher levels of gene transactivation than are longer repeat lengths *(32)*. Moreover, genetic variations in the length of the polyglutamine stretch are implicated in the progressive nature of prostate cancer *(34,35)* and in the neuromuscular degenerative disease described by Kennedy, otherwise known as spinal bulbar muscular atrophy *(36)*. In prostate cancer, the more transcriptionally active AR with fewer polyglutamine residues is associated with higher incidence and faster progression of disease, whereas in spinal bulbar muscular atrophy, abnormally long repeats that exceed 40 glutamine residues are associated with neuronal degeneration.

DNA-Binding Domain

The DNA-binding domain represents a highly conserved, cysteine-rich region that occupies a central location within the structural organization of the various members of the steroid-receptor superfamily (*see* Fig. 3). In the AR, this 66-amino-acid domain is encoded by exons 2 and 3 and shares 70–80% homology of amino acid sequence with the related glucocorticoid (GR) and progesterone (PR) receptors *(26)*. Derivation of the molecular structure of the AR DNA-binding domain is based on previous nuclear magnetic resonance (NMR) and X-ray crystallographic data for the GR. The DNA-binding domain of AR consists of three α-helices organized into two zinc fingers within which four cysteine residues at the base of each finger coordinate zinc in a tetrahedral

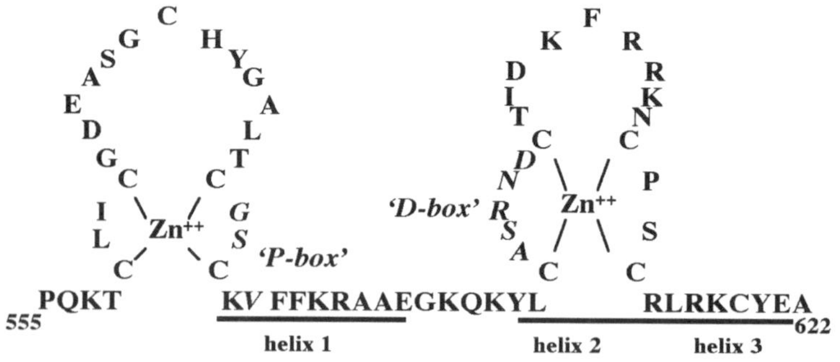

Fig. 3. Amino acid sequence of the human androgen-receptor DNA-binding domain. The single-letter amino acid code is shown for the sequence within the two zinc fingers formed by tetrahedral coordination of zinc by each of four cysteines in the androgen receptor DNA-binding domain. The proximal "P box," comprised of the amino acids G, S, and V, for specific recognition of the androgen response element on DNA is indicated in the first finger and the distal "D box," composed of A, S, R, N, and D, involved in dimerization is indicated in the second finger. Three helices are formed within the structure of the DNA-binding domain, with helices 1 and 3 arranged in perpendicular plane to the DNA.

array *(37)*. The first zinc finger incorporates a perpendicularly oriented α-helix where the amino acid residues gly577, ser578, and val581 at its carboxy terminus form the proximal (P) box, which is conserved in AR, GR, and PR. Mutational analyses showed that this conserved sequence is responsible for the common recognition and binding of these three receptors to a similar DNA steroid response element (SRE) consisting of the consensus palindromic nucleotide sequence, -AGAACAnnnTGTTCT-. The α-helix containing the P box is positioned in the major groove of DNA where the three conserved amino acid residues make base-specific contacts with DNA. The second zinc finger has two α-helices, the first of which forms the distal (D) box, consisting of five amino acids (ala-ser-arg-asn-asp) that form a symmetric interface for homodimerization of the receptor that accompanies its binding to a palindromic SRE, as previously demonstrated for GR. The first and third helices within the DNA-binding domain are perpendicular to each other and form numerous hydrogen bonds.

The critical features of protein–DNA binding that differentially determine the specificity of AR, GR, and PR binding to DNA regulatory sequences, and hence their discriminatory function in steroid-specific gene regulation, are now under scrutiny. Recent experiments have identified genes that are specifically responsive to androgens and analysis of the AR-binding sites in their promoters has revealed SRE motifs that resemble direct nucleotide repeat sequences rather than palindromic, inverted nucleotide repeat sequences *(38)* (*see* Table 1). Further analysis of the binding of AR to these direct-repeat nucleotide binding sites suggested that the dimerization interface within the AR homodimers differed from that observed on inverted-repeat DNA-binding sites. These findings predicted that dimerization of the AR occurred in a head-to-tail orientation of the monomeric AR molecules and that the intermolecular interactions at the dimerization interface involved amino acids in the second zinc finger and the adjoining hinge region *(38)*. Subsequent mutation analysis revealed that three specific amino acids, thr585, gly610, and leu617, are involved in the recognition of the direct nucleotide repeat

Table 1
Classification of Androgen Response Elements

A. High affinity, nonspecific
GRE177   GTTACA aac TGTTCT
C3(1) ARE   AGTACT tga TGTTCT
GRE2 TAT   TGTACA gga TGTTCT
PSA ARE1   AGCACT tgc TGTTCT
SLP-HRE-3   GAAACA gcc TGTTCT

B. High affinity, AR specific
PB-ARE-2   GGTTCT tgg AGTACT
SLP-HRE-2   TGGTCA ggc AGTTCT
SC ARE1.2   GGCTCT ttc AGTTCT

C. Low affinity, nonspecific
PB-ARE-1   ATAGCA tct TGTTCT
MVDP pARE   TGAAGT tcc TGTTCT
GPX5   ATCCTA tgt TGTTCT
CRP2   AGAACA aaa TGTACA

D. Low affinity, AR specific
SC ARE   AGCAGG ctg TGTCCC

Note: Four classes of androgen response elements have been defined by Claessens et al. *(38)* based on gel-shift assays of protein–DNA binding with AR or GR and by transfection experiments in which transcription of an ARE-reporter gene is activated by either AR and/or GR. The androgen response elements (AREs) and glucocorticoid response elements (GREs) are derived from the promoter sequences: GRE177 from the MMTV-LTR; C3(1) ARE from the C3 subunit of the rat prostate prostatein gene; GRE TAT from the mouse liver tyrosine aminotransferase gene; PSA ARE1 from the human prostate-specific antigen gene; SLP-HRE-2 and -3 from the mouse sex-limited protein gene; PB-ARE-1 and -2 from the rat prostate probasin gene; SC ARE1.2 from the human secretory component gene; VDP pARE from the mouse vas deferens protein gene; GPX5 from the mouse epididymal glutathione peroxidase 5 gene; and CRP2 from the cystatin-related protein gene.

that serves as an AR-specific binding site in the rat probasin gene promoter. Further support for this hypothesis will evolve as the AR-binding sites are identified within the promoters of other androgen-responsive genes. In addition, the proximity of binding sites on the DNA of gene promoters for other transcription factors can also modify the specificity for AR binding to adjacent SREs; hence, the transcriptional activity of AR is also dependent on the context of individual promoter elements *(39)*.

Nuclear Localization Signal and the Hinge Region

In the absence of ligand, the AR is primarily localized to the cytoplasm, whereas the addition of androgen induces its rapid translocation to the nucleus *(14)*. A bipartite nuclear targeting signal sequence encoded at the junction between exons 3 and 4 functions to shuttle the AR through nuclear pores. The signal sequence consists of 2 clusters of basic amino acids, separated by 10 amino acids, that reside within the region that joins the DNA-binding domain and the hinge region (40). Amino acid substitutions or deletions in this region bounded by residues 617–633 cause an almost complete cytoplasmic localization of the receptor.

Recent advances in imaging techniques and the in vivo expression of chimeric AR tagged with a modified version of green fluorescent protein have revealed a number of important properties associated with ligand-dependent nuclear translocation of the receptor in live cells (41). First, in the absence of ligand, the AR is predominantly localized to the cellular cytoplasm. Second, upon the addition of androgen, such as DHT, the nuclear translocation of AR is apparent within minutes and is nearly complete within 30 min. The apparent rate and extent of nuclear import is reduced with ligands that display reduced affinity for the receptor or antagonist activity. In the presence of androgens that act as agonists and activate transcription, the nuclear AR appears tightly associated with chromatin and organized within distinct subnuclear compartments. By comparison, when cells are exposed to antagonists, such as the antiandrogens flutamide or bicalutamide, the AR exhibits ligand-dependent migration into the nucleus but does not display a pattern of subnuclear compartmentalization as observed in the presence of androgen. Furthermore, androgen withdrawal releases the receptor from its chromatin association and exports it back into the cytoplasmic compartment for recycling when the steroid is reintroduced. The small nuclear ring finger protein SNURF, which interacts with the AR through a region overlapping the bipartite nuclear localization signal, facilitates AR nuclear import and retards its export upon hormone withdrawal (42). Further details regarding the processes of nuclear import and export are likely to become apparent from additional experiments using sophisticated imaging techniques.

The hinge region has been associated with conformational flexibility induced by the binding of ligand to the carboxy-terminal domain and the binding of the ligand-activated receptor to DNA. Interestingly, a repressor activity is associated with the hinge region in AR. Deletion of amino acid residues 628–646 from the hinge region of AR created a mutant receptor with a twofold higher ligand-dependent transactivation activity than the wild-type receptor (43). Moreover, interaction of the mutant receptor with the p160 coactivator TIF2 was significantly enhanced, as was its effect on AR transactivation. Mutations of the AR involving single-amino-acid substitutions within the hinge region also occur in prostate cancer. Recently, several of these mutant ARs were shown to have increased transcriptional activity when compared with the wild-type AR (44).

Ligand-Binding Domain

Androgen agonists and antagonists bind to the carboxy-terminal ligand-binding domain of AR encoded by exons 4–8 (26). In the absence of ligand, some steroid receptors actually repress gene transactivation by occupying nuclear chromatin sites. By contrast, the AR is predominantly localized to the cytoplasm in the absence of ligand and exists within a large macromolecular complex of chaperone proteins that includes several members of the heat shock family (45). In this state, the AR is maintained in an inactive conformation that is not capable of binding to DNA. Deletion of the ligand-binding domain relieves its repressive function such that the truncated AR protein is able to bind to DNA and is constitutively active as a result of expression of its intrinsic AF-1 activation domain (14). Alternatively, the binding of an androgen agonist causes the inactive macromolecular chaperone complex to dissociate and promotes the nuclear translocation and DNA binding of AR *(46)*. Agonist binding also activates the transactivation function of AF-2 and this coincides with alteration of the AR molecular conformation. The active conformation of the receptor is stabilized by the presence of androgen and AR homodimers bind in the nucleus to androgen response elements (AREs) on DNA *(47)*. Androgens bind to either the nonphosphorylated or phosphorylated forms of AR. Although the significance of posttranslational modification of AR by phosphorylation has not been clearly defined, its role in ligand-independent activation via alternative signal transduction pathways has been inferred from a number of recent studies.

A series of 12 conserved helices form the ligand-binding domain of steroid receptors as revealed by X-ray crystallographic analyses of these receptors conducted in the presence and absence of agonists and antagonists *(48,49)*. The AR ligand-binding-domain crystal structure in the presence of the synthetic ligand, R1881, contains nine α-helices, two 3_{10}-helices, and four short β-strands associated in two antiparallel β-sheets *(50,51)* (*see* Fig. 4). The AR, like PR, has no helix 2, but its helix 12 is longer than those of some other steroid receptors and has an extended carboxy-terminal amino acid chain. The helices are arranged in a "helical sandwich" pattern and helices 4 and 5, and 10 and 11, are contiguous. In the case of AR, helices 10 and 11 are interrupted by a proline residue at position 868 which causes a kink between the helices. As in PR, there is a very short β-sheet formed by the loop between helices 8 and 9 and the carboxy-terminus, which holds helix 12 in the closed agonist conformation, close to and capping the ligand-binding site (*see* Fig. 5). The androgen ligand DHT interacts with helices 3, 5, and 11 within the ligand-binding domain. The AF-2 region resides within helix 12 of the AR and other receptors. When the receptor is occupied by a steroid agonist, helix 12 closes over the ligand-binding pocket to form a surface for interaction with transcriptional coactivators; by contrast, binding of antagonists prevents this interface from forming. Conformational changes that accompany binding of steroid agonists also promote the intramolecular interactions that occur between the amino-terminal transactivation (AF-1) and carboxy-terminal ligand-binding (AF-2) domains in AR, interactions that are critical for receptor transactivation *(29)*. The relatively weaker transactivation effect of the AF-2 domain in AR has been associated with a competition between the internal AF-1 domain and coactivators for interaction with AF-2. It has been suggested that the p160 family of coactivators interact with AR by forming a bridge that links the AF-1 and AF-2 domains *(28–31,52)*.

Steroid Response Elements in DNA

Steroid response elements minimally contain a core recognition motif of six nucleotide basepairs, generally consisting of two core motifs (half-sites) separated by a spacer of variable length *(53,54)* (*see* Table 1). The nucleotide sequence of the core motif is relatively specific for subgroups of receptors; the AR, GR, and PR all bind to hexamer half-sites with the consensus sequence TGTTCT. However, an ARE sequence differs from that for the estrogen receptor, TGACCT, at positions 3 and 4, which determines receptor-specific recognition. The consensus SRE for AR is a 15-bp sequence, AGAACAnnnTGTTCT, organized as an inverted or palindromic repeat of core motifs, but which fails in most circumstances to discriminate among AR, GR, and PR. More recently, the identification of synthetic and naturally occurring direct repeats that specify binding of AR, rather than GR, or PR, have suggested that regulatory regions in the

```
           660                          680                              700
            •              HELIX 1     •                                 •
                           ▄▄▄▄▄▄▄                                       ▄▄▄▄
hAR   EETTQKLTVS   HIEGYECQPI   FLNVLEAIEP   GVVCAGHDNN   QPDSFAALLS
hPR   QALSQRFTFS   PGQDIQLIPP   LINLLMSIEP   DVIYAGHDNT   KPDTSSSLLT
hGR   SENPGNKTIV   PATLPQLTPT   LVSLLEVIEP   EVLYAGYDSS   VPDSTWRIMT
                        720                          740
        HELIX 3           •               HELIX 4    •      HELIX 5
      ▄▄▄▄▄▄▄▄                           ▄▄▄▄▄▄▄▄        ▄▄▄▄▄▄▄
hAR   SLNELGERQL   VHVVKWAKAL   PGFRNLHVDD   QMAVIQYSWM   GLMVFAMGWR
hPR   SLNQLGERQL   LSVVKWSKSL   PGFRNLHIDD   QITLIQYSWM   SLMVFGLGWR
hGR   TLNMLGGRQV   IAAVKWAKAI   PGFRNLHLDD   QMTLLQYSWM   FLMAFALGWR
           760                          780                          800
            •      ꓱ       ꓱ    HELIX 6    •     HELIX 7           •
      ▄▄▄▄   ■■■■■■■  ■■■■                                       ▄▄
hAR   SFTNVNSRML   YFAPDLVFNE   YRMHKSRMYS   QCVRMRHLSQ   EFGWLQITPQ
hPR   EFLCMKVLLL   LNTIPLEGLR   SQTQFEEMRS   SYIRELIKAI   GLRQKGVVSS
hGR   EYLCMKTLLL   LSSVPKDGLK   SQELFDEIRM   TYIKELGKAI   VKREGNSSQN
                        820                          840
        HELIX 8       ꓱ   •                HELIX 9      •
      ▄▄▄▄▄▄▄▄      ■■■■■                 ▄▄▄▄▄▄▄▄        ▄▄▄▄
hAR   EFLCMKALLL   FSIIPVDGLK   NQKFFDELRM   NYIKELDRII   ACKRKNPTSC
hPR   EFLCMFVLLL   LNTIPLEGLR   SQTQFEEMRS   SYIRELIKAI   GLRQKGVVSS
hGR   EYLCMKTLLL   LSSVPKDGLK   SQELFDEIRM   TYIKELGKAI   VKREGNSSQN
           860                          880                          900
        HELIX   •   10                HELIX 11    •          HELIX 12  •
      ▄▄▄▄▄▄▄                        ▄▄▄▄▄▄▄▄▄▄▄▄▄▄             ▄▄▄▄▄▄▄
hAR   SRRFYQLTKL   LDSVQPIARE   LHQFTFDLLI   KSHMVSVDFP   EMMAEIISVQ
hPR   SQRFYQLTKL   LDNLHDLVKQ   LHLYCLNTFI   QSRALSVEFP   EMMSEVIAAQ
hGR   WQRFYQLTKL   LDSMHEVVEN   LLNYCFQTFL   D.KTMSIEFP   EMLAEIITNQ
                   ꓱ          919
      ▄▄▄▄▄▄   ■■■■■■■   •
hAR   VPKILSGKVK   PIYFHTQ
hPR   LPKILAGMVK   PLLFHKK
hGR   IPKYSNGNIK   KLLFHQK
```

Fig. 4. Amino acid primary sequence of the human androgen-receptor ligand-binding domain and its homology with the ligand-binding domains of the human progesterone and glucocorticoid receptors. The single-amino-acid code is shown for each of the receptors and the amino acid residue number is indicated (*) for the androgen receptor. The positions of each of the conserved 11 α-helices (H1–H12) and the 4 β-strands in the AR secondary structure are indicated by the solid and dashed lines, respectively, based on the recently published crystal structures of the androgen receptor. (From refs. *50* and *51*.)

promoters of androgen-responsive genes may utilize these sequence-specific binding sites *(38,55)* (*see* Table 1). As mentioned previously, the dimerization of AR monomers in an antiparallel configuration when bound to DNA may also direct AR-specific transactivation *(38)*.

Transcriptional Activation

Sequence-specific DNA-binding transcription factors, such as AR, interact with other general transcription factors in the control of gene activation. These general factors, in turn, interact with the core promoter elements to induce basal transcription. RNA polymerase II and the general transcription factors form the transcription initiation complex

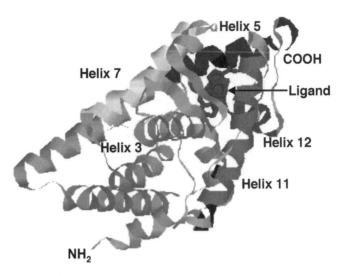

Fig. 5. Tertiary ribbon structure of the human AR ligand-binding domain in the presence of its ligand based on its crystal structure. The ligand, methyltrienolone (R1881), which makes contact with helices 3, 5, and 11 is shown within the binding pocket of the AR, which is capped by helix 12 in the presence of androgen agonists. The AR crystal structure was published by Matias et al. (ref. *50*) and can be viewed at the internet website http://ww.rcsb.org/pdb/ in the Protein Data Bank (PDB) Structure Explorer under the molecule reference number 1E3G.

in conjunction with the TATA-box binding proteins, TATA-binding protein (TBP) and TBP-associated factors ($TAF_{II}s$). Steroid receptors may enhance basal transcription, either by direct interaction with the basal transcription machinery or with $TAF_{II}s$ *(56)*. For example, interaction of the amino terminus of AR with $TF_{II}F$ has been reported *(57)*. Most such interactions between AR and the transcriptional machinery imply direct binding of AR to chromatin. However, AR may not necessarily bind to DNA but rather may bind directly with other sequence specific DNA-binding transcription factors, such as AP-1 and nuclear factor (NF)-κB to modulate gene transcription *(58,59)*.

Coactivators and Corepressors

Coactivators are cellular proteins that interact with the agonist-activated steroid receptor complexes to enhance transactivation of target genes, whereas, in most cases, corepressors have an inverse effect through interaction with antagonist-bound or ligand-free receptors *(60–62)*. A general model for coactivator and corepressor function has evolved. Initially, the repressor protein associates with the receptor on chromatin to maintain a transcriptionally inactive structure by tethering of histone deacetylases to the DNA at sites close to the responsive element for the receptor. Subsequently, binding of hormone by the receptor causes release of the corepressor and recruitment of acetyltransferases, which disrupt the chromatin template by acetylation of histones. Finally, interaction between the activation domains of both the receptor and the recruited coactivator with the basal transcription factors results in gene transcription. Whereas the aforementioned mechanisms may be generally applicable, the ligand-free AR exists predominantly in the cytoplasm in a complex of chaperone proteins and is probably not involved in interactions with corepressors that possess histone deacetylase activity as part of an inactive chromatin-bound complex. However, when steroid antagonists bind to receptors, these complexes can bind to DNA, yet they fail to activate gene transcription. This effect may be the result of failure of coactivators to interact with the antagonist-bound form of the receptor or to the hypothetical binding of a corepressor and associated histone deacetylase. Coactivators may have several roles, including expression of intrinsic histone acetyltransferase (HAT) activity, recruitment of other proteins with HAT activity, and as integrators that enable regulatory molecules to be recruited and assembled at sites of transcriptional activity (60,61).

A number of coactivators are either directly or indirectly involved in chromatin remodeling (60,61). The so-called p160 family of coactivators have been subdivided into three subgroups, represented by SRC-1 (steroid-receptor coactivator-1), SRC-2 which includes TIF2 (transcriptional intermediary factor 2) and GRIP-1 (glucocorticoid-receptor interacting protein 1) and SRC-3, which includes TRAM-1 (thyroid-receptor activator molecule 1), ACTR, and AIB1 (amplified in breast cancer 1). In general, these coactivators interact with the ligand-activated AF-2 regions of different steroid receptors to enhance transcriptional activity. However, for AR, the interaction of these coactivators appears to be predominantly with the AF-1 region and much less with the AF-2 region (30,31). The coactivators possess one or more receptor interaction domains represented by the amino acid sequence motif LXXLL. The coactivators like SRC-1 also interact with integrators such as p300/CBP (cAMP-response element binding [CREB]-binding protein) and pCAF (p300/CBP-associated factor), proteins that possess intrinsic HAT activity, with the overall effect being synergistic for transcriptional activation (60,61).

Other proteins have been identified as coactivators or effectors of transcriptional activity through their specific interaction with AR. Among these are a series of proteins of varying molecular weight that have been reported by Chang et al. The most well-characterized of these proteins is ARA-70 (AR-associated protein, 70 kDa), which interacts in a ligand-dependent manner with AR to increase its transcriptional activity (63). Other members of this group include ARA24, ARA54, ARA55, and ARA160 (64–66). The interaction between AR and other putative coregulator proteins has been reported (67–75). These proteins include ARIP3 (androgen-receptor interacting protein)/PIAS 1 (protein inhibitor of activated STAT), SNURF, ANPK (androgen nuclear protein kinase), BRCA1 (breast cancer susceptibility), BAG-1, Smad3, cyclin E, Ubc9 (ubiquitin E2-conjugating enzyme), and HBO1 (MYST family, human origin recognition complex). The encyclopedia of proteins continues to grow, but the biological relevance of individual protein interactions with AR will require further investigation.

By contrast to molecules that function as coactivators, the corepressors act to repress basal promoter activity in the absence of hormone. Studies of the corepressors, NCo-R (nuclear-receptor corepressor), SMRT (silencing mediator for retinoids and thyroid hormone), and RIP140 (receptor interacting protein, 140 kDa) have provided some general insights into the activities of these molecules (62). The relative activity and interaction of general corepressors on AR transcriptional activity have not been reported, but the PIASy isoform functions in transrepression of AR activity (75).

Ligand-Independent Activation

Steroid receptors, including AR, can also be stimulated to activate gene transcription in the absence of ligand by growth factors, such as insulin-like growth factor I (IGF-I), keratinocyte growth factor (KGF), epidermal growth factor (EGF), luteinizing hormone-releasing hormone (LHRH), neuropeptides, HER-2/neu, interleukin-6 (IL-6) and other agents that directly or indirectly increase intracellular kinase activity or diminish phosphatase activity (76,77). Although the AR is a phosphoprotein, it is unclear whether peptide-activated kinases directly phosphorylate the AR or whether this results in receptor activation, possibly through enhanced binding to DNA. In addition to the AR itself, phosphorylation of coactivators and basal transcription factors could explain the AR ligand-independent transcriptional activity. Importantly, peptide activation of AR activity is synergistic with minimal levels of androgens, thus lowering the androgen threshold concentration required for full AR function. These observations are particularly relevant for androgen-deprivation therapy of patients with prostate cancer, in whom the level of androgen is decreased but not completely ablated, and in androgen-independent tumors, where AR expression is present.

Protein kinase A (PKA) can induce prostate-specific antigen (PSA) mRNA and androgen-responsive reporters in prostate cancer cells, an effect that is blocked by antiandrogens (78). Forskolin directly activates AR transcriptional activity (79). Interestingly, the binding of AR to ARE sequences is increased when nuclear extracts are prepared from forskolin-treated cells, despite the observation that nuclear levels of AR are 10-fold higher in androgen-treated cells. Both cAMP and the activator of protein kinase C (PKC), TPA, act synergistically to enhance androgen-stimulated AR transcriptional activity (80,81). 8-Bromo-cAMP has also been shown to induce phosphorylation of SRC-1 and to facilitate ligand-independent activation (82). IL-6 activates AR in prostate cancer cells through a mechanism that involves crosstalk between AR and PKA, PKC, and/or MAPK via ErbB2 (83). AP-1 is a complex of transcription factors encoded by c-fos and c-jun protooncogenes and has been implicated in cell growth, differentiation, and development with its activity modulated by growth factors, cytokines, oncogenes, and activation of PKC by tumor promoters. The fact that c-jun inhibits AR action in some prostate cells and activates it in others emphasizes possible cell- and/or promoter-specific responses that may be explained by differences in the requirements of a particular promoter for coactivators or by differences between cells in the availability of required coactivators (78,84,85). The HER2/Neu protooncogene has been linked to proliferation of prostate cancer cells and can induce AR transactivation of the PSA gene by the mitogen-activated protein (MAP) kinase-dependent phosphorylation of AR (86,87). Inactivation of the PTEN tumor suppressor gene in prostate cancer allows the AKT/PKB pathway to be constitutively active. Alternatively, activation of PI3 kinase by IGF-I can lead to activation of AKT/PKB (88). AKT binds to and phosphorylates AR. Taken together, these results show that multiple kinase-dependent phosphorylation pathways can be activated in prostate cancer cells, suggesting that phosphorylation events affecting AR, related transcription factors, or coactivators may lead to ligand-independent activation of AR.

ANDROGEN RECEPTOR AND HUMAN PATHOLOGY

Androgen Insensitivity Syndrome

The AR is required for normal male sex differentiation and development. Much of our knowledge regarding AR function is derived from studies of human subjects with mutations of the AR gene and defects in the biological action of androgens that underlie the androgen-insensitivity syndrome (AIS) (89,90). AIS can be either complete in which the phenotype of the external genitalia is female, or partial, in which the external genitalia are phenotypically ambiguous. Although hypospadias is a frequent phenotypic feature of partial AIS, isolated hypospadias is rarely associated with an AR gene mutation *(91)*. Numerous AR gene mutations have been identified in AIS and consist primarily of single nucleotide substitutions that result in amino acid substitutions, termination codons, frame shifts, or alterations of mRNA splicing and relatively few deletions varying from a few nucleotides to the entire gene *(89,90)*. Mutations leading to varying degrees of androgen insensitivity have been reported in each of the eight exons of the AR gene. However, most mutations have been identified in the regions that encode the DNA- and ligand-binding domains.

Prostate Cancer

The AR has been the focus of intensive investigation for its role in the mechanisms that regulate the growth and progression of prostate cancer. AR expression is present in prostate tumors at all stages of the disease and tumor growth often continues despite androgen ablation therapy that includes inhibition of gonadotropin secretion and testicular androgen synthesis, antiandrogens that antagonize AR function, and even castration. Recent research has centered on the possibility that AR mutations may occur in more advanced stages of prostate cancer and contribute to the progression of disease via alteration of cell function and proliferation. Thus, AR mutations may lead to gain of function such that the AR is exquisitely sensitive to very low levels of androgen *(92)*, the ligand specificity of the receptor is altered *(93,94)*, or the receptor is activated in the absence of ligand *(76,77)*. Although somatic mutations of the AR have been identified in prostate tumor specimens, reports on the frequency of such mutations have been highly variable between laboratories and study populations, ranging from less than 10% to almost 50% *(95–97)*. In general, the frequency of mutations appears to increase in tumors from later stages of prostate cancer as disease progresses and in metastatic lesions. Another mechanism involves AR gene amplification that has been detected in up to 30% of advanced cancer specimens and may lead to enhanced levels of AR expression *(98)*. As previously mentioned, ligand-independent activation of AR may result from crosstalk with other signal transduction pathways in the absence of androgen. In addition, alterations in the size of the polyglutamine repeat may affect the transactivation of AR and influence androgen action in prostate cancer *(35,99)*. Finally, enhanced expression or phosphorylation of coactivators may lead to their affect to amplify AR function, especially in an environment of reduced endogenous androgen levels following ablation therapy *(100)*.

Spinal Bulbar Muscular Atrophy

An abnormal expansion of the polyglutamine stretch, encoded by (CAG)nCAA, was identified as the molecular basis for spinal bulbar muscular atrophy (SBMA; Kennedy's disease) *(36)*. In normal individuals, the (CAG)nCAA repeat contains 9–33 CAG-like triplets, whereas 38–75 CAG codons are generally found in the AR genes of subjects with SBMA. Increasing disease severity is correlated with greater length of this repeat. As a disease, SBMA is characterized by progressive muscle weakness and atrophy with clinical symptoms manifest in the third to fifth decade of life *(32,33,36)*. The pathology is associated with a severe depletion of lower motornuclei in the spinal cord and brainstem and distal axonopathy of the dorsal root ganglion cells. In addition, subjects with SBMA frequently exhibit endocrine abnormalities, including testicular atrophy, reduced or absent fertility, gynecomastia, and elevated follicle-stimulating hormone (FSH), LH, and estradiol levels, similar to what is observed in mild forms of AIS. Sex differentiation occurs normally and characteristics of mild androgen insensitivity only appear later in life. This may be related to the combination of reduced AR expression and decreased testosterone level in older men. SBMA is an X-linked disease and occurs only in men. At present it is not known whether disease progression involves the ligand-activated or ligand-free AR. In two cases, an extended period of exogenous testosterone administration had little effect on clinical symptoms.

In transfection studies, the length of the CAG repeat was inversely proportional to the ability of the expressed AR to transactivate an androgen-regulated reporter gene *(32)*. However, other investigators have suggested that reduced transcriptional activity was secondary to reduced stability of AR mRNA and decreased AR protein synthesis *(101)*. The reduction in AR function has also been related to the reduced interaction between coactivators and AR *(102)*. Interestingly, AR with an expanded CAG repeat are more resistant to proteolytic degradation and, in particular, are less susceptible to cleavage by caspase-3 *(103,104)*. The increased length of the polyglutamine tract also results in the formation of nuclear inclusions. These aggregates accumulate in the cytoplasm and nucleus and sequester other cellular proteins such as SRC-1, NEDD8, and Hsp70 and Hsp90 *(105)*. These aggregates appear to be the result of misfolding of protein and defects in proteolytic degradation involving the ubiquitin–proteasome pathway.

Male Infertility

Male infertility has been associated with an abnormal androgen receptor in subjects with mild forms of androgen insensitivity and absence of other phenotypic abnormalities of the external genitalia *(105)*. Mutations in the AR gene have been associated with only a very few cases of isolated azoospermia *(107–109)*. However, recent studies have demonstrated that the glutamine repeat length may be increased in some men with oligospermia and azoospermia *(110)*. Hence, men with longer CAG repeats centered around the norm of 20 glutamine repeats have a greater risk for infertility.

SUMMARY

Androgens play a key role in male sex differentiation and development and in the maintenance of male reproductive function, and the effects of these hormones are an important component in the development of several pathologic conditions. Testosterone and its 5α-reduced metabolite DHT are potent androgens that act upon target cells to initiate and maintain the masculine phenotype. Germline mutations in the androgen receptor and steroid 5α-reductase genes cause the androgen insensitivity syndromes and 5α-reductase deficiency, respectively. The effects of these genetic mutations on male sex differentiation and development have played a key role in elucidating the pathways of androgen action. Androgen receptors transduce the steroid signal within cells, but attempts to correlate differences in receptor levels with various disease states have been relatively unsuccessful. However, molecular studies of AR gene structure have recently provided new insights toward defining a molecular and genetic basis for the pathology associated with diseases—including spinal bulbar muscular atrophy, prostate cancer, and male infertility—affecting middle-aged and older men. Further studies at the molecular level to define the steroid- and DNA-binding properties of androgen receptors, as well as the transcriptional activity and interactions of the receptor with coactivators, corepressors, and integrators within the transcriptional complex, will provide additional insight into the complex nature of androgen action. Moreover, epidemiologic data and molecular genetic analyses of gene structure have led to a new understanding of the interrelationships between environmental and genetic factors that may impact on the incidence of certain pathologic conditions in men.

REFERENCES

1. Griffin JE, Wilson JD. Disorders of the testes and the male reproductive tract. In: Wilson JD, Foster DW, Kronenberg HM, et al., eds. Williams Textbook of Endocrinology. WB Saunders, Philadelphia, PA, 1998, pp. 819–875.
2. Fuh VL, Stoner E. Androgen inhibitors/antiandrogens. In: Knobil E, Neill JD, eds. Encyclopedia of Reproduction. Academic, San Diego, CA, 1998, pp. 166–173.
3. Hammond GL, Bocchinfuso WP. Sex hormone-binding globulin/androgen binding protein: steroid binding and dimerization domains. J Steroid Biochem Mol Biol 1995;53:1–6.
4. Avvakumov GV, Grishkovskaya I, Muller YA, Hammond GL. Resolution of the human sex hormone-binding globulin dimer interface and evidence for two steroid-binding sites per homodimer. J Biol Chem 2001;276:34453–34457.
5. Dunn JF, Nisula BC, Rodbard D. Transport of steroid hormones: binding of 21 endogenous steroids to both testosterone-binding globulin and corticosteroid-binding globulin in human plasma. J Clin Endocrinol Metab 1981;53:58–68.
6. Pardridge WM. Serum bioavailability of sex steroid hormones. Clin Endocrinol Metab 1986;15: 259–278.
7. Rosner W, Hryb DJ, Khan MS, et al. Sex hormone-binding globulin. Binding to cell membranes and generation of a second messenger. J Androl 1992;13:101–106.
8. Russell DW, Wilson JD. Steroid 5α-reductase: two genes/two enzymes. Annu Rev Biochem 1994;63:25–61.
9. Morimoto I, Hawks ED, Horton R. Studies on the origin of androstanediol and androstanediol glucuronide in young and elderly men. J Clin Endocrinol Metab 1981;52:772–778.
10. Brooks, RV. Androgens. Clin Endocrinol Metab 1975;4:503–520.
11. Simpson ER, Zhao Y, Agarwal VR, et al. Aromatase expression in health and disease. Recent Prog Horm Res 1997;52:185–213.
12. Wilson JD, Griffin JE, Russell DW. Steroid 5α-reductase 2 deficiency. Endocr Rev 1993;14:577–593.
13. Zhou Z-X, Wong C-I, Sar M., Wilson EM. The androgen receptor: an overview. Recent Prog Horm Res 1994;49:249–274.
14. Jenster G, vander Korput HAGM, van Vroonhoven C, et al. Domains of the human androgen receptor involved in steroid binding, transcriptional activation and subcellular localization. Mol Endocrinol 1991;5:1396–1404.
15. Lubahn DB, Joseph DR, Sullivan PM, et al. Cloning of human androgen receptor complementary DNA and localization to the X chromosome. Science 1988;240:327–330.
16. Kuiper GGJM, Faber PW, van Rooij HCJ, et al. Structural organization of the human androgen receptor gene. J Mol Endocrinol 1989;2:R1–R4.
17. Faber PW, van Rooij HCJ, Schipper HJ, et al. Two different, overlapping pathways of transcription initiation are active on the TATA-less human androgen receptor promoter. J Biol Chem 1993;268:9296–9301.
18. Chen S, Supakar PC, Vellanoweth RL, et al. Functional role of a conformationally flexible homopurine/homopyrimidine domain of the androgen receptor gene promoter interacting with SP1 and a pyrimidine single strand DNA-binding protein. Mol Endocrinol 1997;11:3–15.
19. Grad JM, Dai JL, Wu S, Burnstein KL. Multiple androgen response elements and a myc consensus site in the androgen receptor (AR) coding region are involved in androgen-mediated up-regulation of AR messenger RNA. Mol Endocrinol 1999;13:1896–1911.
20. Mizokami A, Chang C. Induction of translation by the 5'-untranslated region of human androgen receptor mRNA. J Biol Chem 1994;269:25655–25659.
21. Lubahn DB, Joseph DR, Sar M, et al. The human androgen receptor: complementary deoxyribonucleic acid cloning, sequence analysis, and gene expression in prostate. Mol Endocrinol 1998;2:1265–1275.

22. Gottlieb B, Beitel LK, Trifiro MA. Variable expressivity and mutation databases: the androgen receptor gene mutations database. Hum Mutat 2001;17:382–388.
23. Kemppainen JA, Lane MV, Sar M, Wilson EM. Androgen receptor phosphorylation, turnover, nuclear transport, and transcriptional activation. J Biol Chem 1992;267:968–974.
24. Blok LJ de Ruiter PE, Brinkmann AO. Androgen receptor phosphorylation. Endocr Res 1996;58:569–575.
25. Gao T, McPhaul MJ. Functional activities of the A and B forms of the human androgen receptor in response to androgen receptor agonists and antagonists. Mol Endocrinol 1998;12:654–663.
26. Lubahn DB, Brown TR, Simental JA, et al. Sequence of the intron/exon junctions of the coding region of the human androgen receptor gene and identification of a point mutation in a family with complete androgen insensitivity. Proc Natl Acad Sci USA 1989;86:9534–9538.
27. Doesburg P, Kuil CW, Berrevoets CA, et al. Functional in vivo interaction between the amino-terminal, transactivation domain and the ligand binding domain of the androgen receptor. Biochemistry 1997;36:1052–1064.
28. He B, Kemppainen JA, Voegel JJ, et al. Activation function 2 in the human androgen receptor ligand binding domain mediates interdomain communication with the NH2-terminal domain. J Biol Chem 1999;274:37219–37225.
29. He B, Kemppainen JA, Wilson EM. FXXLF and WXXLF sequences mediate the NH2- terminal interaction with the ligand binding domain of the androgen receptor. J Biol Chem 2000;275:22986–22994.
30. Alen P, Claessens F, Verhoeven G. et al. The androgen receptor amino- terminal domain plays a key role in p160 coactivator-stimulated gene transcription. Mol Cell Biol 1999;19:6085–6097.
31. Bevan Cl, Hoare S, Claessens F, et al. The AF1 and AF2 domains of the androgen receptor interact with distinct regions of SRC1. Mol Cell Biol 1999;19:8383–8392.
32. Trifiro MA, Kazemi-Esfarjani P, Pinsky L. X-Linked muscular atrophy and the androgen receptor. Trends Endocrinol Metab 1994;5:416–421.
33. Choong CS, Wilson EM. Trinucleotide repeats in the human androgen receptor: a molecular basis for disease. J Mol Endocrinol 1998;21:2235–2257.
34. Irvine RA, Yu MC, Ross RK, Coetzee GA. The CAG and GGC microsatellites of the androgen receptor gene are in linkage disequilibrium in men with prostate cancer. Cancer Res 1995;55:1937–1940.
35. Giovannucci E, Stampfer MJ, Krithivas K, et al. The CAG repeat within the androgen receptor gene and its relationship to prostate cancer. Proc Natl Acad Sci USA 1997;94:3320–3323.
36. LaSpada AR, Wilson EM, Lubahn DB. Androgen receptor gene mutations in X-linked spinal and bulbar muscular atrophy. Nature 1991;352:77–79.
37. Freedman LP. Anatomy of the steroid receptor zinc finger region. Endocr Rev 1992;3:29–145.
38. Claessens F. Verrijdt G, Schoenmakers E, et al. Selective DNA binding by the androgen receptor as a mechanism for hormone-specific gene regulation. J Steroid Biochem Mol Biol 2001;76:23–30.
39. Gonzales MI, Robins D. Oct-1 preferentially interacts with androgen receptor in a DNA- dependent manner that facilitates recruitment of SRC-1. J Biol Chem 2001;276:6420–6428.
40. Zhou Z-X, Sar M, Simental JA, et al. Ligand-dependent bipartite nuclear targeting signal in the human androgen receptor. J Biol Chem 1994;269:13115–13123.
41. Tyagi RK, Lavrovsky Y, Ahn SC, et al. Dynamics of intracellular movement and nucleocytoplasmic recycling of the ligand-activated androgen receptor in living cells. Mol Endocrinol 2000;14:1162–1174.
42. Poukka H, Karvonen U, Yoshikawa N, et al. The RING finger protein SNURF modulates nuclear trafficking of the androgen receptor. J Cell Sci 2000;113:2991–3001.
43. Wang Q, Lu J, Yong EL. Ligand- and coactivator-mediated transactivation function (AF2) of the androgen receptor ligand-binding domain are inhibited by the cognate hinge region. J Biol Chem 2001;276:7493–7499.
44. Buchanan G, Yan M, Harris JM, et al. Mutations at the boundary of the hinge and ligand binding domain of the androgen receptor confer increased transactivation function. Mol Endocrinol 2001;15:46–56.
45. Pratt WB. Role of heat-shock proteins in steroid receptor function. In: Parker M, ed. Frontiers in Molecular Biology: Steroid Hormone Action. IRL, Oxford, 1993, pp. 64–93.
46. Wong CI, Zhou Z-X, Sar M, Wilson EM. Steroid requirement for androgen receptor dimerization and DNA binding. J Biol Chem 1993;268:19004–19012.
47. Langley E, Zhou Z-X, Wilson EM. Evidence for an anti-parallel orientation of the ligand- activated human androgen receptor dimer. J Biol Chem 1994;270:29983–29990.
48. Brzozowski AM, Pike ACW, Dauter Z, et al. Molecular basis of agonism and antagonism in the oestrogen receptor. Nature 1997;389:753–758.

49. Williams SP, Sigler PB. Atomic structure of progesterone complexed with its receptor. Nature 1998;393:392–395.

50. Matias PM, Donner P, Coelho R, et al. Structural evidence for ligand specificity in the binding domain of the human androgen receptor. J Biol Chem 2000;275: 26164–26171.

51. Sack JS, Kish KF, Wang C, et al. Crystallographic structures of the ligand-binding domains of the androgen receptor and its T877A mutant complexed with the natural agonist dihydrotestosterone. Proc Natl Acad Sci USA 2001;98:4904–4909.

52. Berrevoets CA, Doesburg P, Sketetee K, et al. Functional interactions of the AF-2 domain core region of the human androgen receptor with the amino-terminal domain and with the transcriptional coactivator TIF-2 (transcriptional intermediary factor-2). Mol Endocrinol 1998;12:1172–1183.

53. Roche PJ, Hoare SA, Parker MA. A consensus DNA-binding site for the androgen receptor. Mol Endocrinol 1992;6:2229–2235.

54. Nelson CC, Hendy SC, Shukin RJ, et al. Determinants of DNA sequence specificity of the androgen, progesterone, and glucocorticoid receptors: evidence for differential steroid receptor response elements. Mol Endocrinol 1999;13:2090–2107.

55. Zhou Z, Corden JL, Brown TR. Identification and characterization of a novel androgen response element composed of a direct repeat. J Biol Chem 1997;272:8227–8235.

56. Ing N, Beekman JM, Tsai SY, et al. Members of the steroid hormone superfamily interact with TFIIB (S300-II). J Biol Chem 1992;267:17617–17623.

57. McEwan I, Gustafsson J-A. Interaction of the human androgen receptor transactivation function with the general transcription factor TFIIF. Proc Natl Acad Sci USA 1997;94:8485–8490.

58. Bubulya A, Wise SC, Shen X-Q, et al. c-Jun can mediate androgen receptor-induced transactivation. J Biol Chem 1996;271:24583–24589.

59. Kallio PJ, Poukka H, Moilanen A, et al. Androgen-receptor mediated transcriptional regulation in the absence of direct interaction with a specific DNA element. Mol Endocrinol 1995;9:1017–1028.

60. Glass CK, Rosenfeld MG. The coregulator exchange in transcriptional functions of nuclear receptors. Genes Dev 2000;14:121–141.

61. Lee KC, Kraus WL. Nuclear receptors, coactivators and chromatin: new approaches, new insights. Trends Endocrinol Metab 2001;12:191–197.

62. Perissi V, Staszewski LM, McInerney EM, et al. Molecular determinants of nuclear receptor–corepressor interaction. Genes Dev 1999;13:3198–3208.

63. Yeh S, Chang C. Cloning and characterization of a specific coactivator, ARA70, for the androgen receptor in human prostate cells. Proc Natl Acad Sci USA 1996;93:5517–5521.

64. Fujimoto N, Yeh S, Kang HY, et al. Cloning and characterization of androgen receptor coactivator, ARA55, in human prostate. J Biol Chem 1999;274:8316–8321.

65. Kang HY, Yeh S, Fujimoto N, Chang C. Cloning and characterization of human prostate coactivator, ARA54, a novel protein that associates with the androgen receptor. J Biol Chem 1999;274:8570–8576.

66. Hsiao PW, Chang C. Isolation and characterization of ARA160 as the first androgen receptor N-terminal-associated coactivator in human prostate cells. J Biol Chem 1999;274:22373–22379.

67. Kotaja N, Aittomaki S, Silvennoinen O, et al. ARIP3 (androgen receptor- interacting protein 3) and other PIAS (protein inhibitor of activated STAT) proteins differ in their ability to modulate steroid receptor-dependent transcriptional activation. Mol Endocrinol 2000;14:1986–2000.

68. Moilanen AM, Karvonen U, Poukka H, et al. Activation of androgen receptor function by a novel nuclear protein kinase. Mol Biol Cell 1998;9:2527–2543.

69. Yeh S, Hu YC, Rahman M, et al. Increase of androgen-induced cell death and androgen receptor transactivation by BRCA1 in prostate cancer cells. Proc Natl Acad Sci USA 2000;97:11256–11261.

70. Froesch BA, Takayama S, Reed JC. BAG-1L protein enhances androgen receptor function. J Biol Chem 1998;273:11660–11666.

71. Kang HY, Lin HK, Hu YC, et al. From transforming growth factor-β signaling to androgen action: identification of Smad3 as an androgen receptor coregulator in prostate cancer cells. Proc Natl Acad Sci USA 2001;98:3018–3023.

72. Yamamoto A, Hashimoto Y, Kohri K, et al. Cyclin E as a coactivator of the androgen receptor. J Cell Biol 2000;150:873–879.

73. Poukka H, Aarnisalo P, Karvonen U, et al. Ubc9 interacts with the androgen receptor and activates receptor-dependent transcription. J Biol Chem 1999;274:19441–19446.

74. Sharma M, Zarnegar M, Li X, et al. Androgen receptor interacts with a novel MYST protein, HBO1. J Biol Chem 2000;275:35200–35208.

75. Gross M, Liu B, Tan JA, et al. Distinct effects of PIAS proteins on androgen-mediated gene activation in prostate cancer cells. Oncogene 2001;20:3880–3887.

76. Klocker H, Culig Z, Ider IE, et al. Mechanism of androgen receptor activation and possible implications for chemoprevention trials. Eur Urol 1999;35:413–419.

77. Culig Z, Hobisch A, Bartsch G, Klocker H. Androgen receptor—an update of mechanisms of action in prostate cancer. Urol Res 2000;28:211–219.

78. Sadar MD. Androgen-independent induction of prostate specific antigen gene expression by crosstalk between the androgen receptor and protein kinase A signal transduction pathways. J Biol Chem 1999;274:7777–7783.

79. Nazareth LV, Weigel NL. Activation of the human androgen receptor through a protein kinase A pathway. J Biol Chem 1996;268:19900–19907.

80. DeRuiter PE, Teuwen R, Trapman J, et al. Synergism between androgens and protein kinase-C on androgen regulated gene expression. Mol Cell Endocrinol 1995;110:1–6.

81. Ikonen T, Palvimo JJ, Kallio PJ, et al. Stimulation of androgen- regulated transactivation by modulators of protein phosphorylation. Endocrinology 1994;135:1359–1366.

82. Rowan BG, Garrison N, Weigel NL, O'Malley BW. 8-Bromo cAMP induces phosphorylation of two sites on SRC-1 that facilitate ligand independent activation of the chicken progesterone receptor and are critical for functional cooperation between SRC-1 and CBP. Mol Cell Biol 2000;20:8720–8730.

83. Qui Y, Ravi L, Kung HJ. Requirement of ErbB2 for signaling by interleukin-6 in prostate carcinoma cells. Nature 1998;393:83–85.

84. Shemshedini L, Knauthe R, Sassone-Corsi P, et al. Cell-specific inhibitory and stimulatory effects of Fos and Jun on transcription activation by nuclear receptors. EMBO J 1991;10:3839–3843.

85. Bubulaya A, Wise SC, Shen X-Q, et al. c-Jun can mediate AR- induced transactivation. J Biol Chem 1996;271:24583–24589.

86. Craft N, Shostak Y, Carey M, Sawyers CL. A mechanism for hormone-independent prostate cancer through modulation of androgen receptor signaling by the HER-2/neu tyrosine kinase. Nature Med 1999;5:280–285.

87. Yeh S, Lin HK, Kang HY, et al. From HER-2/Neu signal cascade to androgen receptor and its coactivators: a novel pathway by induction of androgen target genes through MAP kinase in prostate cells. Proc Natl Acad Sci USA 1999;96:5458–5463.

88. Li P, Nicosia SV, Bai W. Antagonism between PTEN/MMAC1/TEP-1 and androgen receptor in growth and apoptosis of prostate cancer cells. J Biol Chem 2001;276:20444–20550.

89. Quigley CA, DeBellis A, Marschke KB, et al. Androgen receptor defects: historical, clinical and molecular perspectives. Endocr Rev 1995;16:271–321.

90. Brown TR. Androgen insensitivity syndrome. J Androl 1995;16:299–303.

91. Sutherland RW, Wiener JS, Hicks JP, et al. Androgen receptor gene mutations are rarely associated with isolated penile hypospadias. J Urol 1996;156:828–831.

92. Gregory CW, He B, Johnson RT, et al. Androgen receptor stabilization in recurrent prostate cancer is associated with hypersensitivity to low androgen. Cancer Res 2001;61:2892–2898.

93. Veldscholte J, Berrevoets CA, Ris-Staplers C, et al. The androgen receptor in LNCaP cells contains a mutation in the ligand binding domain which affects steroid binding characteristics and response to antiandrogens. J Steroid Biochem1992;41:665–669.

94. Tan J, Sharief Y, Hamil KG, et al. Dehydroepiandrosterone activates mutant androgen receptors expressed in the androgen-dependent human cancer xenograft CRW22 and LNCaP cells. Mol Endocrinol 1997;11:450–459.

95. Tilley WD, Buchanan G, Hickey TE, Bentel JM. Mutations in the androgen receptor gene are associated with progression of human prostate cancer to androgen independence. Clin Cancer Res 1996;2:277–285.

96. Taplin ME, Bubley GJ, Ko YJ, et al. Selection for androgen receptor mutations in prostate cancers treated with androgen antagonist. Cancer Res 1999;59:2511–2515.

97. Marcelli M, Ittmann M, Mariani S. et al. Androgen receptor mutations in prostate cancer. Cancer Res 2000;60:944–999.

98. Koivisto PA, Kononen J. Palmberg C, et al. Androgen receptor gene amplification: a possible mechanism for androgen deprivation therapy failure in prostate cancer. Cancer Res 1997;57: 314–319.

99. Stanford JL, Just JJ, Gibbs M, et al. Polymorphic repeats in the androgen receptor gene: molecular markers of prostate cancer risk. Cancer Res 1997;57:1194–1198.

100. Gregory CW, He B, Johnson RT, et al. A mechanism for androgen receptor-mediated prostate cancer recurrence after androgen deprivation therapy. Cancer Res 2001;61:4315–4319.
101. Choong CS, Kemppainen JA, Zhou Z-X, Wilson EM. Reduced androgen receptor gene expression with first exon CAG repeat expansion. Mol Endocrinol 1996;10:1527–1535.
102. Irvine RA, Ma H, Yu MC, et al. Inhibition of p160- mediated coactivation with increasing androgen receptor polyglutamine length. Hum Mol Genet 2000;9:267–274.
103. Abdullah A. Trifiro MA, Panet-Raymond V, et al. Spinobulbar muscular atrophy: polyglutamine-expanded androgen receptor is proteolytically resistant in vitro and processed abnormally in transfected cells. Hum Mol Genet 1998;7:379–384.
104. Kobayashi Y, Miwa S, Merry DE, et al. Caspase-3 cleaves the expanded androgen receptor protein of spinal and bulbar muscular atrophy in a polyglutamine repeat length-dependent manner. Biochem Biophys Res Commun 1998;252:145–150.
105. Stenoien DL, Cummings CJ, Adams HP, et al. Polyglutamine-expanded androgen receptors form aggregates that sequester heat shock proteins, proteasome components and SRC-1, and are suppressed by the HDJ-2 chaperone. Hum Mol Genet 1999;8:731–741.
106. Aiman J, Griffin JE, Cushard WG, Wilson JD. Androgen insensitivity as a cause of infertility in otherwise normal men. N Engl J Med 1998;300:223–227.
107. Akin JW, Behzadian A, Tho SPT, McDonough PG. Evidence for a partial deletion in the androgen receptor gene in a phenotypic male with azoospermia. Am J Obstet Gynecol 1991;165:1891–1894.
108. Yong EL, Ng SC, Roy AC, et al. Pregnancy after hormonal correction of severe spermatogenic defect due to mutation in androgen receptor gene. Lancet 1994;344:8925–8927.
109. Ghadessy FJ, Lim J, Abdullah AA, et al. Oligospermic infertility associated with an androgen receptor mutation that disrupts interdomain and coactivator (TIF2) interactions. J Clin Invest 1999;103:1517–1525.
110. Tut TG, Ghadessy FJ, Trifiro MA, et al. Long polyglutamine tracts in the androgen receptor are associated with reduced trans-activation, impaired sperm production, and male infertility. J Clin Endocrinol Metab 1997;82:3777–3782.

3 Hypogonadism in Men
An Overview

Stephen R. Plymate, MD

CONTENTS

INTRODUCTION
CLINICAL CHARACTERISTICS OF HYPOGONADISM
PRIMARY HYPOGONADISM
CHEMOTHERAPY
SECONDARY HYPOGONADISM
COMBINED PRIMARY AND SECONDARY HYPOGONADISM
SUMMARY
REFERENCES

INTRODUCTION

Male hypogonadism may be defined as a failure of the testes to produce testosterone or sperm. This may be caused by a failure of the testes, anterior pituitary gland, or hypothalamus. Hypogonadism may also occur if a testicular product is unable to exert an effect, such as in the androgen-resistance syndromes.

CLINICAL CHARACTERISTICS OF HYPOGONADISM

The clinical presentation of hypogonadism depends on whether the onset was *in utero*, prepubertal, or postpubertal. If hypogonadism is present because of a defect that occurred *in utero*, the individual will have ambiguous genitalia. The clinical pictures of testicular androgen failure of prepubertal and postpubertal onset are presented in Tables 1 and 2.

If the hypogonadism is manifest only as infertility, physical findings may be normal. With the development of sensitive assays for testosterone and free or unbound testosterone, an increasing number of circumstances have been described in which serum testosterone levels are lower than normal without any obvious end-organ deficiencies. Examples of this phenomenon are seen in aging or stressed men who have low levels of serum testosterone without definitive evidence of end-organ deficiency. In the case of stress, end-organ deficiency may not be seen, because the period of hypogonadism is transient. It may be difficult to decide whether these men really are androgen deficient or whether they simply are displaying a physiologic response to stress or age. These

From: *Contemporary Endocrinology: Androgens in Health and Disease*
Edited by: C. Bagatell and W. J. Bremner © Humana Press Inc., Totowa, NJ

Table 1
Classification of Male Hypogonadism

Primary Hypogonadism
   Klinefelter syndrome
      XX males
      XY/XO mixed gonadal dysgenesis
      XYY syndrome
      Ullrich–Noonan syndrome
      Myotonia dystrophica
      Sertoli-cell-only syndrome
      Functional prepubertal castrate
   Enzymatic defects involving testosterone biosynthesis
      5α-reductase deficiency
      Luteinizing hormone gonadotropin-resistant testis
      Persistent mullerian duct syndrome
   Male pseudohermaphroditism involving androgen receptor defects
      Testicular feminization
      Reifenstein syndrome
      Infertility resulting from a receptor defect
      After orchitis
      Cryptorchidism
      Leprosy
      Testicular trauma
      Testicular irradiation
      Autoimmune testicular failure
      Chemotherapy
Secondary Hypogonadism
   Hypogonadotropic hypogonadism
   Isolated luteinizing hormone or follicle-stimulating hormone deficiency
      Acquired gonadotropin deficiencies
      Prolactin-secreting pituitary tumors
      Severe systemic illness
      Uremia
      Hemochromatosis
Combined Primary and Secondary Etiology
   Aging
   Hepatic cirrhosis
   Sickle-cell disease

situations pose further difficulties for clinicians who must decide whether androgen replacement is needed. In those situations in which obvious deficiency states are not present, the indication for replacement therapy may not be clear-cut. In some of these patients, the finding of an exaggerated gonadotropin response to gonadotropin-releasing hormone (GnRH) may help to define the presence of testicular failure.

Functionally, the hypogonadal states may be classified according to the level at which the hypothalamic–pituitary–testicular axis is defective. Briefly, the control of testicular function begins with the release, in a pulsatile fashion, of GnRH from the hypothalamus. GnRH, transported by the hypothalamic pituitary portal system, then causes the release of luteinizing hormone (LH) and follicle-stimulating hormone (FSH) from the anterior

Table 2
Manifestations of Testicular Androgen Failure

Prepubertal Testicular Failure
    Clinical characteristics
        Testes, < 2.5 cm long; volume < 5 mL
        Penis, < 3–5 cm long
    Lack of scrotal pigmentation and rugae
    Prepubertal subcutaneous fat distribution over hips, face, and chest
    Eunuchoidal skeletal proportions: crown to pubis/pubis to floor ratio is decreased; arm span
        is considerably greater than height (normally black men have a decreased ratio and
        relatively longer arm span than whites)
        Female escutcheon
        No terminal facial hair; decreased body hair
        No temporal hair recession
        High-pitched voice
        Decreased muscle mass
        Delayed bone age
        Small prostate
    Cross-hatching over skin lateral to the orbits
        Decreased libido
        Osteoporosis later in life
Postpubertal Testicular failure
    Clinical characteristics
        Normal skeletal proportions and penile length
        Loss of libido
        Decrease in strength and muscle mass
        Decrease in rate of growth of facial hair
        Normal distribution of pubic hair
        Testes are soft; volume < 15 mL
    Prostate adult size, although may be smaller than average
        No change in voice
        Diminished aggressivity
        Decreased amount of axillary and pubic hair
        Osteoporosis later in life

pituitary. An optimal rate of pulsation (3.8 pulses every 6 h) appears to be necessary for adequate secretion of both LH and FSH for normal gonadal function. When the rate is slower than optimal, FSH may be preferentially released in greater amounts than normal and LH in lesser amounts. When the pulse frequency of GnRH is more rapid than normal, serum FSH levels may be suppressed and LH preferentially stimulated. LH subsequently binds to the Leydig cell to initiate testosterone synthesis and secretion. FSH binds to the Sertoli cell and stimulates the production of proteins that, with testosterone from the Leydig cell, induce and maintain normal spermatogenesis. LH and FSH release also are regulated by a negative feedback system (i.e., serum testosterone and estradiol). Inhibin, an FSH-stimulated Sertoli cell peptide, can partially block FSH release from the pituitary without influencing LH release. Serum testosterone and inhibin also may affect the release of GnRH from the hypothalamus. However, the precise role of inhibin in the feedback process in men is not completely defined.

In addition to the direct effects of testosterone on sexual tissues, the secretion of androgens is related to other endocrine systems that may affect body habitus during both puberty and adulthood. This is especially true for the somatotropin axis, in which androgens are necessary for normal growth hormone and insulin-like growth factor-1 secretion. Furthermore, in normal men, components of the gonadal axis are regulated by other endocrine systems (e.g., insulin pulsation closely determines the blood levels of sex hormone-binding globulin [SHBG]). Therefore, hypogonadism may result from abnormalities in multiple systems, and its manifestations are evident in most physiologic systems *(1–3)*.

With this understanding of the hypothalamic–pituitary–gonadal axis, male hypogonadal disorders may be classified into two categories. The first is *primary hypogonadism*, in which the dysfunction is in the testis. Primary hypogonadism is manifested by a deficiency in the main testicular products: testosterone or sperm. The basis for the primary hypogonadism is a testicular defect. In states of primary hypogonadism, there is a loss of negative feedback by testicular products such as testosterone or inhibin on the hypothalamus and pituitary, so that serum LH and FSH levels are elevated in the basal state or, despite normal basal gonadotropin levels, there is an exaggerated gonadotropin response to GnRH.

The presence of testosterone alone is not enough to achieve normal male development. A portion of the Y chromosome is needed for normal testicular development and regression. In humans, this testis-determining factor has been mapped to a 35-kilobase (kb) segment on the short arm of the Y chromosome close to the pseudoautosomal region. The gene isolated from this locus that equates with the testis-determining factor has been called sex-determining region Y (SRY) *(4)*. Recent studies have demonstrated that an autosomal gene on chromosome 17, SOX9, can cause complete testicular differentiation when placed in an XX transgenic mouse *(5)*. In humans, mutation of this gene results in the syndrome camplomelic dysplaysia *(5)*. This syndrome consists of chondrodysplastic dwarfism, chrondrocyte tumors, and intersex XY individuals. Most of the XY individuals with this syndrome are either phenotypic females or intersex.

Secondary hypogonadism (i.e., decreased gonadotropin stimulation of potentially normal testes) presents with low serum testosterone levels or decreased sperm production and low serum gonadotropin levels (or values inappropriately low for the level of serum testosterone, sperm production, or both). Since the discovery of GnRH, some authors have divided secondary hypogonadism into pituitary failure and hypothalamic failure ("tertiary hypogonadism"). In this chapter, the division into primary and secondary hypogonadism is used, with the latter including both pituitary and hypothalamic disorders.

PRIMARY HYPOGONADISM

Including infertile men, primary testicular failure affects 5–10% of the male population *(6)*. Although male infertility is commonly considered a problem that exclusively involves seminiferous tubular function and spermatogenesis, evidence in men with varicoceles has demonstrated the presence of the exaggerated response of both serum LH and FSH to GnRH *(7)*. Total serum testosterone levels are normal in these patients, the augmented gonadotropin response to GnRH indicates a failure in both Leydig cell and seminiferous tubular function. Some compensation for the impaired Leydig cells must occur that is sufficient to return testosterone levels to normal under the influence of increased LH stimulation. These findings confirm that infertile men often possess primary gonadal failure of a subtle nature. Because there is a fairly high incidence of male infertility, primary testicular dysfunction in the male population is an important issue.

Klinefelter Syndrome

The chromosomal constitution of 47,XXY epitomizes the classic form of male primary testicular failure. This abnormality is present in about 1 in 400 men. Klinefelter syndrome, first described in 1942, was based on nine male patients who, at puberty, experienced the onset of bilateral gynecomastia, small testes with Leydig cell dysfunction and azoospermia, and increased urinary gonadotropin excretion *(8)*. Later, it was shown that Leydig cell failure was variable in its magnitude. In 1956, the X-chromatin body (Barr body) was found in these individuals, and in 1959, the XXY chromosome constitution was first described, demonstrating that the disease was the result of an extra X chromosome *(9,10)*.

PHENOTYPIC MANIFESTATIONS

The phenotypic manifestations of Klinefelter syndrome are characteristic for the classic form of the disease in which all cells carry the XXY karyotype. Many men with Klinefelter syndrome have a *mosaic* form, in which some cell lines are XXY and others are XY. In these mosaic individuals, all cell lines are from a single zygote, and the XXY cell lines arise from mitotic nondisjunction after fertilization. Manifestation of the disease may not be typical or consistent. Before puberty, the only physical findings are the small testes; in the classic form of Klinefelter syndrome, a gonadal volume of less than 1.5 mL after the age of 6 yr is usual *(11,12)*. A decreased testicular size is the most diagnostic clinical feature of classic Klinefelter syndrome, even in prepubertal patients diagnosed with the syndrome. The cause for the small prepubertal testicular size is a loss of germ cells before puberty; thus, the prepubertal testis is small. In secondary forms of hypogonadism, the number of germ cells is normal and the prepubertal testicular size is indistinguishable from that of normal boys.

Microcephaly also has been described in some cases of Klinefelter syndrome. After puberty, the more characteristic features of the syndrome appear. These include varying degrees of gynecomastia. The gynecomastia is of interest because it is primarily the result of an increase in periductal tissue rather than ductal tissue; increased ductal tissue often is found in gynecomastia of acute onset, whatever the cause. If the gynecomastia were only the result of the increased estrogen production in Klinefelter syndrome, an increase in ductal tissue might be expected. Nonetheless, the histopathologic appearance of the breast tissue is not consistently separable from that of other patients with longstanding gynecomastia.

After puberty, an abnormality in skeletal proportions becomes manifest. There is an exaggerated growth of the lower extremities resulting in a decreased crown-to-pubis:pubis-to-floor ratio, such as that seen in eunuchoid men. Unlike the true eunuchoid proportions, in which the arm span often is at least 6 cm more than the height, in Klinefelter syndrome the arm span : height ratio usually is not abnormal. The reason for the abnormal growth in the lower extremities is unknown. The phenotypic manifestations, such as the gynecomastia, pattern of hair distribution, muscle mass, and subcutaneous fat distribution, vary even between patients with classic Klinefelter syndrome.

Laboratory Findings

In patients with Klinefelter syndrome, serum testosterone levels range from low to well into the normal range *(13,14)*. The relatively decreased serum testosterone is the result of deficient testosterone production (3.27 ± 1.35 mg/24 h vs 7.04 ± 2.47 mg/24 h in normal persons) *(15)*. An increase in SHBG also occurs in Klinefelter syndrome; thus, the bioavailable, or free, testosterone is further suppressed *(13,16)*. As men with Klinefelter syndrome age, a further decline in testicular function often occurs *(17)*.

Patients with Klinefelter syndrome may have serum estradiol levels higher than those of normal men. The increase in estradiol has been shown to come from an augmented peripheral conversion of testosterone to estradiol *(13,15)*. After puberty, serum gonadotropin levels are elevated, even when serum testosterone levels are normal *(14)*. Before puberty, serum gonadotropin levels are normal *(18)*. In spite of the relatively normal masculine appearance of some young men with Klinefelter syndrome, their physical strength often is significantly less than that of their peers because of the deficient androgen action on muscle. Men with Klinefelter syndrome usually do not have the ability to grow a full beard or a mustache; however, like muscle strength, androgen-dependent hair growth is variable.

The abnormal serum testosterone levels and the diminished response of serum testosterone to human chorionic gonadotropin (hCG) is a reflection of the disturbance of Leydig and Sertoli cell function. Of the two compartments in the testes, the seminiferous tubules are the most affected by the presence of the extra X chromosome *(19,20)*. Clinically, this is manifested by azoospermia, which occurs in virtually all patients with classic Klinefelter syndrome. Testicular biopsy specimens consistently demonstrate seminiferous tubule hyalinization and fibrosis. Because the seminiferous tubule basement membrane is so crucial to spermatogenesis, the defect in basement membrane formation may explain why the initial testicular damage is to the seminiferous epithelium.

In some patients with Klinefelter syndrome, usually the mosaic forms, testicular biopsy specimens have demonstrated focal areas of spermatogenesis. On occasion, sperm have been noted in the ejaculate, and these patients may be fertile. However, most of the reported impregnations have been single events occurring early in the individual's reproductive life, with azoospermia developing in later years *(21)*. Is it the lack of normal androgen environment in the testes or the chromosomal abnormality that impairs spermatogenesis? In part, the answer to this question has come from studies of XXY and XX sex-reversed mice in which sperm can develop but are always diploid, with an XX or XY content *(22)*. In these animals, during spermatogonial mitosis, the XY and XX daughter cells are not viable, but an occasional nondisjunctional event takes place and the extra chromosome is lost. Thus, in subsections of the germinal epithelium, a normal haploid germ cell develops and full spermatogenesis may take place. The testicular biopsy specimens of these animals, as well as of patients with Klinefelter syndrome, show focal areas of spermatogenesis. Because the spermatogenesis takes place in the face of decreased intratesticular testosterone levels, these data support the theory that the extra X material is the pivotal factor controlling spermatogenesis. Interestingly, the XXY fetal testis may be unaffected *(23)*.

Psychopathology

Decreased intellectual development and antisocial behavior occur with a high frequency in Klinefelter syndrome *(24–26)*. In this regard, the incidence of Klinefelter syndrome in subsets of the population with mental retardation ranges from about 0.5% to 2.5%. Studies from Denmark, in which the records of all men taller than 184 cm were surveyed, show that the incidence of criminal offense was 9.3% in men with an XY chromosome pattern, 18.8% in men with an XXY chromosome pattern, and 41.7% in men with an XYY chromosome pattern *(27)*. Furthermore, the incidence of criminal behavior was inversely related to the subjects' full intelligence quotient (IQ). Studies of boys with Klinefelter syndrome have found that there is a significant reduction in verbal IQ at the age of 7 yr *(28)*. Interestingly, as the number of X chromosomes increases in the poly-X disorders, the degree of mental retardation also increases. The mechanism by which the extra X chromosome impairs central nervous system (CNS) function has not been delineated, although it is obvious that there is an inverse relationship between the ability to cope and antisocial behavior. Furthermore, although there is decreased androgen production by the Leydig cells, low androgen production does not appear to be responsible for all of the characteristic clinical manifestations of the syndrome (other states of androgen deficiency are not necessarily associated with increased criminal behavior and mental retardation). It appears that the extra X chromosome may affect neuronal function directly, which then leads to behavioral abnormalities related to decreased IQ and other, nondefined factors.

Other areas of psychiatric dysfunction, such as personality traits of timidity, introspective behavior, and social drive, are more clearly related to the androgen deficiency and often improve after androgen replacement *(29)*. The lack of self-restraint and aggressiveness shown by some subjects appears to be related to the effects of the extra X chromosome on CNS function.

Etiology

The development of the XXY chromosome constitution may occur by several mechanisms. The most common of these is *nondisjunction during the first* and *second meiotic division* in parental oogenesis or spermatogenesis. A second possibility for the development of the classic syndrome is *nondisjunction during the first postzygotic mitosis*. Nondisjunction in mitosis after this time results in mosaic forms of Klinefelter syndrome. A third, and rare, mechanism is *anaphase lag during mitosis or meiosis*, with the lagging chromatid included in the daughter nucleus. There are six reports of men with an XXY chromosome pattern (including one set of brothers) whose mothers had XX/XXX chromosomes *(14)*. These family data suggest a *nondisjunctional event during maternal zygotic development*, and this may have been present in a grandparent. The reason for the nondisjunction is not known, although maternal age has been shown to be a factor. The incidence of Klinefelter syndrome increases from 0.6% when the maternal age is 35 yr or less to 5.4% when the maternal age is greater than 45 yr *(30,31)*. Sixty-five percent of patients with Klinefelter syndrome have a maternal origin for their extra X chromosomes. Maternal age is thought to be a factor because of the longer diplotene stage of the ova in older women. The existence of mothers with an XX/XXX chromosome pattern (discussed earlier) and an increased incidence of twins with Klinefelter syndrome as well as the finding of an increased frequency of Klinefelter syndrome in patients with Down's syndrome suggests that some families may have a factor predisposing to chromosomal nondisjunction.

XX Males

Patients with XX chromosomal configurations may appear as normal females, females with gonadal dysgenesis, true hermaphrodites, or males with gonadal dysgenesis. Only those manifesting as phenotypic males are discussed here. These men proceed through puberty and subsequently present with small testes, infertility, and gynecomastia. As in patients with Klinefelter syndrome, serum testosterone levels may be low to normal, but serum gonadotropin levels are invariably elevated *(32,33)*. These patients tend to be shorter than normal men. There is a high incidence of hypospadias, but no mental retardation. The abnormal skeletal proportions and many of the other associated features of Klinefelter syndrome are absent. The incidence of the syndrome ranges from 1 in 9000 to 1 in 20,000 live births.

In about two-thirds of cases, XX males result from the translocation of the SRY gene to the X chromosome. In the remaining cases, no SRY has been detected. In the latter individuals, it is thought that a mutation occurred in an autosome that triggered the same series of events as SRY, leading to testicular development. This is now known to be caused by a mutation in the SOX9 gene on chromosome 17 *(5)*. SOX9 appears to be the gene first activated directly downstream of SRY, and when transfected into XX transgenic mice, it causes complete testicular differentiation. Evidence for this is found in the fact that SRY-negative men with the XX chromosome pattern often have other congenital abnormalities, especially cardiac problems. These abnormalities suggest autosomal mutations close to an SRY-like region of an autosome, although this region has not been identified *(34)*. The treatment of XX males includes surgery for gynecomastia, androgen-replacement therapy, and psychological support, as described for Klinefelter syndrome.

XY/XO Mixed Gonadal Dysgenesis

Patients with XY/XO mixed gonadal dysgenesis who have the 45 XO/46 XY genotype may appear as phenotypic males, although most patients with this chromosomal constitution are phenotypic females *(35)*. They have been considered to be H-Y antigen positive. Before the report of the translocation in XX males, it was suggested that because they were H-Y antigen positive but had gonadal dysgenesis, they must have lost the Y chromosome from the cell in the zygote. However, these patients also may have a mutation in the autosomal sex-determining gene, SOX9 *(5)*. This issue is now somewhat clouded, and these patients need further study.

Usually, the gonads are located within the abdomen. Both testes may be defective, or one may be a streak gonad. Depending on the gestational timing of the arrested gonadal development of the ipsilateral gonad, there may be a paramesonephric duct. In addition, a rudimentary uterus may be present. At birth, the external genitalia may range from female-appearing, with clitoral enlargement, to male-appearing, with some degree of hypospadias. These patients usually have been raised during their prepubertal years as females; they are discovered at the time of puberty, when primary amenorrhea is noted or when, because of the increased pubertal stimulation of the defective testis and subsequent androgen production, marked virilization occurs.

Treatment consists of supporting the sex-of-rearing with appropriate hormone replacement and castration. Castration is done to prevent the development of a malignancy in the defective gonad (20% incidence) and, if the individual has been raised as a female, to prevent the virilization that may occur after puberty. Fertility is extremely rare and should not be considered in the decision to remove an intraabdominal testis. The tumors that develop may be either dysgerminomas, gonadoblastomas, or embryonal cell carcinomas.

XYY Syndrome

Individuals with the XYY syndrome have erroneously been called "supermales"; this is a misnomer, because testicular function may be normal or associated with varying degrees of impaired spermatogenesis *(36–38)*. These individuals, with a mean height of 189 cm, are markedly taller than normal men and are more prone to antisocial behavior. Serum testosterone levels may be normal or elevated. Serum LH and FSH levels are normal unless spermatogenesis is markedly impaired, in which case the FSH levels are elevated. Findings in testicular biopsy specimens have ranged from normal to markedly impaired spermatogenesis, with seminiferous tubules that have undergone hyalinization. The sex chromosomal abnormalities arise from meiotic nondisjunction in the male or from zygotic nondisjunction. The impaired spermatogenesis alone, therefore, may be the result of diploid YY or XY spermatogonia, as has been described for Klinefelter syndrome. There is no specific therapy for these patients unless they have decreased testosterone levels.

Ulrich–Noonan Syndrome

Ullrich–Noonan syndrome (Noonan syndrome) often has been referred to as "male Turner" syndrome *(39)*. This is because of the phenotypic characteristics commonly shared with women who have Turner syndrome: webbed neck, low hairline, short stature, shield chest, and cubitus valgus *(40)*. However, these men have a normal chromosome pattern. In Noonan syndrome, commonly encountered cardiac abnormalities include pulmonary artery stenosis and atrial septal defects. Although testicular function may be normal, there usually is primary gonadal failure. Infertility, if present, generally is associated with cryptorchidism. Serum levels of testosterone, LH, and FSH may be normal or consistent with primary testicular failure (i.e., decreased serum testosterone and increased LH and FSH). Mental retardation, ptosis, hypertelorism, and low-set ears also are prominent in this disorder. Rarely, autosomal dominant transmission may occur. Treatment is directed toward any cardiac abnormalities, and if there is androgen deficiency, testosterone-replacement therapy should be instituted.

Myotonic Dystrophy

Myotonic dystrophy is an autosomal dominant disorder characterized by an inability to relax the striated muscles after contraction (myotonia). The disorder results in muscle atrophy and eventual death. In addition to the myotonia, frontal balding, lenticular opacities, and primary testicular failure are commonly associated abnormalities *(41)*. Because the disease usually is not manifest until after puberty, most commonly in the late thirties and mid-forties, these men do not have a eunuchoid body habitus. The most prominent physical manifestation of their gonadal failure is the small testes and, sometimes, the other signs of postpubertal gonadal failure. Many cases demonstrate low serum levels of testosterone and azoospermia. In such patients, testicular biopsy specimens reveal complete hyalinization of the seminiferous tubules. Although serum testosterone levels usually are decreased, LH is increased in only 50% of the patients *(42)*. Occasionally, only seminiferous tubule failure is present, which is characterized by a monotropic increase in serum FSH with normal testosterone levels.

The pathogenesis of the testicular failure is unknown. There is no available therapy for the seminiferous tubule failure. Studies indicate that testosterone replacement may result in some improvement in muscle mass and strength. However, the duration of this effect and the resultant functional changes are unknown. Therefore, this therapy should be considered experimental *(43)*.

Sertoli-Cell-Only Syndrome

Sertoli-cell-only syndrome (del Castillo syndrome) is a histologic diagnosis that is made only when a testicular biopsy is performed in an infertile man. The characteristic features are complete, or almost complete, absence of germ cells in all seminiferous tubules *(44)*. Occasionally, a focal area of spermatogenesis may be identified. The basement membrane may be slightly thickened and, under electron microscopy, the Sertoli cells are vacuolated *(45)*. Because Leydig cell function is only mildly impaired, these men present clinically with infertility; the testes are slightly smaller than normal but are of normal consistency. The patients have azoospermia and elevated serum levels of FSH. Mean serum testosterone levels are within the normal range, but lower than the mean for fertile individuals. Furthermore, the response of serum testosterone to hCG is diminished and, although serum LH levels are normal, the values tend to cluster in the upper range for normal men. This indicates that there is a relationship between normal seminiferous tubule function and normal Leydig cell function and that in this syndrome, in which seminiferous tubule function is impaired, there is some compromise of testosterone production.

The cause of Sertoli-cell-only syndrome has not been defined; it may be the end result of one of several inciting factors. However, the prevailing theory for most of these cases is congenital absence or early neonatal loss of the germ cells. This may result from abnormal Sertoli cell function that is unable to support the germ cells. The elevated serum LH levels and the abnormal responses to hCG stem from the fact that normal Leydig cell function also requires normal paracrine activity between the Sertoli and Leydig cells. This form of infertility cannot be reversed.

Functional Prepubertal Castrate

The functional prepubertal castrate syndrome (vanishing testes syndrome) is a relatively rare condition that manifests as prepubertal testicular failure. On physical examination, there is a complete lack of any discernible testicular tissue *(46)*. Usually, serum testosterone levels are low, similar to those of castrated men. There is no response to hCG administration. Castrate levels of serum LH and FSH, normal male wolffian derivatives, an absence of müllerian structures, a eunuchoid body habitus, and a normal XY karyotype also are present *(47)*. Infrequently, when a slight testosterone response to hCG occurs, a testicular remnant may be found in the abdomen or inguinal canal. Because there are no müllerian structures, testes must have been present *in utero* to produce antimüllerian hormone and to allow normal wolffian structures to develop. This has led to the hypothesis that events such as torsion of the testes *in utero*, trauma, infection, or an early manifestation of the polyglandular autoimmune deficiency syndrome may be responsible for the disorder.

Regardless of the cause, recognition of this condition is important for two reasons. First, if hCG administration increases serum testosterone levels, a search should be undertaken for the presence of abdominal testes. Usually, testicular remnants can be found in the scrotum. A computed tomographic scan will show this and may alleviate the need for abdominal surgery to determine the source of testosterone production.

However, abdominal testes should be removed because of the potential for malignant degeneration. Second, androgen replacement should be undertaken at the normal time for puberty. Because this syndrome can be recognized before puberty, these boys should not be made to suffer hypogonadism at the chronologic time of adolescence; artificial testes can be placed in the scrotum to facilitate normal scrotal expansion. The infertility is irreversible.

Enzymatic Defects Involving Testosterone Biosynthesis

Defects of testosterone biosynthesis are reviewed only briefly. These defects can be divided into two categories: those that involve steroidogenesis in the production of both testosterone and cortisol and those that involve testosterone biosynthesis alone (48). Suspicion of one of these enzyme deficiencies should be raised for a male pseudohermaphrodite. The sex chromosomal analysis will reveal an XY karyotype. In the case of disorders involving both testosterone and cortisol production (20,22-desmolase deficiency, 3β-dehydrogenase deficiency, 17α-hydroxylase deficiency), the serum cortisol deficiency may be severe, and these infants appear with adrenal crisis soon after birth. The disorders that primarily affect testicular testosterone production include 17,20-desmolase and 17-ketosteroid reductase deficiency. These patients also manifest as male pseudohermaphrodites and may have relatively normal-appearing female external genitalia. Because they can produce cortisol normally, they may not be detected until they are adults, when they present with primary amenorrhea. The 17,20-desmolase deficiency has been shown to involve either the Δ^4 or the Δ^5 pathway.

The 17β-hydroxysteroid dehydrogenase enzyme is responsible for the conversion of androstenedione to testosterone (49–51). The enzyme is present in the testes and in peripheral tissues. Whether the enzyme in the testes is controlled by the same gene as that in the adrenal gland is unknown. Patients with 17β-hydroxysteroid dehydrogenase deficiency present clinically with ambiguous genitalia and usually are raised as females before puberty. However, at puberty, marked virilization occurs. This probably is the result of the marked increase in secretion of androstenedione from the testes and its subsequent peripheral conversion to testosterone. Often, the diagnosis is first made at this time. However, because the patient already has been raised as a female and fertility is not attainable, it is best to remove the testes to decrease the androgen effect and to eliminate the risk of testicular carcinoma if the testes are located within the abdomen. If the specific diagnosis is made before puberty (i.e., by noting an increase in serum androstenedione after hCG administration), castration before puberty is preferable if the child has been raised as a female. Alternatively, if the child has been raised as a male and the testes are in the scrotum, testosterone treatment should be undertaken at puberty to achieve appropriate virilization and to reduce breast enlargement, which is thought to be caused by the conversion of the weak androgen, androstenedione, to estrone (52).

Any of these enzymatic defects should be considered in a male pseudohermaphrodite if no uterus can be demonstrated. The diagnosis can be made before puberty by stimulating the testes with hCG and measuring the precursor steroid for the enzyme that is deficient. For example, in 17-ketosteroid reductase deficiency, Δ^4 androstenedione is elevated because it cannot be further reduced to testosterone. These enzyme deficiencies may not be complete and the disorders may present in a more heterogeneous fashion.

If both testosterone and cortisol pathways are defective, treatment includes cortisol replacement. Testosterone should be given if the genitalia are primarily male or are ambiguous in an individual who has a male gender identity. If the patient is older when the problem is first recognized (as often may be the case if the only defect is in testosterone synthesis) and if the individual has been raised as a female, castration should be considered; subsequently, estrogen replacement can be started. Surgical correction of the external genitalia should be performed to maintain the female identification. Defects in testosterone production also exist in these patients (unlike the situation in congenital adrenal hyperplasia). Consequently, replacement with corticosteroids does not permit fertility to occur because of the inability to reproduce the high intratesticular levels of testosterone.

5α-Reductase Deficiency

The 5α-reductase deficiency syndrome (pseudovaginal perineoscrotal hypospadias, penis at 12 syndrome, type II incomplete androgen resistance) originally was described in 1961 as a defect in the conversion of testosterone to dihydrotestosterone resulting from the absence or lability of the 5α-reductase enzyme (53). This disorder is most prevalent in certain rural villages in the Dominican Republic. However, it has been described sporadically in other countries throughout the world (54). This is an autosomal recessive disorder that occurs in individuals with an XY chromosome pattern. The testes function normally insofar as androgen production and antimüllerian hormone are concerned; consequently, normal wolffian structures are formed and there is complete regression of the müllerian structures. However, because of the deficiency of dihydrotestosterone, the scrotum is usually bifid and the phallus displays severe hypospadias and may even appear as a moderately enlarged clitoris. Furthermore, there may be a blind, vagina-like pouch (the bifid scrotum) that opens just behind the urogenital sinus. The testes may be located anywhere from within the abdomen in the inguinal canal to within the bifid scrotum. At birth, these individuals appear to be girls who have moderately ambiguous genitalia. However, at puberty, testosterone production by the testes is normal. Because there is no receptor problem, the full testosterone effect occurs, and masculinization, manifest by a deepening of the voice, marked phallic enlargement, loss of subcutaneous fat, and an increase in muscle mass, takes place. However, the sexual tissues that respond primarily to dihydrotestosterone, such as the scrotum, prostate, and testes, remain prepubertal. In adults with this syndrome, serum levels of testosterone are normal or mildly elevated, but dihydrotestosterone concentrations are low. Postpubertal serum gonadotropin levels are slightly increased.

The definitive diagnosis is made by the demonstration of an abnormal basal serum testosterone : dihydrotestosterone ratio (55). After puberty, this ratio is less than 20 in normal men, but greater than 35 in men with 5α-reductase deficiency. When the diagnosis is suspected before puberty, it can be confirmed by measuring the testosterone: dihydrotestosterone ratio after hCG stimulation. In such circumstances, normal boys maintain a ratio of less than 20, but boys with this enzyme deficiency develop a ratio of greater than 50.

The 5α-reductase deficiency syndrome has been of particular interest because of the endocrine abnormalities and because several large kindreds have been found in two isolated agricultural villages in the Dominican Republic, where male and female gender roles are well defined *(56)*. This setting has provided a unique opportunity to determine the contribution of androgens to male gender identity. These psychosocial studies have demonstrated that, in the absence of sociocultural factors that could interrupt the change from female to male sexual orientation, the presence of male levels of testosterone overrides the effects of having been raised as a female. At puberty, these men take on traditional male roles.

Unfortunately, because the testes are usually undescended and because dihydro-testosterone levels are low, sperm production is absent or proceeds to completion in only a few focal areas of the gonad. If the diagnosis has been made before puberty and if the children appear to have the female gender identity, they should be raised as females. The testes should be removed and estrogens should be administered at an appropriate pubertal age. If these patients have proceeded through puberty, they usu-ally should be permitted to continue with their current gender identity, assuming that their phenotype is sufficiently male or female and their chosen gender is appropriate for their social situation. Because an undescended testis is at risk for the development of malignancy and because these individuals are infertile, consideration should be given to removal of the testes and replacement with sex steroids appropriate to the identified gender.

The defects in 5α-reductase described thus far have dealt with the most severe form, in which there is an inability of serum testosterone to bind to the enzyme. However, the defect is genetically heterogeneous, and two additional abnormalities in expression of the 5α-reductase enzyme have been described *(57,58)*. These include an unstable 5α-reductase with a decreased affinity for testosterone and an unstable 5α-reductase with a decreased affinity for the cofactor NADPH (nicotinamide adenine dinucleotide phos-phate, reduced form). These two defects result in milder clinical forms of the disease. Patients have more male-appearing genitalia at birth, allowing for an earlier diagnosis.

The Luteinizing Hormone–Gonadotropin-Resistant Testis

The LH–gonadotropin-resistant testis is a rare defect characterized by a lack of recep-tors or receptor response to LH and hCG *(59)*. In general, these patients have genitalia that appear female. Occasionally, they may have more ambiguous structures, including microphallus, severe hypospadias, a bifid scrotum, and a urogenital sinus. If a vagina is present, it ends in a blind pouch, because there has been complete regression of the müllerian structures as a result of the normal presence of antimüllerian hormone from the testes. Because there is no testosterone production *in utero*, the wolffian structures do not develop. Normally, the fetal testes respond to maternal hCG, and the wolffian structures develop. This is evident especially in patients with hypogonadotropic hypogonadism or Kallmann syndrome, in which, *in utero*, the fetus does not produce LH but the fetal testes respond to maternal hCG. Because androgens are necessary for the completion of spermatogenesis, histologic examination of the testes reveals spermatogenic arrest.

These patients have elevated serum gonadotropin levels and no increase in either serum testosterone or 17-OH progesterone levels after the administration of hCG. They can respond to exogenous androgens if these are indicated. For example, if a patient has been raised as male, he should be treated with testosterone. Alternatively, if the patient has been reared as a female, estrogen therapy should be considered. Because exogenous testosterone cannot achieve the intratesticular levels of testosterone that are necessary to support spermatogenesis, these patients are infertile.

Persistent Müllerian Duct Syndrome

Persistent paramesonephric structures often are part of the syndromes described with defective gonads *(60)*. Sometimes, normal-appearing males will be found at the time of herniorrhaphy or laparotomy to have a cervix, uterus, fallopian tubes, or enlarged prostatic utricle. Occasionally, they may have fathered children, although they often have a history of an undescended testis and infertility. The persistence of the paramesonephric system with otherwise normal testicular development suggests an abnormality of Sertoli cell maturation and deficient production of antimüllerian hormone. Although the reported cases are few, the data suggest autosomal recessive inheritance in some families. These men also are at increased risk for testicular tumors and, when identified, should have gonadal examinations at regular intervals.

Male Pseudohermaphroditism Involving Androgen-Receptor Defects

Androgens enter the target cells and bind to the intracellular receptor, which subsequently attaches to the appropriate site on the gene to initiate translation. If there is an absence of this receptor or defect in this receptor, androgenization cannot occur in spite of a normal or supranormal level of testosterone. The complete absence or lack of dihydrotestosterone binding by the receptor results in the complete female phenotype, which is seen in the testicular feminization syndrome. Variants of this syndrome depend on the degree of receptor defect. A summary of mutations that have been described in the androgen receptor leading to hypogonadism can be found on the Internet (http://xanadu.mgh.harvard.edu/receptor/trrfront.html).

Testicular Feminization

Classically, patients with the testicular feminization syndrome appear to be well-developed females who are identified only after they have gone through a normal puberty and are seen for evaluation of amenorrhea. These patients are chromosomally normal males who have a complete absence of androgen receptors *(61,62)*. At puberty, they have normal breast development because of the unopposed estrogen effects *(63,64)*. On physical examination, the clitoris is of normal size, but pelvic examination reveals a blind vaginal pouch. The testes may present as masses in the labia or may be located within the abdomen. At times, the testes are in the canal of Nuck, and patients have what appear to be bilateral inguinal hernias. Because the testes are not in their normal scrotal position, there is a potential for malignancy, and these gonads should be removed *(65)*. In general, these individuals have been raised as females; they do not respond to exogenous androgens and the female gender identity should be continued. Treatment consists of castration and estrogen replacement. Because they have an XY karyotype with testes, antimüllerian hormone is present and müllerian structures are absent. The wolffian structures do not develop. Because the Leydig cells can function normally in these men, testosterone levels are normal or elevated. Serum LH is increased because of the lack of androgen feedback and serum FSH is increased because of seminiferous tubular dysfunction.

The classic form of this disease results in a complete lack of binding of androgens to the receptor. However, multiple defects in the androgen-receptor gene have been described. These defects may be in either the hormone-binding domain or the DNA-binding domain of the receptor; the latter defect accounts for those forms of testicular feminization in which hormone binding is intact *(66)*. These defects in the androgen receptor have been reviewed *(67)*. The inheritance of testicular feminization is X-linked recessive. Although these patients have a more severe biochemical syndrome, they usually have less difficulty with social adjustment than do patients with other types of pseudohermaphroditism because their phenotypic sex is less ambiguous.

REIFENSTEIN SYNDROME

Individuals with Reifenstein syndrome have partial androgen resistance and are detected at birth with variable degrees of pseudohermaphroditism, ranging from hypospadias and undescended testes to a urogenital sinus, with perineal opening of the urethra and complete lack of fusion of the scrotum *(68,69)*. The karyotype is XY. At puberty, when the testes are physiologically stimulated by endogenous gonadotropins to produce testosterone, an incomplete androgen effect may be noted. Subsequently, the penis remains small, the testes usually remain undescended, and the scrotum is poorly developed. Androgen-sensitive hair growth is decreased and muscle mass and strength are diminished in these patients. The estrogen receptors function normally. Therefore, the increased testosterone production at puberty provides an increased sex steroid substrate for the peripheral production of estrogen in either the liver or fat, and marked gynecomastia usually develops. Most commonly, the testes remain within the abdomen. Light-microscopic examination shows an absence of normal spermatogenesis and hyalinization of most seminiferous tubules. The Leydig cells appear normal. Serum levels of testosterone and dihydrotestosterone are normal or elevated. Because there is also a decrease in functional androgen receptors in the pituitary, serum LH and FSH levels are elevated. This experiment of nature further demonstrates that serum testosterone, as well as estradiol, contributes to normal gonadotropin regulation.

Men with Reifenstein syndrome present a difficult problem in gender selection. Unlike their more severely affected counterparts with testicular feminization, these men are usually raised as males. Studies have shown that although there may be some response to exogenous testosterone therapy, very high dosages (e.g., 400 mg of testosterone enanthate intramuscularly each week) are required to achieve an androgenizing effect. Unfortunately, these dosages have not been proven to be safe for long-term treatment; in addition, they provide the sex steroid substrate for estrogen production. Even high dosages of testosterone usually result in only a partial androgenization. Thus, the long-term treatment of these individuals requires adequate psychological support. Consideration should be given to removing testes if they are located within the abdomen because they are prone to malignant transformation.

If patients with Reifenstein syndrome have been reared as females, castration and estrogen-replacement result in a relatively normal phenotypic female and a more satisfactory outcome than does conversion to a male. Castration prevents partial virilization, which may occur at puberty (especially in 17-ketosteroid reductase deficiency).

Reifenstein syndrome has been shown to have a heterogeneous cause, with some patients demonstrating a decreased number of normal receptors and others having receptors that are defective, as evidenced by their decreased affinity for dihydrotestosterone, their heat lability, and their failure to be stabilized by molybdate *(70–73)*. This variability of receptor number or activity may be the result of the varied genetic defects that are found in Reifenstein syndrome *(74,75)*. An X-linked inheritance is predominant, but in some cases, distinction between X-linked and autosomal recessive inheritance is not clear.

Infertility Resulting from an Androgen-Receptor Defect

A group of men with severe oligospermia have been reported to possess unstable androgen receptors (76). These men were described as phenotypically normal, and the condition was found only when they underwent evaluation for infertility with androgen-receptor measurements. Usually, they were noted to have serum testosterone levels in the upper normal range and LH values that were high normal or mildly elevated. The incidence of this syndrome among infertile men has not been determined because screening for abnormal androgen receptors is not usually required in the workup of male infertility. Since the original description of this defect, subsequent investigators have not been able to confirm the results of the original study. Unfortunately, no treatment is available for this problem.

The syndromes associated with androgen-receptor defects have been described as separate entities; however, their mode of inheritance (i.e., autosomal recessive) is similar. Whether these syndromes are distinctly different or simply represent varying degrees of the same disease process awaits identification of the specific causative gene defect.

Postpubertal Orchitis (Epidemic Parotitis)

Although prepubertal mumps is almost never associated with orchitis, men who acquire mumps during or after puberty have about a 25% chance of developing orchitis (77). The orchitis is usually clinically apparent; nevertheless, some men being evaluated for infertility give a history of postpubertal mumps without a recollection of orchitis. Orchitis is commonly unilateral. However, testicular biopsy at the time of the orchitis demonstrates bilateral involvement. Furthermore, both testes are damaged if the patient has abnormal spermatogenesis and infertility. Of those men who have postpubertal mumps orchitis, as many as 60% will be infertile. During the acute infection, these patients demonstrate sloughing of the germinal seminiferous epithelium. On physical examination, they have atrophic testes. At that time, the biopsy shows tubular sclerosis and hyalinization, which may be focal or diffuse. Although the usual testicular consequence of mumps orchitis is seminiferous tubule failure, some of these men also have Leydig cell failure and androgen deficiency. In view of the recent evidence that local paracrine factors from the Sertoli cells are necessary for adequate Leydig cell function, the finding of decreased testosterone production in these patients is not surprising. These patients usually show a monotropic increase in serum FSH levels but may have elevated LH levels, depending on the degree of androgen deficiency. Stimulation tests with GNRH may be necessary to reveal the exaggerated rise in gonadotropins if the testicular damage is mild and the basal FSH levels are normal.

Since the development of a mumps vaccine, the incidence of mumps orchitis has decreased significantly. This means that many individuals who do have mumps are adults who did not receive the vaccine as children and are more prone to orchitis. Treatment with androgens or estrogens during the acute phase of the infection to suppress and protect the germinal seminiferous tubular epithelium has been suggested. However, this approach is of dubious benefit and no definitive studies have been performed (78). Corticosteroid treatment has been shown to decrease the inflammation and severity of the acute orchitis; whether long-term follow-up treatment would diminish the damage to the seminiferous tubules is unknown (79). If spermatogenesis has been severely impaired, there is no successful therapy for the infertility. If androgen is deficient, testosterone-substitution therapy should be instituted. Other viral infections may cause similar problems.

Cryptorchidism

At birth, as many as 10% of male infants have an undescended testis. By 1 yr of age, 70–90% of these testes descend into the scrotum, and after puberty, only 0.3–0.4% of men continue to have one or both undescended testes *(80)*. Undescended testes have been associated with numerous gonadal disorders, including hypogonadotropic hypogonadism, Ullrich–Noonan syndrome, Klinefelter syndrome, and Reifenstein syndrome *(81)*. Nevertheless, most patients with cryptorchidism have no readily discernible endocrine disease. The association of the true cryptorchid testis and the high incidence of infertility with these syndromes indicates that, in most patients, the problem does not lie within the anatomic structures associated with testicular descent but arises from an endocrine-related developmental abnormality. This is particularly true for unilateral cryptorchidism.

In animals made cryptorchid, infertility develops, which further confirms the damage caused by an abdominal testicle. Human cryptorchidism is associated with infertility in about 70% of cases *(82)*. The cryptorchid testicle is treated by bringing it surgically into the scrotum as soon as the abnormality is detected. This decreases the 8% risk of carcinoma of the testis that is associated with this disorder and places the testis in a location where it can more easily be observed. Another reason to bring the testis into the scrotum is to increase the possibility of fertility. Unfortunately, even when the once-cryptorchid testis is placed in the scrotum, infertility is common.

Various nonsurgical maneuvers (e.g., hCG or GnRH administration) have been tried to stimulate the testis to migrate permanently into the scrotum. These maneuvers have not been proven successful *(83)*.

Leprosy

Although leprosy occurs infrequently in the United States, it remains a common problem in many countries and affects many men, who require years of therapy for the disease. The *Mycobacterium leprae* organism has been shown to invade the testis directly and cause primary testicular failure. This occurs in as many as 75% of men with the disease *(84)*. Although leprosy most often affects both testicular compartments and causes infertility and decreased testosterone production with elevated serum gonadotropin levels, the disease may result in selective destruction of either compartment, causing isolated increases in serum LH or FSH levels *(85)*. Most other infectious processes of the testes affect primarily the seminiferous epithelium. In addition, even when serum LH levels are elevated selectively, affected men still have decreased sperm counts. In leprosy, the greatest damage is to the interstitial compartment. Serum testosterone responses to hCG are blunted to a degree that is proportional to the elevation of serum estradiol.

The severity of testicular damage appears to be related somewhat to the type of leprosy, with lepromatous and borderline leprosy causing the greatest degree of Leydig cell failure and tuberculoid leprosy causing the least. The recognition of androgen deficiency is important in a chronic catabolic disease such as this because androgen replacement may hasten the overall rate of recovery.

Testicular Trauma

The traumatic loss of both testes results in hypogonadism (posttraumatic testicular dysfunction) that requires androgen replacement. However, injury to one testicle that disrupts the continuity of the blood–testis barrier also appears to result in damage to the unaffected, contralateral testis. Sometimes, this damage manifests by infertility. The mechanism for the infertility is unknown, but it may be similar to the cause of infertility in the case of a single undescended testis. Clinically, the appearance of the individual depends on the degree of androgen deficiency and whether the injury occurred before or after puberty.

One of the most common reasons for the loss of a testicle before puberty is testicular torsion. This problem, which tends to be recurrent and often is bilateral, results from a developmental defect. The torsion may be reversed and the testis fixed in place. If the testis is not viable, it should be removed. Subsequently, the viability of the testis depends on the length of time the blood supply has been interrupted. Unfortunately, as may occur with an undescended testis, fertility of the unaffected testis may be compromised.

Testicular Irradiation

Irradiation of the testes usually is associated with a treatment program for an associated disease, such as Hodgkin's disease or prostatic carcinoma. Most of the current data regarding the effects of irradiation on seminiferous tubule dysfunction are derived from two investigations in which otherwise normal men who were undergoing vasectomies had semen analyses, testicular biopsies, and serum hormone measurements made before, during, and while recovering from graded doses of X-irradiation *(86,87)*. These studies demonstrated that doses as small as 15 rads may cause a marked fall in the sperm count and that doses of 50 rads may cause azoospermia. After doses as high as 400 rads, sperm counts and testicular biopsy results returned to normal *(88)*. The time required for normalization correlated directly with the radiation dose and depended on the number of type A spermatogonia remaining after irradiation. A failure to recover was noted at doses of 600 rads or more, and the biopsy specimens in these men demonstrated a complete loss of type A spermatogonia. Disappearance of spermatocytes did not occur consistently until doses were in the range of 200 rads. Serum measurements of FSH began to show significant increases at doses greater than 30 rads, and the return of serum FSH levels to normal paralleled the return to normal spermatogenesis. No significant change in the levels of serum LH or testosterone occurred at any of these doses.

If a patient is scheduled to receive therapeutic irradiation, suppression of spermatogenesis with testosterone or testosterone and an GnRH agonist or antagonist has been suggested to protect against infertility, because dividing cells are more sensitive to the effects of irradiation. This preventive treatment has not been tested. The only acceptable methods of preventing the damage are testicular shielding during irradiation or sperm-banking before treatment. Consideration must be given to the increased numbers of chromosomal breaks that will occur during the irradiation, which may lead to an increase in fetal anomalies.

It appears that Leydig cell dysfunction is not seen until doses of greater than 800 rads are administered. However, these are common doses of therapeutic irradiation *(88)*. In studies performed on men who had received therapeutic irradiation for prostate cancer without testicular shielding (the usual procedure), a significant decrease in basal serum testosterone levels, compared with age-matched men, was noted. A single, large dose was more deleterious than were fractional doses of similar total magnitude. Serum LH and FSH levels were found to be significantly increased, indicating primary testicular damage. Treatment of the testosterone deficiency should be considered, because this should improve the anabolic state and enable patients to tolerate chemotherapy. However, in the case of prostate carcinoma, an androgen-responsive tumor, replacement therapy should not be given.

Radioiodine therapy for thyroid cancer also has been associated with testicular dysfunction, primarily a loss of spermatogenesis *(89)*. However, because comprehensive studies have not been done, the frequency of significant damage is unknown.

Autoimmune Testicular Failure

Two types of autoimmune testicular failure have been described. The most common of these is infertility resulting from the production of antibodies to sperm *(90)*. This situation has been described most convincingly after vasovasostomy in men who have had a vasectomy. The antibody reaction may be responsible for the persistence of infertility in spite of normal sperm counts after vasovasostomy.

The presence of antisperm antibodies of the IgA class in semen and of the IgG class in the peripheral blood may be a cause of idiopathic infertility. The mechanism for the appearance of these antibodies in infertile men without histories of testicular damage or genital infections is unknown. However, because of the high incidence of antisperm antibodies in the normal fertile population, this theory may not be valid. Treatment of this form of infertility with high-dose glucocorticoids has been attempted.

The second, and less common, form of autoimmune testicular failure is that which occurs with steroid cell antibodies and subsequent loss of testosterone production *(91)*. This type of steroid cell antibody has been recognized most commonly in women with ovarian failure but is rarely seen in men. Usually, this condition is seen with other endocrine gland autoimmune diseases, especially Addison's disease. The antibody is directed against the microsomal portion of the cell and not against the steroid hormone. Thyroid disease (e.g., Graves' disease, hypothyroidism, or Hashimoto thyroiditis), hypoparathyroidism, pernicious anemia, diabetes mellitus, and alopecia totalis also have been associated with Leydig cell failure resulting from steroid cell antibodies. This form of autoimmune disease has been linked with the HLA-B8 major histocompatibility locus on chromosome 6. Because of the small number of men described with autoimmune Leydig cell failure, specific types of HLA association are unknown. Androgen-replacement treatment is required in these patients.

CHEMOTHERAPY

Similar to radiation exposure, chemotherapy also may damage the testes. Alkylating agents, such as nitrogen mustards, cyclophosphamide, and chlorambucil, consistently harm spermatogenesis in a dose-related fashion *(92,93)*. Other agents, such as procarbazine and various combinations of drugs, also affect spermatogenesis in most individuals *(94)*. The appearance of gynecomastia provides a clue that Leydig cell function may be affected *(95,96)*.

The same recommendations for prevention of damage described in the section on irradiation also apply to chemotherapeutic agents. Sperm-banking may be considered in young men who undergo curative chemotherapy for malignancies such as Hodgkin's disease or germ cell carcinoma. In some of these tumors, especially Hodgkin's disease, testicular function may be affected by the disease itself. The effects of chemotherapy on Leydig cell function have not been well described; however, the association of gynecomastia with chemotherapy suggests a defect in testosterone production.

SECONDARY HYPOGONADISM

Hypogonadotropic Hypogonadism

Hypogonadotropic hypogonadism may be caused by acquired or congenital defects. The presentation of the acquired forms of the disorder varies depending on whether the individual has gone through puberty and whether other anterior or posterior pituitary hormone deficiencies are involved. If the individual acquires the disorder before the onset of puberty, the presentation is that of a prepubertal male, as noted in Table 2. If puberty has occurred before the onset of the disorder, the presentation is with signs and symptoms of postpubertal testicular failure. The acquired forms of the disorder and some congenital forms have additional anterior pituitary deficiencies. If growth hormone is deficient, it is of clinical significance only if the individual is prepubertal and has not reached his adult height. After puberty, when the epiphyses of the long bones have fused and linear growth has ceased, growth hormone deficiency will no longer be apparent.

Classic Hypogonadotropic Eunuchoidism

Just as Klinefelter syndrome has become the prime example of hypergonadotropic hypogonadism, the congenital hypogonadotropic eunuch is the classic example of hypogonadotropic hypogonadism. As originally described by Kallmann and colleagues, this syndrome (Kallmann syndrome) is characterized by isolated gonadotropin deficiency and anosmia or hyposomia resulting from defective development of the olfactory bulbs *(96,97)*. Other findings occasionally described with this disorder include midline cleft palate and lip, congenital deafness, cerebellar seizures, a short fourth metacarpal, and cardiac abnormalities *(98,99)*.

Kallmann syndrome is most commonly associated with autosomal dominant inheritance *(98)*. The associated defects, especially anosmia, have enabled tracing of father-to-son transmission *(100)*. However, kindreds have been reported that suggest an autosomal recessive or X-linked form of inheritance *(101)*. The question of inheritance will be further defined as more men and women with the syndrome become fertile with newer modes of therapy and their progeny are studied.

The incidence of this syndrome is about 1 in 10,000 male births *(98)*. These men present as prepubertal eunuchs. They usually have no evidence of pubertal physical findings and their skeletal proportions are eunuchoid, with the ratio of upper-body segment (pubis to vertex) to lower-body segment (pubis to floor) decreased; the arm span is at least 6 cm greater than the height. These body proportions result from a failure of epiphyseal fusion and continued long-bone growth. Beard and pubic hair growth are absent or minimal. Most patients retain their prepubertal subcutaneous body fat. Hyposmia is present in most cases but may be missed unless specifically tested using appropriate olfactory-sensation materials *(102)*. Muscle mass and strength remain at prepubertal levels. Although some CNS problems have been described *(103)*, mental retardation is not one of them. A small phallus and temporal facial wrinkling caused by hypogonadism are common in this disorder. Gynecomastia may occur; peripheral aromatization of adrenal androgens may be contributory. Testicular development remains at prepubertal levels, with a few patients showing some testicular enlargement at puberty *(104)*. However, unlike Klinefelter syndrome, the testes are of normal prepubertal size because there is no tubular scarring or loss of germ cells. The Leydig cells are immature (as would be seen without LH stimulation), although normal numbers of interstitial cells are present, and the development into mature testosterone-producing Leydig cells occurs with gonadotropin stimulation.

Basal serum gonadotropin levels are low normal or undetectable in these men. However, when multiple samples are taken over a 24-h period, some subjects demonstrate occasional, small pulses of LH *(105)*. When a single bolus dose of gonadotropin-releasing hormone is administered, the response of the pituitary gonadotropins usually is minimal. However, if repeated pulses of gonadotropin-releasing hormone are given, there eventually is a normal rise in serum LH and FSH levels *(106,107)*. These studies indicate that the most likely defect is a deficiency in GnRH secretion by the hypothalamus. Furthermore, autopsy studies have demonstrated anatomically normal pituitary glands *(108)*. Serum testosterone levels remain in the middle of the female range in most patients with this condition before treatment, although they may have shown partial progression through puberty. No other pituitary hormonal defect has been documented in these patients.

About 10% of men with idiopathic hypogonadotropic hypogonadism provide a history of some pubertal development with subsequent regression; this diagnosis should be suspected in any man who has passed the normal pubertal age and remains prepubertal *(105)*. Serum gonadotropin levels are low, testosterone levels are low, and prolactin levels are normal *(109,110)*. If one of the associated abnormalities, such as anosmia, cleft palate, and cleft lip, is present, the diagnosis can be made with some assurance. However, if these findings are absent, differentiating between delayed puberty and idiopathic hypogonadotropic eunuchoidism can be extremely difficult, because puberty does not occur until 18 or 19 yr of age in some normal men. Several maneuvers have been described that purport to differentiate this condition from delayed puberty *(108,111,112)*. These include a subnormal serum prolactin response to thyrotropin-releasing hormone or to phenothiazine, a decreased serum testosterone response to exogenous hCG, and a normal LH response to pulsatile stimulation by GnRH. None of these tests have been consistently reliable. If the differentiation cannot be made and the circumstances warrant, treatment with testosterone or hCG for 3 or 6 mo may be indicated. After this, therapy can be discontinued and the patient observed to see whether spontaneous puberty progresses.

The treatment of idiopathic hypogonadotropic eunuchoidism has two goals: to provide adequate androgen replacement and to achieve fertility. Replacement with androgens does not impair subsequent therapeutic stimulation of spermatogenesis. As opposed to most of the causes of primary testicular failure in which improvement of fertility is not possible, fertility may be initiated, in secondary hypogonadism, and several methods are available.

In addition to the concern regarding fertility in these men, androgen-replacement therapy is needed to develop muscle mass, prevent osteoporosis, provide psychological support, and produce full pubertal development. Any of the methods for inducing spermatogenesis also will replace androgens by stimulating the Leydig cells. However, once fertility has been achieved, exogenous androgen therapy probably is the most satisfactory and economic choice for the patient. Then, if another pregnancy is desired, the patient can be switched back to gonadotropin or GnRH therapy.

Idiopathic hypogonadotropic eunuchoidism may occur in women. The condition may be isolated or inherited as an autosomal dominant or autosomal recessive trait. It presents similarly in women and men, with a failure to proceed through puberty. These patients usually appear as normal prepubertal females and only rarely have had any signs of pubertal development. In addition, they may have other characteristic somatic features, including anosmia, short fourth metacarpals, and midline defects.

Other syndromes manifest as isolated gonadotropin deficiency. Most of these are associated with severe neurologic damage and mental retardation.

Isolated Deficiency of Luteinizing Hormone or Follicle-Stimulating Hormone

The original reports of isolated LH deficiency occurred in eunuchoid men with testicular volumes, suggesting some development greater than that seen in patients with idiopathic hypogonadotropic hypogonadism *(113,114)*. The term *fertile eunuch* was applied to these men, although most are infertile because the low intratesticular concentrations of testosterone do not support complete spermatogenesis *(115)*. In these patients, testicular biopsy specimens reveal some progression of spermatogenesis. The serum testosterone levels are also low, accounting for the eunuchoid body habitus. Therapy with hCG restores normal serum testosterone levels and completes spermatogenesis *(116)*. Because data have shown that some men with classic idiopathic hypogonadotropic hypogonadism and low levels of both serum LH and FSH may have testicular volumes greater than 5 mL and may demonstrate complete spermatogenesis with hCG alone, it is thought that these syndromes most likely are a part of the spectrum of the same disease. A group of older men have been described who manifest impotence, low serum testosterone levels, low LH levels, and normal FSH levels. These men have gone through normal puberty and fathered children, and it has not been determined whether their LH deficiency is acquired or is a late expression of a congenital disorder.

Isolated deficiency of FSH also has been reported *(117,118)*. These men are seen for infertility and are normally androgenized. They are not eunuchoid in appearance, have normal serum testosterone levels, and have sperm counts ranging from azoospermia to oligospermia.

Acquired Forms of Gonadotropin Deficiency

Gonadotropin deficiency may result from numerous acquired disorders. It had been thought that these lesions caused the loss of gonadotropin secretion by compression and necrosis of pituitary tissue. This especially appears to be true in the case of tumors or granulomatous disease. However, it has been shown that some pituitary lesions can cause hypogonadism without anatomically affecting the pituitary tissue. For instance, tumors that produce corticotropin-releasing hormone, cortisol, or prolactin may directly inhibit gonadotropin secretion. Clinically, the appearance of these patients depends on whether they have gone through puberty (*see* Table 2).

Patients who have space-occupying lesions of the sella may lose other pituitary hormones and have symptoms of multiple hormone deficiencies (i.e., hypothyroidism resulting from thyroid-stimulating hormone deficiency, hypoadrenalism resulting from adrenocorticotropic hormone deficiency). Before puberty, growth hormone deficiency may be manifested by short stature. However, short stature caused by growth hormone deficiency is not seen after puberty because maximum growth has already occurred.

Prolactin-Secreting Pituitary Tumors

Prolactin-producing tumors of the pituitary have been divided into microadenomas (<10 mm in diameter) and macroadenomas. In women, more than 80% of the tumors are microadenomas; in men, 80% are macroadenomas *(119,120)*. This difference may result from earlier detection in women (because of the occurrence of galactorrhea or of irregular menstrual cycles) or from a difference in the character of tumor growth between the two sexes. Because galactorrhea occurs so rarely in men, even in men with high serum prolactin levels, early clinical signs of the tumor are not available. Therefore, the tumor may not be manifest until symptoms caused by the mass of the lesion are present *(121)*. In some men, temporal lobe epilepsy has been associated with hyperprolactinemia *(122)*.

The mechanism by which prolactin-producing pituitary adenomas cause hypogonadism has not been well defined. It had been thought that prolactin lowered basal serum LH and FSH levels, but this has been an inconsistent finding. A change in LH pulse amplitude or frequency has occurred in some men *(123)*. Another possibility is that a single neurotransmitter, such as dopamine or γ-aminobutyrate, may be involved. The latter may both stimulate serum prolactin and suppress serum LH, in which case the prolactin itself may have little direct effect on gonadal function *(124)*.

The diagnosis of a prolactinoma requires the finding of an elevated serum prolactin level. Most men with demonstrable prolactinomas have serum prolactin levels greater than 50 ng/mL. Computerized tomography of the sella is the current standard for demonstrating the tumor mass and should be done in men with elevated serum prolactin levels. Although magnetic resonance imaging of the sella may be useful, instruments of less than 1.5 T usually cannot achieve the resolution necessary to define a tumor less than 10 mm in diameter. The exclusion of other causes of hyperprolactinemia (e.g., hypothyroidism, medication, renal failure) is obligatory. As with any large pituitary tumor, the testing of visual fields and other pituitary functions needs to be considered.

Changes in Leydig cell function usually correlate well with reductions in serum prolactin levels, and normal levels of testosterone and potency are associated with a decrease in serum prolactin levels to normal. However, the resumption of spermatogenesis and subsequent fertility have been less consistent; the rate of restored fertility after the treatment of prolactinomas in men is 50% or less. As is the case in many forms of male infertility, the reasons are not entirely clear. Although isolated case reports suggest that a trial of therapy with gonadotropins may be justified, this has not yet been accomplished.

A report of a prolactinoma enlarging during testosterone-replacement therapy suggests that tumor size should be reassessed periodically if androgen replacement is necessary in a man with a prolactinoma *(125)*.

Severe Systemic Illness

Severe systemic illness has a profound effect on gonadal function. Only a few specific entities are examined in this section.

A marked decrease in testosterone is seen early in the course of thermal injury *(126)*. This decrease in serum testosterone is associated with a modest decrease in serum-immunoassayable LH and a marked decrease in serum-bioactive LH. The reason for this difference may be related to the high levels of serum estradiol that are present. Estradiol can cause increased secretion of a form of LH that is not bioactive *(127,128)*. In addition, the high level of cortisol seen with stress may inhibit the output of GnRH. The suppression of testosterone in these men is proportional to the surface area of the burn and, therefore, correlates inversely with survival. Of further interest are the markedly decreased levels of SHBG immediately after the burn; however, the levels of biologically available testosterone also are low because of the extremely low levels of total testosterone. As the patient recovers from the burn and total testosterone rises, there is a rise in SHBG, such that bioavailable testosterone does not increase for a prolonged period after the burn. In these men, the serum LH and FSH responses to exogenous GnRH are normal *(129)*. Autopsy studies of men who have died of burns but did not have scrotal injury reveal disordered spermatogenesis.

The illness may result from physical injury or systemic medical illness. In some circumstances, the defects in testicular function are a result of treatment (e.g., head irradiation for CNS tumors). In most of these situations, the hypogonadism is reversible with resolution of the illness *(130,131)*.

Although obesity is not considered an acute illness, free- and total testosterone levels are decreased in men with a body mass index of 30 or greater. This is accompanied by an attenuated LH pulse amplitude, suggesting that these men may be truly hypogonadal because of their weight *(132)*.

No studies have shown benefit from testosterone treatment of critically ill men. Although it may be tempting to try androgen therapy to reverse their catabolic state, until controlled studies demonstrate benefit, even short-term therapy should not be attempted because it may be harmful (as was the case for thyroid-hormone-replacement therapy in the critically ill).

Uremia

Hypogonadism is a common finding in men undergoing dialysis *(133–135)*. Uremia often is associated with marked hyperprolactinemia, and originally this was thought to be the reason for the hypogonadism. However, if the prolactin level is decreased with bromocriptine, the serum testosterone level remains low, although the libido is improved. Two other factors in uremia may contribute to the hypogonadism. One is zinc deficiency, although zinc replacement has not corrected the hypogonadism completely *(136)*. Androgen replacement in patients with uremia who are receiving dialysis has been a standard practice, primarily as a means of increasing erythrocyte production.

Hemochromatosis

In hemochromatosis, there are excessive tissue iron stores . Usually, hemochromatosis is clinically manifest by the presence of liver disease, and the hypogonadism that occurs in as many as 60% of these men originally was thought to be secondary to the hepatic abnormalities. More recent investigations have shown that the causative lesion resides in the pituitary and is related to the severity of iron overload *(137)*. Serum testosterone, LH, and FSH levels are low. The response of serum gonadotropins to GnRH stimulation decreases as the severity of the systemic disease increases and is totally absent in severe cases of hemochromatosis. However, the testes respond normally to LH. Thus, the primary defect appears to be pituitary failure.

Treatment of the hemochromatosis with phlebotomy in young men results in a partial normalization of hypothalamic–pituitary–gonadal function. However, this improvement occurs in a minority of men and is only partial. The younger the man, the greater is the likelihood of improvement; amelioration of established disease in men older than 40 yr is rare *(138)*.

COMBINED PRIMARY AND SECONDARY HYPOGONADISM

Aging

Women undergo a marked change in gonadal function with age, as evidenced by menopause, but the situation in men is less clear. Early studies demonstrated a well-defined change in total serum testosterone levels with age *(139)*. However, because many of these studies were done on men with systemic illnesses and because these illnesses by themselves may significantly affect gonadal function, the results probably were not representative of the normal aging process without superimposed disease. Studies done on normal, older, healthy men have demonstrated few differences compared to younger men *(140)*. Nevertheless, a small difference persists, especially when diurnal variations in total testosterone are examined. When the bioavailable (non-SHBG-bound) testosterone was measured, a more marked difference between young and elderly populations was discovered. Part of the reason for the greater difference in non-SHBG-bound testosterone than in total testosterone is the slight fall in total serum testosterone that occurs with age and the increase in SHBG, which further decreases the available testosterone. The reason for the increase in SHBG is not well understood. Explanations include stimulation by the increased serum estrogen that occurs with age, possible alteration in response to decreased thyroid hormones, or a change in glycosylation of the SHBG that might prolong the circulating half-life of this protein. This subject has recently been reviewed extensively *(141)*.

Hepatic Cirrhosis

Both cirrhosis and significant ethanol ingestion have major effects on testicular function. Acute ethanol ingestion lowers serum testosterone levels and raises LH levels, suggesting a primary effect on the testes *(142,143)*. One way in which ethanol may acutely inhibit spermatogenesis is by interfering with alcohol dehydrogenase. This enzyme is necessary for the metabolism of retinol, an important substrate for normal spermatogenesis; ethanol has an affinity for this enzyme that is 50 times greater than the affinity for retinol. Therefore, ethanol alone without any secondary damage to the liver may inhibit testicular function. Normal men who ingest significant amounts of ethanol and achieve blood alcohol levels greater than 0.10 mg/dL have a temporary decrease in serum testosterone and a rise in LH.

If the long-term ingestion of ethanol results in cirrhotic changes of the liver, permanent alterations in gonadal function occur. These include suppression of gonadotropin release and decreased testosterone production *(144)*. In addition, a rise in SHBG may lead to a further decrease in bioavailable testosterone. The SHBG in these individuals may be abnormal; inhibition of transport of testosterone is retarded, as would be expected by a rise in SHBG, but no inhibition of estradiol transport occurs *(145)*. Estradiol production is increased and provides an additional explanation for the gynecomastia. Furthermore, although serum testosterone levels are decreased, the increased availability of estradiol also may provide a mechanism for the suppression of gonadotropin output.

Sickle-Cell Disease

Men with sickle cell disease display characteristics of prepubertal hypogonadism *(146,147)*. They have eunuchoid skeletal proportions, small testes, decreased muscle mass, and decreased hair growth. However, because most patients with sickle cell disease are black, their eunuchoid skeletal proportions may not be abnormal. Normal black men may have skeletal proportions that tend to fit the definition of eunuchoid measurements in whites. In some patients with sickle cell disease, serum testosterone levels are low, but LH and FSH levels may be inappropriately normal. GnRH tests have yielded equivocal results.

These findings suggest that there most likely are several possible causes for the hypogonadism, including hypogonadotropic hypogonadism of chronic stress and specific destruction of testicular tissue because of interruption of the blood supply by the sickling process. Hypogonadism also may be caused by malnutrition and, possibly, zinc deficiency. Treatment with androgens has not been studied systematically in these patients.

SUMMARY

This chapter presents a large number of causes for hypogonadism in men, however, the most important aspect in making the diagnosis is to first suspect hypoganism from history and clinical exam, as indicated in Table 2.

REFERENCES

1. Hobbs C, Plymate S, Rosen C, Adler R. Testosterone administration increases insulin-like growth factor I levels in normal men. J Clin Endocrinol Metab 1993;77:776.
2. Peiris A, Stagner J, Plymate S, Vogel R. Relationship between secretory pulses to sex hormone binding globulin in normal men. J Clin Endocrinol Metab 1993;76:279.
3. Weissberger A, Ho K. Activation of the somatotropic axis by testosterone in adult males: evidence for the role of aromatization. J Clin Endocrinol Metab 1993;76:1407.
4. Goodfellow P, Lovell-Badge R. SRY and sex determination in mammals. Annu Rev Genet 1993;27:71.
5. Koopman P, Bullejos M, Bowles J. Regulation of male sexual development by Sry and Sox9. J Exp Zool 2001;290:463.
6. Mosher WD. Infertility trends among U.S. couples: 1965–1976. Family 1982;14:22.
7. Nagao RR, Plymate SR, Berger RE, et al. Comparison of gonadal function between fertile and infertile men with varicoceles. Fertil Steril 1986;46:930.
8. Klinefelter HG Jr, Reifenstein EC Jr, Albright F. Syndrome characterized by gynecomastia, aspermatogenesis without a-Leydigism and increased excretion of follicle-stimulating hormone. J Clin Endocrinol Metab 1942;2:615.
9. Plunkett ER, Barr ML. Cytologic tests of sex in congenital testicular hypoplasia. J Clin Endocrinol Metab 1956;16:829.
10. Lodi A, Monti D, Gaspari G, et al. Klinefelter's syndrome in nontwin brothers and maternal XX/XXX mosaicism. J Endocrinol Invest 1979;2:419.
11. Laron Z, Hochman H. Small testes in prepubertal boys with Klinefelter's syndrome. J Clin Endocrinol Metab 1971;32:671.
12. Ratcliffe SG. The sexual development of boys with the chromosome constitution of 47 XXY (Klinefelter's syndrome). In: Bancroft J, ed. Clinics in Endocrinology and Metabolism, WB Saunders, Philadelphia, PA, 1982, vol. 11, p. 703.
13. Plymate SR, Leonard JM, Paulsen CA, et al. Sex hormone-binding globulin changes with androgen replacement. J Clin Endocrinol Metab 1983;57:645.
14. Plymate SR, Paulsen CA. Klinefelter's syndrome. In: King R, Motulsky A, eds. The Genetic Basis of Common Disease. Oxford University Press, New York, 1989, p. 127.
15. Wang C, Baker HW, Burger HG, et al. Hormonal studies in Klinefelter's syndrome. Clin Endocrinol (Oxf) 1975;4:399.
16. Wieland RG, Zorn EM, Johnson MW. Elevated testosterone-binding globulin in Klinefelter's syndrome. J Clin Endocrinol Metab 1980;51:1199.
17. Gabrilove JL, Freiberg EK, Thornton JC, Nicholis GL. Effect of age on testicular function in Klinefelter's syndrome. Clin Endocrinol (Oxf) 1979;11:343.
18. Ratcliffe SG, Bancroft J, Axworthy D, McCloren W. Klinefelter's syndrome in adolescence. Arch Dis Child 1982;57:6.
19. Nistal M, Santamaria L, Paniagua R. Quantitative and ultrastructural study of Leydig cells in Klinefelter's syndrome. J Pathol 1985;146:323.
20. Sasagawa I, Katayama T. Ultrastructural study of Leydig cells in cases with Klinefelter's syndrome. J Clin Electron Microsc 1985;18:163.

21. Schill WB, Strasser R, Krassnigg F, et al. Spermatological investigation in men with Klinefelter's syndrome. In: Bandmann HJ, Breit R, Perwein E, eds. Klinefelter's Syndrome. Springer-Verlag, New York, 1984, p. 147.

22. Ohno S. Control of Meiotic Processes in the Testis in Normal and Infertile Men. In: Troen P, Nankin H, eds. Raven Press, New York, 1976, p. 1.

23. Jequirer AM, Bullimore NJ. Testicular and epididymal histology in a fetus with Klinefelter's syndrome at 22 weeks' gestation. Br J Urol 1989;11:214.

24. Swanson DW, Stipes AN. Psychiatric aspects of Klinefelter's syndrome. Am J Psychiatry 1969;126:814.

25. Ferguson-Smith MA. The prepubertal testicular lesion in chromatin-positive Klinefelter's syndrome (primary micro-orchidism) as seen in mentally handicapped children. Lancet 1959;1:219.

26. de la Chapelle A. Sex chromosome abnormalities among the mentally defective in Finland. J Ment Defic Res 1963;7:129.

27. Witkin HA, Mednick SA, Schulsinger F, et al. Criminality in XYY and XXY men. Science 1976;193:547.

28. Ratcliffe SG. Klinefelter's syndrome in children: a longitudinal study of 47,XXY boys identified by population screening in Klinefelter's syndrome. In: Bandmann HJ, Breit R, Perwein E, eds. Klinefelter's Syndrome. Springer-Verlag, New York, 1984, p. 38.

29. Becker KL. Clinical and therapeutic experiences with Klinefelter's syndrome. Fertil Steril 1972;23:568.

30. Ferguson-Smith MA, Yates JRW. Maternal age specific rates for chromosome aberrations and factors influencing them. Prenat Diagn 1984;4:5.

31. Carothers AD, Collyer S, de Mey R, Frackiewicz A. Parental age and birth order in the aetiology of some sex chromosome aneuploidics. Ann Hum Genet 1979;41:227.

32. Borelli JB, Bender BG, Puck MH, et al. The meaning of early knowledge of a child's infertility in families with 47,XXY and 45,X children. Child Psychiatry Hum Dev 1984;14:215.

33. Perez-Palacios G, Medina M, Ullao-Aguirre A, et al. Gonadotropin dynamics in XX males. J Clin Endocrinol Metab 1981;53:254.

34. Fechner P, Marcantonio S, Jaswaney V, et al. The role of the sex-determining region Y gene in the etiology of 46, XX maleness. J Clin Endocrinol Metabol 1993;76:690.

35. Davidoff F, Federman DD. Mixed gonadal dysgenesis. Pediatrics 1973;52:725.

36. Philip J, Lundsteen C, Owen D. The frequency of chromosome aberrations in tall men with special reference to 47,XYY and 47,XXY. Am J Hum Genet 1976;28:404.

37. Santen RJ, de Kretser DM, Paulsen CA, Vorhees J. Gonadotrophins and testosterone in the XYY syndrome. Lancet 1970;2:371.

38. Skakkebaek NE, Hulten M, Jacobsen P, Mikkelsen M. Quantification of human seminiferous epithelium. II. Histological studies in eight 47,XYY men. J Reprod Fertil 1973;32:391.

39. Noonan JA. Hypertelorism with Turner phenotype. Am J Dis Child 1968;116:373.

40. Mendez HM, Opitz JM. Noonan syndrome: a review. Am J Med Genet 1985;21:493.

41. Takeda R, Ueda M. Pituitary–gonadal function in male patients with myotonic dystrophy—serum luteinizing hormone, follicle-stimulating hormone and testosterone levels, and histological damage of the testis. Acta Endocrinol (Copenh) 1977;84:382.

42. Sagel J, Distiller LA, Morley JE, Isaacs H. Myotonia dystrophica: studies on gonadal function using gonadotropin-releasing hormone (GNRH). J Clin Endocrinol Metab 1975;40:1110.

43. Wells S, Josefowicz R, Forbes G, Griggs R. Effect of testosterone on metabolic rate and body composition in normal men and men with muscular dystrophy. J Clin Endocrinol Metab 1992; 74:332.

44. de Kretser DM, Burger HG, Fortune D, et al. Hormonal, histological and chromosomal studies in adult males with testicular disorder. J Clin Endocrinol Metab 1972;35:392.

45. de Kretser DM, Kerr JB, Paulsen CA. The peritubular tissue in the normal and pathological human testis: an ultrastructural study. Biol Reprod 1975;12:317.

46. Green AA, Dynsley-Green A, Zachman M, et al. Congenital bilateral anorchia in childhood: a clinical, endocrine, and therapeutic evaluation of 21 cases. Clin Endocrinol (Oxf) 1976;5:381.

47. Bergada C, Cleveland WW, Jones HW, Wilkins L. Variants of embryonic testicular dysgenesis: bilateral anorchia and the syndrome of rudimentary testes. Acta Endocrinol (Copenh) 1962;40:521.

48. Forest MG. Inborn errors of testosterone biosynthesis in the intersex child. In: Josso N, ed. Pediatric and Adolescent Endocrinology, Karger, Basel, 1981, vol 8, p. 133.

49. Goebelsmann U, Horton R, Mestman JH, et al. Male pseudohermaphroditism due to testicular 17β-hydroxysteroid dehydrogenase deficiency. J Clin Endocrinol Metab 1973;36:867.

50. Saez JM, Morera AM, de Peretti E, Bertrand J. Further in vivo studies in male pseudohermaphroditism with gynecomastia due to a testicular 17-ketosteroid defect (compared to a case of testicular feminization). J Clin Endocrinol Metab 1972;34:598.

51. Saez JM, de Peretti E, Morera AM, et al. Familial male pseudohermaphroditism with gynecomastia due to a testicular 17-ketosteroid reductase defect. I. In vivo studies. J Clin Endocrinol Metab 1971;32:604.

52. Castro-Magana M, Angulo M, Uy J. Male hypogonadism with gynecomastia caused by late-onset deficiency of 17-ketosteroid reductase. N Engl J Med 1993;328:1297.

53. Imperato-McGinley JL, Guerrero L, Gautier T, Peterson RE. Steroid 5α-reductase deficiency in man: an inherited form of male pseudohermaphroditism. Science 1974;186:1213.

54. Walsh PC, Madden JD, Harrod MJ, et al. Familial incomplete male pseudohermaphroditism, type 2. Decreased dihydrotestosterone formation in pseudovaginal perineoscrotal hypospadias. N Engl J Med 1974;291:944.

55. Peterson RE, Imperato-McGinley J, Gauiter T, Sturla E. Male pseudohermaphroditism due to steroid 5α-reductase deficiency. Am J Med 1977;62:170.

56. Imperato-McGinley JL, Peterson RE. Male pseudohermaphroditism: the complexities of male phenotypic development. Am J Med 1976;61:251.

57. Leshin M, Griffin JE, Wilson JD. Hereditary male pseudohermaphroditism associated with an unstable form of 5α-reductase. J Clin Invest 1978;62:685.

58. Fisher KL, Kogut MD, Moore RJ, et al. Clinical, endocrinological, and enzymatic characterization of two patients with 5α-reductase deficiency: evidence that a single enzyme is responsible for the 5α-reduction of cortisol and testosterone. J Clin Endocrinol Metab 1978;47:653.

59. David R, Yoon DJ, Landin L, et al. A syndrome of gonadotropin resistance possibly due to a luteinizing hormone receptor defect. J Clin Endocrinol Metab 1984;59:156.

60. Josso N, Fetcke C, Cachin O, et al. Persistence of müllerian ducts in male pseudohermaphroditism and its relationship to cryptorchidism. Clin Endocrinol (Oxf) 1983;19:247.

61. Kovacs WJ, Griffin JE, Weaver DD, et al. A mutation that causes lability of the androgen receptor under conditions that normally promote transformation to the DNA-binding state. J Clin Invest 1984;73:1095.

62. Griffin JE, Wilson JD. The syndromes of androgen resistance. N Engl J Med 1980;302:198.

63. Boyar RM, Moore RJ, Rosner W, et al. Studies on gonadotropin–gonadal dynamics in patients with androgen insensitivity. J Clin Endocrinol Metab 1978;47:1116.

64. MacDonald PC, Madden JD, Brenner PF, et al. Origin of estrogen in normal men and in women with testicular feminization. J Clin Endocrinol Metab 1979;49:905.

65. O'Leary JA. Comparative studies of the gonad in testicular feminization and cryptorchidism. Fertil Steril 1965;16:813.

66. Kaufman M, Pinsky L, Baird PH, McGillivray BC. Complete androgen insensitivity with a normal amount of 5α-dihydrotestosterone-binding activity in labium majus skin fibroblasts. Am J Med Genet 1983;4:401.

67. McPhaul MJ, Marcelli M, Zoppi S, et al. Genetic basis of endocrine disease: the spectrum of mutations in the androgen gene that causes androgen resistance. J Clin Endocrinol Metabol 1993;76:17.

68. Reifenstein EC Jr. Hereditary familial hypogonadism. Clin Res 1947;3:86.

69. Amrhein JA, Klingensmith GJ, Walsh PC, et al. Partial androgen insensitivity: Reifenstein syndrome revisited. N Engl J Med 1977;297:350.

70. Wilson JD, Harrod MJ, Goldstein JL, Griffin JE. Familial incomplete male pseudohermaphroditism, type I. N Engl J Med 1974;290:1097.

71. Griffin JE, Punyashthiti K, Wilson JD. Dihydrotestosterone binding by cultured human fibroblasts: comparison of cells from control subjects and from patients with hereditary male pseudohermaphroditism due to androgen resistance. J Clin Invest 1976;57:1342.

72. Gyorki S, Warne GL, Khalid BAK, Funder JW. Defective nuclear accumulation of androgen receptors in disorders of sexual differentiation. J Clin Invest 1983;72:819.

73. Eil C. Familial incomplete male pseudohermaphroditism associated with impaired nuclear androgen retention. J Clin Invest 1982;71:850.

74. Bremner WJ, Ott J, Moore DJ, Paulsen CA. Reifenstein's syndrome: investigation of linkage to X-chromosomal loci. Clin Genet 1974;6:216.

75. Wooster R, Mangion J, Eeles R, et al. A germline mutation in the androgen receptor gene in two brothers with breast cancer and Reifenstein syndrome. Nat Genet 1992;2:132.

76. Aiman J, Griffin JE, Gazak JM, et al. Androgen insensitivity as a cause of infertility in otherwise normal men. N Engl J Med 1979;300:223.

77. Ballew JW, Masters WH. Mumps, a cause of infertility. I. Present consideration. Fertil Steril 1954;5:536.

78. Savran J. Diethylstilbestrol in prevention of orchitis following mumps. Rhode Island Med J 1946;29:662.

79. Mongon ES. The treatment of mumps orchitis with prednisone. Am J Med Sci 1959;237:749.

80. Charney CW. The spermatogenic potential for the undescended testis before and after treatment. J Urol 1960;83:697.

81. Rajfer J, Walsh PC. Testicular descent: normal and abnormal. Urol Clin North Am 1978;5:223.

82. Albescu JZ, Bergada C, Cullen M. Male fertility in patients treated for cryptorchidism before puberty. Fertil Steril 1971;22:829.

83. Rajfer J, Handelsman DJ, Swerdloff RS, et al. Hormonal therapy of cryptorchidism. A randomized double-blind study comparing human chorionic gonadotropin and gonadotropin releasing hormone. N Engl J Med 1986;314:466.

84. Shilo S, Livshin Y, Sheskin J, Spitz IM. Gonadal function in lepromatous leprosy. Lepr Rev 1981;52:127.

85. Kannan V, Vijaya G. Endocrine testicular functions in leprosy. Horm Metab Res 1984;16:146.

86. Rowley MJ, Leach DR, Warner GA, Heller CG. Effect of graded doses of ionizing radiation in the human testis. Radiat Res 1974;59:665.

87. Paulsen CA. The study of irradiation effects on the human testis, including histologic, chromosomal and hormonal aspects. Final progress report of AEC contract AT(45-1)-2225, Task Agreement 6. RLO-2225-2, 1973.

88. Clifton DK, Bremner WJ. The effect of testicular x-irradiation on spermatogenesis in man. J Androl 1983;4:387.

89. Handelsman DJ, Turtle JR. Testicular damage after radioactive iodine (^{131}I) therapy for thyroid cancer. Clin Endocrinol (Oxf) 1983;18:465.

90. Haas GGJ, Cines DB, Schreiber AD. Immunologic infertility: identification of patients with antisperm antibody. N Engl J Med 1980;303:722.

91. Elder M, Maclaren N, Riley W. Gonadal autoantibodies in patients with hypogonadism and/or Addison's disease. J Clin Endocrinol Metab 1981;52:1137.

92. Schilsky RL, Lewis BJ, Sherins RJ, Young RC. Gonadal dysfunction in patients receiving chemotherapy for cancer. Ann Intern Med 1980;93:109.

93. Shalet SM. Disorders of the endocrine system due to radiation and cytotoxic chemotherapy. Clin Endocrinol (Oxf) 1983;18:637.

94. Chapman RM, Sutcliffe SB, Rees LH, et al. Cyclical combination chemotherapy and gonadal function. Lancet 1979;1:285.

95. Friedman NM, Plymate SR. Leydig cell dysfunction and gynaecomastia in adult males treated with alkylating agents. Clin Endocrinol (Oxf) 1980;12:553.

96. Kallmann FJ, Schoenfeld WA, Barrera SE. The genetic aspects of primary eunuchoidism. Am J Ment Defic 1944;48:203.

97. Takeda T, Takasu N, Yamauchi K, et al. Magnetic resonance imaging of the hypoplasia of the rhinencephalon in a patient with Kallman's syndrome. Intern Med 1992;31:394.

98. Santen RJ, Paulsen CA. Hypogonadotropic eunuchoidism, I. Clinical study of the mode of inheritance. J Clin Endocrinol Metab 1973;36:47.

99. Herzog AG, Seibel MM, Schomer DL, et al. Reproductive endocrine disorders in men with partial seizures of temporal lobe origin. Arch Neurol 1986;43:347.

100. Merriam GR, Beitins IZ, Bode HH. Father-to-son transmission of hypogonadism with anosmia: Kallmann's syndrome. Am J Dis Child 1977;131:1216.

101. Hermanussen M, Sippell WG. Heterogeneity of Kallmann's syndrome. Clin Genet 1985;28:106.

102. Henkin RF, Barter FC. Olfactory thresholds in normal men and in patients with adrenocortical insufficiency. J Clin Invest 1966;45:1631.

103. Schwankhaus JD, Currie J, Jaffe MJ, et al. Neurological findings in men with isolated hypogonadotropic hypogonadism. Neurology 1989;39:223.

104. Yoshimoto Y, Moridera K, Imura H. Restoration of normal pituitary gonadotropin reserve by administration of luteinizing-hormone-releasing hormone in patients with hypogonadotropic hypogonadism. N Engl J Med 1975;292:242.

105. Spratt DI, Finkelstein JS, O'Dea LS, et al. Long-term administration of gonadotropin-releasing hormone in men with idiopathic hypogonadotropic hypogonadism. A model for studies of the hormone's physiologic effects. Ann Intern Med 1986;105:848.

106. Hoffman AR, Crowley WF Jr. Induction of puberty in men by long-term pulsatile administration of low-dose gonadotropin-releasing hormone. N Engl J Med 1982;307:1237.

107. Bremner WJ, Fernando NN, Paulsen CA. The effect of gonadotropin-releasing hormone in hypogonadotrophic eunuchoidism. Acta Endocrinol (Copenh) 1977;85:1.

108. Gauthier G. Olfacto-genital dysplasia (agenesis of the olfactory lobes) with absence of gonadal development at puberty. Acta Neurochir 1960;21:345.

109. Bardin CW, Ross GT, Rifkind AB, et al. Studies of the pituitary–Leydig cell axis in young men with hypogonadotrophic hypogonadism and hyposmia: comparison with normal men, prepubertal boys, and hypopituitary patients. J Clin Invest 1969;48:2046.

110. Boyar RM, Finkelstein JW, Witkin M, et al. Studies of endocrine function in isolated gonadotropin deficiency. J Clin Endocrinol Metab 1973;36:64.

111. Dunkel L. Metoclopramide test in the diagnosis of isolated hypogonadotrophic hypogonadism. Acta Endocrinol (Copenh) 1986;111:241.

112. Winters SJ. How to diagnose delayed puberty? Int J Androl 1984;7:177.

113. Pasqualini RW, Bur GE. Hypoandrogenic syndrome with spermatogenesis. Fertil Steril 1955;6:144.

114. Faiman C, Hoffman RJ, Ryan RJ, Albert A. The "fertile eunuch" syndrome: demonstration of isolated luteinizing hormone deficiency by radioimmunoassay technique. Mayo Clin Proc 1968;43:661.

115. McCullagh EP, Beck JC, Jones HW. A syndrome of eunuchoidism with spermatogenesis, normal urinary FSH and low or normal ICSH (fertile "eunuchs"). J Clin Endocrinol Metab 1953;13:489.

116. Al-Ansari AA, Khalil TH, Kelani Y, Mortimer CH. Isolated follicle-stimulating hormone deficiency in men: successful long-term gonadotropin therapy. Fertil Steril 1984;42:618.

117. Mozaffarian GA, Higley M, Paulsen CA. Clinical studies in an adult male patient with "isolated follicle stimulating hormone (FSH) deficiency." J Androl 1983;4:393.

118. Maroulis G, Parlow AF, Marshall JR. Isolated follicle-stimulating hormone deficiency in man. Fertil Steril 1977;28:818.

119. Rodman EF, Goodman R. Prolactinomas in males. In: Olefsky JM, Robbins RJ, eds. Prolactinomas— Contemporary Issues in Endocrinology and Metabolism, Churchill Livingstone, New York, 1986, vol 2, p. 115.

120. Carter JN, Tyson JE, Tolis G, et al. Prolactin-secreting tumors and hypogonadism in 22 men. N Engl J Med 1978;299:847.

121. Greenspan SL, Neer RM, Ridgway EC, Klibanski A. Osteoporosis in men with hyperprolactinemic hypogonadism. Ann Intern Med 1986;104:777.

122. Spark RF, Wills CA, Royal H. Hypogonadism, hyperprolactinaemia, and temporal lobe epilepsy in hyposexual men. Lancet 1984;1:413.

123. Winters SJ, Troen P. Altered pulsatile secretion of luteinizing hormone in hypogonadal men with hyperprolactinaemia. Clin Endocrinol (Oxf) 1984;21:257.

124. Fuchs E, Mansky T, Stock KW, et al. Involvement of catecholamines and glutamate in gabaergic mechanisms regulatory to luteinizing hormone and prolactin. Neuroendocrinology 1984;38:484.

125. Murray FT, Cameron DF, Ketchum C. Return of gonadal function in men with prolactin-secreting pituitary tumors. J Clin Endocrinol Metab 1984;59:79.

126. Plymate SR, Vaughan GM, Mason AD Jr, Pruitt BA Jr. Central hypogonadism in burned men. Horm Res 1987;27:152.

127. Friedl KE, Plymate SR, Bernhard WN, Mohr LC. Elevation of plasma estradiol in healthy men during a mountaineering expedition. Horm Metab Res 1988;20:239.

128. Veldhuis JD, Sowers JR, Rogol AD, et al. Pathophysiology of male hypogonadism associated with endogenous hyperestrogenism. Evidence for dual defects in the gonadal axis. N Engl J Med 1985;312:1371.

129. Dolecek R, Dvoracek C, Jezek M, et al. Very low serum testosterone levels and severe impairment of spermatogenesis in burned male patients. Correlations with basal levels and levels of FSH, LH and PRL after GNRH + TRH. Endocrinology Exp 1983;17:33.

130. Constine L, Woolf P, Cann D, et al. Hypothalamic–pituitary dysfunction after irradiation for brain tumors. N Engl J Med 1993;328:87.
131. Spratt D, Bigos S, Beitens I, et al. Both hyper- and hypogonadotropic hypogonadism occur transiently in acute illness: bio- and immunoreactive gonadotropins. J Clin Endocrinol Metab 1992;75:1562.
132. Vermeulen A, Kaufman J, Deslypere J, Thomas G. Attenuated luteinizing hormone (LH) pulse amplitude but normal LH pulse frequency, and its relation to plasma androgens in hypogonadism of obese men. J Clin Endocrinol Metab 1993;76:1140.
133. Lim VS, Fang VS. Gonadal dysfunction in uremic men. A study of the hypothalamo–pituitary testicular axis before and after renal transplantation. Am J Med 1975;58:655.
134. Sawin CT, Longcope C, Schmitt GW, Ryan RJ. Blood levels of gonadotropins and gonadal hormones in gynecomastia associated with chronic hemodialysis. J Clin Endocrinol Metab 1973;36:988.
135. Handelsman DJ. Hypothalamic–pituitary gonadal dysfunction in renal failure, dialysis and renal transplantation. Endocr Rev 1985;6:151.
136. Mahajan SK, Abbasi AA, Prasad AS, et al. Effect of oral zinc therapy on gonadal function in hemodialysis patients. A double-blind study. Ann Intern Med 1982;97:357.
137. Duranteau L, Chanson P, Blumberg-Tick J, et al. Non-responsiveness of serum gonadotropins and testosterone to pulsatile GnRH in hemochromatosis suggesting a pituitary defect. Acta Endocrinol (Copenh) 1993;128:351.
138. Cundy T, Butler J, Bomford A, Williams R. Reversibility of hypogonadotrophic hypogonadism associated with genetic haemochromatosis. Clin Endocrinol (Oxf) 1993;38:617.
139. Vermeulen A. Androgen secretion after age 50 in both sexes. Horm Res 1983;18:37.
140. Harman SM, Tsitouras PD. Reproductive hormones in aging men. I. Measurement of sex steroids, basal luteinizing hormone, and Leydig cell response to human chorionic gonadotropin. J Clin Endocrinol Metab 1980;51:35.
141. Matsumoto, AM. Androgens and aging. J Gerontol Med Sci 2002;57A:M76.
142. Galvao-Teles A, Monteiro E, Gavaler JS, Van Thiel DH. Gonadal consequences of alcohol abuse: lessons from the liver. Hepatology 1986;6:135.
143. Ida Y, Tsujimaru S, Nakamaura K, et al. Effects of acute and repeated alcohol ingestion on hypothalamic–pituitary–gonadal and hypothalamic–pituitary–adrenal functioning in normal males. Drug Alcohol Depend 1992;31:57.
144. Bannister P, Handley T, Chapman C, Losowsky MS. Hypogonadism in chronic liver disease: impaired release of luteinising hormone. Br Med J 1986;293:1191.
145. Sakiyama R, Pardridge WM, Judd HL. Effects of human cirrhotic serum or estradiol and testosterone transport into rat brain. J Clin Endocrinol Metab 1982;54:1140.
146. Landefeld CS, Schambelan M, Kaplan SL, Embury SH. Clomiphene-responsive hypogonadism in sickle cell anemia. Ann Intern Med 1983;99:480.
147. el-Hazami M, Bahakim H, al-Fawaz I. Endocrine functions in sickle-cell anemia patients. J Trop Pediatr 1991;38:307.

4

Dihydrotestosterone and 5α-Reductase
Normal Physiology and Inhibition

Paul R. Sutton, MD, PhD, *John K. Amory,* MD,
and Richard V. Clark, MD, PhD

CONTENTS

DIHYDROTESTOSTERONE IN EMBRYOGENESIS AND NORMAL ADULT
   PHYSIOLOGY
INHIBITION OF 5α-REDUCTASE
SUMMARY
REFERENCES

DIHYDROTESTOSTERONE IN EMBRYOGENESIS AND NORMAL ADULT PHYSIOLOGY

In man, 4–8% of testosterone (T) undergoes 5α-reduction, resulting in the formation of the potent androgen dihydrotestosterone (DHT). DHT plays a crucial role in the formation of the external male genitalia and prostate during fetal life. In the adult, however, DHT is associated with a variety of chronic conditions, including benign prostatic hyperplasia, androgenic alopecia, acne vulgaris, and, perhaps, carcinoma of the prostate—making inhibition of DHT production an attractive target for pharmacotherapy. This chapter will review the role of DHT in normal development during fetal life as well as its functions in the adult. We will also discuss pharmaceutical means of reducing DHT synthesis in the treatment of DHT-dependent diseases, with particular emphasis on the emergence of the new class of 5α-reductase inhibitors.

DHT Metabolism

DHT is produced by 5α-reduction from the 4–8 mg of testosterone produced daily by the adult male testes *(1)*. Four to eight percent of this T is 5α-reduced to DHT—mostly in androgen-responsive organs. Approximately 50 µg of DHT is produced from 5α-reduction within the testes, whereas production in other tissues is approx 300 µg daily. Circulating serum DHT levels are 30–86 ng/dL (1.0–2.9 nmol/L) in normal men *(2,3)*.

Tissue DHT levels within androgen-dependent organs are many times higher than DHT concentrations in circulating plasma. In the prostate, for example, tissue DHT concentrations are 10 times higher than plasma concentrations *(4–6)*. Intraprostatic T

From: *Contemporary Endocrinology: Androgens in Health and Disease*
Edited by: C. Bagatell and W. J. Bremner © Humana Press Inc., Totowa, NJ

levels are one-tenth the serum T levels, demonstrating the remarkable *in situ* conversion of T to DHT in this organ. In the testes, both Leydig and Sertoli cells contain 5α-reductase activity and tissue DHT concentrations are also 10 times higher than in the peripheral blood, but only a fraction of tissue T concentration *(7)*. It is interesting to note that testicular 5α-reductase activity may be upregulated in low gonadotropin states (such as the administration of experimental male contraceptive regimens), thereby serving to preserve intratesticular DHT concentration and total androgen bioactivity *(7,8)*.

Most serum DHT, like T, is bound to sex hormone-binding globulin (SHBG) and albumin with only a small percentage as free hormone. In tissue, DHT has a higher affinity for the androgen receptor than T and, once bound, the DHT–androgen receptor complex is more stable and exhibits a more potent stimulus on gene expression than T *(9)*. There are two 5α-reductase isozymes that convert T to DHT. 5α-Reductase type I is found largely in skin and the liver, whereas 5α-reductase type II is located mainly in the male urogenital tract both during fetal and adult life *(10)*. Both T and DHT are metabolized to androstandiol, the 3α-diol of DHT that is rapidly metabolized by glucuronide conjugation and excreted in the urine *(11)*.

DHT Function

During male embryogenesis, the testes differentiate and begin to secrete T 6–8 wk after fertilization. T induces the development and further differentiation of the wolffian ducts, whereas DHT is necessary for differentiation of the urogenital sinus, leading to the formation of the external genitalia and the prostate. The critical period for formation of the external genitalia is during wk 8–12 of embryogenesis. In addition to regulating the differentiation of structures of the urogenital sinus, DHT may also play a role in the development of sexually dimorphic brain structures *(12,13)*. The importance of DHT in male embryogenesis is clearly illustrated by studies of men with mutations in 5α-reductase type II, who have very low levels of DHT during development. In the absence of DHT, these male children are born with a female phenotype, including a bifid scrotum, which can be mistaken for vagina, and a small phallus with severe hypospadias (male pseudohermaphrodism) *(14)*. At puberty, these individuals undergo masculinization, manifested by a deepening of the voice and marked increases in muscle mass and penis size; at this time, most will change their gender role behavior from female to male *(15)*. However, testicular function with impaired spermatogenesis and infertility is characteristic of these individuals after puberty.

During adult life, DHT plays a role in the maintenance of sexual hair as well as having a causative role in acne vulgaris, prostatic hypertrophy, and androgenic alopecia. At puberty, in the axillae, on the face, and in the pubic region, DHT promotes the transformation of *vellus* follicles, which produce small, unpigmented hairs into *terminal* follicles, which form larger, pigmented hairs *(16)*. Paradoxically, DHT has the opposite effect on scalp hairs. Terminal follicles are replaced by vellus ones, leading to androgenic alopecia in some adult males. Inhibition of 5α-reductase type II with finasteride improves hair counts and hair weight in men with androgenic alopecia *(17)*.

In adult life, the prostate continues to depend on DHT for maintenance of its adult size, as inhibition of 5α-reductase decreases prostate size by 20–30%. The administration of a 5α-reductase inhibitor results in a reduction in glandular tissue that appears to be mediated by apoptosis *(18)*. Bone density is decreased in men with hypogonadism, but it is normal in men with 5α-reductase type II deficiency *(19)* and does not decrease with finasteride administration *(20)*. This suggests that T is more important than DHT for the maintenance of bone mineral density in adult men. Finally, 5α-reductase activity is largely absent in skeletal muscle *(10)* and muscle mass is normal in men with 5α-reductase type II deficiency *(15)*, demonstrating that DHT is not required for maintainence of muscle mass in the adult male.

INHIBITION OF 5α-REDUCTASE

Androgens influence the development and/or progression of a variety of chronic disease states: benign prostatic hyperplasia, carcinoma of the prostate, androgenic alopecia, acne vulgaris, and, in women, hirsutism. Both the prostate gland and structures of the skin and pilosebaceous unit are androgen responsive and express 5α-reductase isozymes. The absence of benign protatic hyperplasia (BPH) and androgenic alopecia in males with congenital deficiency of 5α-reductase-type II suggests a causal role for DHT in the etiology and/or progression of these conditions. Recently developed inhibitors of 5α-reductase are proving to be effective therapies for subsets of men with BPH and androgenic alopecia. Whether inhibitors of 5α-reductase reduce the risk of developing prostate cancer is being actively studied.

Benign Prostatic Hyperplasia

Although cellular and molecular details remain obscure, BPH commonly develops in aging men under the influence of androgens *(21,22)*. Huggins and colleagues first demonstrated the androgen dependence of the adult prostate gland in the laboratory dog and humans in the 1940s *(23,24)*. Reduction in androgen effects, either by castration or injection with estrogens, leads to regression of hyperplastic prostatic glandular tissue *(23,24)*. DHT is the androgen primarily responsible for the growth, differentiation, and maintenance of the prostate. This is best illustrated by males with familial male pseudohermaphroditism resulting from deficiencies of 5α-reductase, in whom prostate growth is vestigial and the epithelial component is virtually absent *(25,26)*. Interest in inhibitors of 5α-reductase as a potential therapeutic target in BPH arose from the observation that men with congenital deficiencies of 5α-reductase type II do not develop BPH *(25,27,28)*.

The principal 5α-reductase isozyme in the prostate gland is type II, with a minor contribution by 5α-reductase type I. The type II 5α-reductase enzyme is expressed by stromal cells and cells of the basal epithelium *(29)*. Interestingly, serum and intraprostatic T and DHT levels are not markedly different in patients with BPH compared with normal controls *(30,31)*. Rather, it is believed that BPH develops as a result of coordinate gene expression of growth factors and cytokines under the permissive influence of DHT and the androgen receptor *(32,33)*. Hyperplasia of both stromal and epithelial components of the prostate result in lower-urinary-tract symptoms *(34)*. Untreated, BPH increases the risk for acute urinary retention, detrusor instability, recurrent urinary tract infection, and, rarely, renal failure *(35)*.

Finasteride is the best-studied 5α-reductase inhibitor. It was synthesized among a series of 4-azosteroid derivatives at Merck Laboratories (Rahway, NJ) in the 1980s. Finasteride is a preferential inhibitor of type·II 5α-reductase, resulting in a 80–90% reduction of intraprostatic DHT levels *(36)* and a 70–80% reduction in serum DHT *(37)*. To date, numerous randomized clinical trials comparing finasteride 5 mg daily to placebo in men with BPH have been completed *(38)*. Two key trials in the early 1990s demonstrated that finasteride significantly reduced lower-urinary-tract symptoms (as measured by standardized symptom indices) and increased peak urinary flow over 2 yr of follow-up *(39,40)*. Both trials enrolled men with moderately symptomatic BPH and enlarged prostate glands. A VA Cooperative study compared men with BPH treated according to assignment to one of four groups: terazosin (an α_1-blocker), finasteride, terazosin plus finasteride, and placebo *(41)*. This study, which randomized men with moderately symptomatic BPH without regard to prostate size, found that finasteride did not improve symptoms significantly more than placebo and that the addition of finasteride to terazosin was not significantly better than terazosin alone *(41)*. Subsequent studies of finasteride in BPH shed light on these apparently discrepant results. A recent meta-analysis demonstrated that men with baseline prostate volumes greater than 40 cm^3 by ultrasound enjoyed a statistically significant improvement of urinary symptom scores and peak urinary flow, whereas men with small prostate volumes did not *(42)*. Similarly, patients with increased prostate-specific antigen (PSA) ≥ 1.4 ng/mL and an enlarged prostate gland by digital rectal examination benefit preferentially from finasteride *(43)*.

Finasteride also reduces the risk of the clinically important outcomes of acute urinary retention and requirement for resection of the prostate in men with BPH and enlarged prostates *(44–46)*. According to a meta-analysis of three randomized trials, treatment with finasteride 5 mg daily reduced the risk of acute urinary retention requiring catheterization from 2.7% to 1.1% at 2 yr of follow-up, corresponding to a number needed to treat (NNT) of 62 to prevent 1 episode of acute urinary retention *(46)*. The risk of prostatectomy was reduced from 6.5% to 4.2% (NNT 44) and the risk of either event was reduced from 7.5% to 4.9% (NNT 38) *(46)*. A subsequent trial extended these results to 4 yr of follow-up, with a reduction of acute urinary retention or prostatectomy from 13.2% to 6.6% (NNT 15) *(44)*. Again, men with elevations of PSA ≥ 1.4 ng/mL (and increased prostate volume on digital rectal examination) were significantly more likely to benefit from finasteride than men with lower PSAs and smaller prostate volumes *(45)*.

Treatment with finasteride is associated with apoptosis and regression of the epithelial component of the prostate gland *(47–49)*. Finasteride results in a 20% to 30% decrease in prostate volume *(39,50)*. Whereas clinical improvements in clinical symptom scores and peak urinary flow are maximal after 6 mo of treatment and subsequently stabilize *(51)*, continued involution of the prostatic epithelium occurs with ongoing treatment with finasteride *(52)*. Regression of BPH in men treated with finasteride has been associated with upregulation of insulin-related growth factor binding proteins, transforming growth factor-β, and downregulation of basic fibroblast growth factor *(48,49,53,54)*.

In general, treatment of men with BPH with α_1-blockers results in greater symptomatic improvement than finasteride *(41,55)*. Treatment with α_1-blockers remains the mainstay of medical therapy for BPH. Treatment with α_1-blockers is associated with significant side effects, including dizziness, asthenia, and postural hypotension *(56)*. Tamsulosin, a newer α_1-blocker more selective for α_1-adrenergic receptors in periurethral smooth muscle, may be associated with fewer side effects *(57,58)*. Finasteride is relatively well tolerated, with the most common side effects being decreased libido, ejaculatory dysfunction, erectile dysfunction, and breast tenderness *(38)*. The risk of any sexual side effect occurring was estimated to be 9% *(46)*. Prolonged treatment with finasteride does not affect bone mineral density *(20)*. Finasteride may be indicated for men with BPH and enlarged prostate volume, or in men with BPH who are intolerant of the side effects of α_1-blockers. The recently completed NIH Medical Therapy of Prostatic Symptoms Trial (MTOPS) compared response to doxazosin alone, finasteride alone, both in combination, or placebo over a minimum of 4 yr. Patients were selected on the basis of moderate to severe symptoms of BPH, not prostate size. Preliminary results indicated that combination therapy with both finasteride and doxazosin reduced the risk of clinical progression of BPH with improvement in symptom score and urinary flow more than monotherapy with either drug alone *(59)*. Also, finasteride and the combination of finasteride and doxazosin significantly reduced the risk of acute urinary retention and invasive therapy *(59)*. Inhibitors of 5α-reductase may be particularly useful in treating men who are eager to forestall or avoid prostatectomy. The Federal Drug Administration (FDA) has recently approved dutasteride (GlaxoSmithKline) for the treatment of symptoms and complications associated with BPH. Dutasteride inhibits both type I and type II 5α-reductase and results in greater reductions of serum and tissue DHT, compared with finasteride. Results from clinical studies with dutasteride indicate clinical efficacy comparable to that reported for finasteride *(43,60)*.

Prostate Cancer

Carcinoma of the prostate (CaP) is the most common cancer diagnosed and the second leading cause of cancer death in men in the United States. An estimated 198,000 cases and more than 31,000 deaths occurred in 2001 *(61)*. The androgen responsiveness of CaP is well known. CaP is exceedingly rare in males castrated at an early age. Furthermore, androgen blockade by orchiectomy, gonadopropin-releasing hormone (GnRH) agonists, antiandrogens, and estrogens results in symptomatic improvement and reduction in tumor burden in men with locally advanced or metastatic CaP *(62,63)*.

It has been hypothesized that 5α-reductase inhibitors, such as finasteride or dutasteride, might be effective chemoprevention for the development of CaP *(64,65)*. The Prostate Cancer Prevention Trial (PCPT) randomized 18,000 healthy men over 55 yr of age, with normal digital rectal examinations and PSAs ≤ 3 ng/mL, to 5 mg finasteride daily vs placebo. Patients will be followed for 7 yr with completion of the trial expected in 2004 *(66)*. Data from other studies offer reasons for caution. In a recent observational study of men with elevated PSAs with sextant biopsies negative for the presence of CaP at baseline, CaP developed in 8/27 men (30%) treated for 12 mo with 5 mg finasteride daily compared with 1/25 men (4%) treated with placebo *(67)*. Among men with prostatic intraepithelial neoplasia (PIN), a precancerous lesion, at baseline, CaP developed in 6/8 patients treated with finasteride vs 0/5 men treated with placebo ($p = 0.021$) *(67)*. In this study, serum PSAs were roughly halved during the treatment period, consistent with other studies, and serum T was increased 21% *(67,68)*. Long-term administration of finasteride does not affect the histology of CaP on biopsy specimens *(69)*. These data suggest that finasteride may not prevent the development of CaP in men with elevated PSA or established PIN *(18)*. Importantly, treatment with 5α-reductase inhibitors does not interfere with the detection of prostate cancer by PSA testing. PSA levels decline with the regression of the prostatic epithelium, typically to 50% of baseline value in an individual with BPH. This decrease in PSA stabilizes within 6 mo on therapy with either finasteride or dutasteride. Thereafter, patients can be easily followed for prostate cancer detection by doubling the PSA value on therapy for comparison with pretherapy values (e.g., a PSA of 2.0 on therapy would be equivalent to a pretreatment PSA value of 4.0) *(60,68)*.

Finasteride has also been studied as therapy for men already diagnosed with CaP. In a 12-wk study of 28 asymptomatic men with metastatic CaP (Stage D), finasteride 10 mg daily had no effect on prostatic acid phosphatase, serum testosterone, prostate volume, or lesions on bone scan, although PSA levels were significantly lower in men treated with finasteride *(70)*. In a study of men with elevated PSAs (0.6–10.0 ng/mL) and no evidence of recurrent CaP following radical prostatectomy, 10 mg finasteride daily for 24 mo delayed progressive increases in PSA by an average of 14 mo and did not appear to influence response to subsequent androgen-deprivation therapy in those men in whom recurrent CaP was ultimately diagnosed *(71)*. Recurrent disease was diagnosed in 5/41 men (12%) treated with finasteride and 8/43 men (19%) treated with placebo; although this difference was not statistically significant, it raises the possibility that finasteride treatment reduces or delays recurrence *(71)*. Finasteride has also been proposed as potentially effective "maintenance" therapy for men with CaP who have favorable PSA responses following androgen block-ade with nonsteroidal antiandrogens and/or GnRH agonists *(29)*.

Finasteride is a selective 5α-reductase type II antagonist and incompletely blocks the intraprostatic conversion of T to DHT (approx 80% reduction). It may be that residual intraprostatic DHT is sufficient for the development or progression of prostate cancer. It has also been observed that 5α-reductase type I is upregulated in prostate cancer cell lines in vitro, as well as in many prostate cancer ex vivo samples *(72,73)*. Although it may well be that the upregulation of 5α-reductase type I is an artifact of in vitro culture *(74)* or may be a consequence of dedifferentiation in vivo, it may also be true that CaP develops in a milieu where 5α-reductase type I is the dominant isozyme. Finasteride, a selective inhibitor of 5α-reductase type II, would not be expected to prevent the devel-opment of CaP if this were the case *(75)*. Inhibitors of both 5α-reductase isozymes, such as dutasteride might be better candidates for hormonal chemoprevention of CaP *(29,76)*. Interestingly, results from the phase III clinical trials with dutasteride show a reduction in diagnosed cancer incidence in the treated group compared to placebo, 1.1% (24/2167 patients) on dutasteride vs 1.9% (42/2158 patients) on placebo *(60)*. It may also be true that T, not DHT, is the androgen necessary and sufficient for the pathogenesis of CaP. Testosterone levels are actually increased during treatment with finasteride *(31)*. It may be necessary to reduce both T and DHT levels in order to prevent CaP or prevent the progression of PIN to CaP.

Androgenic Alopecia and Hirsutism

Finasteride is also FDA-approved for the treatment of male pattern baldness, or androgenic alopecia (AGA). Male pattern baldness results from a shortening of the anagen (growth) phase and prolonging the telogen (rest) phase of hair follicles, resulting in progressively finer, shorter hair *(77)*. AGA occurs in 23–87% of adult males and may occur in women as well *(77)*. AGA does not occur in the absence of androgens *(78)*.

The rationale for the use of a 5α-reductase inhibitor in the treatment of AGA again stems from observations of cohorts of patients with familial male pseudohermaphrodit-ism as a result of 5α-reductase type II deficiency, in which AGA does not develop *(25)*. Furthermore, concentrations of DHT in the sebum are higher in bald areas of the human scalp than in areas with hair *(79)*. Both type I and type II 5α-reductase isozymes are found in the male scalp, with the type II isozyme present in hair bulbs and the type I enzyme present in sebaceous glands *(80)*. The distribution of 5α-reductase in the scalp parallels the distribution of DHT, with highest concentrations found in the vertex and lowest in the occipital area *(81)*. No genetic polymorphisms in the two genes that encode 5α-reductase enzymes have been found to explain an inherited predisposition for AGA *(82)*, although polymorphisms in the androgen receptor have been implicated *(83)*.

Five milligrams of finasteride daily was found to reduce the concentration of DHT in scalp biopsy samples from men with AGA *(84)*. Subsequently, a number of carefully performed randomized controlled trials have demonstrated the efficacy of finasteride in reversing alopecia in a subset of men with AGA *(17,85–90)*. Approximately half of treated men enjoy a significant improvement in hair counts when treated with finasteride *(85)*. Improvements in scalp hair counts persist for 5 yr or more with continued treatment *(90)*. Dose ranging studies suggest that 1 mg finasteride daily is the optimal dose *(88)*. Finasteride treatment appears to decrease apoptosis of hair follicles by downregulating caspases and upregulating inhibitors of apoptosis *(91)*. The net result is an increase in anagen hair follicles *(89)*. Finasteride does not affect spermatogenesis or sexual function in these studies *(92,93)*. Finasteride does not increase hair growth or slow progression of hair thinning in postmenopausal women with AGA *(94)*. It remains to be seen whether dutasteride, an inhibitor of both 5α-reductase isozymes, will be more effective than finasteride in men with AGA or whether it will be effective in treating women with AGA.

Finasteride has also been used to treat hirsutism in women. In one study, 5 mg finasteride daily was compared with 100 mg spironolactone daily in 14 hirsute women *(95)*. Although only finasteride had a significant impact on serum hormones, both treatments were effective in decreasing anagen hair diameter in this small study. Similarly, another study compared 5 mg finasteride daily with treatment with spironolactone (100 mg daily), flutamide (250 mg daily), or placebo in 40 hirsute women. Finasteride, spironolactone, and flutamide were all shown to be more effective than placebo after 6 mo of follow-up *(96)*. Concern remains regarding the possible feminization of male fetuses during the first trimester of pregnancy; therefore, fertile women treated with inhibitors of the type II 5α-reductase, such as finasteride or dutasteride, should be counseled to use effective means of contraception (oral contraceptives or intrauterine devices).

Acne

Acne vulgaris occurs commonly during puberty, when it is present in 50% of pubertal girls and as many as 85% of pubertal boys *(97)*. Acne is multifactorial, although it is believed that increases in sebum production contribute to its development *(98)*. Androgen stimulates sebum production, cellular proliferation of sebaceous glands, and an increase in intracellular lipid content *(99)*. Similarly, androgenic progestins increase sebum production. Estradiol reduces sebum production.

The predominant form of 5α-reductase in sebaceous glands is type I *(80)*. Finasteride is a selective inhibitor of the type II isozyme and would not be expected to have significant effects on acne. Indeed, usual doses of finasteride (1–5 mg daily) do not significantly reduce sebum DHT *(100)*. Dual-type inhibitors, such as dutasteride, or a selective inhibitor of type I 5α-reductase may be useful therapies for acne. Concerns regarding feminization of male fetuses in fertile women reduce enthusiasm for an inhibitor of the type II isozyme for the treatment of acne in young women.

SUMMARY

Dihydrotestosterone plays a critical role in the normal development and differentiation of external male genitalia and the prostate gland. DHT is metabolized from T through the action of two principle 5α-reductase isozymes. Type I 5α-reductase is the predominant isozyme in the skin and liver, whereas type II 5α-reductase is found in the male urogenital tract. Males with congenital deficiencies of type II 5α-reductase do not develop benign prostatic hypertrophy or androgenic alopecia.

Inhibitors of 5α-reductase have been approved for the treatment of BPH and AGA. Finasteride, an inhibitor of type I 5α-reductase, and dutasteride, an inhibitor of both 5α-reductase isozymes, have been shown to reduce symptoms and prevent complications of BPH, particularly in men with enlarged prostate glands. Finasteride is effective in improving hair counts in approximately half of men with AGA.

It remains uncertain whether inhibitors of 5α-reductase have a clinically important role in the prevention or treatment of carcinoma of the prostate. Preliminary data have been inconclusive and results of large randomized trials for prostate cancer prevention are expected after 2004. There are at least theoretical reasons to suggest that a non-selective inhibitor of both 5α-reductase isozymes, such as dutasteride, may be more effective than a type-II-specific inhibitor, such as finasteride.

Inhibitors of 5α-reductase may be effective therapies for women with androgenic hirsutism and men and women with acne. Enthusiasm for the treatment of fertile women with medications that inhibit type II 5α-reductase is mitigated by concern for potential feminization of male fetuses during gestation.

REFERENCES

1. Horton R, Testicular steroid transport, metabolism, and effects. In: Becker, KL, ed. Principles and Practice of Endocrinology and Metabolism, Lippencott, Philadelphia, PA, 1992.
2. Ito T, Horton R. The source of plasma dihydrotestosterone in man. J Clin Invest 1971;50(8):1621–1627.
3. Meikle AW, Stringham JD, Wilson DE, et al. Plasma 5 alpha-reduced androgens in men and hirsute women: role of adrenals and gonads. J Clin Endocrinol Metab 1979;48(6):969–975.
4. Forti G, Salerno R, Moneti G, et al. Three-month treatment with a long-acting gonadotropin-releasing hormone agonist of patients with benign prostatic hyperplasia: effects on tissue androgen concentration, 5 alpha-reductase activity and androgen receptor content. J Clin Endocrinol Metab 1989;68(2):461–468.
5. Habib FK, Ross M, Tate R, et al. Differential effect of finasteride on the tissue androgen concentrations in benign prostatic hyperplasia. Clin Endocrinol (Oxf) 1997;46(2):137–144.
6. Monti S, Di Silverio F, Toscano V, et al. Androgen concentrations and their receptors in the periurethral region are higher than those of the subcapsular zone in benign prostatic hyperplasia (BPH). J Androl 1998;19(4):428–433.
7. McLachlan RI, O'Donnell L, Stanton PG, et al. Effects of testosterone plus medroxyprogesterone acetate on semen quality, reproductive hormones, and germ cell populations in normal young men. J Clin Endocrinol Metab 2002;87(2):546–556.
8. Anderson RA, Wallace AM, Wu FC. Comparison between testosterone enanthate-induced azoospermia and oligozoospermia in a male contraceptive study. III. Higher 5 alpha-reductase activity in oligozoospermic men administered supraphysiological doses of testosterone. J Clin Endocrinol Metab 1996;81(3):902–908.
9. Russell DW, Wilson JD. Steroid 5 alpha-reductase: two genes/two enzymes. Annu Rev Biochem 1994;63:25–61.
10. Thigpen AE, Silver RI, Guileyardo JM, et al. Tissue distribution and ontogeny of steroid 5 alpha-reductase isozyme expression. J Clin Invest 1993;92(2):903–910.
11. Horton R. Dihydrotestosterone is a peripheral paracrine hormone. J Androl 1992;13(1):23–27.
12. Grisham W, Tam A, Greco CM, et al. A putative 5 alpha-reductase inhibitor demasculinizes portions of the zebra finch song system. Brain Res 1997;750(1–2):122–128.
13. Lephart ED, Lund TD, Horvath TL. Brain androgen and progesterone metabolizing enzymes: biosynthesis, distribution and function. Brain Res Brain Res Rev 2001;37(1–3):25–37.
14. Wilson JD. The role of androgens in male gender role behavior. Endocr Rev 1999;20(5):726–737.

15. Imperato-McGinley J, Peterson RE, Gautier T, et al. Androgens and the evolution of male-gender identity among male pseudohermaphrodites with 5alpha-reductase deficiency. N Engl J Med 1979;300(22):1233–1237.

16. Randall VA, Hibberts NA, Thornton MJ, et al. The hair follicle: a paradoxical androgen target organ. Horm Res 2000;54(5–6):243–250.

17. Price VH, Menefee E, Sanchez M, et al. Changes in hair weight and hair count in men with androgenetic alopecia after treatment with finasteride, 1 mg, daily. J Am Acad Dermatol 2002;46(4):517–523.

18. Steers WD. 5Alpha-reductase activity in the prostate. Urology 2001;58(6 Suppl 1):17–24; discussion, 24.

19. Frade Costa EM, Prado Arnhold IJ, Inacio M, et al. Normal bone density in male pseudohermaphroditism due to 5alpha- reductase 2 deficiency. Rev Hosp Clin Fac Med Sao Paulo 2001;56(5):139–142.

20. Matsumoto AM, Tenover L, McClung M, et al. The long-term effect of specific type II 5alpha-reductase inhibition with finasteride on bone mineral density in men: results of a 4-year placebo controlled trial. J Urol 2002;167(5):2105–2108.

21. Miller EA, Ellis WJ, Endocrine aspects of benign prostatic hyperplasia. In: Becker, KL, ed. Principles and Practice of Endocrinology and Metabolism, 3rd Edition, Lippencott Williams & Wilkins, Philadelphia, PA, 2001, pp. 1207–1212.

22. McConnell JD. The pathophysiology of benign prostatic hyperplasia. J Androl 1991;12(6):356–363.

23. Huggins C, Clark PJ. Quantitative studies of prostatic secretion: II. The effect of castration and of estrogen injection on the normal and on the hyperplastic prostate glands of dogs. J Exp Med 1940;72:747–761.

24. Huggins C, Stevens RA. The effect of castration on benign hypertrophy of the prostate in man. J Urol 1940;43:705–714.

25. Imperato-McGinley J, Guerrero L, Gautier T, et al. Steroid 5alpha-reductase deficiency in man: an inherited form of male pseudohermaphroditism. Science 1974;186(4170):1213–1215.

26. Walsh PC, Madden JD, Harrod MJ, et al. Familial incomplete male pseudohermaphroditism, type 2. Decreased dihydrotestosterone formation in pseudovaginal perineoscrotal hypospadias. N Engl J Med 1974;291(18):944–949.

27. Imperato-McGinley J, Gautier T, Zirinsky K, et al. Prostate visualization studies in males homozygous and heterozygous for 5 alpha-reductase deficiency. J Clin Endocrinol Metab 1992;75(4):1022–1026.

28. Fratianni CM, Imperato-McGinley J. The syndrome of 5a-reductase deficiency. Endocrinologist 1994;4:302–314.

29. Rittmaster RS. 5Alpha-reductase inhibitors. J Androl 1997;18(6):582–587.

30. Geller J. Effect of finasteride, a 5 alpha-reductase inhibitor on prostate tissue androgens and prostate-specific antigen. J Clin Endocrinol Metab 1990;71(6):1552–1555.

31. McConnell JD, Wilson JD, George FW, et al. Finasteride, an inhibitor of 5 alpha-reductase, suppresses prostatic dihydrotestosterone in men with benign prostatic hyperplasia. J Clin Endocrinol Metab 1992;74(3):505–508.

32. Steiner MS. Review of peptide growth factors in benign prostatic hyperplasia and urological malignancy. J Urol 1995;153(4):1085–1096.

33. Culig Z, Hobisch A, Cronauer MV, et al. Regulation of prostatic growth and function by peptide growth factors. Prostate 1996;28(6):392–405.

34. McConnell JD, Barry MJ, Bruskewitz RC, et al., Benign prostatic hyperplasia: diagnosis and treatment. In: Clinical Practice Guideline, No. 8. Agency for Health Care Policy and Research, Public Health Service, US Department of Health and Human Services, Rockville, MD, 1994.

35. Jacobsen SJ, Girman CJ, Lieber MM. Natural history of benign prostatic hyperplasia. Urology 2001;58(6 Suppl 1):5–16; discussion, 16.

36. Span PN, Voller MC, Smals AG, et al. Selectivity of finasteride as an in vivo inhibitor of 5alpha-reductase isozyme enzymatic activity in the human prostate. J Urol 1999;161(1):332–337.

37. Uygur MC, Arik AI, Altug U, et al. Effects of the 5 alpha-reductase inhibitor finasteride on serum levels of gonadal, adrenal, and hypophyseal hormones and its clinical significance: a prospective clinical study. Steroids 1998;63(4):208–213.

38. Clifford GM, Farmer RD. Medical therapy for benign prostatic hyperplasia: a review of the literature. Eur Urol 2000;38(1):2–19.

39. Gormley GJ, Stoner E, Bruskewitz RC, et al. The effect of finasteride in men with benign prostatic hyperplasia. The Finasteride Study Group. N Engl J Med 1992;327(17):1185–1191.

40. The Finasteride Study Group. Finasteride (MK-906) in the treatment of benign prostatic hyperplasia. Prostate 1993;22(4):291–299.
41. Lepor H, Williford WO, Barry MJ, et al. The efficacy of terazosin, finasteride, or both in benign prostatic hyperplasia. Veterans Affairs Cooperative Studies Benign Prostatic Hyperplasia Study Group. N Engl J Med 1996;335(8):533–539.
42. Boyle P, Gould AL, Roehrborn CG. Prostate volume predicts outcome of treatment of benign prostatic hyperplasia with finasteride: meta-analysis of randomized clinical trials. Urology 1996; 48(3):398–405.
43. Roehrborn CG, Boyle P, Bergner D, et al. Serum prostate-specific antigen and prostate volume predict long-term changes in symptoms and flow rate: results of a four-year, randomized trial comparing finasteride versus placebo. PLESS Study Group. Urology 1999;54(4):662–669.
44. McConnell JD, Bruskewitz R, Walsh P, et al. The effect of finasteride on the risk of acute urinary retention and the need for surgical treatment among men with benign prostatic hyperplasia. Finasteride Long-Term Efficacy and Safety Study Group. N Engl J Med 1998;338(9):557–563.
45. Roehrborn CG, McConnell JD, Lieber M, et al. Serum prostate-specific antigen concentration is a powerful predictor of acute urinary retention and need for surgery in men with clinical benign prostatic hyperplasia. PLESS Study Group. Urology 1999;53(3):473–480.
46. Andersen JT, Nickel JC, Marshall VR, et al. Finasteride significantly reduces acute urinary retention and need for surgery in patients with symptomatic benign prostatic hyperplasia. Urology 1997; 49(6):839–845.
47. Rittmaster RS, Norman RW, Thomas LN, et al. Evidence for atrophy and apoptosis in the prostates of men given finasteride. J Clin Endocrinol Metab 1996;81(2):814–819.
48. Saez C, Gonzalez-Baena AC, Japon MA, et al. Regressive changes in finasteride-treated human hyperplastic prostates correlate with an upregulation of TGF-beta receptor expression. Prostate 1998;37(2):84–90.
49. Thomas LN, Wright AS, Lazier CB, et al. Prostatic involution in men taking finasteride is associated with elevated levels of insulin-like growth factor-binding proteins (IGFBPs)-2, -4, and -5. Prostate 2000;42(3):203–210.
50. Beisland HO, Binkowitz B, Brekkan E, et al. Scandinavian clinical study of finasteride in the treatment of benign prostatic hyperplasia. Eur Urol 1992;22(4):271–277.
51. Ekman P. Maximum efficacy of finasteride is obtained within 6 months and maintained over 6 years. Follow-up of the Scandinavian Open-Extension Study. The Scandinavian Finasteride Study Group. Eur Urol 1998;33(3):312–317.
52. Marks LS, Partin AW, Dorey FJ, et al. Long-term effects of finasteride on prostate tissue composition. Urology 1999;53(3):574–580.
53. Glassman DT, Chon JK, Borkowski A, et al. Combined effect of terazosin and finasteride on apoptosis, cell proliferation, and transforming growth factor-beta expression in benign prostatic hyperplasia. Prostate 2001;46(1):45–51.
54. Saez C, Gonzalez-Baena AC, Japon MA, et al. Expression of basic fibroblast growth factor and its receptors FGFR1 and FGFR2 in human benign prostatic hyperplasia treated with finasteride. Prostate 1999;40(2):83–88.
55. Debruyne FM, Jardin A, Colloi D, et al. Sustained-release alfuzosin, finasteride and the combination of both in the treatment of benign prostatic hyperplasia. European ALFIN Study Group. Eur Urol 1998;34(3):169–175.
56. Barry MJ, Roehrborn CG. Benign prostatic hyperplasia. Br Med J 2001;323(7320):1042–1046.
57. Michel MC, Bressel HU, Mehlburger L, et al. Tamsulosin: real life clinical experience in 19,365 patients. Eur Urol 1998;34(Suppl 2):37–45.
58. Dutkiewics S. Efficacy and tolerability of drugs for treatment of benign prostatic hyperplasia. Int Urol Nephrol 2001;32(3):423–432.
59. McConnell JD. Long term effects of medical therapy on the progression of BPH: results from the MTOPS trial. J Urol 2002;167(Suppl 4):265 (abstract).
60. Roehrborn CG, Boyle P, Nickel CJ, et al. Efficacy and safety of dual inhibitor of 5 alpha reductase types 1 and 2 (dutasteride) in men with benign prostatic hyperplasia (BPH). Urology 2002;60: 434–441.
61. Cancer Facts and Figures. American Cancer Society, Atlanta, GA, 2001, p. 5.
62. Seidenfeld J, Samson DJ, Hasselblad V, et al. Single-therapy androgen suppression in men with advanced prostate cancer: a systematic review and meta-analysis. Ann Intern Med 2000;132(7): 566–577.

63. Seidenfeld J, Samson DJ, Aronson N, et al. Relative effectiveness and cost-effectiveness of methods of androgen suppression in the treatment of advanced prostate cancer. Evid Rep Technol Assess (Summ) 1999(4):i-x, 1-246, I1-36, passim.

64. Gormley GJ. Role of 5 alpha-reductase inhibitors in the treatment of advanced prostatic carcinoma. Urol Clin North Am 1991;18(1):93–98.

65. Brawley OW, Thompson IM. Chemoprevention of prostate cancer. Urology 1994;43(5): 594–599.

66. Feigl P, Blumenstein B, Thompson I, et al. Design of the Prostate Cancer Prevention Trial (PCPT). Control Clin Trials 1995;16(3):150–163.

67. Cote RJ, Skinner EC, Salem CE, et al. The effect of finasteride on the prostate gland in men with elevated serum prostate-specific antigen levels. Br J Cancer 1998;78(3):413–418.

68. Guess HA, Gormley GJ, Stoner E, et al. The effect of finasteride on prostate specific antigen: review of available data. J Urol 1996;155(1):3–9.

69. Yang XJ, Lecksell K, Short K, et al. Does long-term finasteride therapy affect the histologic features of benign prostatic tissue and prostate cancer on needle biopsy? PLESS Study Group. Proscar Long-Term Efficacy and Safety Study. Urology 1999;53(4):696–700.

70. Presti JC, Jr., Fair WR, Andriole G, et al. Multicenter, randomized, double-blind, placebo controlled study to investigate the effect of finasteride (MK-906) on stage D prostate cancer. J Urol 1992;148(4):1201–1204.

71. Andriole G, Lieber M, Smith J, et al. Treatment with finasteride following radical prostatectomy for prostate cancer. Urology 1995;45(3):491–497.

72. Boudon C, Lobaccaro JM, Lumbroso S, et al. 5Alpha-reductase activity in cultured epithelial and stromal cells from normal and hyperplastic human prostates—effect of finasteride (Proscar), a 5 alpha-reductase inhibitor. Cell Mol Biol (Noisy-le-grand) 1995;41(8):1007–1015.

73. Iehle C, Radvanyi F, Gil Diez de Medina S, et al. Differences in steroid 5alpha-reductase iso-enzymes expression between normal and pathological human prostate tissue. J Steroid Biochem Mol Biol 1999;68(5–6):189–195.

74. Smith CM, Ballard SA, Worman N, et al. 5Alpha-reductase expression by prostate cancer cell lines and benign prostatic hyperplasia in vitro. J Clin Endocrinol Metab 1996;81(4):1361–1366.

75. Cilotti A, Danza G, Serio M. Clinical application of 5alpha-reductase inhibitors. J Endocrinol Invest 2001;24(3):199–203.

76. Frye SV, Bramson HN, Hermann DJ, et al. Discovery and development of GG745, a potent inhibitor of both isozymes of 5 alpha-reductase. Pharm Biotechnol 1998;11:393–422.

77. Bergfeld WF. Androgenetic alopecia: an autosomal dominant disorder. Am J Med 1995;98 (1A):95S–98S.

78. Hamilton JB. Male hormone stimulation is a prerequisite and an incitant in common baldness. Am J Anat 1942;71:451–480.

79. Sawaya ME. Biochemical mechanisms regulating human hair growth. Skin Pharmacol 1994;7(1-2):5–7.

80. Kaufman KD. Androgen metabolism as it affects hair growth in androgenetic alopecia. Dermatol Clin 1996;14(4):697–711.

81. Sawaya ME, Price VH. Different levels of 5alpha-reductase type I and II, aromatase, and androgen receptor in hair follicles of women and men with androgenetic alopecia. J Invest Dermatol 1997;109(3):296–300.

82. Ellis JA, Stebbing M, Harrap SB. Genetic analysis of male pattern baldness and the 5alpha-reductase genes. J Invest Dermatol 1998;110(6):849–853.

83. Ellis JA, Stebbing M, Harrap SB. Polymorphism of the androgen receptor gene is associated with male pattern baldness. J Invest Dermatol 2001;116(3):452–455.

84. Dallob AL, Sadick NS, Unger W, et al. The effect of finasteride, a 5 alpha-reductase inhibitor, on scalp skin testosterone and dihydrotestosterone concentrations in patients with male pattern baldness. J Clin Endocrinol Metab 1994;79(3):703–706.

85. Kaufman KD, Olsen EA, Whiting D, et al. Finasteride in the treatment of men with androgenetic alopecia. Finasteride Male Pattern Hair Loss Study Group. J Am Acad Dermatol 1998;39 (4 Pt1):578–589.

86. Brenner S, Matz H. Improvement in androgenetic alopecia in 53–76-year-old men using oral finasteride. Int J Dermatol 1999;38(12):928–930.

87. Leyden J, Dunlap F, Miller B, et al. Finasteride in the treatment of men with frontal male pattern hair loss. J Am Acad Dermatol 1999;40(6 Pt 1):930–937.

88. Roberts JL, Fiedler V, Imperato-McGinley J, et al. Clinical dose ranging studies with finasteride, a type 2 5alpha-reductase inhibitor, in men with male pattern hair loss. J Am Acad Dermatol 1999;41(4):555–563.

89. Van Neste D, Fuh V, Sanchez-Pedreno P, et al. Finasteride increases anagen hair in men with androgenetic alopecia. Br J Dermatol 2000;143(4):804–810.

90. The Finasteride Male Pattern Hair Loss Study Group. Long-term (5-year) multinational experience with finasteride 1 mg in the treatment of men with androgenetic alopecia. Eur J Dermatol 2002;12(1):38–49.

91. Sawaya ME, Blume-Peytavi U, Mullins DL, et al. Effects of finasteride on apoptosis and regulation of the human hair cycle. J Cutan Med Surg 2002;6(1):1–9.

92. Overstreet JW, Fuh VL, Gould J, et al. Chronic treatment with finasteride daily does not affect spermatogenesis or semen production in young men. J Urol 1999;162(4):1295–1300.

93. Tosti A, Piraccini BM, Soli M. Evaluation of sexual function in subjects taking finasteride for the treatment of androgenetic alopecia. J Eur Acad Dermatol Venereol 2001;15(5):418–421.

94. Price VH, Roberts JL, Hordinsky M, et al. Lack of efficacy of finasteride in postmenopausal women with androgenetic alopecia. J Am Acad Dermatol 2000;43(5 Pt 1):768–776.

95. Wong IL, Morris RS, Chang L, et al. A prospective randomized trial comparing finasteride to spironolactone in the treatment of hirsute women. J Clin Endocrinol Metab 1995;80(1):233–238.

96. Moghetti P, Tosi F, Tosti A, et al. Comparison of spironolactone, flutamide, and finasteride efficacy in the treatment of hirsutism: a randomized, double blind, placebo-controlled trial. J Clin Endocrinol Metab 2000;85(1):89–94.

97. Carmina E, Lobo RA, Hirsutism, alopecia, and acne. In: Becker KL, ed. Principles and Practice of Endocrinology and Metabolism, 3rd Edition. Lippincott Williams & Wilkins: Philadelphia, PA, 2001, pp. 991–1008.

98. Luderschmidt C, Pathogenesis of acne vulgaris. In: Hammerstein J, Lachnit-Fixson U, Neumann F, and Plewig G, eds. Androgenization in Women. Excerpta Medica, Amsterdam, 1980, p. 75.

99. Kiraly CL, Alen M, Korvola J, et al. The effect of testosterone and anabolic steroids on the skin surface lipids and the population of Propionibacteria acnes in young postpubertal men. Acta Derm Venereol 1988;68(1):21–26.

100. Schwartz JI, Tanaka WK, Wang DZ, et al. MK-386, an inhibitor of 5alpha-reductase type 1, reduces dihydrotestosterone concentrations in serum and sebum without affecting dihydrotestosterone concentrations in semen. J Clin Endocrinol Metab 1997;82(5):1373–1377.

5

Estrogen Action in Males
Insights Through Mutations in Aromatase and Estrogen-Receptor Genes

Jonathan Lindzey, PhD
and Kenneth S. Korach, PhD

Contents

Introduction
Behavior
Hormones
Testis and Ductule Structures
Accessory Sex Structures
Clinical Presentations
Conclusions
References

INTRODUCTION

Testosterone (T) exerts a wide range of effects that span many life stages and are absolutely critical for successful reproduction in male vertebrates. For instance, T secreted by the embryonic and/or neonatal testes plays a critical role in sexual differentiation of internal and external genitalia *(1)*, accessory sex structures *(2)*, and organization of the central nervous system (CNS) *(3)*. Pubertal increases in T play critical roles in pubertal maturation *(4)* and T continues to play critical roles in activation of sex behaviors *(5)*, regulation of the hypothalamic–pituitary–gonadal axis *(6)* and stimulation of peripheral reproductive structures in adult males *(2)*. In addition, it has become more widely accepted that T also plays critical roles in nonreproductive effects such as bone growth and expression of renal and hepatic enzymes.

At the cellular level, these diverse actions of T can be mediated by several different paths (*see* Fig. 1): (1) interaction of T with androgen receptors (ARs), (2) conversion of T into 5α-dihydrotestosterone (5α-DHT) by 5α-reductase and subsequent interactions with AR, or (3) conversion of T into 17β-estradiol (E_2) by P450aromatase (CYP19) and subsequent interactions with estrogen receptors (ERs) (the "aromatization hypothesis"). For instance, direct activation of AR by T is required for normal development of wolffian derivatives such as the seminal vesicle, whereas conversion to 5α-DHT is required for

From: *Contemporary Endocrinology: Androgens in Health and Disease*
Edited by: C. Bagatell and W. J. Bremner © Humana Press Inc., Totowa, NJ

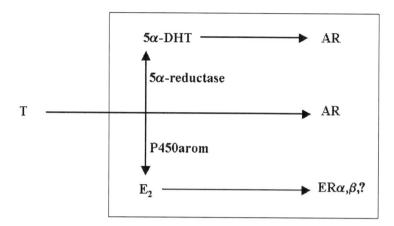

Fig. 1. Cellular paths of action for testosterone (T) in a generalized target cell. T may directly activate androgen receptor (AR) or undergo enzymatic conversion by 5α-reductase or P450aromatase into 5α-dihydrotestosterone (5α-DHT) or 17β-estradiol (E_2). In turn, 5α-DHT can activate AR and E_2 can activate either ERα or ERβ.

normal masculinization of external genitalia derived from the urogenital sinus and tubercle *(2)*. The best examples of T effects via aromatization lay in the masculinization and activation of male-typical behaviors *(3,5)*.

Data supporting the aromatization hypothesis has arisen from classical approaches such as (1) castration and replacement studies, (2) pharmacological receptor blockers, or (3) aromatase blockers. Over the years, these approaches have certainly supported the validity of the "aromatization hypothesis" in explaining some of the effects of T, particularly in the nervous system. Recent characterizations of aromatase-deficient human patients and aromatase knockout (ARKO) mice have further validated the role of aromatization in T actions on male physiology (*see* discussion below).

Historically, estrogens were thought to act via a single nuclear receptor, ERα, or potentially via membrane receptors. However, the discovery of a second nuclear ER, ERβ *(7)*, has expanded the potential paths by which estrogens may act in males or females. Indeed, both ERα and ERβ bind endogenous estrogens with fairly similar affinities and exhibit relatively similar binding specificities except that ERβ exhibits higher affinities for some phytoestrogens *(8)*. These two receptors are expressed preferentially in certain tissues, whereas in other target tissues and cells, these receptors may be coexpressed to varying degrees *(9–11)*. Coexpression of these receptors may prove to be particularly interesting and vexing, as some studies indicate that ERα and ERβ may form functional heterodimers *(12,13)*. Thus, although we can make solid statements as to the need for aromatization in mediating T effects, it is quite difficult to determine whether the E_2 is acting via ERα or ERβ in tissues that coexpress these receptors. The recent synthesis of an ERα specific agonist, propyl pyrazole triol (PPT), and an ERβ-specific antagonist, tetrahydrochrysene (THC), will no doubt facilitate such studies but these compounds were only recently produced and their in vivo efficacy is unknown *(14,15)*. Presently, the ERα knockout (αERKO) *(16)* and ERβ knockout (βERKO) mice *(17)* represent our best nonpharmacologic approaches for delineating ERα-mediated vs ERβ-mediated effects in vivo. Fortunately, disruption of ERα does not appear to obviously alter the patterns or levels of expression of ERβ *(18,19)*. This chapter focuses on more recent insights into the roles of aromatase, ERα, and ERβ in male reproduction through characterization of (1) naturally occurring mutations in aromatase or estrogen receptors and (2) targeted disruptions of aromatase or ER genes in mice (ARKO, αERKO, βERKO).

BEHAVIOR

The CNS is perhaps the best example of an androgen target in which T effects often require aromatization and activation of ER. This is particularly true for normal sexual differentiation or "organization" of hypothalamic nuclei during critical periods of development and subsequent "activation" or regulation of behavioral and neuroendocrine patterns in the adult. For instance, neonatal castration will feminize male rats so that exogenous T treatments of feminized adult males fail to activate male-typical sex behaviors: mounting, intromission and ejaculation. Similarly, T treatments of female pups will masculinize females so that T treatments of masculinized adult females will activate mounting behaviors (3,5). Significantly, neonatal E_2 treatments mimic many of the organizational effects of T on sex behaviors, and adult E_2 treatments will mimic many of the activational effects of T in adults (3,5). Similar E_2 effects have also been observed in a number of different species including mice.

Studies with the ARKO mouse certainly corroborate earlier studies indicating that aromatization plays a critical role in the organization of neural substrates governing mounting and copulatory behaviors. Intact, adult male ARKO mice exhibit significantly reduced mounting and copulatory behaviors and reduced fertility (20,21). Another study reports normal fertility in young males but infertility as males age (22). Interestingly, E_2 treatments of ARKO males result in a dose-dependent restoration of fertility if treatments are begun prior to neonatal day 10 and continued episodically through testing as adults (20). The authors reported that this restoration of fertility occurred without significant increases in mounting behaviors but did not present the details of these behavioral data. Nonetheless, these data suggest that these neonatal treatments either missed a critical prenatal window for organization of behaviors or that E_2 treatments of adults were insufficient to activate behaviors in the adults. These data also suggest that (1) low levels of mounting behavior may be sufficient to ensure fertilization when mice are housed together over long periods and (2) E_2 may have rescued fertility by acting at the level of the testes. This animal model would obviously benefit from a rigorous study examining the importance of E_2 during early "organization" vs adult "activation." These studies would better allow us to assess the importance of aromatase during these different life stages.

Although the ARKO mouse supports the hypothesis that estrogens are required for normal display of male sex behaviors, E_2 could potentially act through ERα, ERβ, or a membrane receptor. Indeed, both ERα and ERβ are expressed in the medial preoptic area (mPOA) of rodents (19,23–26), a region involved in controlling male-typical sex behaviors (5). Despite this "coregionalization," βERKO males exhibit normal mounting and copulatory behaviors (27,28), whereas αERKO males have been reported to exhibit relatively normal (29) to severely reduced mounting behaviors (30), reduced intromissions, and very rare ejaculations (29,30). The discrepancy in mounting data from these two studies may stem simply from differences in testing paradigms that might affect motivational behaviors: neutral arena vs home cage. The presence of mounting behaviors in the Ogawa study (29) also suggests that AR pathways or other estrogen signaling paths may suffice to organize and activate some degree of mounting behavior. Interestingly, a recent study by the same group compared behaviors of αERKO, βERKO, and double knockout (α,βERKO males) (27). This study suggests that whereas βERKO males exhibit a normal repertoire of mounting and copulatory behaviors, the α,βERKO males exhibit even more severe deficits in mounting behaviors than do the αERKO males. The implication is that ERβ may suffice to organize or activate some degree of mounting behavior in the absence of ERα and that the absence of both creates a more severe behavioral phenotype (27). The authors suggest that ERα and ERβ may be somewhat redundant in their actions on mounting behaviors. Nonetheless, in general, these data support the hypothesis that aromatization is necessary for a normal suite of male sex behaviors and that E_2 acts primarily through ERα to mediate the organization and/or activation of sex behaviors. By comparison, ERβ apparently plays little role in male-typical sex behaviors. This generalization, however, should be further tested in other species as ERα- and ERβ-specific agonists and antagonists become available.

Androgen-dependent, intermale aggression is another behavior that has been reported to depend on aromatization of T. Indeed, in a "resident–intruder" design, ARKO residents exhibited no aggressive interactions against an ARKO intruder and wild-type (WT) resident males also exhibited reduced aggression against ARKO intruders compared with WT intruders (31). Neonatal E_2 treatments of ARKO males resulted in a dose-dependent increase in intermale aggression that was most pronounced when E_2 treatments were begun on neonatal day 1 and continued episodically through testing as adults. These data suggest a critical window for organization of E_2 effects but because of experimental design, they fail to distinguish between "organizational" and "activational" effects of E_2 on aggression. Although aggressive behaviors are normal in βERKO males, αERKO and α,βERKO males both exhibit severe deficits in aggressive behaviors toward bulbectomized intruders (27,29). Thus, E_2 and ERα are obviously critical to the normal display of intermale aggression in mice and ERβ does not exert any redundant control over aggression as it may for mounting behaviors (27).

HORMONES

The neural centers that regulate gonadotropin-releasing hormone (GnRH) synthesis and secretion and, ultimately, secretion of gonadotropins are subject to organizational and activational effects of T. Typically, luteinizing hormone (LH) secretion is described as a "tonic" pulsatile background against which a "surge" component can be overlaid. Both males and females possess "tonic" components, whereas only females typically exhibit an estrogen-dependent, preovulatory LH "surge." In some species, such as primates, the ability to "surge" is not sexually differentiated; both the male and female can deliver an LH surge when given the appropriate E_2 treatments. However, in rodents, the ability to deliver an LH surge is sexually dimorphic and one region implicated in sexual differentiation of the LH surge is the anteroventral periventricular nucleus (AvPV). In female rodents, this region is larger, contains more dopaminergic neurons and, furthermore, AvPV lesions abolish LH surges (32,33). Masculinization by neonatal T treatments results in a male-typical AvPV characterized by reduced volume and tyrosine hydroxylase (TH) immunostaining. Although no studies have reported on AvPV nuclei of ARKO mice, analyses of αERKO mice demonstrated that male αERKOs possess an AvPV more typical of female mice—larger and greater numbers of dopaminergic neurons. Thus, it appears that masculinization (or defeminization) of the AvPV requires activation of ERα, presumably during development, in order to induce cell death in the AvPV of male mice *(34)*.

Regulation of the "tonic" pattern of LH secretion in adult male vertebrates clearly relies on negative feedback by T. Castration results in dramatic increases in serum LH, whereas T replacement reinstates or maintains negative feedback on LH synthesis and secretion *(6,35)*. A number of studies demonstrated that E_2 treatments can suppress LH levels in castrated male mice and rats, but dihydrotestosterone (DHT) can also suppress serum LH in some studies in male rodents *(6,35,36)*. Thus, it appears that there may be some degree of redundancy in the receptor paths by which T regulates LH synthesis and secretion.

Characterizations of models of androgen insensitivity, estrogen insensitivity, and estrogen insufficiency further supports the notion of redundant receptor pathways involved in T regulation of LH in males. For instance, serum LH and T levels are elevated in Tfm mice *(37)* and Tfm rats *(38,39)* and there are some cases of androgen insensitivity in humans *(40)*. However, serum LH levels are also elevated in the only known ERα-deficient male patient *(41)* and one aromatase-deficient male patient *(42)*, whereas a second aromatase deficient adult male patient exhibited only slight elevations in serum LH *(43)*. These data suggest that AR pathways play a significant role in mediating the negative feedback effects of T on LH but that aromatization and activation of ERα also plays a role.

Several lines of evidence from the αERKO model further support a role for both ERα and AR in regulating LH. First, serum LH and T levels are only slightly elevated (two-fold) in adult αERKO males despite complete E_2 insensitivity *(35,36)*. Second, castration results in dramatic elevations of LH levels in both WT and αERKO males and E_2 treatments suppress the postcastration rise in serum LH in WT males but not in αERKO males. Third, T or DHT treatments will partly suppress the postcastration rise in serum LH in αERKO males. Thus, AR signaling is sufficient to maintain relatively normal serum LH levels in the absence of intact ERα signaling, but ERα pathways can also effectively suppress synthesis and secretion of LH in WT males. Furthermore, the estrogen insensitivity observed in αERKO males coupled with normal serum LH values in βERKO males suggest that ERβ does not play a significant role in mediating negative feedback effects on LH synthesis and secretion in males.

Testicular feedback regulation of follicle-stimulating hormone (FSH) is more complicated and involves a combination of testicular T and testicular inhibin. It appears that there may be some species differences in the degree of dependence on estrogen and ER vs inhibin regulation of FSH in male rodents and primates. For instance, aromatase-deficient and ERα-deficient humans exhibit elevated FSH *(41,42)*, whereas ARKO and αERKO males exhibit normal serum FSH levels *(22,35,44,45)*. This implies that testicular inhibin may play a more important role in rodent models. Indeed, castration causes significant elevations of serum FSH in both WT and αERKO males, whereas E_2 or T treatments suppress serum FSH only in the castrated WT *(35)*, suggesting that aromatization and activation of ERα plays a role in suppression of FSH in normal WT male mice. The fact that T and DHT treatments failed to suppress serum FSH in castrated αERKO males further suggests that the normal serum FSH levels observed in intact αERKO males are the result of the feedback effects of testicular inhibins *(35)*. Thus, although both inhibins and T regulate FSH in humans and mice, it appears that inhibin feedback more effectively substitutes for deficiencies in estrogen signaling in mice.

TESTIS AND DUCTULE STRUCTURES

The roles of the testes and ductal structures are to synthesize hormones, produce sperm, induce sperm maturation, and transport sperm. There is little doubt that gonadotropins and androgens play critical roles in regulating steroidogenesis and spermatogenesis. However, until recently, the role of estrogens in normal testis functions received little attention despite well-documented evidence that abnormal developmental exposures to E_2 or estrogenic compounds can cause abnormalities in testes and accessory sex structures *(46)*. Indeed critical compartments of the testis and ductule structures express aromatase and/or ERα and ERβ. Studies have detected aromatase in Leydig and Sertoli cells *(47)* and germ cells *(48–50)*, and E_2 levels are very high in rete testis fluid of rats *(51)*. A number of studies consistently report that ERα is expressed in Leydig cells *(52–54)*, whereas ERβ is most often reported in seminiferous tubules *(55)* and/or Sertoli cells *(53,56,57)*. Studies have also detected ERα *(53)* and ERβ *(52,57)* in germ cells at various stages of spermatogenesis. ERα is also expressed in the efferent ductules of mice *(58)*, rats *(54,59)*, and primates *(60,61)*. The presence of aromatase and both ERα and ERβ in testicular and ductal compartments certainly suggests that estrogens might play a critical role in testicular function. Indeed, recent studies demonstrated that estrogens can promote initiation of spermatogenesis in mice *(62)* and prevent apoptosis in human germ cells *(63)*.

Because of the small number of patients and confounding familial azoospermia and infertility in one patient *(43)*, it is presently unknown the extent to which sperm function is compromised in aromatase-deficient adult humans *(42,43)*. However, the single known ERα-deficient human exhibits reduced sperm number and motility *(41)*, suggesting that aromatization and activation of ERα may play a role in production and normal function of human sperm. More convincing support for this hypothesis is found in ARKO and αERKO mice.

Male ARKO mice initially exhibited normal testis and ductal morphologies with normal sperm present in the testis and ductal structures *(22,44)*. These males were also able to sire litters despite reduced male sex behaviors (discussed earlier). It appears that deficits in numbers of mature sperm begin to occur around 4.5 mo. By 1 yr of age, the males experience a dramatic reduction in numbers of round and elongated spermatids despite normal progression of earlier stages of spermatogenesis *(22)*. Coincident with this spermatogenic block, the testis weights and volumes of seminiferous epithelium are also reduced *(22)*. Thus, the onset of infertility is associated with changes in testicular morphology and a spermatogenic block at the transition to round spermatids.

Despite expression of ERβ in multiple cell types in the testis, βERKO males are as fertile as WT littermates and exhibit normal testicular morphology and spermatogenesis *(see* Fig. 2) *(17)*. However, adult αERKO males exhibit complete infertility and progressive testicular dysmorphogenesis that is characterized by relatively normal testes and onset of spermatogenesis during peripubertal stages followed by progressive decreases in spermatogenesis, decreased seminiferous epithelial height, dilated lumens of the seminiferous tubules, and, ultimately, reduced testis weight *(see* Fig. 2) *(45)*. An identical phenotype is also observed in the α,βERKO males, indicating that ERβ plays no role in this progressive testicular dysmorphogenesis *(see* Fig. 2). Significantly, even if αERKO sperm are harvested prior to onset of dramatic testicular changes, these sperm are unable to fertilize eggs in vitro *(45)*. It should be noted that LH and FSH levels are

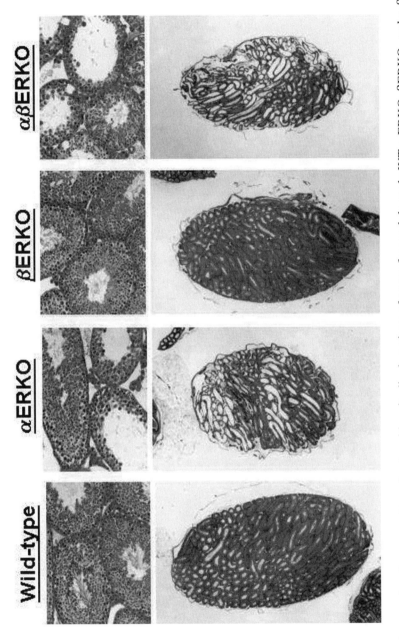

Fig. 2. Photomicrographs of cross-sections (top) and longitudinal sections of testes from adult, male WT, αERKO, βERKO, and α,βERKO mice. Note the normal appearance of WT and βERKO testes, whereas both αERKO and α,βERKO males exhibit the same reduction in testis volume, collapse of seminiferous tubules and epithelium, luminal dilation, and cessation of spermatogenesis. Sections were stained with hematoxylin and eosin and photographed at ×66 and ×13.2 magnification for the cross-section and longitudinal sections, respectively.

sufficient to support normal testis function in these models and, therefore, these testis phenotypes probably arise from deficits in estrogen signaling within the testes or accessory structures.

Superficially, there appear to be similarities between ARKO and αERKO males in that both undergo progressive morphological changes and, ultimately, both are infertile. There are, however, important differences in the levels at which this infertility occur. For instance, mature spermatids from ARKOs are capable of fertilization, as evidenced by the ability of young ARKO males to sire offspring *(44)*, ARKO males do not manifest the profound luminal dilation found in seminiferous tubules of αERKO mice, and spermatogenesis is arrested only at later stages *(22)*. In contrast, αERKO spermatids are not competent at any age and there is profound luminal dilation in αERKO seminiferous tubules followed by collapse of the seminiferous tubules, and almost complete cessation of spermatogenesis in older males *(45)*.

Clearly, failure to complete spermatogenesis in ARKO and αERKO mice will lead to infertility. However, the bases for compromised spermatogenesis seem quite different between these two lines of mice. In ARKO mice, there is an age-dependent, developmental block at later stages of spermatogenesis, whereas in the αERKO, there is a complete collapse of seminiferous tubules and almost compete cessation of all stages of spermatogenesis in older males. In the case of the αERKO male, it appears that the collapse of the tubules and spermatogenesis is the result of defects in the ability of the efferent ductules to absorb fluid passing from the seminiferous tubules through the rete testis and into the efferent ductules *(60,61,64)*. This αERKO phenotype may stem partly from reduced expression of a Na^+/H^+-exchange protein in efferent ductules that, in turn, reduces fluid resorption *(65)*. This creates sufficient "fluid pressure" in the tubules so that the lumens expand, the epithelium regresses, and spermatogenesis effectively ceases. Thus, defects in spermatogenesis appear fairly specific in the ARKO male, whereas the αERKO undergoes a generalized collapse of the tubule anatomy and function that hinges on failure of a supporting somatic tissue (efferent ductules). It is unclear why aromatase-deficient males do not undergo the same dramatic reduction in fluid resorption, collapse of the tubule, and cessation of all stages of spermatogenesis. However, it is possible that dietary estrogens or ligand-independent, growth factor activation of ERα in the efferent ductules may be sufficient to maintain normal fluid resorption even in the absence of E_2.

The fact that αERKO sperm are incompetent to fertilize eggs prior to the onset of gross testicular dysmorphogenesis and reduced spermatogenesis suggests that ERα action is required either within the sperm or in supporting cells such as the Sertoli or ductal cells. Because heterozygote matings yield "knockout" pups, it appears that ERα is not required at the level of the germ cell. Indeed, rescue of αERKO sperm function was recently demonstrated in a study in which αERKO germ cells were transplanted into aspermic, sterile host males. In this study, the αERKO germ cells underwent spermatogenesis and maturation in the WT host and the host was able to sire offspring using the αERKO spermatids *(66)*. This clearly demonstrates that it is not ERα action within the germ cell but ERα action on supporting somatic cells that is required to generate mature, functional sperm. This again raises the question of why ARKO males initially exhibit normal spermatogenesis and sperm competency despite an absence of estrogen. It is possible that dietary estrogens or growth factor activation of ERα may initially support sperm maturation or that continued high levels of androgens may produce some phenotypic effects in older ARKO males.

Although αERKO mice are clearly sterile because of a lack of estrogen action on somatic cells of the testis and/or ductule structures, ARKO mice appear to become infertile as a result of a developmental arrest prior to the round spermatid stage. The fact that αERKO mice do not exhibit such a clear-cut arrest suggests that ERα-independent mechanisms may mediate the effects of estrogen on spermatogenic progression. However, because βERKO males exhibit normal fertility, it is unclear what receptor mechanisms mediate estrogen-dependent progression of spermatogenesis in ARKO mice. It is possible that ERα and ERβ are redundant in their effects on spermatogenic progression or that another estrogen signaling protein is expressed in spermatogonia.

ACCESSORY SEX STRUCTURES

Prostate

Prostate differentiation and function in the adult are clearly dependent on androgens. Based on 5α-reductase-deficient humans, the intracellular production of 5α-DHT is absolutely required for the normal development and function of the prostate (2). Interestingly, prostatic stromal cells express mostly ERα mRNA and protein (67,68), whereas epithelial cells express mostly ERβ in rodents (53,69). Although these data raise the possibility that estrogen may also play a role in prostate physiology, there is currently no evidence that E_2 action is important for normal prostate physiology. Rather, the evidence is that exposure to estrogenic compounds during sensitive windows can lead to prostatic abnormalities later in life (67,68).

The ARKO mouse exhibits enlarged ventral, anterior, and dorsolateral prostate lobes associated with hyperplasia of epithelial and stromal compartments (70). It seems likely that this phenotype stems from chronic exposure to elevated levels of T and prolactin, but despite chronic exposure to these hormones and an absence of E_2, no malignancy developed (70). Adult αERKO males exhibit normal prostate histology despite prolonged exposure to elevated androgens (45,71), whereas reports from one group indicate that βERKO males show some degree of prostatic hyperplasia with increasing age (72). This hyperplasia may be related to an increase in AR observed in the prostates of βERKO males (72). However, it should be noted that other groups have not observed prostatic hyperplasia in βERKO males (73).

Because neonatal exposures to E_2 have been shown to produce permanent alterations in prostate function, a recent study examined the effects of neonatal diethylstilbestrol (DES) exposures in WT, αERKO, and βERKO males (71). This study found that DES exposure results in transient reductions in ERα, downregulation of AR and ERβ, and epithelial dysplasia in prostates from older DES-treated WT males. None of these phenotypes was observed in DES-treated αERKO males, whereas the identical suite of phenotypes was observed in βERKO males (71). These data certainly indicate that ERα is required for the pathological/toxicological effects of estrogen on prostate physiology and that ERβ plays an insignificant role in these phenotypes. This conclusion is strengthened by another study in which tissue recombinants and grafts were made from WT-stromal (S), WT-epithelial (E), αERKO-S, and αERKO-E tissues (74). Following DES challenges of the host animals, squamous metaplasia was observed in recombinants with WT-S and WT-E, but any recombinant that contained an αERKO component failed to exhibit squamous metaplasia. This suggests that ERα is required in both stromal and epithelial compartments of the prostate for estrogenization.

Seminal Vesicle

Similar to the prostate, the seminal vesicle is an heavily androgen-dependent target that is prone to pathological "estrogenization" during critical periods of differentiation. However, E_2 does not appear to play much role in normal seminal vesicles (SV) physiology. It is true that seminal vesicles in ARKO *(22)* and older αERKO males are hypertrophied *(45)* but that βERKO SVs are normal in appearance *(17)*. However, the enlarged SVs appear to stem primarily from the elevated levels of androgens present in males ARKOs and αERKOs, whereas βERKOs have normal T levels and SV weights.

Neonatal DES studies also have demonstrated that DES will estrogenize the SV and cause greatly reduced wet weights. A recent study documented that neonatal DES treatments resulted in dramatically reduced SV weights in WT males but had no effect in αERKO males *(71)*. As with the prostate, these data suggest that ERα mediates the pathological effects of neonatal estrogenization of the seminal vesicles.

CLINICAL PRESENTATIONS

Based on the above discussions, aromatase and ERα deficiencies have profound impacts upon fecundity of mice, whereas, because the small number of patients, the reproductive impact of these deficiencies on human males remains speculative. There are, however, some more overt clinical symptoms that derive from these deficiencies in humans. Both aromatase- and ERα-deficient adult males were found to be above average in height and exhibited continued linear bone growth associated with an absence of epiphysial fusion. Other skeletal phenotypes included osteopenia and increased bone turnover *(41–43)*. Interestingly, these patients also exhibited hyperinsulinemia, reduced glucose tolerance, and abnormal serum lipid profiles *(41–43)*, suggesting a relationship between estrogen deficiency and abnormal metabolic profiles. Male and female αERKO mice have been reported to show phenotypes of obesity, insulin resistance, and reduced glucose tolerance similar to the clinical cases *(75)*. Based on similarities among human patients, ARKO mice, and αERKO mice, it appears that estrogen action via ERα is required for a normal metabolic profile. Thus, a similar suite of skeletal and metabolic phenotypes might reasonably lead a clinician to suspect a problem with estrogen synthesis or signaling. The features that clearly distinguish aromatase deficiency from ERα deficiencies is the very low or absent levels of estrogens in the former vs high estrogen levels and estrogen insensitivity in the latter. Indeed, transdermal E_2 treatments are quite effective in ameliorating some of the skeletal and serum abnormalities in aromatase-deficient males *(76)* but have no effect in an ERα-deficient male *(41)*.

CONCLUSIONS

Successful reproduction in males requires appropriate male sex behaviors, normal hormone profiles, normal spermatogenesis, and support from accessory sex structures. Obviously, deficits at any of these levels can result in partial or complete infertility. Although we have very few models of estrogen deficiency or ER deficiency to examine in humans, evidence suggests that hormone profiles and gametogenesis may be significantly altered in the absence of estrogen or ERα. The ultimate effects of these mutations on human male fertility are not well understood. Detection and characterization of additional aromatase or ERα-deficient patients will further allow us to determine the roles of these two genes in human male reproduction.

Nonetheless, the ARKO and αERKO animal models clearly indicate that normal estrogen signaling and/or ERα are required for (1) normal sex behavior, (2) normal hormone profile, (3) normal gametogenesis, and (4) normal function of accessory sex structures in male mice. The end result of estrogen insufficiency or compromised ERα signaling in these models is infertility as a result of primarily of deficits in behavior, spermatogenesis, or function of accessory sex structures. It does not appear that ERβ plays an obvious or significant role in male reproductive physiology, in contrast to the critical roles of ERβ in female reproductive physiology *(17)*. However, it should be noted that there are species differences in the patterns of expression of ERβ *(9,10,77)* and, thus, it is possible that ERβ plays a more significant role in male reproduction in nonrodent species. Therefore, it will be important to further explore the role of both ERα and ERβ in other species as naturally occurring mutations are found or as ERα- and ERβ-specific ligands become more readily available and better characterized.

REFERENCES

1. Byskov A, Hoyer P. Embryology of mammalian gonads and ducts. In: Knobil E, Neill J, eds. The Physiology of Reproduction, 2nd Edition. Raven, New York, 1994, Vol. 1, pp. 487–540.
2. Luke M, Coffey D. The male accessory tissues:structure, androgen action and physiology. In: Knobil E, Neill J, eds. The Physiology of Reproduction, 2nd Edition. Raven, New York, 1994, Vol. 1, pp. 1435–1488.
3. Gahr M. Brain Structure: causes and consequences of brain sex. In: Short R, Balaban E, eds. The Differences Between the Sexes, Cambridge University Press, Cambridge, 1994, pp. 273–300.
4. Ojeda S, Urbanski H. Puberty in the rat. In: Knobil E, Neill J, eds. The Phsyiology of Reproduction, 2nd Edition. Raven, New York, 1994, Vol. 2, pp. 363–410.
5. Meisel R, Sachs B. The physiology of male sexual behavior. In: Knobil E, Neill J, eds. The Physiology of Reproduction, 2nd Edition. Raven, New York, 1994, Vol. 2, pp. 3–106.
6. Haisenleder DJ, Dalkin AC, Marshall JC. Regulation of gonadotropin gene expression. In: Knobil E, Neill JD, eds. The Physiology of Reproduction, 2nd Edition. Raven, New York, 1994,Vol. 2, pp. 1793–1813.
7. Kuiper GGJM, Enmark E, Pelto-Huikko M, et al. Cloning of a novel estrogen receptor expressed in rat prostate and ovary. Proc Natl Acad Sci USA 1996;93:5925–5930.
8. Kuiper GGJM, Carlsson B, Grandien K, et al. Comparison of the ligand binding specificity and transcript tissue distribution of estrogen receptors a and b. Endocrinology 1997;138(3):863–870.
9. Couse JF, Korach KS. Estrogen receptor null mice: what have we learned and where will they lead us? [published erratum appears in Endocr Rev 1999 Aug;20(4):459]. Endocr Rev 1999;20(3):358–417.
10. Lindzey J. Expression and function of estrogen receptors-a and b. In: Manni A, Verderame M, eds. Selective Estrogen Receptor Modulators. Humana, Totowa, NJ, 2002, pp. 29–56.
11. Shughrue PJ, Scrimo PJ, Merchenthaler I. Evidence for the colocalization of estrogen receptor-beta mRNA and estrogen receptor-alpha immunoreactivity in neurons of the rat forebrain. Endocrinology 1998;139(12):5267–5270.
12. Pettersson K, Grandien K, Kuiper GGJM, Gustafsson J-A. Mouse estrogen receptor b forms estrogen response element binding heterodimers with estrogen receptor a. Mol Endocrinol 1997;11(10):1486–1496.
13. Cowley SM, Hoare S, Mosselman S, Parker MG. Estrogen receptors a and b form heterodimers on DNA. J Biol Chem 1997;272(32):19858–19862.
14. Meyers MJ, Sun J, Carlson KE, et al. Estrogen receptor subtype-selective ligands: asymmetric synthesis and biological evaluation of *cis*- and *trans*-5,11-dialkyl- 5,6,11,12-tetrahydrochrysenes. J Med Chem 1999;42(13):2456–2468.
15. Sun J, Meyers MJ, Fink BE, et al. Novel ligands that function as selective estrogens or antiestrogens for estrogen receptor-alpha or estrogen receptor-beta. Endocrinology 1999;140(2):800–804.
16. Lubahn DB, Moyer JS, Golding TS, et al. Alteration of reproductive function but not prenatal sexual development after insertional disruption of the mouse estrogen receptor gene. Proc Natl Acad Sci USA 1993;90:11162–11166.

17. Krege JH, Hodgin JB, Couse JF, et al. Generation and reproductive phenotypes of mice lacking estrogen receptor beta. Proc Natl Acad Sci USA 1998;95(26):15677–15682.
18. Couse JF, Lindzey J, Grandien K, et al. Tissue distribution and quantitative analysis of estrogen receptor-alpha (ERalpha) and estrogen receptor-beta (ERbeta) messenger ribonucleic acid in the wild-type and ERalpha-knockout mouse. Endocrinology 1997;138(11):4613–4621.
19. Shughrue P, Scrimo P, Lane M, et al. The distribution of estrogen receptor-beta mRNA in forebrain regions of the estrogen receptor-alpha knockout mouse. Endocrinology 1997;138(12):5649–5652.
20. Toda K, Okada T, Takeda K, et al. Oestrogen at the neonatal stage is critical for the reproductive ability of male mice as revealed by supplementation with 17beta-oestradiol to aromatase gene (Cyp19) knockout mice. J Endocrinol 2001;168(3):455–463.
21. Honda S, Harada N, Ito S, et al. Disruption of sexual behavior in male aromatase-deficient mice lacking exons 1 and 2 of the cyp19 gene. Biochem Biophys Res Commun 1998;252(2):445–449.
22. Robertson KM, O'Donnell L, Jones ME, et al. Impairment of spermatogenesis in mice lacking a functional aromatase (cyp 19) gene. Proc Natl Acad Sci USA 1999;96(14):7986–7991.
23. Shughrue PJ, Lane MV, Merchenthaler I. Comparative distribution of estrogen receptor-alpha and -beta mRNA in the rat central nervous system. J Comp Neurol 1997;388(4):507–525.
24. Shughrue P, Lubahn D, Negro-Vilar A, et al. Responses in the brain of estrogen receptor alpha-disrupted mice. PNAS 1997;94:11,008–11,012.
25. Shughrue PJ. Estrogen action in the estrogen receptor alpha-knockout mouse: is this due to ER-beta? Mol Psychiatry 1998;3(4):299–302.
26. Shughrue PJ, Lane MV, Scrimo PJ, Merchenthaler I. Comparative distribution of estrogen receptor-alpha (ER-alpha) and beta (ER-beta) mRNA in the rat pituitary, gonad, and reproductive tract. Steroids 1998;63(10):498–504.
27. Ogawa S, Chester AE, Hewitt SC, et al. Abolition of male sexual behaviors in mice lacking estrogen receptors alpha and beta (alpha beta ERKO). Proc Natl Acad Sci USA 2000;97(26):14737–14741.
28. Ogawa S, Chan J, Chester AE, et al. Survival of reproductive behaviors in estrogen receptor beta gene-deficient (βERKO) male and female mice. Proc Natl Acad Sci USA 1999;96(22):12887–12892.
29. Ogawa S, Lubahn DB, Korach KS, Pfaff DW. Behavioral effects of estrogen receptor gene disruption in male mice. Proc Natl Acad Sci USA 1997;94(4):1476–1481.
30. Wersinger SR, Sannen K, Villalba C, et al. Masculine sexual behavior is disrupted in male and female mice lacking a functional estrogen receptor alpha gene. Horm Behav 1997;32(3):176–183.
31. Toda K, Saibara T, Okada T, et al. A loss of aggressive behaviour and its reinstatement by oestrogen in mice lacking the aromatase gene (Cyp19). J Endocrinol 2001;168(2):217–220.
32. Simerly R, Swanson L, Gorski R. The distribution of monoaminergic cells and fibers in a periventricular preoptic nucleus involved in the control of gonadotropin release: immunohistochemical evidence of a dopaminergic sexual dimorphism. Brain Res 1985;330:55–64.
33. Simerly R, Swanson L, Handa R, Gorski R. Influence of perinatal androgen on the sexually dimorphic distribution of tyrosine hydroxylase-immunoreactive cells and fibers in the anteroventral periventricular nucleus of the rat. Neuroendocrinol 1985;40:501–510.
34. Simerly RB, Zee MC, Pendleton JW, et al. Estrogen receptor-dependent sexual differentiation of dopaminergic neurons in the preoptic region of the mouse. Proc Natl Acad Sci USA 1997;94(25):14077–14082.
35. Lindzey J, Wetsel WC, Couse JF, et al. Effects of castration and chronic steroid treatments on hypothalamic gonadotropin-releasing hormone content and pituitary gonadotropins in male wild-type and estrogen receptor-alpha knockout mice. Endocrinology 1998;139(10):4092–4101.
36. Wersinger SR, Haisenleder DJ, Lubahn DB, Rissman EF. Steroid feedback on gonadotropin release and pituitary gonadotropin subunit mRNA in mice lacking a functional estrogen receptor alpha. Endocrine 1999;11(2):137–143.
37. Naik SI, Young S, Charlton HM, Clayton RN. Pituitary gonadotropin-releasing hormone receptor regulation in mice. I: males. Endocrinology 1984;115(1):106–113.
38. Purvis K, Haug E, Clausen OP, et al. Endocrine status of the testicular feminized male (TFM) rat. Mol Cell Endocrinol 1977;8(4):317–334.
39. Naess O, Haug E, Attramadal A, Aakvaag A, Hansson V, French F. Androgen receptors in the anterior pituitary and central nervous system of the androgen "insensitive" (Tfm) rat: correlation between receptor binding and effects of androgens on gonadotropin secretion. Endocrinology 1976;99(5):1295–1303.
40. Brinkmann AO. Molecular basis of androgen insensitivity. Mol Cell Endocrinol 2001;179(1–2):105–109.
41. Smith EP, Boyd J, Frank G, et al. Estrogen resistance caused by a mutation in the estrogen-receptor gene in a man. N Engl J Med 1994;331:1056–1061.

42. Morishima A, Grumbach MM, Simpson ER, et al. Aromatase deficiency in male and female siblings caused by a novel mutation and the physiological role of estrogens. J Clin Endocrinol Metab 1995;80(12):3689–3698.

43. Carani C, Qin K, Faustini-Fustini M, et al. Effect of testosterone and estradiol in a man with aromatase deficiency. N Engl J Med 1997;337(2):91–95.

44. Fisher CR, Graves KH, Parlow AF, Simpson ER. Characterization of mice deficient in aromatase (ArKO) because of targeted disruption of the cyp19 gene. Proc Natl Acad Sci USA 1998;95(12): 6965–6970.

45. Eddy EM, Washburn TF, Bunch DO, et al. Targeted disruption of the estrogen receptor gene in male mice causes alteration of spermatogenesis and infertility. Endocrinology 1996;137(11):4796–4805.

46. McLachlan JA, Newbold RR, Burow ME, Li SF. From malformations to molecular mechanisms in the male: three decades of research on endocrine disrupters. Apmis 2001;109(4):263–272.

47. Levallet J, Bilinska B, Mittre H, et al. Expression and immunolocalization of functional cytochrome P450 aromatase in mature rat testicular cells. Biol Reprod 1998;58(4):919–926.

48. Hess RA, Bunick D, Bahr JM. Sperm, a source of estrogen. Environ Health Perspect 1995;103(Suppl 7): 59–62.

49. Nitta H, Bunick D, Hess RA, et al. Germ cells of the mouse testis express P450 aromatase. Endocrinology 1993;132:1396–1401.

50. Janulis L, Bahr JM, Hess RA, et al. Rat testicular germ cells and epididymal sperm contain active P450 aromatase. J Androl 1998;19(1):65–71.

51. Free MJ, Jaffe RA. Collection of rete testis fluid from rats without previous efferent duct ligation. Biol Reprod 1979;20(2):269–278.

52. Jefferson WN, Couse JF, Banks EP, et al. Expression of estrogen receptor beta is developmentally regulated in reproductive tissues of male and female mice. Biol Reprod 2000;62(2):310–317.

53. Pelletier G, Labrie C, Labrie F. Localization of oestrogen receptor alpha, oestrogen receptor beta and androgen receptors in the rat reproductive organs. J Endocrinol 2000;165(2):359–370.

54. Fisher JS, Millar MR, Majdic G, et al. Immunolocalisation of oestrogen receptor-alpha within the testis and excurrent ducts of the rat and marmoset monkey from perinatal life to adulthood. J Endocrinol 1997;153(3):485–495.

55. Pelletier G, Luu-The V, Charbonneau A, Labrie F. Cellular localization of estrogen receptor beta messenger ribonucleic acid in cynomolgus monkey reproductive organs. Biol Reprod 1999;61(5): 1249–1255.

56. Saunders PT, Maguire SM, Gaughan J, Millar MR. Expression of oestrogen receptor beta (ER beta) in multiple rat tissues visualised by immunohistochemistry. J Endocrinol 1997;154(3):R13–R16.

57. van Pelt AM, de Rooij DG, van der Burg B, van der Saag PT, Gustafsson JA, Kuiper GG. Ontogeny of estrogen receptor-beta expression in rat testis. Endocrinology 1999;140(1):478–483.

58. Nielsen M, Bjornsdottir S, Hoyer PE, Byskov AG. Ontogeny of oestrogen receptor alpha in gonads and sex ducts of fetal and newborn mice. J Reprod Fertil 2000;118(1):195–204.

59. Hess RA, Gist DH, Bunick D, et al. Estrogen receptor (alpha and beta) expression in the excurrent ducts of the adult male rat reproductive tract. J Androl 1997;18(6):602–611.

60. Hess RA. Oestrogen in fluid transport in efferent ducts of the male reproductive tract. Rev Reprod 2000;5(2):84–92.

61. Hess RA, Bunick D, Lubahn DB, et al. Morphologic changes in efferent ductules and epididymis in estrogen receptor-alpha knockout mice. J Androl 2000;21(1):107–121.

62. Ebling FJ, Brooks AN, Cronin AS, et al. Estrogenic induction of spermatogenesis in the hypogonadal mouse. Endocrinology 2000;141(8):2861–2869.

63. Pentikainen V, Erkkila K, Suomalainen L, et al. Estradiol acts as a germ cell survival factor in the human testis in vitro. J Clin Endocrinol Metab 2000;85(5):2057–2067.

64. Hess RA, Bunick D, Lee KH, et al. A role for oestrogens in the male reproductive system [see comments]. Nature 1997;390(6659):509–512.

65. Zhou Q, Clarke L, Nie R, et al. Estrogen action and male fertility: roles of the sodium/hydrogen exchanger-3 and fluid reabsorption in reproductive tract function. Proc Natl Acad Sci USA 2001; 98(24):14132–14137.

66. Mahato D, Goulding EH, Korach KS, et al. Spermatogenic cells do not require estrogen receptor-alpha for development or function [see comments]. Endocrinology 2000;141(3):1273–276.

67. Prins GS, Birch L. Neonatal estrogen exposure up-regulates estrogen receptor expression in the developing and adult rat prostate lobes. Endocrinology 1997;138(5):1801–1809.

68. Chang WY, Wilson MJ, Birch L, Prins GS. Neonatal estrogen stimulates proliferation of periductal fibroblasts and alters the extracellular matrix composition in the rat prostate. Endocrinology 1999;140(1):405–415.

69. Chang WY, Prins GS. Estrogen receptor-beta: implications for the prostate gland. Prostate 1999;40(2):115–124.

70. McPherson SJ, Wang H, Jones ME, et al. Elevated androgens and prolactin in aromatase-deficient mice cause enlargement, but not malignancy, of the prostate gland. Endocrinology 2001;142(6):2458–2467.

71. Prins GS, Birch L, Couse JF, et al. Estrogen imprinting of the developing prostate gland is mediated through stromal estrogen receptor alpha: studies with alphaERKO and betaERKO mice. Cancer Res 2001;61(16):6089–6097.

72. Weihua Z, Makela S, Andersson LC, et al. A role for estrogen receptor beta in the regulation of growth of the ventral prostate. Proc Natl Acad Sci USA 2001;98(11):6330–6335.

73. Dupont S, Krust A, Gansmuller A, et al. Effect of single and compound knockouts of estrogen receptors alpha (ERalpha) and beta (ERbeta) on mouse reproductive phenotypes. Development 2000;127(19):4277–4291.

74. Risbridger G, Wang H, Young P, et al. Evidence that epithelial and mesenchymal estrogen receptor-alpha mediates effects of estrogen on prostatic epithelium. Dev Biol 2001;229(2):432–442.

75. Heine PA, Taylor JA, Iwamoto GA, et al. Increased adipose tissue in male and female estrogen receptor-α knockout mice. Proc Natl Acad Sci USA 2000;97:12729–12734.

76. Rochira V, Faustini-Fustini M, Balestrieri A, Carani C. Estrogen replacement therapy in a man with congenital aromatase deficiency: effects of different doses of transdermal estradiol on bone mineral density and hormonal parameters. J Clin Endocrinol Metab 2000;85(5):1841–1845.

77. O'Donnell L, Robertson KM, Jones ME, Simpson ER. Estrogen and spermatogenesis. Endocr Rev 2001;22(3):289–318.

6

Alterations of Androgen Action Caused by Mutation of the Human Androgen Receptor

Michael J. McPhaul, MD

CONTENTS

INTRODUCTION
PHENOTYPIC SPECTRUM OF ANDROGEN RESISTANCE CAUSED
BY MUTATIONS OF THE HUMAN ANDROGEN RECEPTOR
HUMAN ANDROGEN RECEPTOR AND ITS FUNCTIONAL DOMAINS
MUTATIONS OF THE ANDROGEN RECEPTOR
ANDROGEN RECEPTOR MUTATIONS CAUSING QUALITATIVE
ABNORMALITIES OF LIGAND BINDING
MUTATIONS OF THE ANDROGEN RECEPTOR ASSOCIATED
WITH NORMAL LEVELS OF ANDROGEN BINDING
IN GENITAL SKIN FIBROBLASTS
ANDROGEN RECEPTOR MUTATIONS RESULTING
IN DECREASED LEVELS OF LIGAND BINDING
MINIMAL DEFECTS OF VIRILIZATION CAUSED BY MUTATIONS
OF THE ANDROGEN RECEPTOR
THE RELATIONSHIP BETWEEN PHENOTYPE AND AR MUTATIONS
VARIATIONS IN PHENOTYPE
VARIATIONS IN THE STRUCTURE OF THE ANDROGEN RECEPTOR GENE
SPINAL AND BULBAR MUSCULAR ATROPHY
AR MUTATIONS IN PROSTATE CANCER
DISTRIBUTION OF AR GENE MUTATIONS
SUMMARY
REFERENCES

INTRODUCTION

In mammals, the complement of sex chromosomes establishes the genotypic sex, which is the principal determinant of the events that take place during sexual development. In particular, the presence or absence of the sex-determining gene, SRY, encoded

From: *Contemporary Endocrinology: Androgens in Health and Disease*
Edited by: C. Bagatell and W. J. Bremner © Humana Press Inc., Totowa, NJ

on the Y chromosome determines whether the primordial gonad will develop as a testis or as an ovary *(1)*. This functional differentiation of the gonad determines the subsequent events in mammalian sexual development *(2,3)*.

In the male embryo, the steroid and polypeptide hormones secreted by the testis mediate the development of the male phenotype, which requires the combined actions of testosterone, 5α-dihydrotestosterone, and müllerian-inhibiting substance (MIS). At approximately the ninth week of development, the Leydig cells of the testes begin to secrete to steroid hormones. The formation of both testosterone and its 5α-reduced metabolite, 5α-dihydrotestosterone, are required to induce the virilization of the internal and external genitalia. In response to these androgens, the external genitalia virilize with the enlargement of the phallus and fusion of the genital ridges to form the scrotum. The wolffian ducts grow to form the pelvic portion of the urogenital sinus and give rise to the seminal vesicles and the epididymis. During this same period, the Sertoli cells of the testes secrete the polypeptide hormone MIS, which mediates the regression of the müllerian duct-derived structures, including the uterus and fallopian tubes *(4)*. In the absence of the actions of these testicular hormones, the uterus and fallopian tubes develop and the upper vaginal segments and urogenital swellings fail to fuse.

Defects in a number of genes that act to alter normal sexual development have been identified and it is clear that defects in male development can be caused by any abnormality that impairs the development of the testes, the normal synthesis of androgen or MIS, or the capacity of tissues to respond to these hormones *(3)*.

PHENOTYPIC SPECTRUM OF ANDROGEN RESISTANCE CAUSED BY MUTATIONS OF THE HUMAN ANDROGEN RECEPTOR

Naturally occurring defects of the human androgen receptor have been identified far more frequently than defects in other members of the nuclear-receptor family. This is likely due to several unique characteristics of the androgen receptor (AR) and the processes that it regulates. First, the androgen receptor gene is located on the X chromosome. As such, normal 46,XY males inherit only a single copy of the gene and disturbances of AR function will be evident phenotypically. Second, although many important processes are modulated by the androgen receptor (virilization of the internal and external male structures, maintenance of bone density, and spermatogenesis), these functions are not required for life. For this reason, even individuals in whom AR function is completely defective are viable and available for ascertainment. Finally, the phenotypes characteristic of androgen insensitivity are often evident at birth (ambiguities of sexual development) or detected at puberty (complete testicular feminization) and precipitate endocrine or genetic analyses.

As a result of these characteristics of the androgen receptor, a wide range of individuals of varying phenotypes are available for study *(5,6)*. In individuals in whom the AR is nonfunctional or is not expressed, internal and external male structures fail to develop. This syndrome has been variously termed "complete testicular feminization" *(7)* or "complete androgen insensitivity." Externally, such patients appear as normal females with developed breasts and normal external female genitalia. Decreased or absent axillary and pubic hair represents a potential clue to the nature of the underlying disorder. Careful evaluation of such individuals will identify testes located either intraabdominally or within the labia majora. Although the tissues of such individuals are incapable of responding to the actions of androgen, the testes secrete MIS normally. Consequently, the müellerian duct-derived structures regress, and the uterus and Fallopian tubes are absent and the vagina is blind-ending.

Individuals with less severe defects of androgen action display a range of intermediate phenotypes (5,6). These phenotypes, characterized by the varying degrees of virilization present, have been referred to by a number of terms, including partial androgen insensitivity, incomplete testicular feminization, and Reifenstein syndrome. At one end of the spectrum, minor degrees of virilization (clitoromegaly, posterior labial fusion) may be evident and the phenotype is predominantly female in character (partial androgen insensitivity, incomplete testicular feminization). In contrast, affected subjects may instead display a phenotype that is predominantly male in character with severe urogenital abnormalities and gynecomastia (Reifenstein phenotype). Quigley et al. have outlined a grading system to permit a more precise categorization of patients with incomplete forms of androgen resistance (6).

In a small number of instances, patients display phenotypes in which male sexual development is normal or near normal, but in whom selected androgen-dependent processes are disturbed. Such individuals may display subtle signs of undervirilization, such as gynecomastia, or may simply exhibit infertility as a manifestation of their AR defect.

HUMAN ANDROGEN RECEPTOR AND ITS FUNCTIONAL DOMAINS

The AR is a member of the nuclear-receptor gene family and is most closely related to the mineralocorticoid and progesterone receptors (8) (see Fig. 1). Like other members of this gene family, the AR is comprised of distinct domains that mediate the high affinity binding of androgen (ligand-binding domain [LBD], residues 676–917) and the recognition of specific DNA sequences (DNA-binding domain [DBD], residues 559–624). The three-dimensional structures of these domains of the human AR have been solved (9,10) or modeled based on the basis of the structures of similar domains of related receptors (11). In addition to motifs responsible for mediating the binding of the receptor to its target DNA sequences and the high-affinity binding of the ligand, regions within and adjacent to the DBD regulate the nuclear localization of the AR (12,13). Finally, the amino terminus of the AR comprises a large portion of the molecule and is required for the maximal activation of responsive genes (14–16).

In addition to these important functional domains, the open reading frame of the human AR also contains several repeat elements within the amino terminus. These regions are comprised of trimeric nucleotide repeats that encode segments of the AR comprised of repeating glutamine, proline, or glycine residues (see Fig. 1). As discussed in the following section, these elements are particularly significant with respect to their involvement in the pathogenesis of specific disease states.

MUTATIONS OF THE ANDROGEN RECEPTOR

Absent Ligand Binding

LARGE-SCALE DELETIONS

In most instances, the absence of detectable levels of androgen-binding assays in genital skin fibroblast-binding assays (ligand binding negative) is associated with phenotype of complete testicular feminization (complete androgen insensitivity).

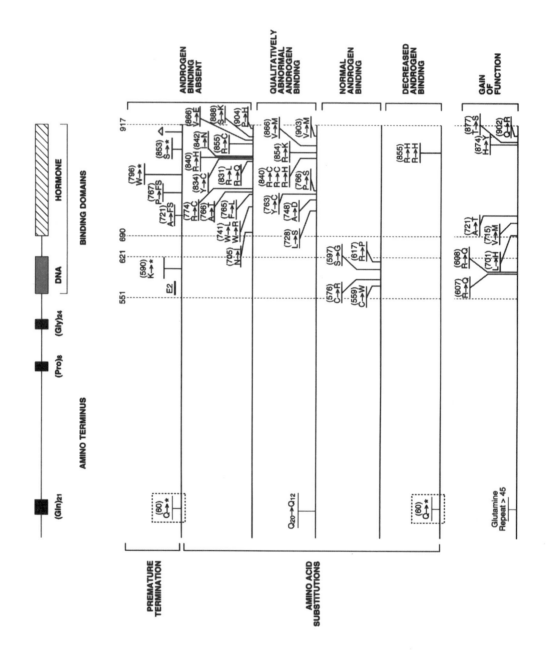

The initial patient in this category in whom a defect of the AR was identified was an individual in whom Southern blotting analysis of genomic DNA samples demonstrated a partial deletion of the AR gene *(17)*. Although additional characterization of this patient has not been reported, mapping of the AR gene using restriction endonucleases suggested that a large portion of the 3' end of the coding segment of the gene had been deleted. Given the large segments of the gene that were removed and the instability of most truncated ARs *(18)*, it is unlikely that an AR protein accumulated in measurable quantities.

Additional families have been identified in which sizable portions of the AR gene have been deleted. Two patients have been characterized in which the entire coding sequence of the AR gene is absent. In one patient, the phenotype was complete androgen insensitivity *(19)*. In contrast, in addition to a phenotype of complete androgen insensitivity, the second patient had additional somatic abnormalities, including mental retardation *(20)*. Although the alterations of gene structure identified in these two patients have proven to be infrequent, both were important in helping to establish the "null" phenotype resulting from a complete absence of AR function. Although this has been deduced by clinicians and from animal models (for the mouse), this information has particular importance with respect to concepts relating to the pathogenesis of spinal and bulbar muscular atrophy (*see* later section). In this regard, it seems likely that the abnormalities of the second patient *(20)* are the result of effects of the deletion on adjacent genetic loci. An additional patient with complete deletion of the AR gene has been reported *(21)*.

Many patients have been identified with partial deletions of the AR gene. In some instances, such deletions span individual exons; in other instances, multiple exons have been deleted. Only a few of these partially deleted AR gene alleles have been completely defined. In some cases, the region(s) deleted have been inferred on the basis of an inability to amplify a region of the gene.

An interesting exception to this is the family described by McClean et al. *(22)*. Unexpectedly, the analysis of affected patients in this pedigree gave evidence for distinct breakpoints within the AR gene. In some instances, portions encompassing exon 5 was deleted, whereas in others, a larger segment that contained both exons 5 and 6 was missing. The authors suggested that their findings were consistent with a region of instability in the region surrounding exon 5 in this pedigree. The source of this instability has not been defined in further detail.

SMALL DELETIONS AND INSERTIONS

Although large-scale deletions of the AR gene are rare relative to the number of reported cases, small-scale alterations of the AR gene structure are more frequent. In a

Fig. 1. Schematic structure of the human AR and representative AR mutations. (Top) A schematic displaying the major functional elements of the human AR. The conserved DNA-binding and ligand-binding domains are indicated, as are the repeat elements contained in the AR amino terminus. (Bottom) The various categories of ligand binding abnormality and representative mutations that have been identified in patients with androgen resistance. In addition to these loss-of-function mutations, alterations of AR structure that result in the gains of function associated with spinal and bulbar muscular atrophy (glutamine repeat expansion) or prostate or breast cancer (substitution mutations) are depicted. (Modified with permission from McPhaul, MJ. Rec Prog Horm Res 2002;57:181–194 © The Endocrine Society.)

number of alleles, deletions have been identified that remove one or several nucleotides. In those instances in which the open reading frame is maintained, the deletion of one or several single amino acids results. In those cases that disrupt the open reading frame, a frame shift and premature termination result.

Insertions occur less frequently than deletions, although the same comments pertain regarding the maintenance of the AR open reading frame. The one formal exception to this generalization is the lengthening of the glutamine repeat in the amino terminus that occurs in patients with X-linked spinal and bulbar muscular atrophy (Kennedy's disease).

ALTERATIONS IN AR STRUCTURE CAUSED BY PREMATURE TERMINATION CODONS

Single nucleotide substitutions that result in the introduction of premature termination codons into the open reading frame of the androgen receptor gene were among the first defects in the AR gene to be identified. Such mutations have been detected in all of the coding exons of the AR gene. Owing to the location of the critical DBD and LBDs at the carboxyl terminus of the receptor protein, in most instances the truncated mutant AR molecules that result lack one or both of these domains and have no activity in assays of androgen binding or transcriptional activation.

Only a single exception to this generalization has been reported. In this instance, a single nucleotide substitution resulted in the premature termination of the AR protein early in the open reading frame (at amino acid 60). As a result of the amino terminal location of this termination codon, translational initiation occurred at a location more carboxyl terminal (methionine 189) and levels of the resulting amino terminal-truncated AR protein were detected using ligand binding and immunoblot assays *(23)*.

ALTERATIONS IN AR STRUCTURE CAUSED BY CHANGES IN AR mRNA SPLICING

In addition to causing truncation of the AR, single-nucleotide substitutions can induce large-scale structural changes of the androgen receptor by impairing the normal processing of AR mRNA. This type of alteration is most frequently the result of mutations that alter the splice donor or acceptor sites used in the splicing of AR mRNA.

Although a number of such mutations have been identified, the work of Ris-Stalpers et al. serves as an illustrative example *(24)*. In this patient with complete androgen resistance, a single nucleotide change mutated the critical GT splice donor site at the 5' end of intron 4 of the AR gene. As a result of this change, the normal processing of AR mRNA was inefficient and an alternate splicing event occurred using an alternate (cryptic) splice donor in intron 4. These changes are predicted to result in the production of an AR protein lacking 41 amino acids of the normal AR coding sequence, including a portion at the 5' boundary of the AR HBD. This deleted AR protein was not functional in assays of ligand binding or transactivation.

In some instances, alterations of AR mRNA splicing can result in incomplete forms of androgen resistance. This has been shown by the work of Ris-Stalpers et al. *(25)*. These investigators identified a large (>6-kb deletion) of intron 2 within the AR gene of the affected subject that began 18 basepairs upstream of the 5' boundary of exon 3. This structural change led to the accumulation of mRNA encoding an AR lacking exon 3. In addition to mRNA encoding this defective AR, analysis of the RNA from this patient also demonstrated that approx 10% of the AR mRNA was correctly spliced using a cryptic site. These authors postulated that this low-level expression of a normal AR protein was sufficient to that account for the partial androgen-insensitivity syndrome (AIS) phenotype.

Taken in the context of the analyses of AR truncations, these studies suggest that alterations of AR mRNA splicing that result in the synthesis of a truncated AR protein will be associated with complete forms of androgen resistance. Such findings also suggest that in those unusual circumstances where a phenotype of partial androgen resistance is observed, a reduced amount of intact AR may still be synthesized that is responsible for mediating the observed virilization.

Amino Acid Substitutions

Absent ligand binding is frequently traced to single-nucleotide substitutions within the open reading frame that result in amino acid replacements within the LBD of the receptor. The substitution mutations associated with absent ligand binding (as measured in patient fibroblasts) fall into two major categories.

Mutations of the first category involve amino acid substitutions at critical sites within the HBD that result in major alterations of the structure of the HBD. These changes are so profound that the resulting mutant AR is no longer capable of binding ligand, even when expressed in heterologous cells or in bacteria. The mutant AR (W739R) is representative of defective receptors of this class (26,27). This type of mutation has been characterized in only a limited number of instances, but it is likely to reflect major alterations in the conformation of the ligand-binding pocket.

Far more frequently, when cDNAs encoding the mutant receptors from androgen-binding negative genital skin fibroblasts are expressed in heterologous cells, it is found that the mutant receptor retains the capacity to bind the ligand, although these receptors invariably bind androgen with reduced stability or affinity. The mutant AR characterized by Marcelli and co-workers serves as an illustrative example. In this work, a single-nucleotide substitution resulted in an amino acid replacement, R774C, in a subject with complete androgen insensitivity (28). In fibroblast-binding assays, this mutant AR was associated with levels of androgen binding that were below the limits of detection. When the mutant AR was expressed in heterologous cells, the expressed receptor was capable of binding androgen. This androgen-binding capacity was not normal, displaying marked lability to thermal denaturation and reduced ligand affinity. As with most mutants within this class, near-normal levels of immunoreactive receptor are detected, although reduced levels of ligand binding are measured in monolayer-binding assays (29). The discordance between the results of the fibroblast binding assays, and similar assays performed in cells transfected with mutant cDNAs appears simply to reflect differences in the sensitivity of the assays employed and differences in the levels of receptor expressed.

ANDROGEN RECEPTOR MUTATIONS CAUSING QUALITATIVE ABNORMALITIES OF LIGAND BINDING

Prior to the development of techniques to measure AR function, a variety of qualitative tests were applied to screen for AR defects when quantitative assays were unrevealing. Such tests have examined the affinity of the receptor for its ligand, the stability of the AR protein expressed (e.g., to thermal denaturation), and the stability of the hormone–receptor complexes (ligand dissociation rate). The number of mutations that have been described is large and the following mutations are presented as illustrative examples.

The first mutation of this type to be characterized at the molecular level was reported by Lubahn et al., who identified a single-amino-acid substitution (V866M) in the HBD of the AR in affected subjects from a family with complete androgen insensitivity *(30)*. Characterization of androgen binding in fibroblast cultures demonstrated that the AR expressed in fibroblasts displayed a reduced affinity of ligand binding. Functional analysis of this mutated AR demonstrated a reduced ability to stimulate a model androgen-responsive reporter gene. This decreased transcriptional capacity was most evident at lower ligand concentrations and was minimized when such assays were conducted at high concentration ranges *(31)* *(see* below).

The effects of increased doses of androgen concentration have been observed on other mutant androgen receptors that have exhibited qualitative abnormalities of androgen binding. In a patient with Reifenstein phenotype, binding studies performed in fibroblasts indicated a normal level of ligand binding but an accelerated dissociation of ligand *(32)*. When analyzed at the molecular level, two mutations were identified in the AR gene in this patient: a tyrosine-to-cysteine substitution at amino acid residue 763 and a shortened glutamine homopolymeric region in the amino terminus *(33)*. When expression plasmids were constructed to examine the effects of these two mutations in eukaryotic cells, the two mutations were found to interact functionally. The tyrosine-to-cysteine substitution was sufficient to cause the mutant AR to exhibit an accelerated dissociation rate and thermal lability. Although the contraction of the glutamine repeat region itself did not cause changes in the receptor stability or ligand dissociation, the mutant receptor containing both mutations exhibited a functional defect more severe than the receptor containing only the amino-acid-substitution mutation. Cooperative effects of these two structural changes were evident in studies of dissociation rate, thermal stability, and transcriptional activation. These findings suggesting that the receptor and the phenotype were the result of the combined effects of both mutations. Interestingly, subsequent biochemical studies have demonstrated a functional interaction between the amino-terminal and carboxyl-terminal segments of the AR protein *(34,35)*.

A large number of different amino-acid-substitution mutations have been described that cause qualitative abnormalities of ligand binding by the androgen receptor. Virtually all are localized to the LBD at residues that exhibit similar positions compared to the distribution of the mutations that result in the absence of ligand binding *(26)*. This observation suggests that the degree to which the structure of the LBD is disrupted is the determinant that dictates the type of ligand-binding abnormality that is observed: those causing more severe disruptions are associated with absent ligand binding, whereas those that cause more subtle perturbations of structure result in qualitative defects of ligand binding. This concept has been reinforced by studies in which different substitution mutations have been identified that have been associated with distinctive abnormalities of ligand binding. Prior et al. *(36)* reported pedigrees in which the same amino acid residue (arginine 774) was substituted with different amino acid residues. Replacement of this arginine by a cysteine residue (R774C) led to undetectable levels of ligand binding in genital skin fibroblasts. If this same arginine residue was replaced, instead, by a histidine, normal levels of androgen binding were detected in fibroblasts from affected individuals, but this binding activity displayed marked thermal instability.

In a similar fashion, other surveys have identified families in which mutant receptors harboring different amino-acid-substitution mutation at the same residue led to discernibly different effects on ligand binding and on receptor function *(37–39)*. In those instances in which replacement of a residue with different amino acids has resulted in different phenotypes, the functional capacity of the mutant AR has varied in parallel with the degree of virilization that was observed.

As noted earlier, in several instances hormone concentrations have been observed to exert effects on the activities of mutant ARs out of proportion to the changes in the activity of the normal AR assayed at physiologic hormone concentrations. This behavior was explored systematically by Marcelli et al., who examined the functional responsiveness to different ligands of a number of AR mutants with different types of qualitative abnormality caused by amino acid substitutions in the HBD *(27)*. When these mutant ARs were assayed in cells capable of metabolizing testosterone and 5α-dihydrotestosterone, it was observed that the concentration, frequency of addition, and type of androgen used had a dramatic effect on the level of AR function measured. These same variables had a much less profound effect on the activity of the normal AR. In each instance, testosterone was the least potent androgen, whereas dihydrotestosterone and mibolerone exhibited higher potencies. These observations permit three conclusions. First, these experiments demonstrate the critical importance of the stability of the hormone–androgen receptor complex. Conditions that favor the formation and stability of these complexes have major effects on the functions of the mutant receptors in functional assays. Second, these findings demonstrate that mutant ARs capable of binding hormone can be manipulated pharmacologically to exhibit near-normal levels of AR function. This possibility has been tested in the clinical realm in only a limited number of cases, but the results of such interventions suggest that this holds true in vivo as well, at least for a subset of AR mutations *(32,40–45)*. Third, these experiments demonstrate the difficulties inherent in measuring the function of mutant ARs that are only partially defective as a result of qualitative defects of ligand binding. Changes in cell type, ligand, or dosing regimen can each have important effects on the extent of functional defect that is measured.

MUTATIONS OF THE ANDROGEN RECEPTOR ASSOCIATED WITH NORMAL LEVELS OF ANDROGEN BINDING IN GENITAL SKIN FIBROBLASTS

In approx 10% of patients with a clinical syndrome consistent with androgen resistance and data that suggests a defect of the AR (family history and/or endocrine studies), no abnormality of ligand binding can be detected. In these families, affected individuals can exhibit phenotypes ranging from complete testicular feminization to that of mild partial androgen insensitivity *(3,5)*. This category had been proposed to represent either subtle defects of the AR or mutations in genes other than the AR that affect the action of androgens.

Analyses of a number of such pedigrees have demonstrated that in those instances in which family history or endocrine testing suggest the presence of an AR defect, mutations of the DBD are frequently identified. Zoppi et al. analyzed the structure of the AR gene in four subjects with this type of androgen resistance *(46)*. In each instance, an amino acid substitution was identified within the DNA-binding region of the AR. When expressed in heterologous eukaryotic cells, the mutant receptors were found to bind ligand with normal or near-normal kinetics. Despite this, the mutant receptors were severely impaired in transcriptional activation of a model androgen-responsive reporter gene. In vitro studies demonstrated that each of the mutant ARs failed to bind normally to target DNA sequences (androgen response elements). A number of such mutations within the AR DBD have now been reported in patients with complete and partial forms of androgen resistance by a number of different laboratories *(47–51)*.

Other structural alterations of the DBD can mimic the effects of amino acid substitutions within this region. In one instance, an in-frame deletion of exon 3 was detected in a patient with complete testicular feminization *(52)*. This exon encodes half of the critical DBD, and although this mutant receptor was shown to bind hormone normally, it was unable to activate the transcription of a target androgen-responsive reporter gene, in a fashion similar to mutants containing amino-acid-substitution mutations within this segment. Similar effects have been reported for single-amino-acid deletions within the DBD of the AR. In aggregate, these studies suggest that regardless of the type of genetic alteration, mutations in the DBD of the AR cause androgen insensitivity by interfering with the capacity of the receptor to recognize specific target DNA sequences. The information from a number of different studies would suggest that, in general, the degree to which DNA binding by a mutant AR is impaired correlates with the degree of phenotypic abnormality observed.

A small number of patients with partial androgen resistance caused by AR DBD mutations suggest an intriguing specific link to the development of breast cancer. Wooster et al. described two brothers with Reifenstein syndrome that developed breast cancer *(53)*. Sequence analysis of the AR gene of these subjects revealed an amino-acid-substitution mutation (R607Q) in the second zinc finger, a part of the segment implicated in determining the specificity of the DNA binding by the receptor *(54)*. The identification of such mutation in a patient with breast cancer could be a causal association or might simply represent the influence of gynecomastia in the predisposition of affected subject to the development of breast cancer. The report by Lobaccaro and co-workers of an unrelated individual with the Reifenstein phenotype who developed breast cancer *(55)* and who harbored an amino acid substitution at the adjacent amino acid residue (R608K) would seem to make a causative role possible. In such a scenario, the mutated amino acid residues might be expected to alter the pattern of gene activation that occurs in response to androgens in these patients and contribute to the development of breast cancer. Subsequent studies by Poujol et al. *(56)* demonstrated that the mutant AR displayed altered DNA-binding specificity in in vitro studies. It remains to determine whether these effects directly contribute to the development of breast cancer or whether these influences are mediated indirectly through the interference with the action of the AR.

ANDROGEN RECEPTOR MUTATIONS RESULTING IN DECREASED LEVELS OF LIGAND BINDING

The first mutation to be characterized from a patient with reduced amounts of androgen receptor was that reported by Zoppi et al. *(23)*. Unexpectedly, immunoblots performed using antibodies directed at the AR amino terminus did not detect the receptor protein, even though the AR immunoblot assay was at least 10-fold more sensitive than the monolayer-binding assay employed. This discordance was explained by the identification of a termination codon in place of amino acid 60. Further investigations using specific antibodies directed at internal epitopes established that the low level of binding detected in the monolayer-binding assays were the result of the downstream initiation at methionine 189. Subsequent experiments demonstrated that this truncated receptor protein (lacking amino acids 1–189) is synthesized in normal cells and is analogous to the A-form of the progesterone receptor *(57)*. Studies in heterologous cells have established that the phenotype observed in affected individuals within this family (complete testicular feminization) is the result of a combination of reduced amounts androgen receptor and a reduced function of the AR that is synthesized *(58)*.

The patient with partial AIS described by Choong et al. identified a completely distinct mechanism by which reduced levels of apparently normal AR could be expressed *(59)*. In this individual, a single-nucleotide substitution was identified that resulted in the replacement of the second amino acid residue of the AR open reading frame (D2K). Using functional and in vitro assays, the authors presented evidence that although a subtle increase in the rate of ligand dissociation was observed, the reduced level of AR expressed as a result of decreased efficiency of translational initiation was the more important determinant of disturbed AR action in this pedigree.

It is likely that mutations identified within this category will be quite heterogeneous, as the mutations may result in reduced quantities of normal AR. Alternatively, samples placed within this category may express reduced levels of AR that exhibits subtle alterations not detected in monolayer-binding assays performed on fibroblast cultures.

MINIMAL DEFECTS OF VIRILIZATION CAUSED BY MUTATIONS OF THE ANDROGEN RECEPTOR

A small number of AR mutations have been identified in patients exhibiting more subtle disturbances of androgen action. These generally have been associated with either a more subtle phenotype (undervirilized male) or infertility.

Tsukada et al. were the first to report an AR mutation in such a pedigree with androgen resistance and undervirilization and preserved fertility *(60)*. These workers identified an amino acid substitution (L790F) in the LBD of the AR. In ligand-binding assays, the mutant receptor displayed thermal instability and altered kinetics of androgen binding. When analyzed in transfection assays, AR function was observed to be only slightly reduced compared to the normal AR. As would be expected for a mutation causing a qualitative abnormality of the AR (*see* above discussion), the defective function of this mutant AR was most pronounced at lower hormone concentrations.

Among the most intriguing of AR defects are those implicated in causing isolated defects of spermatogenesis. To date, only a small number of such mutant ARs have been reported. In each instance, these mutations have been identified during the evaluation of patients presenting with azoospermia or oligospermia *(61–63)*. In each instance, the mutant AR was found to exhibit only slightly diminished function using transfection assays. In one instance, the mutation was found to cause decreased association of the ligand-activated mutant AR with the coactivator TIF2 in two-hybrid assays *(62,63)*. The mutations identified are diverse (R788S, Q798E, M886V) and none are directly in the formation of the ligand-binding pocket. Two of the substitutions are positioned in helix 7 (R788S, Q798E) and one (M886V) is located at the carboxyl-terminal end of helix 10/11 of the AR LBD. The only property that is clearly shared by these mutations is that each results in only small decreases of AR function. It is interesting to note that no mutations in the DBD of the AR have been described that cause such a phenotype.

In addition to substitution mutations in the AR LBD, increases in the length of the glutamine repeat in the amino terminus of the AR have been associated with an increased risk of impaired spermatogenesis *(64–68)*. This association has been identified in studies of patient populations evaluated for causes azooligospermia or oligospermia. The mechanism responsible for this association is postulated to represent the effects of the decreased function of the AR that has been associated with increases in the length of this segment.

THE RELATIONSHIP BETWEEN PHENOTYPE AND AR MUTATIONS

Although AR-binding assays provided a useful tool with which to classify patients with AR defects, it was clear that no precise correlation existed between with the extent of virilization and the type of binding abnormality *(5)*. The existence of information defining the molecular defects in a large number of patients with different forms of androgen insensitivity has permitted an examination of whether such a correlation exists when the answer is sought using more precise measurements of AR abundance or function.

A number of generalizations can now be made. First, with few exceptions, truncations of the AR protein result in the phenotype of complete androgen insensitivity (complete testicular feminization). This is observed because most truncations of the receptor protein either remove essential functional domains (the LBD or DBD) or result in greatly reduced levels of AR protein *(18,29)*. This stands in contrast to amino-acid-substitution mutations, which have been associated with the complete range of androgen-resistant phenotypes.

Second, although there is broad agreement between the degree of defect that is defined in functional assays of receptor function (and abundance) and the phenotype that is observed in individual patients; at times, this relationship is clearer than at others. In circumstances in which the AR is absent or the genetic defect completely inactivates the receptor, it is not difficult to understand the association with the clinical phenotype of complete testicular feminization. In contrast to these clear-cut situations, when the receptor is not completely defective, precise quantitation of the degree of AR impairment can be more difficult. In such circumstances, the results can be subject to considerable variability introduced by the methods that are used to assess AR function. An example of how such methodological changes could affect measures of AR function was demonstrated by Marcelli et al., who demonstrated that variations in hormone dosing could dramatically alter the levels of receptor function that were measured *(27)*. One avenue to circumvent the effects of transfection is the use of an adenovirus to deliver a model androgen-responsive reporter gene directly into patient fibroblasts. Such a method permits the measurement of AR function and represents one way to minimize the artifacts inherent in assays performed using transfection into heterologous cells *(69)*.

VARIATIONS IN PHENOTYPE

In some syndromes of hormone resistance, such as the generalized resistance to thyroid hormone, identical genotypes have been associated with considerable phenotypic variation. By contrast, similar phenotypes are usually observed in pedigrees in which androgen resistance is caused by mutation of the AR.

Exceptions to this statement clearly exist. In most such instances, the degrees of phenotypic variation have been relatively minor and are seen in patients with intermediate phenotypes, such as the Reifenstein phenotype *(70–72)*. When analyzed at the molecular level, the mutant receptors are only partially defective. Contributions to the extent of this variation have not been exhaustively studied, but have been postulated to include the contribution of factors such as variations in androgen levels *(72)* and the levels of expression of 5α-reductase 2 *(70)*.

A completely different mechanism that could contribute to variations in phenotype has been suggested by the report of Holterhus et al. *(73)*. These authors identified a termination codon in a patient affected with a partial form of androgen resistance, a phenotype inconsistent with that observed for most patients expressing truncated ARs. This apparent discrepancy was explained when studies established that the subject was a genetic mosaic of two AR genes: a normal AR gene and one harboring the truncation mutation. The partial virilized phenotype was a consequence of the expression of a normal AR in a proportion of the patients' fibroblasts. It is not yet established with what frequency this finding can be generalized to other instances in which phenotypic variation occurs.

VARIATIONS IN THE STRUCTURE
OF THE ANDROGEN RECEPTOR GENE

The human AR is unusual in that it contains three separate motifs composed of elements encoding direct repeats of single-amino-acid residues: glutamine, glycine, and proline. Although uncommon, such repeats are not unique to the AR and have been identified in genes encoding other transcription factors, including other members of the nuclear-receptor family.

Each of these elements shows different degrees of sequence variation in the general population. The proline homopolymeric repeat is constant in length and no sequence-length polymorphisms have been reported. In like fashion, the glycine repeat appears to be relatively invariant, although length polymorphisms have been identified in some analyses *(74)*.

In contrast to the proline and glycine repeats, the glutamine homopolymeric domain is highly polymorphic. This has become evident in the course of identifying mutations within AR genes of a number of different pedigrees, as well as from population studies focused on determining the frequency with which this trinucleotide repeat is polymorphic *(33,75,76)*. Although a wide range of lengths are present in the normal population, in most instances this repeat encodes a segment containing 20–23 glutamine residues. This segment of the human AR gene is sufficiently polymorphic in the general population that it has been possible to use it to trace the inheritance of specific AR alleles in family studies.

In addition to their importance as polymorphic markers, it appears that variations in the length of the glutamine homopolymeric segment of the human androgen receptor have functional implications as well. As noted in the following section, alterations in the length of this repeated element have been implicated in the pathogenesis of spinal and bulbar muscular atrophy and have been associated with an increased risk of oligospermia and of developing aggressive forms of prostate cancer.

SPINAL AND BULBAR MUSCULAR ATROPHY

One of the most unexpected alterations of AR structure to be reported was the identification of size variations of the segment encoding the glutamine repeat of the human AR as the genetic change responsible for the development of X- linked spinal and bulbar muscular atrophy (Kennedy's disease). Males carrying this genetic change develop normally and exhibit normal sexual function early in life. During middle age, males carrying a single mutant allele begin to exhibit phenotypic changes characteristic of mild androgen resistance (such as gynecomastia). In this same time frame, neurological symptoms appear as a result of a progressive loss of motor neurons from spinal and bulbar nuclei. Seminal work by La Spada and colleagues *(77)* traced the pathogenesis of this disorder to the expansion of the glutamine homopolymeric domain within the amino terminus of the AR gene (>45 in affected individuals, compared to approx 20 in normal controls). The mechanisms by which these expansions of the glutamine repeat cause the androgen resistance and the neurological symptoms that are observed are still under active investigation. It is clear that this glutamine expansion is somehow responsible for both a partial loss of function (with respect to the activity of the androgen receptor) and for a toxic gain of function (that is responsible for the appearance of the neurological symptoms) *(78,79)*.

AR MUTATIONS IN PROSTATE CANCER

Unexpected responses of the LNCaP cell line to AR antagonists led to the discovery of a mutation within the LBD of the AR that resulted in an apparent relaxation of the ligand responsiveness of the androgen receptor expressed in this cell line *(80)*. In the case of this mutation (T877A), although responsiveness to agonists is preserved (activation in response to dihydrotestosterone or testosterone), the T877A AR is also responding to a variety of agents that cannot activate the normal human AR.

Such somatic mutations may well contribute to the "androgen-independent" growth that is characteristic of advanced prostate cancer. It appears that such mutations are rare in early forms of prostate cancer *(81,82)* and are more frequent in more advanced stages of the disease *(83–85)* (reviewed in ref. *86*). Furthermore, when mutant receptors of this type have been examined in detail, they are found to display altered specificities. Such mutant ARs can be activated by ligands that are unable to activate the normal androgen receptor *(83,84,87–89)*.

It is possible to place such "gain-of-function" alterations of ligand specificity into a conceptual framework pertaining to the appearance and progression of prostate cancer. This is not as easy for a number for other alterations of the AR gene that have been identified in prostate cancer, including amplification of the AR gene and sequence variations in the untranslated segments of the AR *(90–94)*.

DISTRIBUTION OF AR GENE MUTATIONS

A large number of mutations causing a number of different types of androgen-resistant phenotype have now been reported, permitting tentative conclusions to be drawn regarding the relationship between the type of genetic alterations in AR gene and the degree of androgen resistance that is observed. First, it is clear that androgen resistance can be caused a variety of different types of mutation that interrupt the integrity of the AR open reading frame, including complete or partial gene deletions, insertions, premature termination, and abnormalities of AR mRNA splicing. Despite the diversity of potential defects, the common mechanism is the production of a defective receptor protein or the accumulation of the reduced quantity of functional AR. In each instance, the phenotype is that of complete androgen insensitivity (complete testicular feminization).

Nucleotide replacements that result in the substitution of the single-amino-acid residue within the AR protein are the most frequent and interesting defects causing androgen resistance. These mutations are localized to the hormone-binding or DNA-binding domains of the receptor. The sites within the open reading frame where these mutations have been identified do not appear to represent regions of increased rates of mutagenesis (e.g., CG islands), but, instead, represent regions within the AR that are critical enough to be functionally affected by single-amino-acid replacements. More recently, the insights from the solution of the crystal structures of the DBD and LBDs of the AR and related receptors have led to the recognition of structural correlates to the functional abnormalities caused by some of the mutations of the human AR *(9–11)*.

It is also interesting to consider the relative lack of mutations that have been localized to the amino terminus of the receptor protein. The few mutations that have been identified within the amino terminus are those that result—directly or indirectly—in the premature termination or inefficient synthesis of the receptor protein. This is likely because the functions of the amino terminus are more diffuse compared to other segments of the receptor protein (e.g., the DBD and LBD). This concept would fit well with the conclusions of in vitro mutagenesis studies conducted by a number of investigators, namely that although the integrity of the amino terminus is critical for full receptor function, important regions are spread over large portions of the amino terminus *(14–16)*.

SUMMARY

A large body of information has now been derived from the analyses of patients with different types of AR mutation. The behavior of most of the mutations encountered in patients presenting with disorders of sexual development are consistent with a simple "loss-of-function" type of mechanism; that is, the type of mutation is not as important as the effect that the mutation has on the level of AR function or the level of AR expression. Although such assessments will always be imperfect, it appears that a broad agreement exists between the phenotypes that are observed in patients and measures of AR abundance and function in cell culture and in in vitro assays. Those cases where discordance has been observed between individuals carrying the same AR mutation (between pedigrees or between affected members of a single pedigree) likely represent instances where variations in the activity of the receptor or in the levels of androgen are sufficient to account for the variations observed. Understanding these differences may well provide important insights into the influences that serve as modifiers of androgen action.

It has become apparent in recent years that alterations of AR structure have significance beyond the realm of androgen resistance. Alterations in the length of the glutamine repeat within the amino terminus of the human AR have been implicated in the pathogenesis of two diseases: spinal and bulbar muscular atrophy and prostate cancer. Although the mechanisms by which such changes in AR structure contribute to the biology of these diseases are still under active investigation, it appears that, in both diseases, the genetic alterations of the receptor result in the acquisition of novel properties (gain-of-function mutation). In spinal and bulbar muscular atrophy, the glutamine repeat expansion causes the degenerations of specific sets of neurons, whereas in prostate cancer, contraction of this same element is associated with an increased risk of developing aggressive forms of prostate cancer. In the same vein, the identification of somatic mutations of the androgen receptor in advanced prostatic malignancies that display altered ligand responsiveness (particularly in the context of treatment with antiandrogens) suggests that the appearance of such genetic alterations in the tumor cells may well play a role in the progression of this disease as well.

REFERENCES

1. Koopman P. Sry and Sox9: mammalian testis-determining genes. Cell Mol Life Sci 1999;55:839–856.
2. Jost A, Vigier B, Prepin J, Perchellet JP. Studies on sex differentiation in mammals. Recent Prog Horm Res 1973;29:1–41.
3. Quigley CA. Disorders of Sex Determination and Differentiation. In: Jameson, JL, ed. Principles of Molecular Medicine. Humana Totowa, NJ, 1998.
4. Lane AH, Donahoe PK. New insights into mullerian inhibiting substance and its mechanism of action. J Endocrinol 1998;158:1–6.
5. Griffin JE, McPhaul MJ, Russell DW, Wilson JD. The androgen resistance syndromes: steroid 5α-reductase 2 deficiency, testicular feminization, and related disorders. In: Scriver CR, Beaudet AL, Sly WS, et al., eds. The Metabolic and Molecular Bases of Inherited Disease. 7th Edition. McGraw-Hill, New York, 1995, Vol. II, pp 2967–2998.
6. Quigley CA, De Bellis A, Marschke KB, et al. Androgen receptor defects: historical, clinical, and molecular perspectives Endocr Rev 1995;16:271–321.
7. Morris JM. The syndrome of testicular feminization in male pseudohermaphrodites. Am J Obstet Gynecol 1953;65:1192–1211.
8. Mangelsdorf DJ, Thummel C, Beato M, et. al. The nuclear receptor superfamily: the second decade. Cell 1995;83:835–839.
9. Matias PM, Donner P, Coelho R, et al. Structural evidence for ligand specificity in the binding domain of the human androgen receptor. Implications for pathogenic gene mutations. J Biol Chem 2000;275:26164–26171.
10. Sack JS, Kish KF, Wang C, et al. Crystallographic structures of the ligand-binding domains of the androgen receptor and its T877A mutant complexed with the natural agonist dihydrotestosterone. Proc Natl Acad Sci USA 2001;98:4904–4909.
11. Poujol N, Lobaccaro JM, Chiche L, et al. Functional and structural analysis of R607Q and R608K androgen receptor substitutions associated with male breast cancer. Mol Cell Endocrinol 1997;130:43–51.
12. Zhou ZX, Sar M, Simental JA, et al. A ligand-dependent bipartite nuclear targeting signal in the human androgen receptor. Requirement for the DNA-binding domain and modulation by NH2-terminal and carboxyl-terminal sequences. J Biol Chem 1994;269:13115–13123.
13. Jenster G, Trapman J, Brinkmann AO. Nuclear import of the human androgen receptor. Biochem J 1993;293:761–768.
14. Simental JA, Sar M, Lane MV, et al. Transcriptional activation and nuclear targeting signals of the human androgen receptor. J Biol Chem 1991;266:510–518.
15. Jenster G, van der Korput HA, van Vroonhoven C, et al. Domains of the human androgen receptor involved in steroid binding, transcriptional activation, and subcellular localization. Mol Endo 1991;5:1396–1404.
16. Gao TS, Marcelli M, McPhaul MJ. Transcriptional activation and transient expression of the human androgen receptor. J. Steroid Biochem Mol Biol 1996;59:9–20.
17. Brown TR, Lubahn DB, Wilson EM, et al. Deletion of the steroid -binding domain of the human androgen receptor gene in one family with complete androgen insensitivity syndrome: evidence for further genetic heterogeneity in the syndrome. Proc Natl Acad Sci USA 1988;85:8151–8155.
18. Avila DM, Wilson CM, Nandi N, et al. Immunoreactive androgen receptor (AR) in genital skin fibroblasts from subjects with androgen resistance and undetectable levels of AR in ligand binding assays. J Clin Endo Metab 2002;87:182–188.
19. Quigley CA, Friedman KJ, Johnson A, et al. Complete deletion of the androgen receptor gene: definition of the null phenotype of the androgen insensitivity syndrome and determination of carrier status. J Clin Endo Metab 1992;74:927–933.
20. Trifiro M, Gottlieb B, Pinsky L, et al. The 56/58 kDa androgen-binding protein in male genital skin fibroblasts with a deleted androgen receptor gene. Mol Cell Endocrinology 1991;75:37–47.
21. Ahmed SF, Cheng A, Dovey L, et al. Phenotypic features, androgen receptor binding, and mutational analysis in 278 clinical cases reported as androgen insensitivity syndrome. J Clin Endocrinol Metab 2000;85:658–665.
22. MacLean HE, Chu S, Warne GL, Zajac JD. Related individuals with different androgen receptor gene deletions. J Clin Invest 1993;91:1123–1128.
23. Zoppi S, Wilson CM, Harbison MD, et al. Complete testicular feminization caused by an amino-terminal truncation of the androgen receptor with downstream initiation. J Clin Invest 1993;91:1105–1112.

24. Ris-Stalpers C, Kuiper GG, Faber PW, et al. Aberrant splicing of androgen receptor mRNA results in synthesis of a nonfunctional receptor protein in a patient with androgen insensitivity. Proc Natl Acad Sci USA 1990;87:7866–8670.

25. Ris-Stalpers C, Verleun-Mooijman MC, de Blaeij TJ, et al. Differential splicing of human androgen receptor pre-mRNA in X-linked Reifenstein syndrome, because of a deletion involving a putative branch site. Am J Hum Genet 1994;54:609–617.

26. McPhaul MJ, Marcelli M, Zoppi S, et al. Mutations in the ligand-binding domain of the androgen receptor gene cluster in two regions of the gene. J Clin Invest 1992;90:2097–2101.

27. Marcelli M, Zoppi S, Wilson CM, et al. Amino acid substitutions in the hormone-binding domain of the human androgen receptor alter the stability of the hormone receptor complex. J Clin Invest 1994;94:1642–1650.

28. Marcelli M, Tilley WD, Zoppi S, et al. Androgen resistance associated with a mutation of the androgen receptor at amino acid 772 (ArggCys) results from a combination of decreased messenger ribonucleic acid levels and impairment of receptor function. J Clin Endocrinol Metab 1991;73:318–325.

29. Wilson CM, Griffin JE, Wilson JD, et al. Immunoreactive androgen receptor expression in patients with androgen resistance. J Clin Endocrinol Metab 1992;75:1474–1478.

30. Lubahn DB, Brown TR, Simental JA, et al. Sequence of the intron/exon junctions of the coding region of the human androgen receptor gene and identification of a point mutation in a family with complete androgen insensitivity. Proc Natl Acad Sci USA 1989;86:9534–9538.

31. Brown TR, Lubahn DB, Wilson EM, et al. Functional characterization of naturally occurring mutant androgen receptors from subjects with complete androgen insensitivity. Mol Endocrinol 1990;4:1759–1772.

32. Grino PB, Isidro-Gutierrez RF, Griffin JE, Wilson JD. Androgen resistance associated with a qualitative abnormality of the androgen receptor and responsive to high dose androgen therapy. J Clin Endo Metab 1989;68:578–584.

33. McPhaul MJ, Marcelli M, Tilley WD, et al. Molecular basis of androgen resistance in a family with a qualitative abnormality of the androgen receptor and responsive to high-dose androgen therapy. J Clin Invest 1991;87:1413–1421.

34. Langley E, Zhou ZX, Wilson EM. Evidence for an anti-parallel orientation of the ligand-activated human androgen receptor dimmer. J Biol Chem 1995;270:29983–29990.

35. Doesburg P, Kuil CW, Berrevoets CA, et al. Functional in vivo interaction between the amino-terminal, transactivation domain and the ligand binding domain of the androgen receptor. Biochemistry 1997;36:1052–1064.

36. Prior L, Bordet S, MA Trifiro, et al. Replacement of arginine 773 by cysteine or histidine in the human androgen receptor causes complete androgen insensitivity with different receptor phenotypes. Am J Hum Genet 1992;51:143–155.

37. Beitel LK, Kazemi-Esfarjani P, Kaufman M, et al. Substitution of arginine-839 by cysteine or histidine in the androgen receptor causes different receptor phenotypes in cultured cells and coordinate degrees of clinical androgen resistance. J Clin Invest 1994;94:546–554.

38. P Kazemi-Esfarjani, Beitel LK, Trifiro M, et al. Substitution of valine-865 by methionine or leucine in the human androgen receptor causes complete or partial androgen insensitivity, respectively with distinct androgen receptor phenotypes. Mol Endocrinol 1993;7:37–46.

39. Ris-Stalpers C, Trifiro MA, Kuiper GG, et al. Substitution of aspartic acid-686 by histidine or asparagine in the human androgen receptor leads to a functionally inactive protein with altered hormone-binding characteristics. Mol Endocrinol 1991;5:1562–1569.

40. Tincello DG, Saunders PT, Hodgins MB, et al. Correlation of clinical, endocrine and molecular abnormalities with in vivo responses to high-dose testosterone in patients with partial androgen insensitivity syndrome. Clin Endocrinology 1997;46:497–506.

41. Yong EL, Ng SC, Roy AC, et al. Pregnancy after hormonal correction of severe spermatogenic defect due to mutation in androgen receptor gene Lancet 1994;344:826–827.

42. Ong YC, Wong HB, Adaikan G, Yong EL. Directed pharmacological therapy of ambiguous genitalia due to an androgen receptor gene mutation Lancet 1999;354:1444–1445.

43. Tincello DG, Saunders PT, Hodgins MB, et al. Correlation of clinical, endocrine and molecular abnormalities with in vivo responses to high-dose testosterone in patients with partial androgen insensitivity syndrome. Clin Endocrinol 1997;46:497–506.

44. Radmayr C, Culig Z., Hobisch A, et al. Analysis of a mutant androgen receptor offers a treatment modality in a patient with partial androgen insensitivity syndrome. Eur Urol 1998;33:222–226.

45. Weidemann W, Peters B, Romalo G, et al. Response to androgen treatment in a patient with partial androgen insensitivity and a mutation in the deoxyribonucleic acid-binding domain of the androgen receptor. J Clin Endocrinol Metab 1998;83:1173–1176.

46. Zoppi S, Marcelli M, Deslypere JP, et al. Amino acid substitutions in the DNA-binding domain of the human androgen receptor are a frequent cause of receptor-binding positive androgen resistance. Mol Endocrinol 1992;6:409–415.

47. Beitel LK, Prior L, Vasiliou DM, et al. Complete androgen insensitivity due to mutations in the probable alpha-helical segments of the DNA-binding domain in the human androgen receptor. Hum Mol Genet 1994;3:21–27.

48. De Bellis A, Quigley CA, Marschke KB, et al. Characterization of mutant androgen receptors causing partial androgen insensitivity syndrome. J Clin Endocrinol Metab 1994;78:513–522.

49. Sultan C, Lumbroso S, Poujol N, et al. Mutations of androgen receptor gene in androgen insensitivity syndromes. J Steroid Biochem Mol Biol 1993;46:519–530.

50. Lumbroso S, Lobaccaro JM, Belon C, et al. A new mutation within the deoxyribonucleic acid-binding domain of the androgen receptor gene in a family with complete androgen insensitivity syndrome. Fertil Steril 1993;60:814–819.

51. Mowszowicz I, Lee HJ, Chen HT, et al. A point mutation in the second zinc finger of the DNA-binding domain of the androgen receptor gene causes complete androgen insensitivity in two siblings with receptor-positive androgen resistance. Mol Endo 1993;7:861–869.

52. Quigley CA, Evans BAJ, Simental JA. Complete androgen insensitivity due to deletion of exon C of the androgen receptor gene highlights the functional importance of the second zinc-finger of the androgen receptor in vivo. Mol Endocrinol 1992;6:1103–1112.

53. Wooster R, Mangion J, Eeles R, et al. A germline mutation in the androgen receptor gene in two brothers with breast cancer and Reifenstein syndrome. Nat Genet 1992;2:132–134.

54. Evans RM. The steroid and thyroid hormone receptor superfamily. Science 1988;240:889–895.

55. Lobaccaro JM, Lumbroso S, Belon C, et al. Androgen receptor gene mutation in male breast cancer. Hum Mol Genet 1993;2:1799–1802.

56. Poujol N, Lobaccaro JM, Chiche L, et al. Functional and structural analysis of R607Q and R608K androgen receptor substitutions associated with male breast cancer. Mol Cell Endocrinology 1997;130:43–51.

57. Wilson CM, McPhaul MJ. A and B forms of the androgen receptor are present in human genital skin fibroblasts. Proc Natl Acad Sci USA 1994;91:1234–1238.

58. Gao TS, McPhaul MJ. Functional activities of the A- and B- forms of the human androgen receptor in response to androgen receptor agonists and antagonists. Mol Endo 1998;12:654–663.

59. Choong CS, Quigley CA, French FS, Wilson EM. A novel missense mutation in the amino-terminal domain of the human androgen receptor gene in a family with partial androgen insensitivity syndrome causes reduced efficiency of protein translation. J Clin Invest 1996;98:1423–1431.

60. Tsukada T, Inoue M, Tachibana S, et al. An androgen receptor mutation causing androgen resistance in undervirilized male syndrome. J Clin Endocrinol Metab 1994;79:1202–1207.

61. Wang Q, Ghadessy FJ, Trounson A, et al. Azoospermia associated with a mutation in the ligand-binding domain of an androgen receptor displaying normal ligand binding, but defective transactivation. J Clin Endocrinol Metab 1998;83:4303–4309.

62. Lim J, Ghadessy FJ, Abdullah AAR, et al. Human androgen receptor mutation disrupts ternary interactions between ligand, receptor domains, and the coactivator TIF2 (transcription intermediary factor 2). Mol Endocrinol 2000;14:1187–1197.

63. Ghadessy FJ, Lim J, Abdullah AAR, et al. Oligospermic infertility associated with an androgen receptor mutation that disrupts interdomain and coactivator (TIF2) interactions. J Clin Invest 1999;103:1517–1525.

64. Patrizio P, Leonard DGB, Chen KL, et al. Larger trinucleotide repeat size in the androgen receptor gene of infertile men with extremely severe oligozoospermia. J Androl 2001;22:444–448.

65. Mifsud A, Sim CKS, Boettger-Tong H, et al. Trinucleotide (CAG) repeat polymorphisms in the androgen receptor gene: molecular markers of risk for male infertility. Fertility Sterility 2001;75:275–281.

66. Tut TG, Ghadessy FJ, Trifiro MA, et al. Long polyglutamine tracts in the androgen receptor are associated with reduced trans-activation, impaired sperm production, and male infertility. J Clin Endocrinol Metab 1997;82:3777–3782.

67. Yong EL, Lim LSE, Wang Q, et al. Androgen receptor polymorphisms and mutations in male infertility. J Endocrinol Invest 2000;23:573–577.

68. Dowsing AT, Yong EL, Clark M, et al. Linkage between male infertility and trinucleotide repeat expansion in the androgen-receptor gene Lancet 1999;354:640–643.

69. McPhaul MJ, Schweikert H-U, Allman. DR Assessment of androgen receptor function in genital skin fibroblasts using a recombinant adenovirus to deliver an androgen-responsive reporter gene. J Clin Endo Metab 1997;82:1944–1948.

70. Evans BA, Hughes IA, Bevan CL, et al. Phenotypic diversity in siblings with partial androgen insensitivity syndrome. Arch Dis Child 1997;76:529–531.

71. Boehmer AL, Brinkmann AO, Nijman RM, et al. Phenotypic variation in a family with partial androgen insensitivity syndrome explained by differences in 5alpha dihydrotestosterone availability. J Clin Endocrinol Metab 2001;86:1240–1246.

72. Holterhus PM, Sinnecker GH, Hiort O. Phenotypic diversity and testosterone-induced normalization of mutant L712F androgen receptor function in a kindred with androgen insensitivity. J Clin Endocrinol Metab 2000;85:3245–3250.

73. Holterhus PM, Bruggenwirth HT, Hiort O, et al. Mosaicism due to a somatic mutation of the androgen receptor gene determines phenotype in androgen insensitivity syndrome. J Clin Endo Metab 1997;82:3584–3589.

74. Sleddens HF, Oostra BA, Brinkmann AO, Trapman J. Trinucleotide (GGN) repeat polymorphism in the human androgen receptor (AR) gene. Hum Mol Genet 1993;2:493.

75. Sleddens HF, Oostra BA, Brinkmann AO, Trapman J. Trinucleotide repeat polymorphism in the androgen receptor gene (AR). Nucleic Acids Res 1992;20:1427.

76. Edwards A, Hammond HA, Jin L, et al. Genetic variation at five trimeric and tetrameric tandem repeat loci in four human population groups. Genomics 1992;12:241–253.

77. La Spada AR, Wilson EM, Lubahn DB, et al. Androgen receptor gene mutations in X-linked spinal and bulbar muscular atrophy. Nature 1991;352:77–79.

78. Brooks BP, Fischbeck KH. Spinal and bulbar muscular atrophy: a trinucleotide-repeat expansion neurodegenerative disease. Trends Neurosci 1995;18:459–461.

79. Neuschmid-Kaspar F, Gast A, Peterziel H, et al. CAG-repeat expansion in androgen receptor in Kennedy's disease is not a loss of function mutation. Mol Cell Endocrinol 1996;117:149–156.

80. J Veldscholte, Ris-Stalpers C, Kuiper GG, et al. A mutation in the ligand binding domain of the androgen receptor of human LNCaP cells affects steroid binding characteristics and response to anti-androgens. Biochem Biophys Res Commun 1990;173:534–540.

81. Newmark JR, Hardy DO, Tonb DC, et al. Androgen receptor gene mutations in human prostate cancer. Proc Natl Acad Sci USA 1992;89:6319–6323.

82. Evans BA, Harper ME, Daniells CE, et al. Low incidence of androgen receptor gene mutations in human prostatic tumors using single strand conformation polymorphism analysis. Prostate 1996;28:162–171.

83. Taplin ME, Bubley GJ, Shuster TD, et al. Mutation of the androgen-receptor gene in metastatic androgen-independent prostate cancer. N Engl J Med 1995;332:1393–1398.

84. Tilley WD, Buchanan G, Hickey TE, Bentel JM. Mutations in the androgen receptor gene are associated with progression of human prostate cancer to androgen independence. Clin Cancer Res 1996;2:277–285.

85. Marcelli M, Ittmann M, Mariani S, et al. Androgen receptor mutations in prostate cancer. Cancer Res 2000;60:944–949.

86. McPhaul MJ, Avila DM, Zoppi S, McPhaul MJ. The androgen receptor (AR) in syndromes of androgen insensitivity and in prostate cancer. J Steroid Biochem Mol Biol 2001;76:135–142.

87. Culig Z, Hobisch A, Cronauer MV, et al. Mutant androgen receptor detected in an advanced-stage prostatic carcinoma is activated by adrenal androgens and progesterone. Mol Endo 1993;7:1541–1550.

88. Elo JP, Kvist L, Leinonen K, et al. Mutated human androgen receptor gene detected in a prostatic cancer patient is also activated by estradiol. J Clin Endo Metab 1995;80:3494–3500.

89. Peterziel H, Culig Z, Stober J, et al. Mutant androgen receptors in prostatic tumors distinguish between amino-acid-sequence requirements for transactivation and ligand binding. Int J Cancer 1995;63:544–550.

90. Suzuki H, Sato N, Watabe Y, et al. Androgen receptor gene mutations in human prostate cancer. J Steroid Biochem Mol Biol 1993;46:759–765.

91. Suzuki H, Akakura K, Komiya A, et al. Codon 877 mutation in the androgen receptor gene in advanced prostate cancer: relation to antiandrogen withdrawal syndrome. Prostate 1996;29:153–158.

92. Koivisto P, Kononen J, Palmberg C, et al. Androgen receptor gene amplification: a possible molecular mechanism for androgen deprivation therapy failure in prostate cancer. Cancer Res 1997;57:314–319.
93. Crocitto LE, Henderson BE, Coetzee GA. Identification of two germline point mutations in the 5'UTR of the androgen receptor gene in men with prostate cancer. J Urol 1997;158:1599–1601.
94. Paz A, Lindner A, Zisman A, Siegel Y. A genetic sequence change in the 3'-noncoding region of the androgen receptor gene in prostate carcinoma. Eur Urol 1997;31:209–215.

7

Androgen Excess Disorders in Women

Richard S. Legro, MD

CONTENTS

INTRODUCTION
VIRILIZATION
HIRSUTISM
NONCLASSICAL CONGENITAL ADRENAL HYPERPLASIA
CUSHING'S SYNDROME
ANDROGEN EXCESS WITHOUT A PHENOTYPE
TREATMENT OF ANDROGEN EXCESS
SUMMARY
ACKNOWLEDGMENT
REFERENCES

INTRODUCTION

Androgen excess disorders are common in women and may represent the most common endocrinological reason for a physician visit. They are a heterogeneous group of disorders that can produce a common phenotype, and the current differential diagnosis most commonly arrives at polycystic ovary syndrome (PCOS) as the diagnosis of choice. Circulating levels of androgens rarely track into the male range—usually only in cases of virilizing forms of congenital adrenal hyperplasia and androgen-secreting tumors (including many forms of Cushing's syndrome) (*see* Fig. 1). For the more common forms of androgen excess, there is a fine line between normal and elevated androgen levels, with marked peripheral phenotypic signs of androgen excess in a women at circulating testosterone levels of 100–150 ng/dL. This is still only half the lower limit of normal for males, for whom the normal range is approx 300–1000 ng/dL.

Circulating levels of androgens remain a poor diagnostic tool for the source of androgen excess and are only one facet of androgen's action on the body (*see* Fig. 2). They are commonly investigated as the source of androgenic stigmata, but increased androgen production is just one facet of androgen action. Both the adrenal glands and ovaries contribute to the circulating androgen pool in women. The adrenal preferentially secretes weak androgens such as DHEA (dehydroepiandrosterone) or its sulfated "depot" form DHEA-S (up to 90% of adrenal origin). These hormones, in addition to androstenedione (often elevated in women with PCOS), may serve as prohormones for more potent androgens such as testosterone or dihydrotestosterone (DHT). The ovary

From: *Contemporary Endocrinology: Androgens in Health and Disease*
Edited by: C. Bagatell and W. J. Bremner © Humana Press Inc., Totowa, NJ

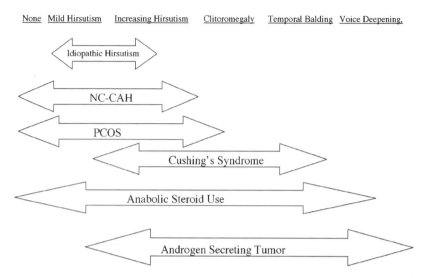

Fig. 1. The spectrum of phenotypes for various androgen excess disorders.

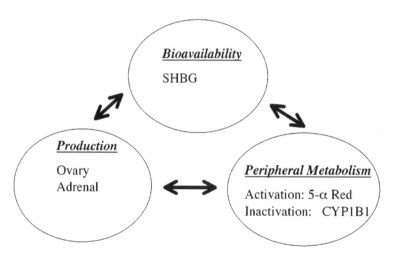

Fig. 2. The triumvirate of androgen action. SHBG, sex hormone-binding globulin; 5–α Red, 5α-reductase; CYP1B1, cytochrome P450, subfamily 1, polypeptide 1.

is the preferential source of testosterone, and it is estimated that 75% of circulating testosterone originates from the ovary (mainly through peripheral conversion of prohormones by liver, fat, and skin, but also through direct ovarian secretion). Androstenedione, largely of ovarian origin, is the only circulating androgen that is higher in premenopausal women than men, yet its androgenic potency is only 10% of testosterone. DHT is the most potent androgen, although it circulates in negligible quantities, and results primarily from the intracellular 5α-reduction of testosterone. In the past, measurement of 3α-androstanediol glucuronide, a peripheral metabolite of DHT was used as a circulating marker of androgen excess in the skin (hirsutism and acne), but its clinical use is negligible.

Table 1
Differential Diagnosis
of Androgen Excess in Women

Congenital adrenal hyperplasia (CAH)
Cushing's syndrome
Androgen-producing tumor—ovary or adrenal
Exogenous anabolic/sex steroids
Hyperprolactinemia
Severely insulin-resistant states
Polycystic ovary syndrome (PCOS)

In addition to increased production of androgens by the ovaries and adrenal glands, increased androgen action may be realized by suppression of binding globulins, primarily sex hormone-binding globulin (SHBG) but also insulin-like growth factor (IGF)-binding globulins, leading to increased bioavailable androgen and free IGF. There may be enhanced local tissue sensitivity to circulating androgens, as has been proposed in the case of idiopathic hirsutism with greater 5α-reductase activity. Additionally, there are a variety of peripheral tissues that can potentiate or inactivate the circulating androgen pool to modify androgen action (i.e., fat and liver).

There are a variety of conditions that can cause androgen excess (*see* Table 1). Some such as prolactin excess tend to be more apocryphal than daily clinical occurrences (abnormal forms or marked elevation of prolactin may have gonadotropin-like effects on androgen secretion). PCOS is probably the most common etiology of androgen excess and it remains the diagnosis of exclusion. It affects 5% of women in the developed world *(1)*.

Although there is no consensus to the definition of PCOS, the diagnostic criteria from the 1990 NIH–NICHD conference on PCOS will be used: hyperandrogenism and/or hyperandrogenemia, oligo-ovulation, and exclusion of other potential causes such as congenital adrenal hyperplasia, hyperprolactinemia, Cushing's syndrome, and androgen-secreting tumors *(2)*. Thus, PCOS represents unexplained hyperandrogenic chronic anovulation and is a diagnosis of exclusion. This chapter will focus on various androgenic phenotypes and their clinical management that occur in reproductive-age women: from virilization to minimal clinical signs of androgen excess.

VIRILIZATION

Clinical Presentation

Virilization in an adult women is a rare disorder and must be separated from more common and less severe causes of androgen excess in women, such as PCOS. Virilization includes the common signs of acne and hirsutism, but it is also accompanied by other peripheral effects such as temporal balding, clitoromegaly, deepening of the voice, breast atrophy, and changes in body contour. A rapid presentation of the virilization often leads to a speedy evaluation and diagnosis, whereas the more lingering forms may be overlooked until there is marked masculinization. Virilization is never "idiopathic" and all cases need to be investigated until a cause is discovered. PCOS or nonclassical congenital adrenal hyperplasia (NC-CAH) rarely causes virilization.

Virilization presents with a variety of peripheral effects. Acne and hirsutism are invariably present. In virilization balding in women tends to present with centripetal balding and frontal recession more characteristic of androgenic alopecia in men, as opposed to the more indolent presentation of androgenic alopecia in women with a generalized thinning of the crown region *(3)*. A deepening of the voice has been reported in women with androgen-secreting tumors or undergoing exogenous androgen treatment (this does not necessarily improve after removal of the androgen excess). Increase in the size of the larynx is one factor in the voice change. Clitoromegaly is defined as a clitoral index greater than 35 mm^2 (the clitoral index is the product of the sagittal and transverse diameters of the glans of the clitoris) *(4)*. In normal women, these diameters are in the range of 5 mm each. The degree of clitoral enlargement correlates with the degree of androgen excess. Androgens can lead to body composition changes especially in the upper body, with increased muscle mass and decreased fat mass. This is accompanied by breast atrophy.

Differential Diagnosis

The differential diagnosis of androgen excess leading to virilization, especially combined with a sudden onset and rapid progression will always begin and end with tumors or dysfunctional states, usually of the ovary and, less commonly, of the adrenal. The most common androgen-producing tumor in a premenopausal woman is a Sertoli–Leydig cell tumor. Any large ovarian tumor can produce androgens indirectly by causing hyperplasia of the surrounding normal stroma (i.e., benign cystic teratomas, dysgerminomas, epithelial tumors). The vast majority of ovarian androgen-secreting tumors are benign. Adrenal tumors are rare, with an estimated incidence of two cases per one million persons per year, these are equally divided among adenomas and carcinomas. The age of onset in adults peaks in the fifth decade. Virilization can accompany both tumors primarily producing androgens and tumors primarily producing cortisol (Cushing's syndrome). A long history of symptoms, as in the case with an ovarian tumor does not exclude the presence of an adrenocortical neoplasm.

Dysfunctional states of the ovary, primarily hyperthecosis may also result in marked androgen excess. In stromal hyperthecosis, most of the ovarian androgen overproduction results from hyperplasia of the ovarian stroma and not from the accumulation of small follicles, as is the case with PCOS. Most women with stromal hyperthecosis have severe hyperinsulinemia, which may be the stimulus for stromal androgen overproduction. It has been reported in both premenopausal and postmenopausal women, often with coexisting sequelae of the insulin-resistance syndrome such as dyslipidemia and glucose intolerance. Surgery, consisting of oophorectomy, usually results in restoration of both normal insulin levels and androgen levels in the acquired late presentations of stromal hyperthecosis.

Extreme elevations in insulin levels occur in individuals with insulin-receptor defects. A substantial number of such defects have now been identified although their overall prevalence is low. In such individuals, the elevated insulin levels may stimulate excess ovarian androgen production, resulting in what has been described as the HAIR-AN syndrome, which represents the coexistence of hyperandrogenism, insulin resistance, and acanthosis nigricans *(5)*. Also in the differential of androgen excess in an adult female are the use of exogenous androgens, anabolic steroids in a bodybuilder for example, or an overdose of androgens in postmenopausal women. Severe hirsutism and even virilization that occurs during pregnancy has its own unique differential, including benign ovarian sources such as hyperreactio luteinalis (i.e., gestational ovarian theca-lutein cysts) or luteomas. Even more rare are such fetoplacental sources such as aromatase deficiency resulting in androgen excess and even virilization in the mother, because of the placental inability to convert precursor androgens into estrogens.

HIRSUTISM

Mechanisms of Hirsutism

The pilosebaceous unit (PSU) is the common skin structure that gives rise to both hair follicles and sebaceous glands and are found everywhere on the body except the palms and soles. The density is greatest on the face and scalp (400–800 glands/cm^2) and lowest on the extremities (50 glands/cm^2). The number of PSUs does not increase after birth (about 5 million), but they can become more prominent through activation and differentiation. Before puberty, the body hair is primarily fine, unpigmented, vellus hair. After puberty and stimulated by the increased androgens, some of these hairs (mainly midline hair) are transformed into coarser, pigmented, terminal hairs. A similar mechanism may explain the increase in acne with puberty with increased sebum production by the sebaceous glands. One of the central paradoxes is that androgens can exert opposite effects (vellus to terminal, terminal to vellus), depending on the site of the hair follicle (*see* Fig. 3).

Hirsutism is defined as excess body hair in undesirable locations, and, as such, it is a subjective phenomenon that makes both diagnosis and treatment difficult. Hirsutism should be viewed much as polycystic ovaries, as a sign rather than a diagnosis *(6)*. Most commonly, hirsutism is associated with androgen excess, or what is referred to as androgen-dependent hirsutism. This tends to be a midline predominant hair growth. It is important to note that factors other than androgen action may contribute to the development of hirsutism. Hyperinsulinemia, which accompanies many benign forms of virilization, can also stimulate the PSU directly, or indirectly by contributing to hyperandrogenemia. Although insulin resistance is not one of the diagnostic criteria for PCOS, women with PCOS appear to be uniquely insulin resistant *(7)*. Insulin resistance in the periphery, primarily skeletal muscle, which utilizes approx 85–90% of circulating insulin, is compensated for by excess insulin section by the β-cells of the pancreas. The compensatory hyperinsulinemia may contribute to androgen excess by directly stimulating androgen production in the adrenal glands and ovaries, as well as suppressing the production of key binding globulins such as SHBG (with corresponding increased bioactivity of circulating androgens) or IGF-binding globulins (leading to increased IGF action in key target tissues such as the ovary). Insulin also has myriad effects on cellular metabolism, including amino acid and electrolyte transport, stimulating lipogenesis, and serving as a mitogenic factor. Overall, the net effects are storage of energy in the form of carbohydrate, protein, and fat.

Differential Diagnosis of Hirsutism

The differential diagnosis of hirsutism includes the disorders of androgen excess included in the virilization section, but, more commonly, it involves PCOS, NC-CAH, or idiopathic cases. Idiopathic hirsutism was coined to identify the presence of hirsutism in a eumenorrheic women with normal circulating androgens, but this may reflect our limited ability to assess androgen action in the peripheral compartment. When thor-

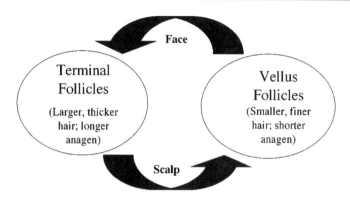

Fig. 3. The paradox of androgen excess on pilosebaceous units of the face vs the scalp.

oughly investigated for androgen excess, most idiopathic cases disappear *(8)*. Hirsutism must also be differentiated from other causes of hair growth. Androgen-independent hirsutism may be a familial tendency (familial hypertrichosis) or the result of medications, such as cyclosporin, diazoxide, minoxidil, and so forth. These medications often result in hypertrichosis, a generalized increase in body hair rather than the midline development of marked terminal hair growth. Also in the differential of androgen excess in an adult female is the use of exogenous androgens, anabolic steroids in a bodybuilder for example, or an overdose of androgens in a postmenopausal women. Severe hirsutism and even virilization that occurs during pregnancy has its own unique differential, including benign ovarian sources such as hyperreactio luteinalis (i.e., gestational ovarian theca–lutein cysts) or luteomas, and extremely rare fetoplacental sources such as aromatase deficiency resulting in androgen excess as a result of the placental inability to convert precursor androgens into estrogens.

Polycystic Ovary Syndrome

Polycystic ovary syndrome tends to develop shortly after menarche and last for most of the reproductive life—although questions persist about its natural history during the reproductive years. It has been proposed that premature pubarche may be the earliest recognizable PCOS phenotype and affected girls display hyperinsulinemia, and elevated DHEA-S levels, and after menarche they become oligomenorrheic *(9)*. At the other end of the reproductive spectrum, both menstrual irregularity *(10)* and hyperandrogenemia *(11)* appear to normalize as women with PCOS approach their late thirties to early forties. In addition to hirsutism, women with PCOS are plagued with a variety of other ailments.

INFERTILITY: CHRONIC ANOVULATION

The most common reason that women with PCOS present to the gynecologist is because of infertility, resulting from chronic anovulation *(12)*. As a general rule, women with PCOS represent one of the most difficult groups to induce ovulation both successfully and safely. Many women with PCOS are unresponsive to clomiphene citrate and human menopausal gonadotropins, and this is exacerbated by the underlying obesity. On the other end of the spectrum are women with PCOS who overrespond to both of these medications. Women with PCOS are at especially increased risks of ovarian hyperstimulation syndrome, a syndrome of massive enlargement of the ovaries and transudation of ascites into the abdominal cavity that can lead to rapid and symptomatic enlargement of the abdomen, intravascular contraction, hypercoagulability, and systemic organ dysfunction (13). They are also at increased risk for multiple pregnancy. There is also emerging evidence that baseline hyperinsulinemia may contribute to the increased ovarian hyperstimulation syndrome (OHSS) risk (14,15).

Gynecological Cancers

Many gynecological cancers have been reported to be more common in women with PCOS, including ovarian, breast, and endometrial cancer. The best case of an association between PCOS and cancer can be made for endometrial cancer. Many risk factors for endometrial cancer, including obesity, chronic anovulation, hypertension, and type 2 diabetes overlap with the PCOS phenotype (16). It is unknown how many induced withdrawal bleeds/yr are necessary to provide adequate prophylaxis against the development of uterine cancer in the PCOS population.

Type 2 Diabetes Mellitus

Women with PCOS have been found to be profoundly insulin resistant at the skeletal muscle. The mechanism is unknown. This baseline insulin resistance combined with the worsening effect of obesity (which may affect up to 50% of the American PCOS population) places these women at increased risk for impaired glucose tolerance and type 2 diabetes. About 30–40% of obese reproductive-age women with PCOS have been found to have impaired glucose tolerance, and about 10% have type 2 diabetes based on a 2-h glucose level > 200 mg/dL (17,18). Of note is that only a small fraction of women with PCOS with either impaired glucose tolerance (IGT) or type 2 diabetes display fasting hyperglycemia consistent with type 2 diabetes by the 1997 American Diabetes Association criteria (fasting glucose ≥ 126 mg/dL) (19). The conversion rate to glucose intolerance over time is uncertain, which makes recommendations for frequency of screening for glucose intolerance difficult. The level of insulin resistance found in women with PCOS based on dynamic measures of insulin action has, in other populations (i.e., children of parents with diabetes), been associated with a marked increased risk of developing type 2 diabetes mellitus.

Cardiovascular Disease

Many of the studies suggesting an increased incidence of cardiovascular disease in PCOS are inferential and are based on risk-factor models. Women with PCOS appear to form a subset of the insulin-resistance syndrome. The insulin-resistance syndrome, which consists of a constellation of symptoms, including insulin resistance, hypertension, and lipid abnormalities, has been linked to increased risk for diabetes and cardiovascular disease (20). In individuals with essential hypertension, insulin resistance results from impairment of insulin action in peripheral tissues, primarily muscle (21). Several reasons in addition to the abnormalities in glucose metabolism discussed here have been suggested to account for this relationship between hyperinsulinemia and hypertension, including sodium retention, overactivity of the sympathetic nervous system, impairment of membrane transport, and stimulation of vascular smooth muscle cells (22).

Other effects of hyperinsulinemia and insulin resistance include the development of an atherogenic plasma lipid profile resulting from insulin enhancement of synthesis of small high-density atherogenic low-density lipoprotein (LDL) subclasses and hypertriglyceridemia. Many women with PCOS have significant dyslipidemia. Studies have shown that women with PCOS have lower high-density lipoprotein (HDL) and higher triglyceride and LDL levels than age-, sex-, and weight-matched controls (23). This elevation in LDL levels *per se* (as opposed to subclasses) is not one of the characteristic findings of the insulin-resistance syndrome, but it contributes to increased cardiovascular risk. Epidemiological studies have shown that hyperlipidemia, including hypertriglyceridemia (especially in women) and elevated LDL/HDL ratios, are associated with an increased risk of atherogenesis.

Hypertensive individuals are more likely to be hyperinsulinemic than controls who are normotensive (21). Insulin resistance persists in these individuals despite successful antihypertensive medication. However, hypertension has not been consistently associated with PCOS, at least not in women of reproductive age (24,25). This is a significant factor that prevents lumping all women with PCOS under the insulin-resistance syndrome. Long-term follow-up of women with PCOS may reveal an increased incidence of hypertension compared to age- and weight-matched controls. This may represent a later sequelae of prolonged insulin resistance. Recent studies have documented other interim risk factors (e.g., increased carotid artery intimal thickness) to suggest that these women have evidence of atherosclerotic disease at an earlier and more advanced stage than appropriate control women (26). Confirmation of this based on actual cardiovascular events such as stroke or myocardial infarction in women with PCOS has not yet appeared.

NONCLASSICAL CONGENITAL ADRENAL HYPERPLASIA

The CYP21 (21-hydroxylase) gene is the most commonly mutated gene in humans, as it is tightly linked to the human leukocyte antigen (HLA) locus on the short arm of chromosome 6, a frequent site of genetic recombination. It is estimated to be present in less than 1% of unselected hirsute women (27). CAH occurs with the highest frequency in the US population among Native Americans in Alaska. Other populations with high carrier status are Ashkenazi Jews (3.7%), Latinos (1.9%), Yugoslavs (1.6%), and Italians (0.3%) (28). Because of the lack of 21-hydroxylation, 17-hydroxyprogesterone accumulates. Because of the lack of cortisol synthesis, ACTH levels increase resulting in overproduction and accumulation of cortisol precursors. These, in turn, can be shunted to androgen biosynthetic pathways, which causes excessive production of androgens, resulting in virilization. NC-CAH can be screened for with a fasting 17-OHP level in the morning. A value less than 2 ng/mL is normal, and, recently, cutoffs as high as 4 ng/mL have been proposed if obtained in the morning and during the follicular phase (29). Values above the cutoff should be screened with an ACTH stimulation test. This is performed in the early morning by giving 250 μg of Cortrosyn, a synthetic form of ACTH, intravenously after baseline 17-OHP analysis and then obtaining a 1-h value. Results are interpreted according to the nomogram of New et al. (30). In affected patients, 1-h values are generally > 10 ng/mL. Phenotype is largely the result of the amount of functional enzymatic activity of the allelic variants, and those with NC-CAH have 10–20% activity (31). About 70% will have oligomenorrhea, 80% hirsutism, and 40% polycystic ovaries on ultrasound (32). Patients also appear to lack the insulin resistance of PCOS. Treatment strategies focus primarily on suppression of adrenal function (*see* the section Treatment of Androgen Excess).

CUSHING'S SYNDROME

Like PCOS, Cushing's syndrome or glucocorticoid excess most commonly occurs in the reproductive years and predominantly affects women. However, the prevalence of 2–5 cases/million is a fraction of the high prevalence of PCOS *(33)*. Nevertheless, it must be considered in the differential of androgen excess. Coexisting signs of Cushing's syndrome, including a moon facies, buffalo hump, abdominal striae, centripetal fat distribution, and hypertension, should be sought and further screened for this cause. Most cases of Cushing's syndrome (about 70%) are the result of a pituitary ACTH-secreting tumor (Cushing's disease) *(34)*. Cortisol excess can be screened with a 24-h urine for free cortisol (which better quantifies excess cortisol production than random spot blood levels; normal values < 100 μg/24 h) or an overnight dexamethasone suppression test.

ANDROGEN EXCESS WITHOUT A PHENOTYPE

It is possible that there may be no external identifying characteristics of androgen excess in a female, and she may present with other associated phenomena, such as polycystic ovaries or chronic anovulation. Polycystic ovary morphology is usually determined by ultrasound, with multiple 2- to 8-mm subcapsular follicles forming a "black pearl necklace" sign *(35)*. Polycystic ovaries are distinct from polycystic ovary syndrome; up to 25% of an unsolicited population may have polycystic ovaries on ultrasound examination and many of these are normoandrogenic, regularly cycling females *(36)*. The differential diagnosis of polycystic ovaries is quite extensive and contains a number of diagnoses unrelated to androgen metabolism (*see* Table 2). Chronic anovulation may be the only signs of androgen excess in some populations. For instance, minimal hirsutism has been noted in Asian women with PCOS , but they have similar degrees of hyperandrogenism and insulin resistance as other ethnic groups affected with PCOS *(37)*.

TREATMENT OF ANDROGEN EXCESS

Overview

The treatment section will focus primarily on PCOS, the most common cause of androgen excess. We are currently changing from a symptom-oriented treatment approach to PCOS, based on either suppression of the ovaries (for hirsutism and menstrual disorders) or stimulation of the ovaries (for infertility), to one that improves insulin sensitivity *(38)*. Multiple studies have shown that improving insulin sensitivity, be it from lifestyle modifications or from pharmacologic intervention, can result in lowered circulating androgens (primarily mediated through increased SHBG and less bioavailable androgen, but also through decreased total testosterone), spontaneous ovulation, and spontaneous pregnancy. However, long-term studies documenting decreases in such sequelae as diabetes or endometrial cancer with improvements in insulin sensitivity are lacking.

Most medical methods for treating hirsutism, although improving hirsutism, do not produce the dramatic results patients desire. In general, combination therapies appear to produce better results than single-agent approaches, response with medical therapies often take 3–6 mo to notice improvement, and adjunctive mechanical removal methods are often necessary. However, the majority of women will experience improvement in

Table 2
Syndromes or Disease Entities That Have Been Associated with Polycystic Ovaries

---

Hyperandrogenism
    Steroidogenic enzyme deficiencies (CAH, aromatase deficiency, etc.)
    Androgen-secreting tumors
        Ovarian
        Adrenal
    Exogenous androgens
        Anabolic steroids
        Transsexual hormone replacement
Hyperandrogenism and Insulin Resistance
    Congenital
        Type A syndrome
        Type B syndrome
        Leprechaunism
        Lipoatrophic diabetes
        Rabson—Mendenall
        Polycystic ovary syndrome (?)
    Acquired
        Cushing's syndrome
Insulin Resistance
    Glycogen storage diseases
Other
    Central nervous system
        Trauma/lesions
        Hyperprolactinemia
    Nonhormonal medications
        Valproate
    Heriditary angioedema
    Bulimia
    Idiopathic
        (includes normoandrogenic women with cyclic menses)

---

their hirsutism. There are, unfortunately, no universally accepted techniques for assessing hirsutism and response to treatment. Trials have been hampered by the above methodology concerns as well as by the small number of subjects. For instance, although spironolactone has had a long and extensive use as an antiandrogen and multiple clinical trials have been published showing a benefit, the overall quality of the trials and small numbers enrolled have limited the ability of a meta-analysis to document its benefit in the treatment of hirsutism (39).

Lifestyle Modifications

Obesity has become epidemic in our society and contributes substantially to reproductive and metabolic abnormalities in PCOS. Unfortunately, there are no effective treatments that result in permanent weight loss, and it is estimated that 90–95% of patients who experience a weight decrease will relapse (40). For obese patients with hirsutism, weight loss is frequently recommended as a potential benefit. Increases in SHBG through improved insulin sensitivity from weight loss may lower bioavailable androgen levels. In one study, about 50% of these women who lost weight experienced improvement in their hirsutism *(41)*. Unfortunately, there have been few studies on the effect of exercise alone on insulin action in hyperandrogenic women *(42)*. It is reasonable to assume that exercise would have the same beneficial effects in women with PCOS as women with type 2 diabetes *(43)*. There is much hype about the beneficial effects of diets of varying composition on insulin sensitivity, with many popular sources advocating a high-protein diet as the diet of choice in women with PCOS. There are few studies to support this, and there are theoretical concerns about the adverse effects of high protein on renal function in a population at high risk for diabetes, as well as the adverse effects of the increased fat composition of these diets on dyslipidemia.

Ornithine Decarboxylase Inhibitors

Ornithine decarboxylase is necessary for the production of polyamines and is also a sensitive and specific marker of androgen action in the prostate *(44)*. Inhibition of this enzyme limits cell division and function. Recently, a potent inhibitor of this enzyme, eflornithine, has been tested and found to be effective as a facial creme against hirsutism and has been Food and Drug Administration (FDA)-approved for this indication. It is given as a 13.9% creme of eflornithine hydrochloride and is applied to affected areas twice a day. In clinical trials, 32% of patients showed marked improvement after 24 wk compared to 8% of placebo-treated and benefit was first noted at 8 wk. It is pregnancy category C. It appears to be well tolerated. A variety of adverse skin conditions occurred in 1–3% of subjects.

Ovarian Suppressive Therapies

Women with documented hyperandrogenemia would theoretically benefit most from this form of therapy. Suppressing the ovary has been achieved with either oral contraceptives, depot progestins, or gonadotropin-releasing hormone (GnRH) analog treatment. Oral contraceptives both inhibit ovarian steroid production through lowering of gonadotropins and raise SHBG through their estrogen effect, thus further lowering bioavailable testosterone. They also may inhibit dihydrotestosterone binding to the androgen receptor and 5α-reductase activity and increase hepatic steroid clearance (because of stimulation of the P450 system). These myriad actions contribute to improving hirsutism *(45)*. There are theoretical reasons for choosing an oral contraceptive using a less androgenic progestin, but few studies to show a clinical difference between different types of progestin. Although a triphasic oral contraceptive containing norgestimate has been shown to improve acne and has received an FDA indication for this, other pills also offer similar results.

A GnRH agonist may cause greater lowering of circulating androgens, but comparative trials against other agents and combined agent trials have been mixed and have not shown a greater benefit to one or the other or combined treatment *(46–49)*. A GnRH agonist given alone results in unacceptable bone loss *(49)*. Glucocorticoid suppression of the adrenal also offers theoretical benefits, but deterioration in glucose tolerance is problematic for women with PCOS, and long-term effects such as osteoporosis are of significant concern. It may be useful as adjunctive therapy in inducing ovulation with clomiphene citrate.

Insulin-Sensitizing Agents

Drugs developed initially to treat type 2 diabetes have also been utilized to treat PCOS. None of these agents are currently FDA-approved for the treatment of PCOS or for related symptoms such as anovulation, hirsutism, or acne. These include metformin *(50–52)*, thiazolidinediones, and an experimental insulin sensitizer drug *d-chiro*-inositol *(53)*.

METFORMIN

The longest and most varied published experience with any agent that improves insulin sensitivity in women with PCOS has been with metformin. Metformin was approved for the treatment of type 2 diabetes by the FDA in 1994, but was used clinically for close to 20 yr before that in other parts of the world. Metformin is a biguanide that works primarily by suppressing hepatic gluconeogenesis, but it also improves insulin sensitivity in the periphery. Metformin has no known human teratogenic risk or embryonic lethality in humans. There have been no reported abnormalities associated with its use during pregnancy in women with diabetes *(54–56)* or to a women with marked hyperandrogenism during pregnancy *(57)*, or to the small number of women with PCOS who have conceived during treatment *(58–60)*. Some clinicians advocate its use during early pregnancy to reduce the miscarriage rate, but the documentation for this claim is poor. Studies of longer duration with metformin in PCOS suggest long-term improvement in ovulatory function in about half of the patients *(61)*. Unfortunately, there have been few well-designed studies that test the effect of metformin on hirsutism.

THIAZOLIDINEDIONES

Thiazolidinediones are PPAR-γ (peroxisome proliferator-activating receptor) agonists and are thought to improve insulin sensitivity through a postreceptor mechanism. It is difficult to separate the effects of improving insulin sensitivity from that of lowering serum androgens, as any "pure" improvement in insulin sensitivity can raise SHBG and, thus, lower bioavailable androgen. Given the long onset of action for improving hirsutism, longer periods of observation are needed. In a large multicenter trial, troglitazone has been shown to have a dose-response effect in improving ovulation and hirsutism *(62)*. This appeared to be mediated through decreases in hyperinsulinemia and decreases in free-testosterone levels. Troglitazone has subsequently been removed from the worldwide market because of hepatotoxicity. Newer thiazolidinediones such as rosiglitazone and pioglitazone appear to be safer in terms of hepatotoxicity, but they have been associated with embryotoxicity in animal studies (both pregnancy category C) and little has been published on their effects in women with PCOS.

Antiandrogens

ANDROGEN-RECEPTOR ANTAGONISTS

These compounds antagonize the binding of testosterone and other androgens to the androgen receptor (AR). As a class, therefore, they are teratogenic and pose risk of feminization of the external genitalia in a male fetus should the patient conceive. Spironolactone, a diuretic and aldosterone antagonist, also binds to the androgen receptor with 67% of the affinity of dihydrotestosterone *(63)*. It has other mechanisms of action, including inhibition of ovarian and adrenal steroidogenesis, competition for ARs in hair follicles, and direct inhibition of 5α-reductase activity. There is a dose-response effect and a long period of onset—6 mo or more. About 20% of the women will experience increased menstrual frequency and this is one reason for combining this therapy with the oral contraceptive *(64)*. Because it can cause and exacerbate hyperkalemia, it should be used cautiously in patients with renal impairment. The medication also has potential teratogenicity as an antiandrogen, although exposure has rarely resulted in ambiguous genitalia in male infants *(65)*. Acne has also been successfully treated with spironolactone *(66)*. Thus, much of the treatment basis is empiric. Cyproterone acetate, not available commercially in the United States, is a progestogen with antiandrogen properties, that has seen widespread use in hyperandrogenic women in other parts of the world. It is frequently combined in an oral contraceptive. A related compound, dropirenone, has recently been approved in a combination oral contraceptive with ethinyl estradiol in the United States, although its effects in hyperandrogenic women have not been studied extensively to date. Flutamide is another nonsteroidal antiandrogen that has been shown to be effective against hirsutism *(67)*. There is greater risk of teratogenicity with this compound and contraception should be used.

ANTIANDROGENS: 5α-REDUCTASE INHIBITORS

There are two forms of the enzyme 5α-reductase: Type 1 is found predominantly in the skin and type II is predominantly found in the prostate and reproductive tissues. Both forms are found in the pilosebaceous unit and may contribute to hirsutism, acne, and balding. Finasteride inhibits both forms. It has been found to be effective for the treatment of hirsutism in women *(68,69)*. Finasteride is better tolerated than other antiandrogens, but it has the highest and clearest risk for teratogenicity in a male fetus and adequate contraception must be used. Randomized trials have found that spironolactone, flutamide, and finasteride all have similar efficacy in improving hirsutism *(70,71)*.

Other Methods

Minoxidil has mild efficacy in increasing hair growth in women with alopecia. Ketoconazole is an inhibitor of the P450 enzyme system and, thus, inhibits androgen biosynthesis, but has hepatotoxicity. Others have given aromatase inhibitors to induce ovulation and lower circulating androgens, although hirsutism has not been the primary focus to date.

Mechanical hair removal (shaving, plucking, waxing, depilatory creams, electrolysis, and laser vaporization) can control hirsutism, and these methods often are the front-line treatment used by women. Laser vaporization is receiving increasing attention. Hair is damaged using the principle of selective photothermolysis with wavelengths of light well absorbed by follicular melanin and pulse durations that selectively thermally damage the target without damaging surrounding tissue. Patients with dark hair and light skin are ideal candidates. This therapy appears to be most effective during anagen.

Surgical Options

The beneficial influence of treatment on sequelae of PCOS, especially destructive ovarian interventions such as wedge resection or ovarian drilling, has been suggested but not proven. Many argue that the best monotherapy results for the endocrine abnormalities in PCOS can be obtained through surgical destructive processes of the ovary, wedge resection, or ovarian drilling *(72–74)*. The value of laparoscopic ovarian drilling as a primary treatment for subfertile patients with anovulation (failure to ovulate) and PCOS is undetermined according to a Cochrane review *(75)*. There is insufficient evidence to determine whether laparoscopic surgery is more beneficial than gonadotropin therapy as the next treatment step in clomiphene-resistant women *(75)*. None of the various drilling techniques appear to offer obvious advantages, and some have promoted unilateral drilling *(75)*. The results of the ovarian drilling may, in some cases, also be temporary *(76)*. Surgery, consisting of total abdominal hysterectomy and bilateral salpingo-oophorectomy, is not a usual initial treatment option for androgen excess, but may be indicated in some cases of refractory ovarian hyperandrogenism, especially in perimenopausal or postmenopausal women.

SUMMARY

Androgen excess is common, but it is poorly understood. Most cases fall into a heterogeneous category known as polycystic ovary syndrome. No clear molecular or genetic mechanism has been identified to date to explain the vast majority of cases. Diagnostic evaluation focuses on separating causes of virilization from milder forms of androgen excess. Treatment tends to be symptom based. In PCOS, improving insulin sensitivity appears to improve both ovulation and hirsutism.

ACKNOWLEDGMENT

This work was supported by PHS grants U54 HD34449 The National Cooperative Program in Infertility Research (NCPIR). K24 HD01476, a GCRC grant MO1 RR 10732 to Pennsylvania State University, and U10 HD 38992 The Reproductive Medicine Network.

REFERENCES

1. Knochenhauer ES, Key TJ, Kahsar-Miller M, et al. Prevalence of the polycystic ovary syndrome in unselected Black and White women of the Southeastern United States: a prospective study. J Clin Endocrinol Metab 1998;83:3078–3082.
2. Dunaif A, Givens JR, Haseltine FP, et al. Polycystic ovary syndrome. Current Issues in Endocrinology and Metabolism. Blackwell Scientific, Boston, MA, 1992.
3. Ludwig E. Classification of the types of androgenetic alopecia (common baldness) occurring in the female sex. Br J Dermatol 1977;97:247–254.
4. Tagatz GE, Kopher RA, Nagel TC, Okagaki T. The clitoral index: a bioassay of androgenic stimulation. Obstet Gynecol 1979;54:562–564.
5. Barbieri RL, Smith S, Ryan KJ. The role of hyperinsulinemia in the pathogenesis of ovarian hyperandrogenism. Fertil Steril 1988;50:197–212.
6. Givens JR, Kurtz BR. Understanding the polycystic ovary syndrome. Prog Clin Biol Res 1986;225: 355–376.
7. Dunaif A. Insulin resistance and the polycystic ovary syndrome: mechanism and implications for pathogenesis. Endocr Rev 1997;18:774–800.
8. Azziz R, Waggoner WT, Ochoa T, et al. Idiopathic hirsutism: an uncommon cause of hirsutism in alabama. Fertil Steril 1998;70:274–278.
9. Ibanez L, de Zegher F, Potau N. Anovulation after precocious pubarche: early markers and time course in adolescence. J Clin Endocrinol Metab 1999;84:2691–2695.
10. Elting MW, Korsen TJ, Rekers-Mombarg LT, Schoemaker J: Women with polycystic ovary syndrome gain regular menstrual cycles when ageing. Hum Reprod 2000;15:24–28.
11. Winters SJ, Talbott E, Guzick DS, Zborowski J, McHugh KP. Serum testosterone levels decrease in middle age in women with the polycystic ovary syndrome. Fertil Steril 2000;73:724–729.
12. Goldzieher JW, Axelrod LR: Clinical and biochemical features of polycystic ovarian disease. Fertil Steril 1963;14:631–653.

13. Elchalal U, Schenker JG. The pathophysiology of ovarian hyperstimulation syndrome—views and ideas. Hum Reprod 1997;12:1129–1137.
14. Fulghesu AM, Villa P, Pavone V, et al. The impact of insulin secretion on the ovarian response to exogenous gonadotropins in polycystic ovary syndrome. J Clin Endocrinol Metab 1997;82:644–648.
15. Dale PO, Tanbo T, Haug E, Abyholm T. The impact of insulin resistance on the outcome of ovulation induction with low-dose follicle stimulating hormone in women with polycystic ovary syndrome. Hum Reprod 1998;13:567–570.
16. Dahlgren E, Friberg LG, Johansson S, et al. Endometrial carcinoma; ovarian dysfunction—a risk factor in young women. Eup J Obstet Gynecol Reprod Biol 1991;41:143–150.
17. Legro RS, Kunselman AR, Dodson WC, Dunaif A. Prevalence and predictors of risk for type 2 diabetes mellitus and impaired glucose tolerance in polycystic ovary syndrome: a prospective, controlled study in 254 affected women. J Clin Endocrinol Metab 1999:84;165–169.
18. Ehrmann DA, Barnes RB, Rosenfield RL, et al. Prevalence of impaired glucose tolerance and diabetes in women with polycystic ovary syndrome. Diabet Care 1999;22:141–146.
19. Anonymous. American Diabetes Association: clinical practice recommendations 1997. Diabetes Care 1997;20(Suppl 1): S1–S70.
20. Reaven GM. Banting lecture 1988. Role of insulin resistance in human disease. Diabetes 1988;37:1595–1607.
21. Haffner SM, Miettinen H, Gaskill SP, Stern MP: Metabolic precursors of hypertension. The San Antonio Heart Study . Arch Intern Med 1996;156:1994–2001.
22. Lind L, Lithell H, Pollare T. Is it hyperinsulinemia or insulin resistance that is related to hypertension and other metabolic cardiovascular risk factors? J Hypertens 1993;11(Suppl): S11–S16
23. Talbott E, Clerici A, Berga SL, et al. Adverse lipid and coronary heart disease risk profiles in young women with polycystic ovary syndrome: results of a case-control study. J Clin Epidemiology 1998;51:415–422.
24. Zimmermann S, Phillips RA, Dunaif A, et al. Polycystic ovary syndrome: lack of hypertension despite profound insulin resistance. J Clin Endocrinol Metab 1992;75:508–513.
25. Holte J, Gennarelli G, Berne C, et al. Elevated ambulatory day-time blood pressure in women with polycystic ovary syndrome: a sign of a pre-hypertensive state? Hum Reprod 1996;11:23–28.
26. Talbott EO, Guzick DS, Sutton-Tyrrell K, et al. Evidence for association between polycystic ovary syndrome and premature carotid atherosclerosis in middle-aged women. Arterio Thromb Vasc Biol (Online) 2000:20(11):2414–2421.
27. Chetkowski RJ, DeFazio J, Shamonki I, et al. The incidence of late-onset congenital adrenal hyperplasia due to 21-hydroxylase deficiency among hirsute women. J Clin Endocrinol Metab 1984;58:595–598.
28. New MI, Speiser PW. Genetics of adrenal steroid 21-hydroxylase deficiency. Endocr Rev 1986;7:331–349.
29. Azziz R, Hincapie LA, Knochenhauer ES, et al. Screening for 21-hydroxylase-deficient nonclassic adrenal hyperplasia among hyperandrogenic women: a prospective study. Fertil Steril 1999;72:915–925.
30. New MI, Lorenzen F, Lerner AJ, et al. Genotyping steroid 21-hydroxylase deficiency: hormonal reference data. J Clin Endocrinol Metab 1983;57:320–326.
31. Speiser PW, Dupont J, Zhu D, et al. Disease expression and molecular genotype in congenital adrenal hyperplasia due to 21-hydroxylase deficiency. J Clin Invest 1992;90:584–595.
32. Azziz R, Dewailly D, Owerbach D. Clinical review 56: nonclassic adrenal hyperplasia: current concepts. J Clin Endocrinol Metab1994;78:810–815.
33. Cizza G, Chrousos GP. Adrenocorticotrophic hormone-dependent Cushing's syndrome. Canc Treat Res 1997;89:25–40.
34. Plotz CM, Knowlton AL, Ragan C. The natural history of Cushing's syndrome. Am J Med 1952;13:597–605.
35. Polson DW, Adams J, Wadsworth J, et al. Polycystic ovaries—a common finding in normal women. Lancet 1988;1:870–872.
36. Farquhar CM, Birdsall M, Manning P, et al. The prevalence of polycystic ovaries on ultrasound scanning in a population of randomly selected women. Aust NZJ Obstet Gynaecol 1994;34:67–72.
37. Carmina E, Koyama T, Chang L., et al. Does ethnicity influence the prevalence of adrenal hyperandrogenism and insulin resistance in polycystic ovary syndrome? Am J Obstet Gynecol 1992;167:1807–1812.
38. Nestler JE. Role of hyperinsulinemia in the pathogenesis of the polycystic ovary syndrome, and its clinical implications. Semin Reprod Endocrinol 1997;15:111–122.

39. Lee O, Farquhar C, Toomath R, Jepson R. Spironolactone versus placebo or in combination with steroids for hirsutism and/or acne. Cochrane Database of Systematic Reviews CD000194, 2000.

40. Rosenbaum M, Leibel RL, Hirsch J. Obesity. N Engl J Med 1997;337:396–407.

41. Pasquali R, Antenucci D, Casimirri F, et al. Clinical and hormonal characteristics of obese amenorrheic hyperandrogenic women before and after weight loss. J Clin Endocrinol Metab 1989;68:173–179.

42. Jaatinen TA, Anttila L, Erkkola R, et al. Hormonal responses to physical exercise in patients with polycystic ovarian syndrome. Fertil Steril 1993;60:262–267.

43. Braun B, Zimmermann MB, Kretchmer N. Effects of exercise intensity on insulin sensitivity in women with non-insulin-dependent diabetes mellitus. J Appl Physiol 1995;78:300–306.

44. McCann PP, Pegg AE. Ornithine decarboxylase as an enzyme target for therapy. Pharmacol Therapeut 1992;54:195–215.

45. Givens JR, Andersen RN, Wiser WL, et al. The effectiveness of two oral contraceptives in suppressing plasma androstenedione, testosterone, LH, and FSH, and in stimulating plasma testosterone-binding capacity in hirsute women. Am J Obstet Gynecol 1976;124:333–339.

46. Azziz R, Ochoa TM, Bradley EL Jr, et al. Leuprolide and estrogen versus oral contraceptive pills for the treatment of hirsutism: a prospective randomized study. J Clin Endocrinol Metab 1995;80:3406–3411.

47. Heiner JS, Greendale GA, Kawakami AK, et al. Comparison of a gonadotropin-releasing hormone agonist and a low dose oral contraceptive given alone or together in the treatment of hirsutism. J Clin Endocrinol Metab 1995;80:3412–3418.

48. Elkind-Hirsch KE, Anania C, Mack M, Malinak R: Combination gonadotropin-releasing hormone agonist and oral contraceptive therapy improves treatment of hirsute women with ovarian hyperandrogenism. Fertil Steril 1995;63:970–978.

49. Carr BR, Breslau NA, Givens C, et al. Oral contraceptive pills, gonadotropin-releasing hormone agonists, or use in combination for treatment of hirsutism: a clinical research center study. J Clin Endocrinol Metab 1995;80:1169–1178.

50. Velazquez EM, Mendoza S, Hamer T, et al. Metformin therapy in polycystic ovary syndrome reduces hyperinsulinemia, insulin resistance, hyperandrogenemia, and systolic blood pressure, while facilitating normal menses and pregnancy. Metabol 1994;43:647–654.

51. Nestler JE, Jakubowicz DJ. Lean women with polycystic ovary syndrome respond to insulin reduction with decreases in ovarian p450c17 alpha activity and serum androgens. J Clin Endocrinol Metab 1997;82:4075–4079.

52. Nestler JE, Jakubowicz DJ, Evans WS, Pasquali R. Effects of metformin on spontaneous and clomiphene-induced ovulation in the polycystic ovary syndrome. N Engl J Med 1998;338:1876–1880.

53. Nestler JE, Jakubowicz DJ, Reamer P, et al. Ovulatory and metabolic effects of d-chiro-inositol in the polycystic ovary syndrome. N Engl J Med 1999;340:1314–1320.

54. Coetzee EJ, Jackson WP. Metformin in management of pregnant insulin-independent diabetics. Diabetologia 1979;16:241–245.

55. Callahan TL, Hall JE, Ettner SL, et al. The economic impact of multiple-gestation pregnancies and the contribution of assisted-reproduction techniques to their incidence. N Engl J Med 1994;331:244–249.

56. Coetzee EJ, Jackson WP. Pregnancy in established non-insulin-dependent diabetics. A five-and-a-half year study at Groote Schuur Hospital. S Afric Med J 1980;58:795–802.

57. Sarlis NJ, Weil SJ, Nelson LM. Administration of metformin to a diabetic woman with extreme hyperandrogenemia of nontumoral origin: management of infertility and prevention of inadvertent masculinization of a female fetus. J Clin Endocrinol Metab 1999;84:1510–1512.

58. Diamanti-Kandarakis E, Kouli C, Tsianateli T, Bergiele A. Therapeutic effects of metformin on insulin resistance and hyperandrogenism in polycystic ovary syndrome. Eur J Endocrinol 1998;138:269–274.

59. Velazquez E, Acosta A, Mendoza SG: Menstrual cyclicity after metformin therapy in polycystic ovary syndrome. Obstet Gynecol 1997;90:392–395.

60. Vandermolen DT, Ratts VS, Evans WS, et al. Metformin increases the ovulatory rate and pregnancy rate from clomiphene citrate in patients with polycystic ovary syndrome who are resistant to clomiphene citrate alone . Fertil Steril 2001;75:310–315.

61. Moghetti P, Castello R, Negri C, et al. Metformin effects on clinical features, endocrine and metabolic profiles, and insulin sensitivity in polycystic ovary syndrome: a randomized, double-blind, placebo-controlled 6-month trial, followed by open, long-term clinical evaluation. J Clin Endocrinol Metab 2000;85:139–146.

62. Azziz R, Ehrmann D, Legro RS, et al. Troglitazone improves ovulation and hirsutism in the polycystic ovary syndrome: a multicenter, double blind, placebo-controlled trial. J Clin Endocrinol Metab 2001;86:1626–1632.

63. Eil C, Edelson SK. The use of human skin fibroblasts to obtain potency estimates of drug binding to androgen receptors. J Clin Endocrinol Metab 1984;59:51–55.

64. Helfer EL, Miller JL, Rose LI. Side-effects of spironolactone therapy in the hirsute woman. J Clin Endocrinol Metab 1988;66:208–211.

65. Groves TD, Corenblum B. Spironolactone therapy during human pregnancy. Am J Obstet Gynecol 1995;172:1655–1656.

66. Muhlemann MF, Carter GD, Cream JJ, Wise P. Oral spironolactone: an effective treatment for acne vulgaris in women. Br J Dermatol 1986;115:227–232.

67. Fruzzetti F, De Lorenzo D, Ricci C, Fioretti P. Clinical and endocrine effects of flutamide in hyperandrogenic women. Fertil Steril 1993;60:806–813.

68. Moghetti P, Castello R, Magnani CM, et al. Clinical and hormonal effects of the 5 alpha-reductase inhibitor finasteride in idiopathic hirsutism. J Clin Endocrinol Metab 1994;79:1115–1121.

69. Fruzzetti F, de Lorenzo D, Parrini D, Ricci C. Effects of finasteride, a 5 alpha-reductase inhibitor, on circulating androgens and gonadotropin secretion in hirsute women. J Clin Endocrinol Metab 1994;79:831–835.

70. Moghetti P, Tosi F, Tosti A, et al. Comparison of spironolactone, flutamide, and finasteride efficacy in the treatment of hirsutism: a randomized, double blind, placebo-controlled trial. J Clin Endocrinol Metab 2000;85:89–94.

71. Wong IL, Morris RS, Chang L, et al. A prospective randomized trial comparing finasteride to spironolactone in the treatment of hirsute women. J Clin Endocrinol Metab 1995;80:233–238.

72. Katz M, Carr PJ, Cohen BM, Millar RP: Hormonal effects of wedge resection of polycystic ovaries. Obstet Gynecol 1978;51:437–444.

73. Greenblatt E, Casper RF. Endocrine changes after laparoscopic ovarian cautery in polycystic ovarian syndrome. Am J Obstet Gynecol 1987;156:279–285.

74. Adashi EY, Rock JA, Guzick D, et al. Fertility following bilateral ovarian wedge resection: a critical analysis of 90 consecutive cases of the polycystic ovary syndrome. Fertil Steril 1981;36:320–325.

75. Farquhar C, Vandekerckhove P, Arnot M, Lilford R. Laparoscopic "drilling" by diathermy or laser for ovulation induction in anovulatory polycystic ovary syndrome. Cochrane Database of Systematic (2), CD001122, 2000.

76. Donesky BW, Adashi EY. Surgically induced ovulation in the polycystic ovary syndrome: wedge resection revisited in the age of laparoscopy. Fertil Steril 1995;63:439–463.

8

Androgen Pharmacology
and Delivery Systems

Christina Wang, MD
and Ronald S. Swerdloff, MD

CONTENTS

INTRODUCTION
PHARMACOLOGY OF ANDROGENS
ANDROGEN PREPARATIONS AND DELIVERY SYSTEMS
SELECTION OF THE ANDROGEN DELIVERY SYSTEM
ACKNOWLEDGMENT
REFERENCES

INTRODUCTION

Historically, testis extracts from animals and then men were used as a rejuvenation mixture with poor success. Testosterone was first synthesized in the 1930s, providing for the first time a means to provide sufficient testosterone to treat hypogonadal men. Initially, testosterone pellets were developed for subcutaneous implant and the methyl derivative (methyltestosterone) was administered as an orally active agent. In the 1950s, the testosterone esters (propionate, enanthate, and cypionate) became available and have continued to be used for testosterone-replacement therapy in androgen deficiency (1–4). During the peak era of steroid chemistry, modifications of the testosterone molecule were made to achieve orally active bioactivity and for the "anabolic" effects such as increased nitrogen retention, muscle protein synthesis, muscle strength, and mass. Methyltestosterone and fluoxymesterone were prescribed as oral preparations for hypogonadism, but the former was criticized for its hepatotoxicity and the latter was a weak androgen. In the 1970s, oral testosterone undecanoate was marketed with wide acceptance in Europe, Australia, and Asia but was not available in the United States. In the past 10 yr, there has been a resurgence in the interest of development of new formulations and delivery systems of testosterone for potential new indications such as androgen replacement in elderly men, male contraception, severe wasting diseases, and androgen replacement in gonadectomized or postmenopausal females.

From: *Contemporary Endocrinology: Androgens in Health and Disease*
Edited by: C. Bagatell and W. J. Bremner © Humana Press Inc., Totowa, NJ

PHARMACOLOGY OF ANDROGENS

Testosterone is the major androgen produced by the Leydig cells of the testis and acts directly or through its conversion to 5α-dihydrotestosterone (DHT) on androgen receptors present in reproductive and nonreproductive tissues. The major target organs for testosterone include the testis, derivatives of the wolffian ducts (epididymis, seminal vesicles), muscle, liver, bone marrow, and, possibly, bone and brain. Some tissues (e.g., prostate, external genitalia, and skin) have high levels of the 5α-reductase enzyme and greater specificity for DHT. Alternatively, testosterone is converted to estradiol (E_2) both in the testis and peripherally via the aromatase enzyme and acts through interaction with estrogen receptors. The presumptive target organs of E_2 include the liver, brain, adipose tissue and bone and the accessory reproductive organs (efferent ducts).

In androgen-deficiency states, it is desirable that the androgen be aromatizable to estrogens to achieve the full beneficial effects on bone and lipoproteins. In animals, estrogens are necessary for sexual dimorphic behavior, with androgenic effects mediated through aromatization to estradiol in the brain. In humans, there is little evidence that conversion of testosterone to E2 is required for sexual function and male behavior. Although conversion of testosterone to DHT is important for male external genitalia development, DHT is not required in adult man to maintain external genitalia or sexual function. Recent studies demonstrating low bone mass and severe osteoporosis in male patients with estrogen-receptor or aromatase enzyme gene mutations suggest the important role of estrogens in attaining and maintaining peak bone mass in men *(5–7)*. There are no data to indicate that estrogens are required to maintain bone mass in adult or elderly men. Correlation studies suggest, however, that serum bioavailable estradiol concentrations show the better correlation with bone mineral density than serum total- or bioavailable-testosterone levels in elderly men *(8,9)*.

Natural testosterone is available in several formulations for therapeutic use: transdermal patch or gel, implants, bioadhesive tablets, or as cyclodextrins. Testosterone esters such as testosterone enanthate, cypionate, decanoate, or undecanoate are synthesized by esterification at the 17β position with fatty acids of varying lengths. The duration of the testosterone ester depends on the length and type of the fatty acid. These 17β-testosterone esters are rapidly metabolized by the liver to release both testosterone and the fatty acid side chain. Further modifications of the 17β-testosterone esters with addition of a methyl group at the 19 position produces long-acting 19 nor-testosterone esters such as nandrolone decanoate or phenylproprionate. These testosterone esters are aromatizable to estrogens and can be reduced by the 5α-reductase enzyme. Modification of the testosterone molecule with a 17α-methyl group led to the synthesis of orally active methyltestosterone. Other 17α-alkyl testosterone derivatives include fluoxymesterone, oxandrolone, stanozole, and danazole. These 17α-alkyl derivatives of testosterone are not aromatizable to estrogens and not converted to testosterone. A derivative of DHT (mesterolone) is a weak androgen but is orally active. All of these derivatives are synthesized based on modification of the testosterone molecule.

ANDROGEN PREPARATIONS AND DELIVERY SYSTEMS (*SEE* TABLE 1)

Oral Preparations

When administered orally, nonmodified testosterone is absorbed by the gastrointestinal tract but is very rapidly cleared and metabolized by the liver. For this reason,

Table 1
Androgen Preparation and Delivery Systems

Oral/buccal
    Testosterone
    Buccal testosterone[a]
    Bioadhesive buccal testosterone[a]
    Testosterone cyclodextrin[a]
    Testosterone undecanoate[b]
    Selective androgen-receptor-modulators[c] (SARMs)
Injectables
    Testosterone enanthate
    Testosterone cypionate
    Testosterone undecanoate[a]
    Testosterone buciclate[a]
    Testosterone decanoate[a]
    Testosterone microspheres[a]
Transdermal
    Testosterone patch
    Testosterone gel
    DHT gel[a]
Implants
    Testosterone pellets
    7α-methyl nor-testosterone[a] (MENT)

[a]In phase II or III clinical trials.
[b]Oral testosterone undecanoate is available in some countries.
New formulation is undergoing phase II/III clinical trials.
[c]In preclinical development or early clinical studies.

hundreds of milligrams of testosterone have to be ingested in multiple doses for androgen replacement; thus, oral testosterone has not been used very successfully in practice. To overcome this problem and avoid first-pass effects of androgens on the liver, transbuccal preparations of oral androgen formulations have been created. One such effort involves the preparation of a sublingually administered testosterone enclosed in a carbohydrate ring (cyclodextrin); the latter facilitates absorption in the oral cavity. Clinical studies show high peak levels of testosterone are attained about 30 min after administration of 5 or 10 mg of sublingual testosterone cyclodextrin. The levels fall rapidly to reach the basal state in about 3–4 h *(10)*. Despite the peaks and troughs of serum testosterone levels, administration of 5 or 10 mg testosterone cyclodextrin three times per day resulted in improvement in sexual function and mood and significant increases in lean body mass and bone turnover markers *(11,12)*. Apparently because of the short half-life and frequent administration, this preparation is not yet available in the market. Buccal testosterone tablets give a similar pharmacokinetic profile to testosterone cyclodextrin *(13)*. A bioadhesive buccal testosterone tablet that gellifies when applied to the gums is also undergoing clinical efficacy trials. On contact with the gums, the tablet forms a bioadhesive gel and attains a relatively steady state of serum testosterone for 12 h. The bioadhesive table is not an irritant to the gums and is applied twice per day *(14)*.

The 17α-alkyl esters of testosterone were the first orally active forms of testosterone to be synthesized. These 17α-alkyl derivatives are not converted to testosterone in the body but fit the androgen receptor directly. Thus, monitoring of therapy requires the measurement of the administered steroids by gas chromatograph–mass spectroscopy, which is not generally available to clinicians. Methyltestosterone has been reported to be associated with cholestatic jaundice. Other 17α-alkyl derivatives are used as "anabolic" steroids for wasting diseases and, in the past, for the treatment of aplastic and refractory anemias. When used in high doses, hepatic toxicity has been reported *(15,16)*. These modified orally active 17α-alkyl derivatives are not aromatized to estrogens. In addition, because of the first-pass effect through the liver, these agents cause significant increases in serum low-density lipoprotein (LDL)-cholesterol and decreases in high-density lipoprotein (HDL)-cholesterol *(17)*. For the above reasons, 17α-alkyl androgens are not often recommended for long-term androgen-replacement therapy. Despite concerns about potential toxicity, these orally active steroids are commonly used by athletes for bodybuilding and enhancing muscle strength.

Other non-17α-alkylated oral androgens are approved for use in the United States and/or other countries. Mesterolone is an α-methyl derivative of DHT. Available in Europe and Asia, mesterolone is a weak androgen and has not been found useful for androgen-replacement therapy. Oral testosterone undecanoate has been marketed over 15 yr for clinical use in Europe, Asia, Australia, South America, and some countries in North America (Mexico and Canada). This ester has a very long side chain and is lipophilic. When administered orally, it is absorbed by the lymphatics and then to the systemic circulation. Thus, the absorption of testosterone undecanoate may be affected by the amount of fat in the diet. The peak serum testosterone levels in circulation occurred 4–5 h after administration and the levels gradually declined to baseline in 8–10 h *(18,19)*. There is very large variability in the time to achieve peak serum testosterone levels. The serum DHT levels are relatively high after testosterone undecanoate oral administration. The usual dose is 80 mg (two capsules) bid or tid and the preparation must be taken with meals. Despite a high intrasubject and intersubject variation in serum testosterone levels after oral testosterone undecanoate administration, the preparation is well accepted by many patients. Long-term studies have demonstrated its safety as androgen replacement for hypogonadal men *(20)*. Because of the ease of administration, testosterone undecanoate has also been used for the induction of puberty in boys with constitutional delayed growth and development.

Injectables

Testosterone propionate maintains testosterone levels only for 2–3 d after an intramuscular (im) injection and is impractical for androgen replacement. Testosterone enanthate or cypionate are longer acting and have been widely used for androgen-replacement therapy. The pharmacokinetics of testosterone enanthate are well defined *(21,22)* (*see* Fig. 1, right panel). The usual recommended dose for testosterone replacement in an adult man is 200 mg im every 2 wk (*see* Table 2). Peak serum testosterone levels may reach above the physiological range 1–3 d after the injection and return to baseline levels by 10–14 d. Some patients may experience fluctuations in mood and energy with the peaks and troughs of serum testosterone. To lessen these complaints, testosterone enanthate can be administered in lower doses more frequently (e.g., 100 mg every 7–10 d). Testosterone enanthate has been administered to patients over a wide age

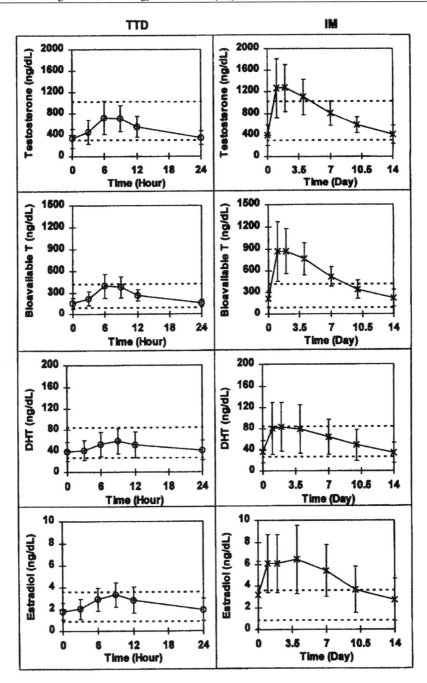

Fig. 1. Steady-state pharmacokinetic profiles of testosterone (T), bioavailable T (BT), DHT, and E$_2$ profiles during nightly applications of TTD systems ($n = 27$; left panels) and biweekly im injections of testosterone enanthate ($n = 29$, right panels) measured at wk 16. Dashed lines denote upper and lower limits of normal range based on morning serum samples (T, 306–1031 ng/dL; BT, 92–420 ng/dL; DHT, 28–85 ng/d; E$_2$, 0.9–3.6 ng/dL). Error bars denote ±SD. [From Dobs AS, Meikle AW, Arver S, Sanders SW, Caranelli KE, Mazer NA. Pharmacokinetics, efficacy, and safety of a permeation enhanced testosterone transdermal system in comparison with biweekly injections of testosterone enanthate for treatment of hypogonadal men. J Clin Endocrinol Metab 1999;84(10):3469–3478. © The Endocrine Society.]

Table 2
Dose and Frequency of Administration of Commonly Used Androgens

Preparation	Route	Dose/frequency
Testosterone undecanoate	Oral	80 mg bid or tid
Testosterone enanthate or cypionate	Intramuscular injection	200 mg once every 2 wk or 100 mg once every 1–10 d
Testosterone patches	Transdermal	5 mg/d
Testosterone gel	Transdermal	5, 7.5, or 10 g gel/d
Testosterone implants	Subcutaneous	200 mg pellets—either 6 for up to 6 mo or 4 for up to 4 mo

range (infants to elderly men) with good safety profiles. Combinations of several testosterone esters with different pharmacokinetics, including testosterone propionate, decanoate and enanthate, have been marketed in Europe but offer no advantage over testosterone enanthate injections.

There have been efforts to develop longer-acting testosterone preparations. Studies in China first demonstrated that testosterone undecanoate, when formulated in tea seed oil and administered intramuscularly as 500- or 1000-mg injections, resulted in peak serum testosterone levels between 7 and 14 d. Serum testosterone levels remained within the normal adult range for 4–6 wk with the 500-mg dose and as long as 12 wk with 1000-mg doses (23,24) (see Fig. 2). Subsequent studies in Europe confirmed that 1000 mg of testosterone undecanoate administered intramuscularly could maintain serum testosterone levels within the normal range for 12 wk (24,25). Although this preparation has been shown to be an effective androgen-replacement therapy in hypogonadal men, it has not yet been approved for use nor marketed in Europe and North America. At present, its clinical use is limited to China.

Nandrolone esters can also be administered as im injections for androgenic replacement, but its use has been principally limited to chronic debilitating illnesses and surreptitious use by bodybuilders and athletes to increase muscle mass and strength and improve athletic performance. Nandrolone has also been used in small-scale male contraceptive trials.

A long-acting ester of testosterone, testosterone buciclate can maintain normal serum levels in hypogonadal men for up to 20 wk with a single im injection (26). Toxicological studies of the buciclate side chain are underway and there have been no further reports of results from clinical studies.

Testosterone can be incorporated into microspheres of a lactide : glycolide copolymer. A single im injection of testosterone microspheres can maintain serum testosterone levels within the normal range for 70 d (27). The development of testosterone microspheres has not progressed until recently because of problems of instability and nonuniformity of the testosterone-containing microspheres. A recent study reaffirmed that a single subcutaneous injection of testosterone in biodegradable polylactide–coglycolide normalized serum testosterone for up to 10–11 wk. There is, however, a pronounced early peak followed by a prolonged period of low-normal serum total testosterone concentrations after im administration (28).

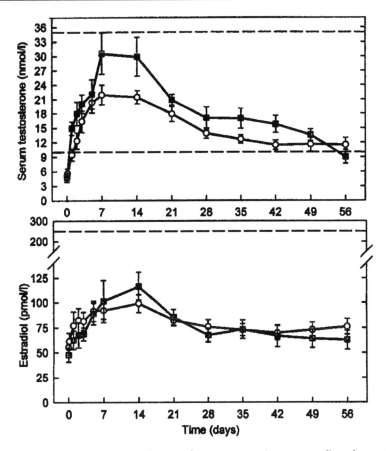

Fig. 2. Serum concentrations (mean ± SEM) of testosterone (upper panel) and estradiol (lower panel) after single-dose im injections of 1000 mg testosterone undecanoate in tea seed oil in 7 hypogonadal men (study I, squares) or caster oil in 14 hypogonadal men (study II, circles). Broken lines indicate normal range of testosterone and upper normal limit of estradiol. [From Behre HM, Abstragen K, Oettel M, Hubler D, Nieschlag E. Intramuscular injection of testosterone undecanoate for the treatment of male hypogonadism: phase I studies. Eur J Endocrinol 140:414–419. © Society of the European Journal of Endocrinology.]

Implants

Testosterone can also be provided as long-lasting implants. Crystalline testosterone has been fused to form testosterone pellets (75 mg in the United States, 100 or 200 mg in Europe and Australia) that can be inserted subcutaneously into the abdominal wall with a trocar under local anesthesia. Testosterone pellets are commonly used for androgen-replacement therapy in Australia and the United Kingdom and they have been shown to correct symptoms of androgen deficiency. Detailed pharmacokinetics of serum testosterone after testosterone pellet insertion are available *(29,30)*. In hypogonadal men, insertion of six 200-mg pellets can maintain serum testosterone levels in the adult normal range for 5–6 mo. Serum testosterone levels peaked 2–4 wk after implant insertion and then gradually decreased. The main drawbacks with the testosterone pellets are the requirement of a minor surgical procedure by an experienced provider and the reported 5–10% rate of extrusion *(31)*.

The steroid 7α-methyl-19 nor-testosterone (MENT) is also formulated as an implant. This androgen is about 10 times as potent as testosterone in the suppression of gonadotropins and maintenance of levator ani muscle but only 4 times as potent on testosterone in promoting prostate growth in castrated rats *(32)*. A reduced stimulation of prostate growth relative to many other target organs has also been demonstrated in monkeys *(33)*. The prostate-sparing effects are explained by the demonstration that MENT is not reduced by 5α-reductase and thus have fewer androgenic effects on the prostate, hair follicles, and the skin. MENT is being formulated as a subcutaneous implant inserted in the subcutaneous tissue of the upper arm and also as a transdermal gel preparation. A two-center study showed when administered as a subcutaneous implant, the MENT acetate (containing 115 mg active compound releasing 350–400 g/d MENT) had similar effects as testosterone enanthate injections on restoration of sexual function and improvement of mood states in hypogonadal men *(34)*. Large-scale clinical studies have not yet been conducted.

Transdermal Preparations

In the mid-1990s, a transdermal scrotal patch releasing 6 mg testosterone per day was developed. The application of the patch to scrotal skin required hair clipping or shaving to optimize adherence. This daily patch (Testoderm) produced steady-state serum testosterone levels in the lower normal range in hypogonadal men *(35,36)*. The use of the scrotal skin patch has been superseded by the development of nonscrotal skin patches. The permeation-enhanced testosterone patch (Androderm) delivers 5 mg/d testosterone and can be applied to the body (*see* Fig. 1, left panel). It produces serum testosterone levels in the normal range, mimicking the diurnal variation of testosterone *(37,38)*. The application is associated with skin irritation in up to 60% of the subjects, with 10–15% of users discontinuing application because of the skin irritation *(39)*. Preapplication of corticosteroid cream to the skin has been reported to decrease the severity of the skin irritation. The other available nonscrotal patch (Testoderm TTS) causes minimal skin irritation (about 12% itching and 3% erythema) but may have a problem adhering to the skin. These transdermal testosterone patches provide steady-state delivery of testosterone to the body and have been shown to reverse the signs and symptoms of male hypogonadism and andropause *(40,41)*.

Recently, a 1% hydroalcoholic gel (Androgel) containing 25 or 50 mg testosterone in 2.5 or 5 g gel, delivering approx 2.5 or 5 mg testosterone to the body per day, has been approved for clinical use in hypogonadism. The pharmacokinetic profile of serum testosterone levels after application of 5–10 g of the testosterone gel compared to 5 mg of a permeation-enhanced testosterone patch is shown in Fig. 3. After application of 5 or 10 g of gel containing 50 or 100 mg testosterone, serum testosterone levels rose gradually and a steady state was achieved after 2–3 d. About 9–14% of the testosterone in the gel is bioavailable *(42)*. After long-term application, serum testosterone is maintained in the mid-normal range with 5 g of gel and in the upper normal range with 10 g of gel. After testosterone gel application, dose-proportionate increases in serum DHT and E_2 are observed *(43)*. This testosterone-gel preparation has been demonstrated to improve sexual function and lean body mass, muscle mass, and bone mineral density while decreasing fat mass in hypogonadal men *(44,45)*. The advantages of the testosterone gel over the testosterone patch are the absence of skin irritation, the ease of application, and the ability to deliver testosterone in the low, mid, or upper normal range. A potential complication of testosterone-gel application is the transfer of testosterone to

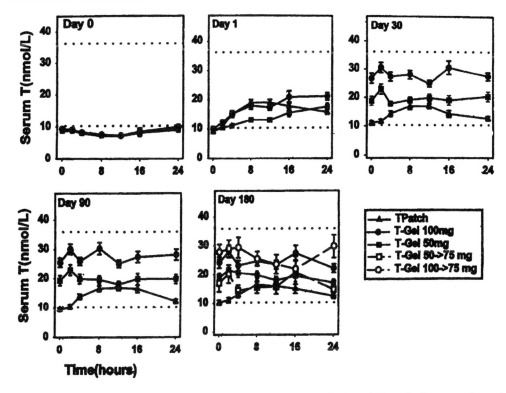

Fig. 3. Serum testosterone (T) concentrations (mean ± SE) befor (d 0) and after transdermal testosterone applications on d 1, 30, 90, and 180. Time 0 h was 0800 h, when blood sampling usually began. On d 90, the dose in the subjects applying T gel 50 or 100 was uptitrated or downtitrated if their preapplication serum testosterone levels were below or above the normal adult male range, respectively, The dotted lines denote the adult male normal range and the dashed lines and open symbols represent subjects whoe T-gel dose were adjusted. [From Swerdloff RS, Wang C, Cunningham G, Dobs A, Iranmanesh A, Matsumoto AM, Synder PJ, Weber T, Longstreth J, Berman N, Testosterone Gel Study Group. Long term pharacokinetics of transdermal testosterone gel in hypogonadal men. J Clin Endocrinol Metab 2000; 85:4500–4510. © The Endocrine Society.]

women or children upon close contact with the skin. Transfer of transdermal testosterone from the skin can be avoided by wearing clothing or showering after application. This preparation has gained a significant market share of androgen formulations in the United States, although it is marketed at a slightly higher price than the patches.

In addition to delivering testosterone through the skin, DHT gels have been marketed in some countries in Europe. DHT cannot be converted to E_2 and will not produce gynecomastia. It has been hypothesized that administration of DHT may have less effect on prostate growth because it is not aromatizable. A decrease in estrogen levels may decrease prostate growth because both estrogens and androgens are required for the development of benign prostatic hyperplasia in dogs and possibly in humans. DHT gel has been reported to be useful in the treatment of hypogonadal young and elderly men *(46–49)*. The DHT gel has been reformulated and the pharmacokinetics of DHT at different doses (16, 32, and 64 mg applied to the skin) have been reported to give total testosterone plus DHT levels in the low, mid, and high normal adult range *(50)*.

The inability of DHT to be converted to estrogens may be problematic. The issues with the use of DHT in androgen replacement include, first, whether DHT can maintain bone mass and whether it will cause greater suppression of HDL cholesterol or decrease LDL cholesterol levels. Such issues have to be addressed in comparative studies between testosterone and DHT and in long-term follow-up studies after DHT treatment of androgen-deficient men *(51)*.

SELECTIVE ANDROGEN RECEPTOR MODULATORS

Recent understanding of the molecular structure of the androgen receptor and the modulation of its activity by coactivators or corepressors allows molecular drug modeling to develop AR agonists and antagonists. Screened by high-throughput in vitro cell culture systems, a large number of these compounds have been synthesized and are undergoing testing in several pharmaceutical companies *(52,53)*. Some of the SARM have been developed with the goal of achieving the beneficial effects of androgens on sexual function, mood, muscle mass, and strength and bone mineral density without adversely promoting growth of the prostate gland or allowing a high-androgen microenvironment that could theoretically (although unproven) promote the conversion of histological to clinical prostate cancer. These agents may be steroidal or nonsteroidal compounds and are developed as orally active agents. Although the steroidal SARM may be aromatizable to estrogens (e.g., MENT), the nonsteroidal compounds would not be converted to DHT and estradiol and may have more tissue-specific effects than testosterone. These agents have not been tested in phase II/III clinical trials.

SELECTION OF THE ANDROGEN DELIVERY SYSTEM

The selection of which androgen delivery system will provide adequate replacement for hypogonadal men depends on the goals of therapy and the clear understanding of the pharmacokinetics of each preparation. Different target tissues may have different responsiveness to the same dose of androgen. Experiments in animals and men show that the maintenance of sexual function and mood appears to require low normal serum testosterone concentrations *(12,54,55)*. Once threshold serum testosterone levels are achieved, further elevation of serum testosterone to the higher normal range does not appear to further improve sexual function or mood. In contrast, lean body mass and muscle mass appear to be dependent on the dose of testosterone administered and the serum testosterone levels achieved. Recent studies by Bhasin et al. *(55)* reported that normal men rendered hypogonadal by gonadotropin-releasing hormone (GnRH) agonist treatment showed a dose-related increase in lean body mass (measured by dual-energy X-ray absorptiometry) and muscle mass (by magnetic resonance imaging) in response to exogenous testosterone enanthate injections. It is likely also that bone mineral density is also dependent on the dose of testosterone replacement in hypogonadal men *(45)*. The increase in hematocrit and hemoglobin levels as well as the decrease in serum HDL cholesterol levels are also proportional to the serum concentration of testosterone *(55)*. Thus, the beneficial effects of more androgen delivered to the body must be weighed against the potential risks of the associated increase in hematocrit/hemoglobin. It should be noted that it is generally believed that the suppression of gonadotropins is dependent on the dose of exogenous of testosterone administered. For male contraception, preparations capable of delivering higher doses of testosterone are usually required.

Administration of agents providing steady-state serum levels of testosterone has been proposed to be associated with fewer adverse effects, such as development of acne or fluctuation of mood and libido. On the other hand, clinical reports show that oral testosterone undecanoate or testosterone cyclodextrin is well tolerated and accepted by many men with improvement in sexual function and mood and without increased adverse effects despite the unfavorable pharmacokinetics with peaks and troughs after each oral administration. Although generally accepted that the steady-state serum levels are desirable, preparations producing variations of serum testosterone are also effective as androgen-replacement therapy (11,12,56).

Thus, the selection of androgen preparations should be individualized depending on the goals of therapy, the preference of the subjects, affordability, and availability of the delivery systems for the patients. The recent development of transdermal and new injectable testosterone preparations in the future availability of selective androgen-receptor modulators will allow the physician to tailor the therapy according to the needs of the patient.

ACKNOWLEDGMENT

This work was supported by NIH grant no. M01-RR-00425 to the GCRC at Harbor–UCLA Medical Center.

REFERENCES

1. Bhasin S, Gabelnick HL, Spieler JM, et al. Pharmacology, Biology and Clinical Applications of Androgen. Wiley–Liss, New York, 1996.
2. Nieschlag E, Behre HM. Testosterone: Action, Deficiency, Substitution, 2nd Edition. Springer-Verlag, Berlin, 1998.
3. Wang C, Swerdloff RS. Androgen replacement therapy. Ann Med 1997;29:365–370.
4. Wang C, Swerdloff RS. Androgen replacement therapy, risks and benefits. In: Wang C, ed. Male Reproductive Function. Kluwer Academic, Norwell, MA, 1999, pp. 157–172.
5. Smith EP, Boyd J, Frank GR, et al. Estrogen resistance caused by a mutation in the estrogen-receptor gene in a man. N Engl J Med 1994;331:1056–1061.
6. Morishima A, Grumback MM, Simpson ER, et al. Aromatase deficiency in male and female siblings caused by a novel mutation and the physiological role of estrogens. J Clin Endocrinol Metab 1995;80: 3689–3698.
7. Carani C, Oin K, Simoni M, Faustini-Fustini M, et al. Effect of testosterone and estradiol in a man with aromatase deficiency. New Engl J Med 1997;337:91–95.
8. Greendale G, Edelstein S, Barrett-Connor E. Endogenous sex steroids and bone mineral density in older women and men. The Rancho Bernardo Study. J Bone Miner Res 1997;12:1833–1841.
9. Khosla S, Melton LJ, Atkinson EJ, et al. Relationship of serum sex steroid levels and bone turnover markers with bone mineral density in men: a key role for bio-available estrogen. J Clin Endocrinol Metab 1998;83:2266–2275.
10. Salahian B, Wang C, Alexander G, et al. Pharmacokinetics, bioefficacy, and safety of sublingual testosterone cyclodextrin in hypogonadal men: comparison to testosterone enanthate. J Clin Endocrinol Metab 1995;80:3567–3575.
11. Wang C, Eyre DE, Clark R, et al. Sublingual testosterone replacement improves muscle mass and strength and decrease bone resorption and increases bone formation markers in hypogonadal men: A Clinical Research Center Study. J Clin Endocrinol Metab 1996;81:3654–3662.
12. Wang C, Alexander G, Berman N, et al. Testosterone replacement therapy improves mood in hypogonadal men—a Clinical Research Center study. J Clin Endocrinol Metab 1996;81:3578–3583.
13. Dobs AS, Hoover DR, Chen M-C, Allen R. Pharmacokinetic characteristics, efficacy, and safety of buccal testosterone in hypogonadal males: a pilot study. J Clin Endocrinol Metab 1998; 83:330–339.
14. Drewe J, Levine H, Larsen F, Mair S. Pharmacokinetics of a new transdermal formulation, COL-1621, for hormonal replacement in males. Results of a single dose study in healthy females. 82nd Annual Meeting, Endocrine Society, 2000, Abstract 2250.

15. De Lorimier AA, Gordon GS, Lower RC, Carbone JV. Methyltestosterone, related steroids, and liver function. Arch Intern Med 1965;116:289–294.
16. Nadell J, Kosek J. Peliosis hepatis. Twelve cases associated with oral androgen therapy. Arch Pathol Lab Med 1977;101:405–410.
17. Friedl KE, Hannan CJJ, Jones RE, Plymate SR. High-density lipoprotein cholesterol is not decreased if an aromatizable androgen is administered. Metabolism 1990;39:69–74.
18. Nieschlag E, Mauss J, Coert A, Kicovic PM. Plasma androgen levels in men after oral administration of testosterone or testosterone undecanoate. Acta Endocrinol (Copenh) 1975;79:366–374.
19. Schumeyer T, Wickings E, Freischem C, Nieschlag E. Saliva and serum testosterone following oral testosterone undecanoate administration in normal and hypogonadal men. Acta Endocrinol (Copenh) 1983;102:456–462.
20. Gooren LJ. A ten-year safety study of the oral androgen testosterone undecanoate. J Androl 1994;15:212–215.
21. Snyder PJ, Lawrence DA. Treatment of male hypogonadism with testosterone enanthate. J Clin Endocrinol Metab 1980;51:1335–1339.
22. Sokol RZ, Palacios A, Campfield LA, et al. Comparison of the kinetics of injectable testosterone in eugonadal and hypogonadal men. Fertil Steril 1982;37:425–430.
23. Zhang GY, Gu YO, Wang XH, et al. Pharmacokinetic study of injectable testosterone undecanoate in hypogonadal men. J Androl 1998;19:761–768.
24. Behre HM, Abshagen K, Oettel M, et al. Intramuscular injection of testosterone undecanoate for the treatment of male hypogonadism: Phase I studies. Eur J Endocrinol 1999;140:414–419.
25. Nieschlag E, Buckter D, von Eckardstein S, et al. Repeated intramuscular injections of testosterone undecanoate for substitution therapy in hypogonadal men. Clin Endocrinol 1999;51:757–763.
26. Behre HM, Nieschlag E. Testosterone buciclate (20 Aet-1) in hypogonadal men: pharmacokinetics and pharmacodynamics of the new long-acting androgen ester. J Clin Endocrinol Metab 1992;75:1204–1210.
27. Bhasin S, Swerdloff RS, Steiner B, et al. A biodegradable testosterone microcapsule formulation provides eugonadal levels of testosterone for 10–11 weeks in hypogonadal men. J Clin Endocrinol Metab 1992;74:75–83.
28. Amory JK, Anawalt BD, Blaskovich PD, et al. Testosterone release from a subcutaneous, biodegradable microcapsule formulation (Viatrel) in hypogonadal men. J Androl 2002;23:84–91.
29. Handelsman DJ, Conway AJ, Boylan LM. Pharmacokinetics and pharmacodynamics of testosterone pellets in man. J Clin Endocrinol Metab 1990;71:216–222.
30. Handelsman DJ, Mackey MA, Howe C, et al. An analysis of testosterone implants for androgen replacement therapy. Clin Endocrinol (Oxf) 1997;47:311–316.
31. Kelleher S, Turner L, Howe C, et al. Extrusion of testosterone pellets: a randomized controlled clinical study. Clin Endocrinol (Oxf) 1999;51:469–471.
32. Kumar N, Didolkar AK, Monder C, et al. The biological activity of 7 alpha-methyl-19-nortestosterone is not amplified in male reproductive tract as is that of testosterone. Endocrinology 1992;130:3677–3683.
33. Cummings DE, Kumar N, Bandin CW, et al. Prostate-sparing effects in primates of the potent androgen 7α-methyl-19nortestosterone: a potential alternative to testosterone for androgen replacement and male contraception. J Clin Endocrinol Metab 1998;83:4212–4219.
34. Anderson RA, Martin CW, Kung AWC, et al. 7α-Methyl-19-nortestosterone maintains sexual behavior and mood in hypogonadal men. J Clin Endocrinol Metab 1999;84:3556–3562.
35. Bals-Pratsch M, Knuth UA, Yoon YD, Nieschlag E. Transdermal testosterone substitution therapy for male hypogonadism. Lancet 1986;2:943–946.
36. Cunningham GR, Cordero E, Thornby JI. Testosterone replacement with transdermal therapeutic systems. Physiological serum testosterone and elevated dihydrotestosterone levels. JAMA 1989;261:2525–2530.
37. Meikle AW, Mazer NA, Moellmer JF, et al. Enhanced transdermal delivery of testosterone across nonscrotal skin produces physiological concentrations of testosterone and its metabolites in hypogonadal men. J Clin Endocrinol Metab 1992;74:623–628.
38. Meikle AW, Arver S, Dobs AS, et al. Pharmacokinetics and metabolism of a permeation-enhanced testosterone transdermal system in hypogonadal men: influence of application siteCa clinical research center study. J Clin Endocrinol Metab 1996;81:1832–1840.
39. Brocks DR, Meikle AW, Boike SC, et al. Pharmacokinetics of testosterone in hypogonadal men after transdermal delivery: influence of dose. J Clin Pharmacol 1996;36:732–739.

40. Arver S, Dobs AS, Meikle AW, et al. Long-term efficacy and safety of a permeation-enhanced testosterone transdermal system in hypogonadal men. Clin Endocrinol 1997;47:727–737.
41. Dobs AS, Meikle AW, Arver S, et al. Pharmacokinetics, efficacy, and safety of a permeation-enhanced testosterone transdermal system in comparison with biweekly injections of testosterone enanthate for the treatment of hypogonadal men. J Clin Endocrinol Metab 1999;84:3469–3478.
42. Wang C, Berman N, Longstreth JA, et al. Pharmacokinetics of transdermal testosterone gel in hypogonadal men: application of gel at one site versus four sites. J Clin Endocrinol Metab 2000;85:964–969.
43. Swerdloff RS, Wang C, Cunningham G, et al. Comparative pharmacokinetics of two doses of transdermal testosterone gel versus testosterone patch after daily application for 180 days in hypogonadal men. J Clin Endocrinol Metab 2000;85:4500–4510.
44. Wang C, Swerdloff RS , Iranmanesh A, et al. Transdermal testosterone gel improves sexual function, mood, muscle strength, and body composition parameters in hypogonadal men. J Clin Endocrinol Metab 2000;85:2839–2853.
45. Wang C, Swerdloff RS, Iranmanesh A, et al. Effects of transdermal testosterone gel on bone turnover markers and bone mineral density in hypogonadal men. 2001;54:739–750.
46. Schaison G, Nahonl K, Couzinet B. Percutaneous dihydrotestosterone (DHT) treatment. In: Nieschlag E, Behre HM, eds. Testosterone: Action Deficiency, Substitution. Springer-Verlag, Berlin, 1990, pp. 155–164.
47. De Lignieres B. Transdermal dihydrotestosterone treatment of "andropause." Ann Med 1993;25:235–241.
48. Ly LP, Jimenez M, Zhuang TN, et al. A double-blind, placebo-controlled, randomized clinical trial of transdermal dihydrotestosteronegel on muscular strength, mobility and quality of life in older men with partial androgen deficiency. J Clin Endocrinol Metab 2001;86:4078–4088.
49. Kunelius P, Lukkainen O, Hannuksela ML, et al. The effects of transdermal dihydrotestosterone in the aging male: a prospective, randomized, double blind study. J Clin Endocrinol Metab 2000;87:1467–1472.
50. Wang C, Iranmanesh A, Berman N, et al. Comparative pharmacokinetics of three doses of percutaneous dihydrotestosterone gel in healthy elderly men B A Clinical Research Center Study. J Clin Endocrinol Metab 1998;83:2749–2757.
51. Wang C, Swerdloff RS. Should the non-aromatizable androgen dihydrotestosterone be considered as an alternative to testosterone in the treatment of andropause? J Clin Endocrinol Metab 2002;87:1462–1466.
52. Edwards JP, Zhi L, Poolay CL, et al. Preparation, resolution, and biological evaluation of 5-aryl-1, 2-dihydro-5H-chromeno [3,4-f] quinolines:potent, orally active, nonsteroidal progesterone receptor agonists. J Med Chem 1998;41:2779–2785.
53. Hamann LG, Higuchi RI, Zhi L, et al. Syntheses and biological activity of a novel series of nonsteroidal, peripherally selective androgen receptor antagonists derived from 1,2-dihydropyridono [5,6-g] quinolines. J Med Chem 1998;41:623–639.
54. Buena F, Swerdloff RS, Steiner BS, et al. Sexual function does not change when serum testosterone levels are pharmacologically varied within the normal range. Fertil Steril 1993;59:1118–1123.
55. Bhasin S, Woodhouse L, Casaburi R, et al. Testosterone dose-response relationships in healthy young men. Am J Physiol 2001;281:E1172–E1181.
56. Skakkebaek NE, Bancroft J, Davidson DW, Warner P. Androgen replacement with oral testosterone undecanoate in hypogonadal men: a double-blind controlled study. Clin Endocrinol (Oxf) 1981;14:49–61.

II ANDROGEN EFFECTS ON PHYSIOLOGIC SYSTEMS

9

Androgen Signaling in Prostatic Neoplasia and Hyperplasia

Marco Marcelli, MD, Dolores J. Lamb, PhD,
Nancy L. Weigel, PhD,
and Glenn R. Cunningham, MD

Contents

Introduction
Prostate Cancer
Benign Prostatic Hyperplasia
Treatment Based On Hormonal Manipulation
Androgen-Replacement Therapy
References

INTRODUCTION

The prostate gland is possibly the best-characterized androgen target organ. Circulating androgens and a functioning androgen receptor (AR) are necessary for the development and maintenance of this gland throughout a male's life, and they probably are essential for the development of both prostate cancer and benign prostatic hyperplasia (BPH). Prostate cancer represents the second most common cause of cancer deaths in men *(1)*. In 2003, approx 220,900 American men are expected to be diagnosed with prostate cancer, and it is estimated that prostate cancer would cause 28,900 deaths. Although mortality rates as a result of BPH are < 0.5/100,000 *(2)*, this disease affects the quality of life of many men over age 65 and it costs more than $4 billion/yr in health care costs.

Abnormal steroidogenesis, mutations in the 5α-reductase type II gene or inactivating mutations of AR during embryologic development are associated with failure or inappropriate prostatic development. Lack of a testosterone (T) surge at the time of puberty is associated also with development of a rudimentary gland. A subnormal level of T after successful completion of puberty causes involution of the gland. Thus, normal circulating androgen levels and normal androgen action at target tissues are *essential* for normal development and function of the prostate.

The prostate is comprised of stromal and epithelial cells, and both types of cells have ARs. Functional ARs in the stroma are essential for the development of the prostate.

From: *Contemporary Endocrinology: Androgens in Health and Disease*
Edited by: C. Bagatell and W. J. Bremner © Humana Press Inc., Totowa, NJ

Differentiated stromal and epithelial cells communicate via growth factors. Although ARs are present in both stromal cells and epithelial cells, the stroma is necessary for stimulation of many aspects of epithelial function in an in vitro system *(3)*. Exocrine prostatic secretions appear to nourish and protect ejaculated sperm as well as to provide the liquid that permits ejaculation. In view of the fact that all phases of prostatic development depend on a normally functioning AR and on physiologic concentrations of circulating androgens, this review will provide an in-depth discussion of androgen-regulated signaling pathways in prostate cancer and BPH.

Overview of the Androgen-Regulated Signaling Pathway and of Its Function in the Prostate

Testosterone (T) is the principal circulating androgen secreted by the Leydig cells of the testis *(see* Fig. 1). Most T circulates bound to two proteins (sex hormone-binding globulin [SHBG] and albumin) that maintain a dynamic equilibrium with unbound hormone. Free T represents about 1–2% of the total T in the serum *(4)*.

After entering the target cell through passive diffusion *(5)*, T can be converted to 5α-dihydrotestosterone (DHT) by the enzyme 5α-reductase. T and DHT are the major steroids that bind to the androgen receptor. In some target organs, such as the prostate, the primary androgen bound to the AR is DHT *(6)*; whereas in other tissues, such as the wolffian duct and, possibly, the testis, T is the natural ligand. Nevertheless, only one AR cDNA has been identified, despite the tissue-specific differential preference for one of these two ligands.

Androgen Receptors

Immunohistochemical studies of human and rat prostate tissues have shown that AR is present in the nucleus of the epithelial cells of the prostate *(7,8)*. However, many of the prostatic stromal cells (fibroblasts and smooth muscle) also contain nuclear ARs, and these cells are, therefore, likely targets for androgen action as well.

The AR is a member of the steroid–thyroid–retinoid superfamily of nuclear receptors *(9–14)*, and the protein is expressed in the cytoplasm of androgen-responsive tissues. After binding ligand, the AR becomes activated with an associated change in conformation, translocates to the nucleus, and binds DNA, ultimately regulating the transcription of androgen-responsive target genes. The AR gene is localized on the long arm of the X chromosome at Xq11-q12 and spans a minimum of 54 kb *(15,16)*. Because it is X linked, males have only one copy of the AR gene, whereas females have two X chromosomes and, thus, two copies of the gene (one copy undergoes X inactivation). The open reading frame of AR is encoded by 8 exons and is composed of approx 919 amino acids. The general structure of AR is similar to that of other steroid-receptor family members. It consists of a highly conserved DNA-binding domain (DBD) (encoded by exons 2 and 3), a less highly conserved C-terminal ligand-binding domain (LBD) (encoded by exons 4–8), and a rather poorly conserved N-terminal region (encoded by exon 1) *(17)* *(see* Fig. 2). The N-terminal region contains glutamine, proline, and glycine homopolymeric sequences. There is some degree of variability in the size of AR because of the presence of the polymorphic regions, such as the polyglutamine (polyQ) region in exon 1 *(18)*.

Androgen-receptor mutations are involved in unique clinical disorders. Some of these disorders, such as the syndromes of androgen insensitivity and prostate cancer, involve typical androgen target organs. Other disorders, such as Kennedy's disease, involve less

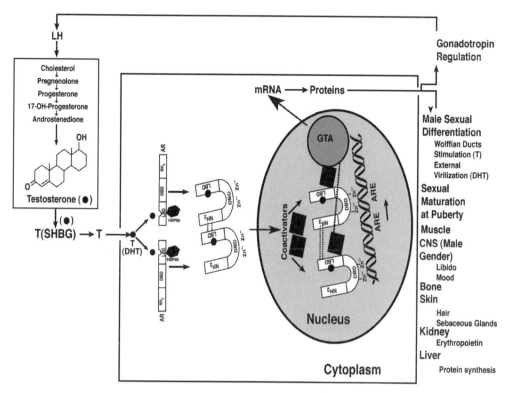

Fig. 1. Mechanism of AR action. Testosterone is the main androgen in circulation. Once inside the cell, T can be 5α-reduced into DHT by the enzyme 5α-reductase. Both T and DHT can bind AR, but DHT binds with greater affinity. Upon ligand binding, the receptor dissociates from heat shock proteins and undergoes a conformational change, phosphorylation, dimerization, and nuclear translocation. Eventually the AR–ligand complex binds DNA and interacts with a number of coactivators that function as docking molecules between the AR and the general transcription apparatus (GTA). The AR functions as a transcription factor and interacts with response elements located in the promoter region upstream of androgen-dependent genes to regulate their transcription. The spectrum of biological activities regulated by AR includes male sexual differentiation, development of the male sexual phenotype at puberty, and regulation of gonadotropin secretion and maintenance of these effects after puberty. Abbreviations: ARE, androgen-responsive element; DBD, DNA-binding domain; GTA, general transcription apparatus; LBD, ligand-binding domain.

typical androgen target tissues, such as the central nervous system, and are associated with an expansion of the polyQ tract located in the N-terminus. Characterization of AR mutants has resulted in the identification of regions of the molecule that regulate additional functions, including nuclear import *(19)*, binding to the nuclear matrix *(20)*, transcriptional activation, dimerization, ligand binding, and DNA binding *(21–25)*.

AR Coactivators

Although it was originally thought that steroid receptors interact directly through transcriptional activation functions (TAF) with proteins in the general transcription complex to stimulate transcription of target genes, studies in recent years have shown that most of these functional interactions are mediated by proteins termed "coactivators."

These coactivator proteins typically interact with the receptor through either the amino terminal or the carboxyl terminal, serving as bridges between the receptor and the proteins of the transcription complex. This is an active area of research and the number of coactivators and the activities associated with them is expanding rapidly. Current models suggest that coactivators form complexes of multiple proteins, some of which have intrinsic enzyme activities that enhance transcription (reviewed in ref. 26). One of the most important coactivator functions is the histone acetyltransferase (HAT) activity that facilitates acetylation of histones that are bound to target genes and that open chromatin structure (27).

The coactivators can be broadly categorized into three groups: (1) those that modulate the activity of a wide variety of transcription factors, (2) those that stimulate the activity of nuclear receptors and few if any other transcription factors, and (3) those that activate one or a few of the nuclear receptors.

CREB-binding protein (CBP) is a coactivator that falls in the group of coactivators that modulate a wide variety of transcription factors. First described as a protein that modulates the activity of cAMP-response elements binding protein (CREB) (28), CBP serves as a coactivator for AR, as well as for other nuclear receptors.

The p160 family of coactivators is an example of those coactivators that interact with most, if not all, nuclear receptors. The nearly simultaneous discovery of the coactivators in different species and the existence of a number of splice variants have led to numerous names for closely related proteins. Three genes have been identified in this family. The first was SRC-1 (29) also called NcoA-1, followed by the other p160 coactivator family members, TIF2/GRIP (SRC-2) (30,31) and p/CIP/RAC3/ ACTR/AIB-1/TRAM (SRC-3) (32–34). These proteins interact in an agonist-dependent manner with the hormone-binding domains of steroid receptors through LXXLL motifs within the coactivators (26). Subsequent studies revealed that there are also substantial interactions with the amino-terminal activation domains of the nuclear receptors. In the case of the androgen receptor, several studies suggest that the most important interactions with AR occur through the amino-terminal domain (35,36). Some of these coactivators are, themselves, HATs, and they recruit P/CAF, another HAT, enhancing histone acetylation at target genes (26).

A plethora of other proteins have been identified that interact with AR and enhance transcriptional activity. In some cases, the specificity of their actions remains to be determined. These include the androgen-receptor-associated (ARA) proteins identified by Chang's group by yeast two hybrid screening as interacting either with the hormone-binding domain or with the N-terminus. Many of these proteins have been cloned previously, and their alternate names are included in parentheses. The ARA proteins include ARA70 (RFG, ELE1), ARA55 (hic5), ARA54, and ARA24 (a Ras-related nuclear protein) (37–40). Other candidates include retinoblastoma protein (Rb) (41), SNURF (small nuclear ring finger protein) (42), Tip60 (also a coactivator for human immunodeficiency virus TAT protein) (43), CAK (cdk-activating kinase) (44), and FHL2 (DRAL) (44). The relative contributions of these proteins to AR action remain to be determined. Some coactivators enhance each other's activity, whereas others appear to be redundant, as the proteins can substitute for each other. These roles will be clarified as mice null for one or more of the coactivators are produced. The SRC-1-null mouse exhibits a reduction in size/development of a number of reproductive tissues, including the prostate, suggesting that it plays a role in vivo in the activity of the reproductive hormone receptors (45).

Although loss of coactivator interactions may lead to a reduction in activity, there is evidence from transient transfection studies indicating that some coactivators may broaden the ligand specificity of AR. Studies from the Chang laboratory indicate that ARA70 cotransfected with AR in DU145 prostate cancer cells that are AR negative causes estradiol and some of the AR antagonists to act as agonists *(46)*. In addition, a recent report has shown that the majority of recurrent prostate cancers express high levels of the androgen receptor and two nuclear receptor coactivators, transcriptional intermediary factor 2 and steroid receptor coactivator 1. Overexpression of these coactivators increases AR transactivation at physiological concentrations of adrenal androgen, thus providing a mechanism for AR-mediated prostate cancer recurrence *(47)*.

Collectively, these studies suggest that coactivators play a critical role in normal AR function. Abnormalities in coactivator structure or in regions of AR that interact with coactivators will have profound effects on androgen action.

PROSTATE CANCER

Epidemiology

The prevalence of prostate cancer at autopsy is considerably higher than its clinical incidence. The epidemiology of prostate cancer is complicated by histological evidence that the prevalence of prostate cancer at autopsy (latent prostate cancer) increases progressively in aging men. It occurs in 15–20% of men 40–50 yr of age and in >50% of men 60–70 yr of age *(48,49)*. The factors responsible for causing a latent prostate cancer to become a clinical prostate cancer are poorly understood.

The clinical incidence of prostate cancer varies greatly, dependent on ethnic background and country of residence. In the United States, it has been estimated that approx 75% of prostate cancers (the occult prostate cancers) will never become diagnosed *(50)*. There is more than a 10-fold difference in the incidence rates of clinical prostate cancer in different countries. This is in sharp contrast with the prevalence of latent prostate cancer, which is roughly the same worldwide *(51)*. Epidemiological observations suggest that diet, genetic susceptibility, environmental carcinogens, and endocrine function may influence the development of prostate cancer. The fact that Japanese and Chinese males immigrating to the United States experience a sharp increase in prostate cancer prevalence in the first and second generation indicates the importance of environmental factors *(52)*. Notably, data on diet and prostate cancer have revealed a strong correlation between per capita fat intake and prostate cancer incidence and mortality *(53)*. Thus, significant ethnic differences in the incidence of clinical prostate cancer seem to provide opportunities for learning more about the pathogenesis of this disease. Potential differences in sex steroid levels have been the focus for many studies.

The incidence and mortality rates from prostate cancer vary among different ethnic groups in the United States. They are higher in African-American (224 and 55/100,000 persons/yr), intermediate among white (150 and 24/100,000), and lowest among Asian-American (82 and 10/100,000) *(1)*. Therefore, investigators have evaluated African-Americans, European-Americans, Asian-Americans, and Asians living in Asia.

Correlation Between Prostate Cancer Epidemiology and Serum Hormonal Levels

Serum hormone levels at the time when prostate cancer is diagnosed may not be representative of those that occur during the development of prostate cancer, so investigators have examined racial differences at different times in a male's life. Recognizing that steroids have the potential to "imprint" target tissues during development, one approach has been to measure serum androgens in pregnant women in an effort to estimate *in utero* exposure to sex steroids. The most frequently cited study showed that serum levels of T were 47% higher in black women and estradiol levels were 37% higher than those in white women *(54)*. SHBG levels were similar. Although we have not been able to identify another study that compared circulating T levels in black and white pregnant women, it is important to note that this may be a simplistic approach to estimating the concentration of androgen in the fetal prostate.

There is a progressive increase in maternal serum T levels throughout pregnancy. The increase in serum total T is primarily the result of the increase in SHBG levels and a decrease in metabolic clearance rates during the first 28 wk and to an increase in production rates after 28 wk *(55)*. Maternal T levels are higher in women with male fetuses from 7 to 14 wk, and they are similar in women with male and female fetuses after 14 wk *(56)*. It is thought that maternal levels may be influenced by fetal androgens or androgen precursors. The fetal testis begins to develop between wk 7 and 8, and Leydig cells differentiate by wk 12. It is thought that human clorionic hyperplasia (hCG) stimulates the Leydig cells to secrete T in the fetus. This is supported by the presence of hCG in the fetal circulation and by observations that the testis does develop in anencephalic fetuses. Peak concentrations of total T are seen at 11–16 wk gestational age in male fetuses *(57,58)*. When the fetus is male, amniotic fluid and fetal plasma T levels are higher from 15 to 23 wk gestation *(58,59)*. Fetal serum levels of luteinizing hormone (LH) and follicle-stimulating hormone (FSH) are much higher in females than males from wk 17 to term, and LH levels vary inversely with free T levels from wk 21 to 24 *(60)*. Chorionic gonadotropin levels were higher at midterm, and free T levels were similar at term. Interestingly, fetal plasma DHT levels at midpregnancy and term were similar in male and female fetuses *(61)*.

The fetal prostate develops in this changing hormonal environment. Prostatic T levels are approx 50 pg/mg wet wt at 16 wk, and they fall to approx 1.5 pg/mg at term. Prostatatic DHT levels are approx 2.5-fold higher at each time-point *(62)*. The predominant estrogen in the fetal prostate is estriol. Estriol levels are higher than DHT levels at 16 wk, and they do not change throughout the remainder of gestation. Estradiol levels are approx 40 pg/mg wet wt at 16 wk, and they decrease to approx 10 pg at term *(62)*. Data are not available to address the question as to whether the prostates in African-American male fetuses are exposed to more T and DHT at critical stages of prostate development.

Testosterone levels are higher in males during the neonatal period and early infancy. Maternal SHBG levels are 21-fold higher than cord blood (fetal) SHBG levels, and levels are similar in male and female fetal cord blood *(63)*. Forest and Cathiard *(64)* found peripheral levels of T to be higher in males during the immediate hours following delivery. Furthermore, plasma total and free-T levels are higher in the male during the first 3 mo of life *(57)*. We have not found reports that compared serum total and free-T levels or estradiol levels in males of different races during the neonatal period or early infancy. It is possible that T and estrogen can imprint the prostate and other organs at this stage of development. Thus, we do not know if imprinting of the prostate during fetal development or early infancy could account for racial differences in the rates of prostate cancer.

Sex steroid hormone levels also have been examined in young men (early twenties). Serum total-T levels were 19% higher and free-T levels were 21% higher in young

African-American men as compared with young European-American men, and serum estrone levels were 16% higher in the black men *(65)*. The increase in total testosterone levels in young adult African-Americans over those of Caucasian men was confirmed by Winters and colleagues *(66)*, but free-T levels were similar in each group. The difference was because of an increase in SHBG levels in the African-American men. These authors postulate that SHBG may stimulate CAMP-dependent protein kinase A and protein kinase A is a coactivator of the AR. In a follow-up study, Ross found serum T levels in young Japanese men to be intermediate between the other two groups *(67)*. Moreover, their SHBG levels were lower than white men. Thus, it is unlikely that differences in total-T levels are causally related to ultimate differences in the incidence of prostate cancer. Whether differences in SHBG levels contribute to the higher incidence of prostate cancer in African-Americans is unknown at this time.

Ethnic differences in male hair distribution suggest differences in serum androgen levels or in androgen effects on androgen-sensitive hair follicles and the prostate, because DHT is the major androgen for both hair follicles and the prostate. Lookingbill and colleagues *(68)* evaluated 184 Caucasian and Chinese subjects. Mean chest hair scores using a scale of 0–4 were 3.0 vs 0.8 ($p < 0.0001$), Caucasian vs Chinese. Serum levels of total and bioavailable T did not differ, but serum levels of precursor androgens were higher in Caucasians, and levels of 5α-reduced androgen products were higher in Caucasians. Santner et al. *(69)* conducted a follow-up study and found no evidence of reduced 5α-reducatase activity, but they did observe a significant reduction of total androgenic ketosteroids excretion in Chinese men living in Beijing compared to Caucasians living in Pennsylvania. Furthermore, Chinese men living in Beijing had lower total serum T, lower SHBG, and lower T production rates when compared to Chinese living in Pennsylvania. No differences in T levels or metabolism were noted between Chinese and Caucasians living in Pennsylvania. Thus, ethnic differences in chest hair are not the result of differences in circulating levels of T. These studies also suggest that differences in national rates for prostate cancer probably cannot be attributed to differences in serum T levels during early adulthood.

A third approach has been to conduct nested case/control studies. A number of prospective studies have correlated prostate cancer risk to sex hormone levels *(70–72)*. When serum T levels are correlated with subsequent development of prostate cancer, these studies have not demonstrated an association. In one study, 222 men who provided plasma in 1982 and developed prostate cancer by 1992 were compared to 390 controls *(73)*. When T and SHBG levels were adjusted simultaneously, a strong trend of increasing prostate cancer risk was observed with increasing levels of T, and an inverse trend was seen with increasing levels of SHBG. Although this may be important, it is unusual to obtain higher total T with lower SHBG levels, as noted in this chapter. Some studies have reported differences in the T/DHT ratio suggesting increased 5α-reductase, but no differences were noted in $3\alpha,17\beta$-androstanediol levels, a major metabolite of DHT. A recent meta-analysis found that men in the highest quartile of serum T had a 2.34-fold increased risk of developing prostate cancer *(74)*. This correlation is based on only two studies *(73,75)*, and differences were observed only after adjusting for BMI, other steroids and SHBG. Differences in serum DHT and estradiol were not significant, but serum insulin-like growth factor (IGF)-1 levels also were associated with a twofold increased risk each of three prospective studies. Thus, there is conflicting evidence that both supports and refutes the hypothesis that men who develop prostate cancer are exposed to increased serum levels of sex steroids.

AR in Prostate Cancer

Radical prostatectomy is the main curative treatment for men with organ-confined disease. Most men with non-organ-confined disease will receive palliative therapy with radiation or androgen ablation. Androgen ablation successfully shrinks primary and metastatic lesions by inducing apoptosis of androgen-dependent prostate cancer cells (76) in up to 80% of cases (77). Unfortunately, whereas the treatment is effective initially, the tumors eventually progress to androgen independence. Prostate cancer may contain foci of both androgen-dependent and androgen-independent cells (78) at the time of diagnosis. Androgen-ablation therapy selects for the growth of androgen-independent clones that can escape the apoptosis induced by androgen ablation (79) and by many cytotoxic drugs. The cells continue to proliferate and produce overwhelming disease that represents the most direct threat to patient survival.

The Role of the AR in Androgen-Independent Prostate Cancer

The molecular basis of progression to androgen-independent disease is not clearly understood. There is evidence that AR is expressed in all stages of prostate cancer evolution, including prostatic intraepithelial neoplasia (PIN) (80), primary disease (8,81–83) and metastatic disease (84,85) both before and after androgen-ablation therapy. Few prostate cancers are AR negative (86). Even the androgen-independent tumors express the AR protein. In addition, recent studies by Tilley et al. support the concept that increased AR immmunoreactivity in early-stage prostate cancer is associated with disease progression following prostatectomy (Tilley, personal communication). A role for AR-stimulated growth of androgen-independent prostate cancer is thus supported by its expression (87,88), together with the overexpression of androgen-regulated genes (89). That AR can play an important role in causing growth of prostatic epithelium is confirmed by the finding of PIN in a recently developed transgenic murine model overexpressing AR in the prostate (90).

In view of these observations, investigators have hypothesized a number of possible "AR-related" mechanisms that could explain progression to androgen-independent growth:

1. Amplification of the AR gene, enhancing AR function and tumor growth at very low concentrations of the ligand (91–93)
2. Superactive androgen receptors resulting from point mutations (94)
3. A promiscuous mutant receptor protein that is activated by ligands other than androgen (95–98)
4. Inactivating mutations of AR generating undifferentiated prostate cancer cells with a malignant and aggressive phenotype (99)
5. Signal transduction crosstalk with activation of growth-stimulating signaling pathways bypassing AR-regulated growth and differentiation (100,101)
6. Increased stimulation by androgen with decreasing length of the polyglutamine repeat of AR (102–105)
7. Increased (or decreased) intraprostatic bioavailability of DHT to activate AR (106,107)
8. Androgen-independent activation of AR (108–113)
9. Modulation of AR signaling with altered availability of different coactivators or corepressors (40,46,47,114)
10. Overexpression of molecules, such as caveolin, that influence AR sensitivity (115)
11. Stabilization of AR in recurrent prostate cancer, which would be associated with hypersensitivity to subphysiological concentration of androgen (116)

Detection of Mutant AR in Prostate Cancer

There is considerable controversy concerning the frequency and nature of these mutations in prostate cancer. Molecular analysis of the AR was conducted in 724 cases of clinically detectable prostate cancer (*see* Table 1). In these 724 cancers, a total of 59 mutations (53 somatic mutations, 2 germline mutations, 4 changes of the polyQ tract) were detected for an overall frequency of 8%. The stage of the disease was described for 660 patients. Early-stage prostate cancer (i.e., stage A or B disease) is rarely associated with mutations of AR (7 mutations [2 somatic mutations, 2 germline mutations, and 3 changes of the polyQ tract] in 336 cases [frequency 0.6%]) *(117–128)*. Primary lesions from patients with more advanced prostate cancer (stages C and D) are more likely to contain mutations of AR. However, the overall incidence is still low (27 somatic mutations and 1 change of the polyQ tract in 238 cases [11.3%]) *(88,91,92,96,117–119,121–124,126,127,129,130)*. Finally, the prevalence of AR mutations is more substantial in metastatic prostate cancer [24 in 97 cases (24%) *(118,127,128,131–133)*]. Thus, mutations of AR are not early events leading to neoplastic degeneration of prostatic tissue, rather they are late developments that may affect biologic behavior and/or response to treatment.

Takahashi and colleagues investigated latent prostate cancers for the prevalence of AR mutations (*see* Table 2) *(137)*. They suggested that inactivating mutations of AR, which are frequent in latent prostate cancer in Japanese men and absent in American men, might prevent the evolution of latent subclinical prostate cancer into a clinically detectable entity. This difference in the prevalence of AR mutations may account for the different incidence of prostate cancer among Americans and Japanese men.

Functional Consequences of AR Mutations in Prostate Cancer

Functional analyses of AR mutants detected in prostate cancer have characterized several different phenotypes that may play different roles in the development of androgen-independent disease.

Mutations Causing "Gain-of-Function"

Androgen-receptor gain-of-function mutations also have been called "promiscuous receptors" *(138)*. The first AR gene mutation with gain-of-function was described in the prostate cancer cell line LNCaP *(95)*, and resulted from the replacement of T at 877 with A. Transfection studies with this receptor showed increased binding affinities for progestens and estradiol. Transcription was activated by these ligands at concentrations that were not sufficient for activation of the wild-type receptor. Interestingly, the T877A AR mutant was also activated by antiandrogens such as hydroxyflutamide, nilutamide, and cyproterone acetate, but not bicalutamide *(139)*. A subset of other AR mutations detected in prostate cancer exhibits a phenotype similar to the T877A variant with enhanced transcriptional activation of AR by several ligands, including the antiandrogens hydroxyflutamide *(97,98,140)* and nilutamide *(97)*, weak agonists like the adrenal precursors dehydroepiandrosterone (DHEA) and androstenedione *(98,140)*, the androgen metabolites androsterone and androstanediol *(140)*, and the glucocorticoid agonist cortisol *(141)*.

Another interesting group of superactive mutants are located at the boundary between the hinge and the LBD (residues 668–671) *(94)*. Compared to wild-type AR, these receptors are 2- to 10-fold more active than wild-type AR upon stimulation with DHT, E2, P,

Table 1
Androgen Receptor Mutations in Prostate Cancer

Ref.	No. of cases		Stage	No. of mutations
117	26		B	1
117	2		D	0
118	8	Primary 8 Mets (16 Metastatic specimens)	D	1 (both in primary and met)
118	7		B	0
119	8		B	0
119	1		C	1
119	1		D	1
96	7		D	1
134	9		C	0
134	6		D	0
129	24		D	6
120	36		B	0
120	4		B	1
121	52		B	0
121	27		D	0
122	17		B	1
122	6		D	0
122	6		D	0
134	64			0
131	10	Bone marrow mets	D	5
91	7		D	0
123	21		B	0
123	9		C	0
123	22		D	2
124	44		16-B 28-D	1
135	13		D	1
88	4		D	0
125	12		B	0
126	5		A	0
126	12		B	2[a]
126	6		C	1[b]
126	13		D	2
130	25		C-D	11
127	14 + 3	Lymph nodes	D	1 (in primary and met)
127	15		B	0
132	5	(in 28 Metastatic deposits)	D	0
133	33	Micro-metastases	D	6
128	99		B	0
128	38		D	11
136	6		B	1

(continued)

Table 1 (continued)

Ref.	No. of cases	No. of mutations	
Stage A and B CaP	336	2	Somatic mutations,
		2	germline mutations,
		and 3	changes of poly Q tract
Stage C and D	238	27	Somatic mutations,
primary CaP		1	change of the poly Q tract
Metastases	97	24	Somatic mutations

Note: It should be noticed that some mutations not inserted in the table have been identified in cell lines *(139,268)* and xenografts *(98)* derived from clinical specimens, or from the prostates of TRAMP mice *(269)*. The total number of cases examined is 724. In 64 of these *(137)*, it was not possible to deduce the disease stage from the study. Thus, the total number of prostate cancer examined for AR mutations in which it is possible to deduce the disease state is 660. From 11 of these patients, specimens were obtained from the primary cancer and metastatic tissue *(118,127)*. (*See* footnote below for explanation of A, B, C, and D staging system.)

Table 2
Androgen Receptor Mutations in Latent Prostate Cancer

Ref.	No. of cases	No. of mutations
137	74 Japanese	18
137	43 American	0
Total	117	18

DHEA, androstenedione, and androgen antagonists. These mutant ARs may be activated by a low circulating level of androgens, resulting in the stimulation of cancer growth in patients previously treated with antiandrogens or with conventional androgen ablation.

The functional consequences of these mutations have several implications, and they help to explain the molecular basis of hormone refractory prostate cancer. Most patients with metastatic cancer undergo treatments that remove testicular, but not adrenal androgens, or they receive potentially agonistic "antiandrogens." Prostate cancers carrying mutations of the gain-of-function type may be resistant to these therapies. A clinical correlate to the activation of AR by hydroxyflutamide in vitro is the so-called "flutamide withdrawal syndrome." These patients with advanced disease experienced an unexpected decrease in serum prostate-specific antigen (PSA) following withdrawal of antiandrogen treatment *(142)*. This syndrome has now been extended to withdrawal syndromes observed after discontinuation of nilutamide, bicalutamide (Casodex), diethylstilbestrol, megestrol acetate, and chlormadinone acetate *(143–147)*.

A1: Well-differentiated, impalpable lesion involving less than 5% of the gland. A2: Impalpable microscopic disease involving more than 5% of gland. B1: Palpable nodule confined to single lobe. B2: Palpable nodules. C: Localized but extraglandular disease. D1: Pelvic lymph nodes involved. D2: Osseous metastases or distant spread to viscera.

A molecular explanation for the flutamide withdrawal syndrome is suggested by the study of Taplin and colleagues *(133)*. This group observed that a larger number of AR mutations (5/16) occurred in micrometastases obtained from patients undergoing complete androgen ablation with luteinizing hormone-releasing hormone (LHRH) agonists and flutamide, as opposed to patients treated with LHRH monotherapy (1/17). Interestingly, mutations in the first group were all localized to codon 877 (T877A or T877S) and were strongly stimulated by hydroxyflutamide, whereas the mutated AR in the second group (D890N) was not stimulated by hydroxyflutamide. When the patients of the first group were switched to bicalutamide (which does not activate the T877A AR), PSA levels decreased. Thus, many gain-of-function mutations may be the result of selective pressure from an AR antagonist, such as flutamide. In addition to AR mutations, coactivators may provide other mechanisms for antiandrogens to activate the AR and possibly maintain growth. Chang and colleagues *(148)* demonstrated that hydroxyflutamide had the ability to activate the transcription of wild-type or T877A AR in the presence of the coactivator ARA70.

In conclusion, gain-of-function AR mutations may offer one mechanism for prostate cancer cells to survive in the androgen-deprived environment of these patients. Furthermore, some "antiandrogens" can act as agonists. In view of these observations, the effectiveness of these agents in the treatment of prostate cancer should be evaluated carefully.

MUTATIONS CAUSING LOSS-OF-FUNCTION

Loss-of-function mutations of the AR have been detected in genomic DNA microdissected from metastatic lymph nodes of patients with prostate cancer *(128)*. Functional analysis of these mutations demonstrated a complete loss of transcriptional activation in cotransfection experiments.

Activation of AR has been considered necessary to sustain growth of prostatic epithelium *(149)*, so it may be surprising that inactivating AR mutations are associated with prostate cancer. However, evidence for a pure growth stimulatory role of AR in prostatic cancer epithelium is controversial, and loss of AR function may be associated with progressive loss of differentiated functions and with a faster replication rate of the cell.

The possibility that declining androgen levels associated with aging contribute to human prostate carcinogenesis and the possibility that androgen supplementation might lower the incidence of the disease is a controversial hypothesis that is based, in part, on this observation *(150)*.

MUTATIONS CAUSING POLYMORPHISMS IN THE NUMBER OF THE POLYQ REPEATS

As described previously for SMBA, the length of the polyQ tract in exon 1 affects the transcriptional activity of AR. An expanded polyQ tract is associated with reduced AR activity *(24,102,103,151)*. Some *(102,103,152)* but not all *(24)* authors have concluded that there is an inverse correlation between polyQ size and transcriptional activity. The inhibitory effect of the polyQ tract on transcription may be exerted, either directly *(102,151)* or indirectly, through effects on AR mRNA stability *(152)* or cellular protein concentration and/or availability.

The relatively low frequency of AR mutations in prostate cancer has led authors to postulate that the role of androgen in prostate cancer must be mediated by the normal, wild-type AR receptor *(105)*. Thus, data have been generated in which the number of Q repeats was compared with the incidence of prostate cancer. A shorter polyQ tract was associated with an increased risk of developing the disease *(105,132,153–156)*. In support of this observation, AR with a reduced polyQ tract has increased transcriptional activity *(102,103,151)*, and enhanced capability to stimulate prostate growth *(157–159)*. It was suggested that the CAG repeat length might be related to the age of the patient at diagnosis and to the response to endocrine therapy rather than to prostate cancer risk *(160)*. However, other authors have failed to detect an increased risk of prostate cancer with the shorter CAG repeat *(161)*. Thus, at this time, the polymorphisms in the CAG repeat length in AR cannot be used to predict a prostate cancer. Some studies have detected an association between a shorter polyQ repeat and the presence of metastatic disease *(132,153)*, high histologic grade *(153)*, and younger age of onset *(162)*. A correlation between the shorter number of Qs *(18)* and the increased incidence, higher mortality, and more aggressive nature of prostate cancer in the African-American population also has been proposed *(163,164)*.

The length of the polyglutamine and polyglycine tracts may also facilitate (or potentiate) the adverse effects of other pre-existing risk factors. The PSA gene has a polymorphic androgen-response element sequence (alleles A and G). One polymorphism, the PSA GG genotype increases the risk for advanced, but not for localized, prostate cancer, whereas the combination of a short CAG allele and PSA GG increases the prostate cancer risk fivefold *(165)*.

Although the increased prostate cancer risk with a shorter repeat is still debated, the notion that smaller polyQs in the AR N-terminal correlates to earlier age onset and to poorer tumor response to endocrine therapy is generally accepted *(160)*. However, some studies in patients with familial prostate cancer did not exhibit shorter repeats *(166)*.

Alternative Pathways of AR Activation

LIGAND-INDEPENDENT ACTIVATION

A possible mechanism for AR activation in patients who underwent androgen-ablative treatments could be mediated by growth-factor-induced transcriptional activation. The possibility that a steroid receptor could be activated by nonsteroid hormone has been observed in studies of the chicken progesterone receptor (cPR) and the human estrogen receptor. These receptors were activated in the absence of steroids by growth factors, neurotransmitters, and other agents that directly or indirectly increase intracellular kinase activity or decrease phosphatase activity *(167–169)*. Culig et al. have reported that the AR can be activated by keratinocyte growth factor, IGF, and epidermal growth factor *(170)*. Nazareth and Weigel reported that the AR can be activated through a protein kinase A signaling pathway *(109)*, and Her-2-neu activates AR signaling when overexpressed in cell lines *(111,112)*. This last observation is interesting in view of two recent observations: First, Her-2-neu is overexpressed in advanced prostate cancer (171) and, second, Her-2-neu signals through Akt to activate AR via phosphorylation of serine 213 and 791 *(113)*. Another intracellular kinase pathway involved in ligand-independent activation of AR is the mitogen-activated protein (MAP) kinase pathway *(172)*. According to these investigators, MAP kinase kinase 1 (MEKK1) induces apoptosis in AR+, but not AR–, prostate cancer cell lines and induces transcriptional activation of AR both in the presence and absence of steroids. Further evidence coupling intracellular kinase pathways with AR action comes from the observation that PTEN, a tumor suppressor gene frequently inactivated in prostate cancer, appears to transcripitonally inhibit AR action *(173)*.

The above data support the possibility that AR can be activated in a nonsteroid hormone-dependent way and still is able to support (or inhibit) transcription of typical AR-dependent genes.

Nongenomic Effects of AR Activation

The dogma of the steroid-receptor mechanism of action is that following ligand binding, the receptor translocates to the nucleus, where it functions as a transcription factor. However, there is increasing evidence that estrogens and progestins, acting through their cognate receptor (174,175) activate nongenomic pathways. These pathways are known to stimulate cellular proliferation and survival. Evidence has now accumulated that the AR also works at least in part by stimulating alternative pathways leading to activation of various protein kinases. Using primary cells obtained from genital skin, prostatic smooth muscle cells, and established prostate cancer cell lines, Peterzile and colleagues demonstrated that DHT leads to a rapid activation of the extracellular signal-regulated kinases (ERKs) ERK-1 and ERK-2. These observations were confirmed and expanded recently (176,177). Migliaccio (174) and collaborators identified activation of a Src/Raf-1/Erk-2 pathway in prostate cancer LNCaP cells by the androgen agonist R1881. Stimulation of this pathway was associated with cell proliferation. Kousteni et al. (177) showed that DHT or estradiol, acting on the AR, estrogen receptor (ER)α or ERβ of osteoblast, osteocyte, embryonic fibroblasts, and HeLa cells, had the ability to activate a Src/Shc/ERK pathway and to inhibit apoptosis. This is a novel way to look at apoptosis that follows hormone withdrawal. It could provide a model for androgen-ablation-induced apoptosis in prostatic epithelium. Efforts to identify apoptotic genes induced by androgen ablation in prostatic epithelium have not been successful, so far (see below). It may be that both nongenomic and genomic mechanisms determine whether a cell undergoes apoptosis.

BENIGN PROSTATIC HYPERPLASIA

The prostate on average weighs 20 g in normal 21- to 30-yr-old men, and the weight changes little thereafter unless the man develops BPH (178). However, because of the prevalence of this disorder, the mean prostate weight at autopsy increases after age 50. The prevalence of histologically diagnosed prostatic hyperplasia increases from 8% in men aged 31–40, to 40–50% in men aged 51–60, and to over 80% in men older than age 80.

A major difficulty in comparing the prevalence of clinical BPH among different populations has been the lack of a common definition. As an example, in a community-based group of 502 men aged 55–74 yr without prostate cancer, the prevalence of BPH was 19% using the criteria of a prostate volume above 30 mL and a high International Prostate Symptom Score (IPSS) (179). However, the prevalence was only 4% if the criteria were a prostate volume above 30 mL, a high score, a maximal urinary flow rate below 10 mL/s, and a postvoid residual urine volume greater than 50 mL. Although symptoms are a major factor in the diagnosis and treatment of BPH, one must recognize that aging men and women have similar urinary symptom scores even though they differ greatly in bladder outlet obstruction (180). For this reason, it is more useful to conduct population-based studies evaluating BPH that rely more on measurements of prostate volume than on symptoms.

One study compared prostate volumes in Japanese men with that in American men, 40–79 yr of age (181). Prostate size increased 6ml/decade in American men, as compared with 3 mL/decade for the Japanese men. Thus, the age-specific prevalence of prostate enlargement was somewhat lower in the Japanese. However, an autopsy study of men who lived in Beijing and Shanghai found that the frequency of histological BPH was similar to that in Western countries *(182)*.

It is thought that diet may contribute to differences in the rates of symptomatic BPH. Saturated fats and zinc may increase and fruits may decrease the risk *(183)*. Asian men consume high-vegetable diets that are high in plant estrogens *(184)*.

Race has some influence on the risk for BPH severe enough to require surgery. Although the age-adjusted relative risk of surgically treated BPH is similar in black and white men, black men less than 65 yr old may need treatment more often than white men *(184)*. In the American Male Health Professional Study, men of Asian ancestry were less likely (relative risk 0.41, 95% confidence interval [CI] 0.21–0.82) to undergo surgery for BPH when compared with white men, and black men had a similar risk as white men *(184)*.

Benign prostatic hyperplasia develops primarily in the periurethral or transitional zone of the prostate. Hyperplastic nodules are composed primarily of stromal components and, to a lesser degree, of epithelial cells; stereologic measurements have revealed a fourfold increase in stroma and a twofold increase in glandular components *(185)*. In one immunohistochemical study, stroma comprised 62% of the volume, epithelium 15%, and glandular lumens 23%; the stroma-to-epithelium ratio was 4.6 *(186)*.

Androgen and BPH

Older age and the presence of hormonally active testes are essential for the development of BPH. Thus, BPH is very rare in untreated hypogonadal men with onset before age 40. The importance of androgen is illustrated by induction of BPH in dogs *(187,188)* and by partial regression of BPH volume when serum levels of T are decreased *(189)*.

Plasma and tissue concentrations of DHT are similar in men with and without BPH. The Physicians' Health Study found similar serum T concentrations at the initial examination in 320 men who developed BPH requiring surgical treatment during the following 9 yr and 320 men who did not develop symptomatic BPH or prostate cancer *(190)*. Walsh and colleagues found similar tissue concentrations of DHT in BPH nodules and in normal prostatic tissue BPH *(191)*. Thus, excess intraprostatic conversion of T to DHT is not responsible for the development of BPH. There are, however, changes in androgen receptors in the BPH prostate. These receptors are primarily located in epithelial cells in normal prostatic tissue, as compared with a more heterogeneous distribution (epithelial and stromal cells) in hyperplastic prostatic tissue *(192)*, and increased transcriptional activity is suggested by recent evidence indicating that risk of surgery for BPH increased with decreased CAG repeats *(193)*.

Estrogen and BPH

There is some evidence that estrogen may contribute to the development of BPH. First, induction of the disorder in dogs is potentiated by the addition of estrogen *(187,188)*. This effect has been partially explained by estrogen induction of ARs. Second, the finding of an increase in the ratio of estrogen to androgen in the serum in older men suggests a role for estrogen in the maintenance, but not necessarily the causation, of BPH. The Physicians' Health Study demonstrated a strong trend for increasing risk of BPH across quintiles for serum estradiol concentrations and a weak inverse trend for serum estrone concentrations in the 320 men who developed BPH necessitating surgery up to 9 yr later *(187)*. The age-related increase in the serum estrogen/androgen ratio is associated with an increase in the estrogen/androgen ratio in prostatic tissue, especially in the stroma *(194)*. Prostatic stromal cells contain estrogen receptors, but the concentrations are lower in hyperplastic than in normal prostatic tissue *(195)*. The concentrations of progesterone receptors in the two types of tissue are similar. Treatment of men with BPH with atamestane, an aromatase inhibitor, reduced serum estrogen concentrations but did not relieve symptoms, increase the urine flow rate, or reduce prostatic size *(196)*. However, another aromatase inhibitor, mepartricin, has been reported to reduce symptoms and increase peak flow rates without changing prostate volume or PSA levels *(196)*. In summary, there is only suggestive evidence that estrogen may contribute to human BPH.

Growth Factors and BPH

Because BPH is primarily a disease of the stroma, the stroma could have intrinsic properties that would enable it to proliferate and also to induce hyperplasia of the epithelium. In the presence of androgen, mesenchymal tissue derived from the urogenital sinus can induce differentiation of epithelium *(197)*. In contrast, stroma lacking functional ARs cannot induce differentiation of normal epithelium. These observations emphasize the importance of the stroma in prostate development. It has been suggested that BPH occurs because prostatic tissue reverts to an embryonic-like state in which it is unusually sensitive to various growth factors. Tissue concentrations of several growth factors are increased in hyperplastic prostatic tissue as compared with normal prostatic tissue. The most consistent increases are in fibroblast growth factors (FGF) 2, 7, 8, or 9, and IGF-II and transforming growth factor-β (TGF-β) and the mRNAs for these substances *(198–203)*. In vitro, epidermal growth factor (EGF), TGF-α, basic FGFs 2–10, IGF-I, and IGF-II stimulate and TGF-β inhibits prostatic epithelial cell growth. Most of these factors stimulate stromal cell growth.

In summary, there is considerable evidence that the androgen signaling pathway contributes to the development of BPH. Differences in androgen signaling and estrogen signaling during normal prostate development may be important. Androgen appears to be required for pathological prostate enlargement, and many of its effects are mediated by growth factors. The growth factors act by both autocrine and paracrine mechanisms to enhance cell proliferation and reduce apoptosis. Estrogen may contribute to this process. Although both epithelial and stromal cells are increased in BPH, the increase in stromal cells dominates in most glands with macronodular BPH.

TREATMENT BASED ON HORMONAL MANIPULATION

Androgen-Ablation-Induced Apoptosis

The precise mechanisms causing apoptosis of prostatic epithelium following castration are not clear. However, a significant amount of information has been generated during the last few years, and many of the intracellular events associated with induction of apoptosis have been clarified. Two major apoptotic pathways originating from two separate subcellular compartments have been identified *(204)* *(see* Fig. 2). The receptor-mediated (or extrinsic) pathway originates at the level of the plasma membrane *(205)*, following interaction of death receptors with their ligands. The mitochondrial (or intrinsic) pathway originates from the mitochondria following activation by proapoptotic Bcl-2 family members *(206)*. Although each pathway is initially centered around unique

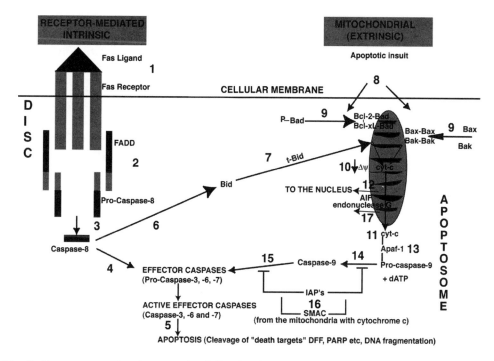

Fig. 2. Receptor-mediated apoptosis: following interaction between a death receptor and its ligand (in this case, the fas receptor and the fas ligand) *(1)*, pro-caspase-8 is recruited to the DISC (death-inducing signaling complex), which consists of the receptor, the adaptor molecule FADD (Fas-associated death-domain-containing molecule), and pro-caspase-8 *(2)*. An active form of caspase-8 emerges from the DISC *(3)* and induces apoptosis by two mechanisms. On one side *(4)*, it directly activates the effector caspases (caspase-3, -6, and -7). These, in turn, cleave various substrates essential for cell survival and induce the typical biochemical and morphological phenotype of apoptosis *(5)*. Alternatively, caspase-8 cleaves the proapoptotic Bcl-2 family member Bid *(6)*. Truncated Bid (t-Bid) complexes to the mitochondrial membrane *(7)* and converges to the mitochondrial pathway. A variety of cellular insults converge to functionally incapacitate the mitochondria *(8)*. These insults are responsible for posttranslational changes of the proapoptotic Bcl-2 family members Bad (which becomes unphosphorylated), Bax, and Bak *(9)*. As a result, Bad will become mitochondrial bound and inactivate through heterodimerization the antiapoptotic Bcl-2 and Bcl-xL. Bax and Bak will homodimerize on the mitochondrial surface and force functional incapacitation of the mitochondria with obliteration of the transmembrane potential ($\Delta\Psi_m$) *(10)*, and translocation to the cytosol of lethal mitochondrial factors such as cytochrome-*c* *(11)*, AIF *(12)*, SMAC *(16)*, and endonuclease G *(17)*. In the presence of APAF-1 and ATP *(13)*, cytochrome-*c* induces activation of pro-caspase-9 into its active form, caspase-9 *(14)*, which, in turn, converges into the effector caspases pathway *(15)*. The IAP proteins inhibit caspase activation and they are inhibited by Smac *(16)*, a mitochondrial protein that follows cytochrome-*c* in the cytosol during apoptosis.

events and each activates a specific apical caspase (i.e., caspase-8 is activated by the extrinsic pathway, and caspase-9 by the intrinsic pathway), the final phase of apoptosis is thought to be common *(204)*. It includes the activation of caspase-3 and caspase-7 and destruction of substrates critical for cell survival *(207)*. It is not completely clear which of these two pathways is activated during castration-induced apoptosis, although observations by Buttyan and collaborators strongly suggest involvement of the mitochondrial pathway (discussed next) *(208)*.

Three major phases have been described for the mitochondrial pathway. In the premitochondrial phase, there is disruption of survival pathways that inactivate proapoptotic molecules (209–212) or facilitate the formation of new antiapoptotic factors *(213,214)*. In the mitochondrial phase, proapoptotic members of the Bcl-2 family of factors (such as Bak and Bax) become mitochondrial bound *(215–218)*, cause loss of mitochondrial transmembrane potential *(219)*, and release apoptotic molecules such as cytochrome-c *(220)*, the apoptosis-inducing factor (AIF) *(221)*, Smac *(222)*, and endonuclease-G *(223)* into the cytosol. Finally, in the postmitochondrial phase, there is the assembling of the apoptosome *(224)*, activation of caspase-9 and then of the executioner caspases *(207)*, disintegration of cellular contents and subsequent absorbtion by neighboring cells.

The leading model to study androgen-ablation-induced apoptosis has been the rat ventral prostate *(225)*. A more complete understanding of the molecular basis for androgen-ablation-induced apoptosis has been slowed by the lack of a cell-line model. Although treatment with androgens induces proliferation or differentiation in cell lines derived from prostatic epithelium *(226–228)*, androgen removal usually is not associated with induction of apoptosis in these models. Nevertheless, investigators have identified a significant number of genes regulated by the addition or removal of androgens in various AR+ cell lines, or AR+ CaP-derived xenografts using ddPCR and microarray technology. Although manipulation of androgen levels in the medium of these experimental models is not followed by apoptosis, some of the genes identified using these approaches have been found to regulate apoptotic functions, and this has furthered our understanding of the possible mechanisms regulating androgen-ablation induced apoptosis.

ANDROGEN-ABLATION-INDUCED APOPTOSIS IN THE RAT VENTRAL PROSTATE

Epithelial cells with apoptotic features appear at 24 h and peak at 48–72 h postcastration *(229)*. By 2 wk postcastration, the wet weight of the ventral prostate is dramatically decreased, and approx 85% of the epithelial cells have undergone apoptosis *(230)*. The morphological events associated with androgen-ablation-induced apoptosis of the ventral prostate secretory epithelium have been carefully described and are similar to those observed in other models of apoptosis. They include blebbing of the apical membrane followed by cell shrinkage, chromatin condensation, formation of apoptotic bodies, and detachment from the basal membrane and neighboring cells *(231)*.

A number of genes induced or repressed during castration-induced apoptosis have been identified. Genes upregulated in the rat ventral prostate after castration include testosterone-repressed prostate message-2 (TRPM-2 or clusterin) *(232)*, TFG-β, c-fos *(233)*, c-myc *(233)*, a 70-kDa heat shock protein *(233)*, fas *(234)*, the rat ventral prostate gene 1 (RVP.1) *(235)*, a matrix carboxy-glutamic acid protein *(235)*, glutathione-S-transferase *(236)* and Nur77/TR3 *(237)*. A proapoptotic role has been clearly defined for some of these molecules (i.e., fas, TFG-β, c-myc, c-fos, Nur77); however, others, such as clusterin, are presumed to work by protecting prostatic epithelial cells from undergoing apoptosis *(238)*, indicating the complexity of the interaction of androgen with the survival and death machinery of a cell. The relationship between the other genes upregulated by castration and androgen-ablation-induced apoptosis has not been established. Among the prostatic genes downregulated by castration, EGF *(239)* is of potential interest. Castration-induced apoptosis may result from a reduction in EGF, a mitogenic factor, and increased expression of TGF-β.

Studies examining changes in the expression of various proapoptotic and antiapoptotic Bcl-2 family members *(208)* have demonstrated the importance of the Bax/Bcl-2 ratio as a determinant of apoptosis. When the ratio was in favor of Bax, usually immediately after castration, cells were undergoing apoptosis. In contrast, no apoptosis was evident after longer intervals, and this was associated with a Bax/Bcl-2 ratio in favor of Bcl-2. Because Bax is one of the most powerful inducers of the mitochondrial pathway of apoptosis, the upregulated Bax/Bcl-2 ratio supports the concept that castration activates this pathway. The rat ventral prostate regenerates after androgen replacement. Evaluating the regenerating prostate before and after androgen replacement is an additional useful model for identifying and studying the function of genes that are induced, or repressed, following treatment with androgens. Because these genes are identified in a regenerating tissue, one would assume that they are involved in antiapoptotic and, possibly, proliferative functions. Using a polymerase chain reaction (PCR)-based cDNA subtraction method with rat ventral prostates from castrated and androgen-replaced rats, Wang identified 25 upregulated and 4 downregulated transcripts *(240)*. One of these, calreticulin, is an important modulator of apoptosis. Calreticulin works by protecting the cell from apoptosis induced by calcium overload. The importance of calreticulin as an antiapoptotic factor has been demonstrated in LNCaP cells. In this cell line, calreticulin increases intracellular Ca^{2+}-buffering capacity and prevents increased intracellular calcium and apoptosis induced by the Ca^{2+} ionophore A23187. In contrast, downregulation of this protein following use of antisense primers permits A23187-induced apoptosis *(241)*. Finding a calcium-binding protein that is androgen stimulated in prostatic epithelium is a potentially important observation. Androgen-ablation-induced apoptosis has been reported to occur follow perturbations of intracellular calcium levels *(242)*. In addition, known inducers of apoptosis of prostatic epithelium, such as thapsigargin, work by disregulating the intracellular levels of calcium *(243,244)*. Based on these observations, one could speculate that under normal circumstances, androgen stimulates calreticulin production. This enables the cell to buffer changes in intracellular Ca^{2+} and to prevent apoptosis. When calreticulin levels fall after castration, the ability to buffer changes in intracellular Ca^{2+} decreases and the cell becomes more prone to undergo apoptosis.

Castration is followed by a 50% reduction in blood flow to the rat ventral prostate within 24 h *(245)*. Interestingly, castration was not associated with blood-flow changes in other androgen-dependent tissues, and testosterone replacement prevented castration-induced blood flow changes in the rat prostate *(245)*. Castration-induced blood-flow changes are associated with apoptosis of the vascular endothelium and, subsequently, of the secretory epithelium. Some authors have hypothesized that prostatic epithelium loss results from hypoxic/ischemic conditions within the prostate *(246)*. Such a novel hypothesis has been preliminaryly validated after observing that hypoxic biomarkers, such as the presence of hydroxyprobe 1 adducts or increased expression of the hypoxia-inducible factor-1α *(247)*.

CONTRIBUTION OF PROSTATE CANCER CELL LINES TO THE UNDERSTANDING OF ANDROGEN ABLATION INDUCTION OF APOPTOSIS

Because LNCaP cells contain AR and secrete PSA in response to androgen stimulation, they are widely used as an androgen-dependent (and well-differentiated) in vitro model of prostate cancer. LNCaP cells undergo growth arrest but not apoptosis in response to androgen deprivation; however, upon androgen removal, they are more likely to undergo apoptosis when treated with a variety of apoptotic substances. LNCaP cells have been used to identify AR-regulated genes. Several of these genes have subsequently been characterized and found to be involved in the regulation of apoptosis. Chang and colleagues *(248)* used ddPCR analysis of androgen-independent and androgen-dependent LNCaP sublines and identified a novel gene, GC79, which is expressed to a higher degree in androgen-dependent cells. GC79 was repressed by physiologic levels (0.1 nM) of androgens only in the androgen-dependent LNCaP–FGC cell line. This molecule seems to have many of the features of a factor that could regulate apoptosis in the prostate. Its expression was increased in the regressing rat ventral prostate after castration, and transfection and induction of this factor in both COS-1 and LNCaP cells led to an apoptotic index eightfold higher than that observed in noninduced transfected cells.

Despite the plethora of information that has been created regarding the interaction between the apoptotic pathway and androgen ablation, the overall understanding of how androgen ablation induces apoptosis is not completely clear. Another subject of extreme interest will be to unravel the antiapoptotic/survival signals that become dominant and prevent full completion of the apoptotic pathway in men treated with androgen ablation who have developed androgen-insensitive disease.

Antihormonal Treatment of CaP

Men with metastatic prostate cancer (CaP) have been treated with androgen ablation since the seminal observation that removal of androgen by castration induces temporary remission of the disease in up to 80% of patients. Androgen ablation is the primary treatment for men with disease outside of the prostate. Although castration is an effective means for removing testicular androgens, it is not acceptable to many men. Treatment with estrogen or with a LHRH agonist also reduces testicular androgen secretion. Eighty-five percent of men having metastatic prostate cancer treated with diethylstilbesterol (3 mg/d) had an objective remission as compared to 86% of men treated with leuprolide *(249)*. Some prostate cancer cells proliferate in the presence of a very low concentration of androgen, and the median time for a clinical relapse is 12–18 mo. Seventy percent of men with androgen-independent tumors eventually die of prostate cancer. Recent years have witnessed an effort to extend the symptom-free period and survival period by total androgen blockade. Because the quality of life is impaired by androgen ablation and because it can be hypothesized that intermittent androgen ablation might be more effective, there also has been interest in intermittent androgen ablation.

Maximum, complete or total androgen blockade has been evaluated in many clinical trials, both in North America and Europe. Because the adrenals can secrete weak androgens that can be converted in part to T, this approach seeks to reduce not only testicular androgens but also to block the effect of adrenal androgens. There were 5710 patients and 3283 deaths in a meta-analysis of 22 randomized trials in which data were available for individual patients *(250)*. These trials compared conventional medical or surgical castration with castration plus prolonged use of antiandrogens (flutamide, cyproterone acetate, or nilutamide). Crude mortality rates were 45% for castration alone and 56% for maximum androgen blockade. The 5-yr survival rates were 22.8% and 26.2%. The improvement of 3.5% (95% CI: 0–7) was not significant. Log rank time-to-death analyses failed to detect significant heterogeneity between trials or significant differences between the effects of various types of maximum androgen blockade. The authors concluded that maximum androgen blockade did not result in longer survival than castration alone. A more recent report provides a 10-yr follow-up comparing goesrelin acetate alone with goesrelin plus flutamide *(251)*. The study involved 589 patients, 55% of whom had metastatic disease at the outset. The hazard ratio to survival was 0.88 (95% CI: 0.68–1.25).

The side effects of androgen blockade are significant, and differences are noted in cost-effectiveness. Bilateral orchiectomy may cause psychological trauma, and antiandrogens may cause tumor flare, hot flashes, gynecomastia, and anemia *(251)*. Long-term, castration, and antiandrogen therapies may cause osteoporosis. Estrogen administration may increase cardiovascular complications, but anemia and osteoporosis are less problematic. Orchiectomy is the most cost-effective, and maximum androgen blockade is the least cost-effective treatment *(252)*.

It has been hypothesized that intermittent androgen blockade may prolong survival and reduce symptoms associated with androgen deprivation *(253)*. Forty-three patients with M1b prostate cancer were treated for 12 mo in a nonrandomized study with androgen deprivation *(254)*. Treatment was stopped until the PSA exceeded 20 ng/mL or when local failure or new bone metastases were detected. In the second treatment period, seven patients experienced hormone-independent tumor growth and died with a mean survival time of 27 mo. Thirty-five patients were responders. In another study, androgen ablation was administered until PSA levels became undetectable or plateaued *(255)*. The time of therapy decreased as the number of treatment cycles increased. The follow-up ranged from 7 to 60 mo (mean: 30 mo), and an average of 45% of the time was spent not receiving androgen ablation. It should be recognized that T levels may be suppressed for extended periods in older men after androgen suppression is stopped. Serum T levels were prospectively measured at 3-mo intervals in 68 men after stopping androgen-deprivation therapy *(256)*. T levels >270 ng/dL were observed in 28%, 48%, and 74% of men at 3, 6, and 12 mo, respectively. Thus, this approach may save money and avoid some side effects; however, patients may not be hormonally normal between treatment periods. Randomized trials are ongoing to determine if intermittent androgen blockade has merit.

It has been hypothesized that antiandrogen treatment prior to radical prostatectomy or prior to radiation treatment of localized disease may improve cure rates *(257)*. Neoadjuvant hormonal therapy decreased the rate of positive margins in six of seven randomized prospective studies *(258)*. Seminal vesicle invasion was not reduced in four studies and only one of four showed a reduction in lymph node metastases. There also was no difference in the time to a rise in PSA levels. Follow-up for these studies is limited to 48 mo, so long-term survival rates are not yet available. However, neoadjuvant therapy does not seem to improve surgical outcomes. In these studies, antiandrogen treatment was given for 3 mo prior to radical prostatectomy. A recent, nonrandomized study suggests that longer (8 mo) antiandrogen treatment prior to surgery may be beneficial *(259)*.

Management of patients who undergo radical prostatectomy and pelvic lymphadenectomy and are found to have positive lymph nodes is a challenge. Timing of antiandrogen therapy has been evaluated in a multicenter study *(260)*. Ninety-eight patients were randomized to observation or to androgen suppression. After a median follow-up of 7.1

yr, survival was improved by immediate androgen suppression. These findings need to be confirmed in larger populations.

Combining androgen ablation with radiation therapy is being evaluated in several studies. D'Amico and colleagues *(261)* at the Dana Farber Cancer Institute conducted a retrospective study of 1586 men with prostate cancer who were treated between January 1989 and August 1999. Men were treated with 3-*d*-conformal radiation therapy alone (*n* = 1310) or in combination with androgen suppression (*n* = 276). Androgen suppression was given for 6 mo (2 mo before, during, and after radiation). They found that patients categorized as intermediate or high risk had a lower PSA failure rate when treated with androgen suppression. Prospective, randomized trials, which are ongoing, are needed to confirm these findings.

Antihormonal Treatment of BPH

Antihormonal therapy for BPH is only modestly effective for mild or moderately symptomatic BPH. Once BPH is established, agents that reduce DHT levels *(262)*, T and DHT levels *(189)* or androgen effects *(263)* reduce prostate volume only by 20–30%, diminish symptoms moderately, and increase urine flow only by an average of < 2 mL/s. Reduction of prostatic DHT levels can prevent progression of the disease *(264)*; however, lowering prostatic DHT does not provide good therapy for moderate to severe BPH. The reasons for the limited effectiveness of therapies that reduce DHT and/or T are poorly understood. Although ARs are present in the secretory epithelial and stromal cells of the prostate, only the former appear to undergo apoptosis in patients treated with a 5α-reductase inhibitor *(261)*. Thus, 5α-reductase inhibitors may be most useful in preventing enlargement of the prostate and development of lower urinary tract symptoms (LUTS).

ANDROGEN-REPLACEMENT THERAPY

Both aging and hypogonadism are associated with an increase in body fat, a decrease in lean body mass and skeletal muscle, a reduction in bone mineral density, loss of libido and erectile function, and a reduction in body hair. Mean serum total T levels fall significantly after the seventh decade of life, and mean free T levels fall a decade earlier. The increase in SHBG levels that occurs with aging tends to mask the fall in free or bioavailable T. Approximately 20% of men aged 60–70 yr have total T levels less than 300 ng/dL and 30% of men aged 70–80 have total levels less than 300 ng/dL *(265)*. The percentages of men in these age groups with low free T indexes are 34% and 68%, respectively!

Testosterone replacement in aging men improves body composition and bone mineral density, and it may improve mood, sense of well-being, cognition, and quality of life; however, there are potential adverse effects on the prostate of aging men *(263,264)*. The possibility that T replacement will cause latent prostate cancers to become a clinical prostate cancers is of concern. Whether long-term androgen replacement in aging men will require more frequent invasive therapy for BPH is not known. As expected, Snyder detected a few clinical prostate cancers in both placebo and T treatment. However, studies by Snyder, et al. *(266)* were not powered to address effects of testosterone-replacement therapy on prostate cancer or BPH. A large clinical trial will be required to address these risks. Until such information is available, we cannot fully assess the risks of testosterone replacement on the prostate in aging men.

REFERENCES

1. Jemal A, Murray T, Samuels A, Ghafoor A, Ward E, Thun M. Cancer statistics, 2003. CA Cancer J Clin 2003;53:5–26.
2. La Vecchia C, Levi F, Lucchini F. Mortality from benign prostatic hyperplasia: worldwide trends 1950–92. J Epidemiol Community Health 1995;49:379–384.
3. Cunha GR. Mesenchimal–epithelial interaction in sex differentiation. Hum Gen 1981;58:68–77.
4. Pardridge WM. Serum bioavailability of sex steroid hormones. Clin Endocrinol Metab 1986;15: 259–278.
5. Lasnitzki I, Franklin HR, Wilson JD. The mechanism of androgen uptake and concentration by rat ventral prostate in organ culture. J Endocrinol 1974;60:81–90.
6. Bruchovsky N, Wilson JD. The intranuclear binding of testosterone and 5-alpha-androstan-17-beta-ol-3-one by rat prostate. J Biol Chem 1968;243:5953–5960.
7. Prins GS, Birch L, Greene GL. Androgen receptor localization in different cell types of the adult rat prostate. Endocrinology 1991;129:3187–3199.
8. Mohler JL, Chen Y, Hamil K, et al. Androgen and glucocorticoid receptors in the stroma and epithelium of prostatic hyperplasia and carcinoma. Clin Cancer Res 1996;2:889–895.
9. Chang CS, Kokontis J, Liao ST. Structural analysis of complementary DNA and amino acid sequences of human and rat androgen receptors. Proc Natl Acad Sci USA 1988;85:7211–7215.
10. Chang CS, Kokontis J, Liao ST. Molecular cloning of human and rat complementary DNA encoding androgen receptors. Science 1988;240:324–326.
11. Lubahn DB, Joseph DR, Sar M, et al. The human androgen receptor: complementary deoxyribonucleic acid cloning, sequence analysis and gene expression in the prostate. Mol Endocrinol 1988;2:1265–1275.
12. Lubahn DB, Joseph DR, Sullivan PM, et al. Cloning of human androgen receptor complementary DNA and localization to the X chromosome. Science 1988;240:327–330.
13. Tilley WD, Marcelli M, Wilson JD, McPhaul JM. Characterization and cloning of a cDNA encoding the human androgen receptor. Proc Natl Aca Sci USA 1989;86:327–331.
14. Trapman J, Klaassen P, Kuiper GG, et al. Cloning, structure and expression of a cDNA encoding the human androgen receptor. Biochem Biophys Res Commun 1988;153:241–248.
15. Lubahn DB, Brown TR, Simental JA, et al. Sequence of the intron/exon junctions of the coding region of the human androgen receptor gene and identification of a point mutation in a family with complete androgen insensitivity, Proc Natl Acad Sci USA 1989;86:9534–9538.
16. Marcelli M, Tilley WD, Wilson CM, et al. Definition of the human androgen receptor gene permits the identification of mutations that cause androgen resistance: premature termination codon of the receptor protein at amino acid residue 588 causes complete androgen resistance. Mol Endocrinol 1990;4:1105–1116.
17. Mangelsdorf DJ, Thummel C, Beato M, et al. The nuclear receptor superfamily: the second decade. Cell 1995;83:835–839.
18. Edwards A, Hammond HA, Jin L, et al. Genetic variation at five trimeric and tetrameric tandem repeat loci in four human population groups. Genomics 1992;12:241–253.
19. Jenster G, Trapman J, Brinkmann AO. Nuclear import of the human androgen receptor. Biochem J 1993;293:761–768.
20. van Steensel B, Jenster G, Damm K, et al. Domains of the human androgen receptor and glucocorticoid receptor involved in binding to the nuclear matrix. J Cell Biochem 1995;57:465–478.
21. Simental JA, Sar M, Lane MV, et al. Transcriptional activation and nuclear targeting signals of the human androgen receptor. J Biol Chem 1991;266:510–518.
22. Simental JA, Sar M, Wilson EM. Domain functions of the androgen receptor. J Steroid Biochem Mol Biol 1992;43:37–41.
23. Jenster G, van der Korput JA, Trapman J, Brinkmann AO. Functional domains of the human androgen receptor. J Steroid Biochem Mol Biol 1992;41:671–675.
24. Gao T, Marcelli M, McPhaul M. Transcriptional activation and transient expression of the human androgen receptor. J Steroid Biochem Molec Biol 1996;59:9–20.
25. Jenster G, van der Korput HA, Trapman J, Brinkmann AO. Identification of two transcription activation units in the N-terminal domain of the human androgen receptor. J Biol Chem 1995; 270:7341–7346.

26. McKenna NJ, Lanz RB, O'Malley BW. Nuclear receptor coregulators: cellular and molecular biology. Endocr Rev 1999;20:321–344.

27. Spencer TE, Jenster G, Burcin MM, et al. Steroid receptor coactivator-1 is a histone acetyltransferase. Nature 1997;389:194–198.

28. Kwok RP, Lundblad JR, Chrivia JC, et al. Nuclear protein CBP is a coactivator for the transcription factor CREB [see comments]. Nature 1994;370:223–226.

29. Onate SA, Tsai SY, Tsai MJ, O'Malley BW. Sequence and characterization of a coactivator for the steroid hormone receptor superfamily. Science 1995;270:1354–1357.

30. Voegel JJ, Heine MJ, Zechel C, et al. TIF2, a 160 kDa transcriptional mediator for the ligand-dependent activation function AF-2 of nuclear receptors. Embo J 1996;15:3667–3675.

31. Hong H, Kohli K, Trivedi A, et al. GRIP1, a novel mouse protein that serves as a transcriptional coactivator in yeast for the hormone binding domains of steroid receptors. Proc Natl Acad Sci USA 1996;93:4948–4952.

32. Chen H, Lin RJ, Schiltz, RL, et al. Nuclear receptor coactivator ACTR is a novel histone acetyltransferase and forms a multimeric activation complex with P/CAF and CBP/p300. Cell 1997;90:569–580.

33. Suen CS, Berrodin TJ, Mastroeni R, et al. A transcriptional coactivator, steroid receptor coactivator-3, selectively augments steroid receptor transcriptional activity. J Biol Chem 1998; 273:27645–27653.

34. Anzick SL, Kononen J, Walker RL, et al. AIB1, a steroid receptor coactivator amplified in breast and ovarian cancer. Science 1997;277:965–968.

35. Bevan CL, Hoare S, Claessens F, et al. The AF1 and AF2 domains of the androgen receptor interact with distinct regions of SRC1. Mol Cell Biol 1999;19:8383–8392.

36. Alen P, Claessens F, Verhoeven G, et al. The androgen receptor amino-terminal domain plays a key role in p160 coactivator-stimulated gene transcription. Mol Cell Biol 1999;19:6085–6097.

37. Hsiao PW, Lin DL, Nakao R, Chang C. The linkage of Kennedy's neuron disease to ARA24, the first identified androgen receptor polyglutamine region-associated coactivator. J Biol Chem 1999;274: 20229–20234.

38. Kang HY, Yeh S, Fujimoto N, et al. Cloning and characterization of human prostate coactivator ARA54, a novel protein that associates with the androgen receptor. J Biol Chem 1999;274:8570–8576.

39. Fujimoto N, Yeh S, Kang HY, et al. Cloning and characterization of androgen receptor coactivator, ARA55, in human prostate. J Biol Chem 1999;274:8316–8321.

40. Yeh S, Chang C. Cloning and characterization of a specific coactivator, ARA70, for the androgen receptor in human prostate cells. Proc Natl Acad Sci USA 1996;93:5517–5521.

41. Yeh S, Miyamoto H, Nishimura K, et al. Retinoblastoma, a Tumor Suppressor, Is a Coactivator for the Androgen Receptor in Human Prostate Cancer DU145 Cells. Biochem Biophys Res Commun 1998;248:361–367.

42. Moilanen AM, Poukka H, Karvonen U, et al. Identification of a novel RING finger protein as a coregulator in steroid receptor-mediated gene transcription. Mol Cell Biol 1998;18:5128–5139.

43. Brady ME, Ozanne DM, Gaughan L, et al. Tip60 is a nuclear hormone receptor coactivator. J Biol Chem 1999;274:17599–17604.

44. Lee DK, Duan HO, Chang C. From androgen receptor to the general transcription factor TFIIH. Identification of cdk activating kinase (CAK) as an androgen receptor NH(2)-terminal associated coactivator. J Biol Chem 2000;275:9308–9313.

45. Xu J, Qiu Y, DeMayo FJ, et al. Partial hormone resistance in mice with disruption of the steroid receptor coactivator-1 (SRC-1) gene. Science 1998;279:1922–1925.

46. Yeh S, Miyamoto H, Shima H, Chang C. From estrogen to androgen receptor: a new pathway for sex hormones in prostate. Proc Natl Acad Sci USA 1998;95:5527–5532.

47. Gregory CW, He B, Johnson RT, et al. A Mechanism for Androgen Receptor-mediated Prostate Cancer Recurrence after Androgen Deprivation Therapy. Cancer Res 2001;61:4315–4319.

48. Carter HB, Piantadosi S, Isaacs JT. Clinical evidence for and implications of the multistep development of prostate cancer. J Urol 1990;143:742–746.

49. Holund B. Latent prostatic cancer in a consecutive autopsy series. Scan J Urol 1980;14:29–35.

50. Etzioni R, Cha R, Feuer EJ, Davidov O. Asymptomatic incidence and duration of prostate cancer. Am J Epidemiol 1998;148:775–785.

51. Yatani R, Shiraishi T, Nakakuki K, et al. Trends in frequency of latent prostate carcinoma in Japan from 1965–1979 to 1982–1986. J Natl Cancer Inst 1988;80:683–687.

52. Cook LS, Goldoft M, Schwartz SM, Weiss NS. Incidence of adenocarcinoma of the prostate in Asian immigrants to the United States and their descendants. J Urol 1999;161:152–155.

53. Giovannucci E, Rimm EB, Colditz GA, et al. A prospective study of dietary fat and risk of prostate cancer. J Natl Cancer Inst 1993;85:1571–1579.

54. Henderson BE, Ross R, Bernstein L. Estrogens as a cause of human cancer: The Richard and Hinda Rosenthal Foundation award lecture. Cancer Res 1988;48:246–253.

55. Bammann BL, Coulam CB, Jiang NS. Total and free testosterone during pregnancy. Am J Obstet Gynecol 1980;137:293–298.

56. Klinga K, Bek E, Runnebaum B. Maternal peripheral testosterone levels during the first half of pregnancy. Am J Obstet Gynecol 1978;131:60–62.

57. Forest MG, Sizonenko PC, Cathiard AM, Bertrand J. Hypophyso-gonadal function in humans during the first year of life. 1. Evidence for testicular activity in early infancy. J Clin Invest 1974;53:819–828.

58. Takagi S, Yoshida T, Tsubata K, et al. Sex differences in fetal gonadotropins and androgens., J Steroid Biochem 1977;8:609–620.

59. Rodeck CH, Gill D, Rosenberg DA, Collins WP. Testosterone levels in midtrimester maternal and fetal plasma and amniotic fluid. Prenat Diagn 1985;5:175–181.

60. Beck-Peccoz P, Padmanabhan V, Baggiani AM, et al. Maturation of hypothalamic-pituitary-gonadal function in normal human fetuses: circulating levels of gonadotropins, their common alpha-subunit and free testosterone, and discrepancy between immunological and biological activities of circulating follicle-stimulating hormone. J Clin Endocrinol Metab 1991;73:525–532.

61. Abramovich DR, Herriot R, Stott J. Dihydrotestosterone levels at midpregnancy and term: a comparison with testosterone concentrations. Br J Obstet Gynaecol 1983;90:232–234.

62. Zondek T, Mansfield MD, Attree SL, Zondek LH. Hormone levels in the foetal and neonatal prostate. Acta Endocrinol (Copenh) 1986;112:447–456.

63. Anderson DC, Lasley BL, Risher RA, et al. Transplacental gradients of sex-hormone-binding globulin in human and simian pregnancy. Clin Endocrinol (Oxf) 1976;5:657–669.

64. Forest MG, Cathiard AM. Pattern of plasma testosterone and delta4-androstenedione in normal newborns: Evidence for testicular activity at birth. J Clin Endocrinol Metab 1975;41:977–980.

65. Ross R, Bernstein L, Judd H, et al. Serum testosterone levels in healthy young black and white men. J Natl Cancer Inst 1986;76:45–48.

66. Winters SJ, Brufsky A, Weissfeld J, et al. Testosterone, sex hormone-binding globulin, and body composition in young adult African American and Caucasian men. Metabolism 2001;50:1242–1247.

67. Ross RK, Bernstein L, Lobo RA, et al. 5-alpha-reductase activity and risk of prostate cancer among Japanese and US white and black males. Lancet 1992;339:887–889.

68. Lookingbill DP, Demers LM, Wang C, et al. Clinical and biochemical parameters of androgen action in normal healthy Caucasian versus Chinese subjects. J Clin Endocrinol Metab 1991;72:1242–1248.

69. Santner SJ, Albertson B, Zhang GY, et al. Comparative rates of androgen production and metabolism in Caucasian and Chinese subjects. J Clin Endocrinol Metab 1998;83:2104–2109.

70. Heikkila R, Aho K, Heliovaara M, et al. Serum testosterone and sex hormone-binding globulin concentrations and the risk of prostate carcinoma: a longitudinal study. Cancer 1999;86:312–315.

71. Eaton NE, Reeves GK, Appleby PN, Key TJ. Endogenous sex hormones and prostate cancer: a quantitative review of prospective studies. Br J Cancer 1999;80:930–934.

72. Mikkola AK, Aro JL, Rannikko SA, Salo JO. Pretreatment plasma testosterone and estradiol levels in patients with locally advanced or metastasized prostatic cancer. FINNPROSTATE Group. Prostate 1999;39:175–181.

73. Gann PH, Hennekens CH, Ma J, et al. Prospective study of sex hormone levels and risk of prostate cancer: A prospective, population-based study of androstenedione, estrogens, and prostatic cancer. J Natl Cancer Inst 1996;88:1118–1126.

74. Shaneyfelt T, Husein R, Bubley G, Mantzoros CS. Hormonal predictors of prostate cancer: a meta-analysis. J Clin Oncol 2000;18:847–853.

75. Hsing AW, Comstock GW. Serological precursors of cancer: serum hormones and risk of subsequent prostate cancer. Cancer Epidemiol Biomarkers Prev 1993;2:27–32.

76. Kyprianou N, English H, Isaacs J. Programmed cell death during regression of PC-82 human prostate cancer following androgen ablation. Cancer Res 1990;50:3748–3753.

77. Koivisto P, Komer M, Visakorpi T, Kallionemi O-P. Androgen receptor gene and hormonal therapy failure of prostate cancer. Am J Pathol 1998;152:1–9.

78. Isaacs J, Coffey D. Adaptation vs selection as the mechanism responsible for the relapse of prostatic cancer to androgen ablation as studied in the Dunning R-3327 H adenocarcinoma. Cancer Res 1981;41:5070–5075.
79. Isaacs J, Lundmo P, Berges R, et al. Androgen regulation of programmed cell death of normal and malignant prostatic cells. J Androl 1992;13:457–464.
80. Van-der-Kwast T, Tetu B. Androgen receptors in untreated and treated prostatic intraepithelial neoplasia. Eur Urol 1996;30:265–268.
81. Sadi MV, Walsh PC, Barrack ER. Immunohistochemical study of androgen receptors in metastatic prostate cancer. Cancer 1991;67:3057–3064.
82. Tilley WD, Lim-Tio SS, Horsfall DJ, et al. Detection of discrete androgen receptor epitopes in prostate cancer by immunostaining: measurement by color video image analysis. Cancer Res 1994;54:4096–4102.
83. Gil-Diez de Medina S, Salomon L, Colombel M, et al. Modulation of cytokeratin subtype, EGF receptor, and androgen receptor expression during progression of prostate cancer. Hum Pathol 1998;29:1005–1012.
84. Hobisch A, Culig Z, Radmayr C, et al. Androgen receptor status of lymph node metastases from prostate cancer. Prostate 1996;28:129–135.
85. Hobisch A, Culig Z, Radmayr C, et al. Distant metastases from prostatic carcinoma express androgen receptor protein. Cancer Res 1995;55:3068–3072.
86. Van-der-Kwast TH, Schalken J, Ruizeveld-de-Winter JA, et al. Androgen receptors in endocrine-therapy resistant human prostate cancer. Int J Can 1991;48:189–193.
87. Ruizeveld-de-Winter JA, Trapman J, Brinkmann AO, et al. Androgen receptor heterogeneity in human prostatic carcinomas visualized by immunocytochemistry. J Pathol 1990;161:329–332.
88. de Vere White R, Meyers F, Chi, S G, et al. Human androgen receptor expression in prostate cancer following androgen ablation. Eur Urol 1997;31:1–6.
89. Gregory CW, Hamil KG, Kim D, et al. Androgen receptor expression in androgen-independent prostate cancer is associated with increased expression of androgen-regulated genes. Cancer Res 1998;58:5718–5724.
90. Stanbrough M, Leav I, Kwan PW, et al. Prostatic intraepithelial neoplasia in mice expressing an androgen receptor transgene in prostate epithelium. Proc Natl Acad Sci USA 2001;98: 10823–10828.
91. Visakorpi T, Hyytinen E, Koivisto P, et al. In vivo amplification of the androgen receptor gene and progression of human prostate cancer. Nat Genet 1995;9:401–406.
92. Koivisto P, Kononen J, Palmberg C, et al. Androgen receptor gene amplification: a possible molecular mechanism for androgen deprivation therapy failure in prostate cancer. Cancer Res 1997;57:314–319.
93. Linja MJ, Savinainen KJ, Saramaki OR, et al. Amplification and overexpression of androgen receptor gene in hormone- refractory prostate cancer. Cancer Res 2001;61:3550–3555.
94. Buchanan G, Yang M, Harris JM, et al. Mutations at the boundary of the hinge and ligand binding domain of the androgen receptor confer increased transactivation function. Mol Endocrinol 2001;15:46–56.
95. Veldscholdte J, Ris-Stalpers C, Kuiper GGJM, et al. A mutation in the ligand binding domain of the androgen receptor of LnCAP cells affects steroid binding characteristics and response to anti-androgens. Biochem Biophys Res Commun 1990;173:534–540.
96. Culig Z, Hobisch A, Cronauer MV, et al. Mutant androgen receptor detected in an advanced stage prostatic carcinoma is activated by adrenal androgens and progesterone. Mol Endocrinol 1993;7:1541–1550.
97. Fenton MA, Shuster TD, Fertig AM, et al. Functional characterization of mutant androgen receptors from androgen-independent prostate cancer [in process citation]. Clin Cancer Res 1997;3: 1383–1388.
98. Tan J, Sharief Y, Hamil KG, et al. Dehydroepiandrosterone activates mutant androgen receptors expressed in the androgen-dependent human prostate cancer xenograft CWR22 and LNCaP cells. Mol Endocrinol 1997;11:450–459.
99. Nazareth LV, Stenoien DL, Bingman III WE, et al. A C619Y Mutation in the Human Androgen Receptor Causes Inactivation and Mislocalization of the Receptor with Concomitant Sequestration of SRC-1. Mol Endocrinol 1999;13:2065–2075.
100. Voeller H, Wilding G, Gelmann E. v-rasH expression confers hormone-independent in-vitro growth to LnCAP prostate carcinoma cells. Mol Endocrin 1991;5:209–216.

101. Papandreou CN, Usmani B, Geng Y, et al. Neutral endopeptidase 24.11 loss in metastatic human prostate cancer contributes to androgen-independent progression. Nat Med 1998;4:50–57.
102. Kazemi-Esfarjani P, Trifiro MA, Pinsky L. Evidence for a repressive function of the long polyglutamine tract in the human androgen receptor: possible pathogenetic relevance for the (CAG)n-expanded neuronopathies. Hum Mol Genet 1995;4:523–527.
103. Chamberlain NL, Driver ED, Miesfeld RL. The length and location of CAG trinucleotide repeats in the androgen receptor N-terminal domain affect transactivation function. Nucleic Acids Res 1994;22:3181–3186.
104. Choong CS, Kemppainen JA, Zhou ZX, Wilson EM. Reduced androgen receptor gene expression with first exon CAG repeat expansion. Mol Endocrinol 1996;10:1527–1535.
105. Hakimi JM, Schoenberg MP, Rondinelli RH, et al. Androgen receptor variants with short glutamine or glycine repeats may identify unique subpopulations of men with prostate cancer. Clin Cancer Res 1997;3:1599–1608.
106. Makridakis N, Ross RK, Pike MC, et al. A prevalent missense substitution that modulates activity of prostatic steroid 5alpha-reductase. Cancer Res 1997;57:1020–1022.
107. Ross RK, Pike MC, Coetzee GA, et al. Androgen metabolism and prostate cancer: establishing a model of genetic susceptibility. Cancer Res 1998;58:4497–4504.
108. Culig Z, Hobisch A, Hittmair A, et al. Expression, structure, and function of androgen receptor in advanced prostatic carcinoma. Prostate 1998;35:63–70.
109. Nazareth L, Weigel N. Activation of the human androgen receptor through a protein kinase A signaling pathway. J Biol Chem 1996;271:19900–19907.
110. Hobisch A, Eder IE, Putz T, et al. Interleukin-6 regulates prostate-specific protein expression in prostate carcinoma cells by activation of the androgen receptor. Cancer Res 1998;58:4640–4645.
111. Yeh S, Lin HK, Kang HY, et al. From HER2/Neu signal cascade to androgen receptor and its coactivators: a novel pathway by induction of androgen target genes through MAP kinase in prostate cancer cells. Proc Natl Acad Sci USA 1999;96:5458–5463.
112. Craft N, Shostak Y, Carey M, et al. A mechanism for hormone-independent prostate cancer through modulation of androgen receptor signaling by the HER-2/neu tyrosine kinase. Nature Med 1999;5:280–285.
113. Wen Y, Hu MC, Makino K, et al. HER-2/neu promotes androgen-independent survival and growth of prostate cancer cells through the Akt pathway. Cancer Res 2000;60:6841–6845.
114. Miyamoto H, Yeh S, Wilding G, Chang C. Promotion of agonist activity of antiandrogens by the androgen receptor coactivator, ARA70, in human prostate cancer DU145 cells. Proc Natl Acad Sci USA 1998;95:7379–7384.
115. Nasu Y, Timme T, Yang G, et al. Suppression of caveolin expression induces androgen sensitivity in metastatic androgen-insensitive mouse prostate cancer. Nature Med 1998;4:1062–1064.
116. Gregory CW, Johnson RT Jr, Mohler JL, et al. Androgen receptor stabilization in recurrent prostate cancer is associated with hypersensitivity to low androgen. Cancer Res 2001;61:2892–2898.
117. Newmark JR, Hardy DO, Tonb DC, et al. Androgen receptor gene mutations in human prostate cancer. Proc Nat Aca Sci USA 1992;89:6319–6323.
118. Suzuki H, Sato N, Watabe Y, et al. Androgen receptor gene mutations in human prostate cancer. J Steroid Biochem Molec Biol 1993;46:759–765.
119. Castagnaro M, Yandell DW, Dockhorn-Dworniczak B, et al. Androgen receptor gene mutations and p53 gene analysis in advanced prostate cancer. Verh Dtsch Ges Pathol 1993;77:119–123.
120. Schoenberg MP, Hakimi JM, Wang SP, et al. Microsatellite mutation (CAG24->18) in the androgen receptor gene in human prostate cancer. Bioch Biophys Res Commun 1994;198:74–80.
121. Ruizeveld-de-Winter JA, Janssen PJA, Sleddens HMEB, et al. Androgen receptor status in localized and locally progressive hormone refractory human prostate cancer. Am J Pathol 1994;144:735–746.
122. Elo JP, Kvist L, Leinonen K, et al. Mutated human androgen receptor gene detected in a prostatic cancer patient is also activated by estradiol. J Clin Endocrinol Metab 1995;80:3494–3500.
123. Suzuki H, Akakura K, Komiya A, et al. Codon 877 mutation in the androgen receptor gene in advanced prostate cancer: relation to antiandrogen withdrawal syndrome. Prostate 1996;29:153–158.
124. Evans BA, Harper ME, Daniells CE, et al. Low incidence of androgen receptor gene mutations in human prostatic tumors using single strand conformation polymorphism analysis. Prostate 1996;28:162–171.
125. Paz A, Lindner A, Zisman A, Siegel Y. A genetic sequence change in the 3'-noncoding region of the androgen receptor gene in prostate carcinoma. Eur Urol 1997;31:209–215.

126. Watanabe M, Ushijima T, Shiraishi T, et al. Genetic alterations of androgen receptor gene in Japanese human prostate cancer. Jpn J Clin Oncol 1997;27:389–393.

127. Wang C, Uchida T. Androgen receptor gene mutations in prostate cancer. Nippon Hinyokika Gakkai Zasshi 1997;88:550–556.

128. Marcelli M, Ittmann M, Mariani M, et al. Androgen receptor mutations in prostate cancer. Can Res 2000;60:944–949.

129. Gaddipati JP, McLeod DG, Heidenberg HB, et al. Frequent detection of codon 877 mutation in the androgen receptor gene in advanced prostate cancers. Cancer Res 1994;54:2861–2864.

130. Tilley W, Buchanan G, Hickey T, Bentel J. Mutations of the androgen receptor gene are associated with progression of human prostate cancer to androgen independence. Clin Cancer Res 1996;2:277–285.

131. Taplin M-E, Bubley GJ, Shuster T, et al. Mutation of the androgen-receptor gene in metastatic androgen-independent prostate cancer. N Engl J Med 1995;332:1393–1398.

132. Hakimi J, Ahmed R, Isaacs W, Bova W, Barrack E. Mutational analysis of the androgen receptor gene in hormone refractory metastases of prostate cancer. Eighty-ninth annual meeting of the american Association for Cancer Research, 1998.

133. Taplin ME, Bubley GJ, Ko YJ, et al. Selection for androgen receptor mutations in prostate cancers treated with androgen antagonist. Cancer Res 1999;59:2511–2515.

134. Culig Z, Klocker H, Eberle J, et al. DNA sequence of the androgen receptor in prostatic tumor cell lines and tissue specimens assessed by means of the polymerase chain reaction. Prostate 1993;22:11–22.

135. Koivisto P, Visakorpi T, Rantala I, Isola J. Increased cell proliferation activity and decreased cell death are associated with the emergence of hormone-refractory recurrent prostate cancer. J Pathol 1997;183:51–56.

136. Koivisto PA, Schleutker J, Helin H, et al. Androgen receptor gene alterations and chromosomal gains and losses in prostate carcinomas appearing during finasteride treatment for benign prostatic hyperplasia. Clin Cancer Res 1999;5:3578–3582.

137. Takahashi H, Furusato M, Allsbrook WC Jr, et al. Prevalence of androgen receptor gene mutations in latent prostatic carcinomas from Japanese men. Cancer Res 1995;55:1621–1624.

138. Wilson J. The promiscuous receptor. Prostate cancer comes of age. New Engl J Med 1995;332:1440–1441.

139. Veldscholte J, Berrevoets CA, Ris-Stalpers C, et al. The androgen receptor in LNCaP cells contains a mutation in the ligand binding domain which affects steroid binding characteristics and response to antiandrogens. J Steroid Biochem Mol Biol 1992;41:665–669.

140. Peterziel H, Culig Z, Stober J, et al. Mutant androgen receptors in prostatic tumors distinguish between amino- acid-sequence requirements for transactivation and ligand binding. Int J Cancer 1995;63:544–550.

141. Zhao XY, Malloy PJ, Krishnan AV, et al. Glucocorticoids can promote androgen-independent growth of prostate cancer cells through a mutated androgen receptor. Nat Med 2000;6:703–706.

142. Scher H, Kelly W. Flutamide withdrawal syndrome: its impact on clinical trials in hormone-refractory prostate cancer. J Clin Oncol 1993;11:1566–1572.

143. Nieh PT. Withdrawal phenomenon with the antiandrogen casodex. J Urol 1995;153:1070–1072; discussion, 1072–1073.

144. Huan SD, Gerridzen RG, Yau JC, Stewart DJ. Antiandrogen withdrawal syndrome with nilutamide. Urology 1997;49:632–634.

145. Akakura K, Akimoto S, Furuya Y, Ito H. Incidence and characteristics of antiandrogen withdrawal syndrome in prostate cancer after treatment with chlormadinone acetate. Eur Urol 1998;33:567–571.

146. Small EJ, Carroll PR. Prostate-specific antigen decline after casodex withdrawal: evidence for an antiandrogen withdrawal syndrome [see comments]. Urology 1994;43:408–410.

147. Bissada NK, Kaczmarek AT. Complete remission of hormone refractory adenocarcinoma of the prostate in response to withdrawal of diethylstilbestrol. J Urol 1995;153:1944–1945.

148. Yeh S, Miyamoto H, Chang C. Hydroxyflutamide may not always be a pure antiandrogen [letter]. Lancet 1997;349:852–853.

149. Zegarra-Moro OL, Schmidt LJ, Huang H, et al. Disruption of androgen receptor function inhibits proliferation of androgen-refractory prostate cancer cells. Cancer Res 2002;62:1008–1013.

150. Prehn RT. On the prevention and therapy of prostate cancer by androgen administration. Cancer Res 1999;59:4161–4164.

151. Mhatre AN, Trifiro MA, Kaufman M, et al. Reduced transcriptional regulatory competence of the androgen receptor in X-linked spinal and bulbar muscular atrophy. Nat Genet 1993;5:184–188.

152. Choong CS, Wilson EM. Trinucleotide repeats in the human androgen receptor: a molecular basis for disease. J Mol Endocrinol 1998;21:235–257.
153. Giovannucci E, Stampfer MJ, Krithivas K, et al. The CAG repeat within the androgen receptor gene and its relationship to prostate cancer [published erratum appears in Proc Natl Acad Sci USA 1997;94(15):8272]. Proc Natl Acad Sci USA 1997;94:3320–3323.
154. Ingles SA, Ross RK, Yu MC, et al. Association of prostate cancer risk with genetic polymorphisms in vitamin D receptor and androgen receptor [see comments]. J Natl Cancer Inst 1997;89:166–170.
155. Stanford JL, Just JJ, Gibbs M, et al. Polymorphic repeats in the androgen receptor gene: molecular markers of prostate cancer risk. Cancer Res 1997;57:1194–1198.
156. Irvine RA, Yu MC, Ross RK, Coetzee GA. The CAG and GGC microsatellites of the androgen receptor gene are in linkage disequilibrium in men with prostate cancer. Cancer Res 1995;55:1937–1940.
157. Correa-Cerro L, Wohr G, Haussler J, et al. (CAG)nCAA and GGN repeats in the human androgen receptor gene are not associated with prostate cancer in a French-German population. Eur J Hum Genet 1999;7:357–362.
158. Jin B, Beilin J, Zajac J, Handelsman DJ. Androgen receptor gene polymorphism and prostate zonal volumes in Australian and Chinese men. J Androl 2000;21:91–98.
159. Kantoff P, Giovannucci E, Brown M. The androgen receptor CAG repeat polymorphism and its relationship to prostate cancer. Biochim Biophys Acta 1998;1378:C1–C5.
160. Bratt O, Borg A, Kristoffersson U, et al. CAG repeat length in the androgen receptor gene is related to age at diagnosis of prostate cancer and response to endocrine therapy, but not to prostate cancer risk. Br J Cancer 1999;81:672–676.
161. Lange EM, Chen H, Brierley K, et al. The polymorphic exon 1 androgen receptor CAG repeat in men with a potential inherited predisposition to prostate cancer. Cancer Epidemiol Biomarkers Prev 2000;9:439–442.
162. Hardy DO, Scher HI, Bogenreider T, et al. Androgen receptor CAG repeat lengths in prostate cancer: correlation with age of onset. J Clin Endocrinol Metab 1996;81:4400–4405.
163. Ross RK, Paganini-Hill A, Henderson BE. The etiology of prostate cancer: what does the epidemiology suggest? Prostate 1983;4:333–344.
164. Morton RA Jr. Racial differences in adenocarcinoma of the prostate in North American men. Urology 1994;44:637–645.
165. Xue W, Irvine RA, Yu MC, et al. Susceptibility to prostate cancer: interaction between genotypes at the androgen receptor and prostate-specific antigen loci. Cancer Res 2000;60:839–841.
166. Miller EA, Stanford JL, Hsu L, et al. Polymorphic repeats in the androgen receptor gene in high-risk sibships. Prostate 2001;48:200–205.
167. Denner LA, Weigel NL, Maxwell BL, et al. Regulation of progesterone receptor-mediated transcription by phosphorylation. Science 1990;250:1740–1743.
168. Power RF, Mani SK, Codina J, et al. Dopaminergic and ligand-independent activation of steroid hormone receptors. Science 1991;254:1636–1639.
169. Kato S, Endoh H, Masuhiro Y, et al. Activation of the estrogen receptor through phosphorylation by mitogen-activated protein kinase. Science 1995;270:1491–1494.
170. Culig Z, Hobish A, Cronauer MV, et al. Androgen receptor activation in prostatic tumor cell lines by insulin-like growth factor I, Keratinocyte growth factor, and epidermal growth factor. Cancer Res 1994;54:5474–5478.
171. Signoretti S, Montironi R, Manola J, et al. Her-2-neu expression and progression toward androgen independence in human prostate cancer. J Natl Cancer Inst 2000;92:1918–1925.
172. Abreu-Martin MT, Chari A, Palladino AA, et al. Mitogen-activated protein kinase kinase kinase 1 activates androgen receptor-dependent transcription and apoptosis in prostate cancer. [in process citation]. Mol Cell Biol 1999;19:5143–5154.
173. Li P, Nicosia SV, Bai W. Antagonism between PTEN/MMAC1/TEP-1 and androgen receptor in growth and apoptosis of prostatic cancer cells. J Biol Chem 2001;276:20,444–20,450.
174. Migliaccio A, Piccolo D, Castoria G, et al. Activation of the Src/p21ras/Erk pathway by progesterone receptor via cross-talk with estrogen receptor. EMBO J 1998;17:2008–2018.
175. Migliaccio A, Di Domenico M, Castoria G, et al. Tyrosine kinase/p21ras/MAP-kinase pathway activation by estradiol-receptor complex in MCF-7 cells. EMBO J 1996;15:1292–1300.
176. Migliaccio A, Castoria G, Di Domenico M, et al. Steroid-induced androgen receptor-oestradiol receptor beta-Src complex triggers prostate cancer cell proliferation. EMBO J 2000;19:5406–5417.

177. Kousteni S, Bellido T, Plotkin LI, et al. Nongenotropic, sex-nonspecific signaling through the estrogen or androgen receptors: dissociation from transcriptional activity. Cell 2001;104: 719–730.

178. Berry SJ, Coffey DS, Walsh PC, Ewing LL. The development of human benign prostatic hyperplasia with age. J Urol 1984;132:474–479.

179. Bosch JL, Hop WC, Kirkels WJ, Schroder FH. Natural history of benign prostatic hyperplasia: appropriate case definition and estimation of its prevalence in the community. Urology 1995;46:34–40.

180. Madersbacher S, Pycha A, Klingler CH, et al. The International Prostate Symptom score in both sexes: a urodynamics-based comparison. Neurourol Urodyn 1999;18:173–182.

181. Tsukamoto T, Kumamoto Y, Masumori N, et al. Prevalence of prostatism in Japanese men in a community-based study with comparison to a similar American study. J Urol 1995;154:391–395.

182. Gu F L, Xia TL, Kong XT. Preliminary study of the frequency of benign prostatic hyperplasia and prostatic cancer in China. Urology 1994;44:688–691.

183. Lagiou P, Wuu J, Trichopoulou A, et al. Diet and benign prostatic hyperplasia: a study in Greece. Urology 1999;54:284–290.

184. Denis L, Morton MS, Griffiths K. Diet and its preventive role in prostatic disease. Eur Urol 1999;35:377–387.

185. Rohr HP, Bartsch G. Human benign prostatic hyperplasia: a stromal disease? New perspectives by quantitative morphology. Urology 1980;16:625–633.

186. Shapiro E, Becich MJ, Hartanto V, Lepor H. The relative proportion of stromal and epithelial hyperplasia is related to the development of symptomatic benign prostate hyperplasia. J Urol 1992;147:1293–1297.

187. Barrack ER, Berry SJ. DNA synthesis in the canine prostate: effects of androgen and estrogen treatment. Prostate 1987;10:45–56.

188. Walsh PC, Wilson JD. The induction of prostatic hypertrophy in the dog with androstanediol. J Clin Invest 1976;57:1093–1097.

189. Eri LM, Haug E, Tveter KJ. Effects on the endocrine system of long-term treatment with the luteinizing hormone-releasing hormone agonist leuprolide in patients with benign prostatic hyperplasia. Scand J Clin Lab Invest 1996;56:319–325.

190. Gann PH, Hennekens CH, Longcope C, et al. A prospective study of plasma hormone levels, nonhormonal factors, and development of benign prostatic hyperplasia. Prostate 1995;26:40–49.

191. Walsh PC, Hutchins GM, Ewing LL. Tissue content of dihydrotestosterone in human prostatic hyperplasis is not supranormal. J Clin Invest 1983;72:1772–1777.

192. Chodak GW, Kranc DM, Puy LA, et al. Nuclear localization of androgen receptor in heterogeneous samples of normal, hyperplastic and neoplastic human prostate. J Urol 1992;147:798–803.

193. Giovannucci E, Stampfer MJ, Chan A, et al. CAG repeat within the androgen receptor gene and incidence of surgery for benign prostatic hyperplasia in U.S. physicians. Prostate 1999;39: 130–134.

194. Krieg M, Nass R, Tunn S. Effect of aging on endogenous level of 5 alpha-dihydrotestosterone, testosterone, estradiol, and estrone in epithelium and stroma of normal and hyperplastic human prostate. J Clin Endocrinol Metab 1993;77:375–381.

195. Barrack ER, Bujnovszky P, Walsh PC. Subcellular distribution of androgen receptors in human normal, benign hyperplastic, and malignant prostatic tissues: characterization of nuclear salt-resistant receptors. Cancer Res 1983;43:1107–1116.

196. Gingell JC, Knonagel H, Kurth KH, Tunn UW. Placebo controlled double-blind study to test the efficacy of the aromatase inhibitor atamestane in patients with benign prostatic hyperplasia not requiring operation. The Schering 90.062 Study Group. J Urol 1995;154:399–401.

197. Cunha GR, Donjacur AA, Cooke PS, et al. The endocrinology and developmental biology of the prostate. Endocrine Rev 1987;8:338–362.

198. Mydlo JH, Michaeli J, Heston WD, Fair WR. Expression of basic fibroblast growth factor mRNA in benign prostatic hyperplasia and prostatic carcinoma. Prostate 1988;13:241–247.

199. Begun FP, Story MT, Hopp KA, et al. Regional concentration of basic fibroblast growth factor in normal and benign hyperplastic human prostates. J Urol 1995;153:839–843.

200. Ropiquet F, Giri D, Lamb D, Ittmann M. FGF7 and FGF2 are increased in benign prostatic hyperplasia and are associated with increased proliferation. J Urol 1999;162:595–599.

201. Giri D, Ropiquet F, Ittmann M. Alterations in expression of basic fibroblast growth factor (FGF) 2 and its receptor FGFR-1 in human prostate cancer. Clin Cancer Res 1999;5:1063–1071.

202. Wang Q, Stamp GW, Powell S, et al. Correlation between androgen receptor expression and FGF8 mRNA levels in patients with prostate cancer and benign prostatic hypertrophy. J Clin Pathol 1999;52:29–34.

203. Monti S, Di Silverio F, Lanzara S, et al. Insulin-like growth factor-I and -II in human benign prostatic hyperplasia: relationship with binding proteins 2 and 3 and androgens. Steroids 1998;63:362–366.

204. Mehmet H. Caspases find a new place to hide [news]. Nature 2000;403:29–30.

205. Ashkenazi A, Dixit V. Death receptors: signaling and modulation. Science 1998;281:1305–1308.

206. Green D, Reed J. Mitochondria and apoptosis. Science 1998;281:1309–1312.

207. Thornberry N, Lazebnick Y. Caspases: enemies within. Science 1998;281:1312–1316.

208. Perlman H, Zhang X. Chen MW, et al. An elevated bax/bcl-2 ratio corresponds with the onset of prostate epithelial cell apoptosis. Cell Death Differ 1999;6:48–54.

209. Zha J, Harada H, Yang E, et al. Serine phosphorilation of death agonist BAD in response to survival factor results in binding to 14-3-3 not Bcl-xl. Cell 1996;87:619–628.

210. Brunet A, Bonni A, Zigmond MJ, et al. Akt promotes cell survival by phosphorylating and inhibiting a Forkhead transcription factor. Cell 1999;96:857–868.

211. Cardone MH, Roy N, Stennicke HR, et al. Regulation of cell death protease caspase-9 by phosphorylation. Science 1998;282:1318–1321.

212. Pekarsky Y, Hallas C, Palamarchuk A, et al. Akt phosphorylates and regulates the orphan nuclear receptor Nur77. Proc Natl Acad Sci USA 2001;98:3690–3694.

213. Zong WX, Edelstein LC, Chen C, et al. The prosurvival Bcl-2 homolog Bfl-1/A1 is a direct transcriptional target of NF-kappaB that blocks TNFalpha-induced apoptosis. Genes Dev 1999;13:382–387.

214. Wang CY, Mayo MW, Korneluk RG, et al. NF-kappaB antiapoptosis: induction of TRAF1 and TRAF2 and c-IAP1 and c- IAP2 to suppress caspase-8 activation. Science 1998;281:1680–1683.

215. Goping IS, Gross A, Lavoie JN, et al. Regulated targeting of BAX to mitochondria. J Cell Biol 1998;143:207–215.

216. Desagher S, Osen-Sand A, Nichols A, et al. Bid-induced conformational change of Bax is responsible for mitochondrial cytochrome c release during apoptosis. J Cell Biol 1999;144:891–901.

217. Eskes R, Desagher S, Antonsson B, Martinou JC. Bid induces the oligomerization and insertion of Bax into the outer mitochondrial membrane. Mol Cell Biol 2000;20:929–935.

218. Griffiths GJ, Dubrez L, Morgan CP, et al. Cell damage-induced conformational changes of the pro-apoptotic protein Bak in vivo precede the onset of apoptosis. J Cell Biol 1999;144:903–914.

219. Zamzami N, Marchetti P, Castedo M, et al. Sequential reduction of mitochondrial transmembrane potential and generation of reactive oxygen species in early programmed cell death. J Exp Med 1995;182:367–377.

220. Liu X, Kim C, Yang J, et al. Induction of apoptotic program in cell-free extracts: requirement for dATP and cytochrome c. Cell 1996;86:147–157.

221. Susin S, Lorenzo H, Zamzani N, et al. Molecular characterization of mitochondrial apoptosis-inducing factor. Nature 1999;397:441–446.

222. Du C, Fang M, Li Y, et al. Smac, a mitochondrial protein that promotes cytochrome c-dependent caspase activation by eliminating IAP inhibition. Cell 2000;102:33–42.

223. Li LY, Luo X, Wang X. Endonuclease G is an apoptotic DNase when released from mitochondria. Nature 2001;412:95–99.

224. Li P, Nijhawan D, Budihardjo I, et al. Cytochrome c and dATP-dependent formation of Apaf-1/caspase-9 complex initiates an apoptotic protease cascade. Cell 1997;91:479–489.

225. Kyprianou N, Isaacs, J. Activation of programmed cell death in the rat ventral prostate after castration. Endocrinology 1988;122:552–562.

226. Geck P, Maffini MV, Szelei J, et al. Androgen-induced proliferative quiescence in prostate cancer cells: the role of AS3 as its mediator. Proc Natl Acad Sci USA 2000;97:10,185–10,190.

227. Lee C, Sutkowski D, Sensibar J, et al. Regulation of proliferation and production of prostate specific antigen in androgen-sensitive prostate cancer cells, LNCaP, by dihydrotestosterone. Endocrinology 1995;136:796–803.

228. Sonnenschein C, Olea N, Pasanen M, et al. Negative controls of cell proliferation: human prostate cancers and androgens. Cancer Res 1989;49:3474–3481.

229. Sandford NL, Searle JW, Kerr JF. Successive waves of apoptosis in the rat prostate after repeated withdrawal of testosterone stimulation. Pathology 1984;16:406–410.

230. English HF, Drago JR, Santen RJ. Cellular response to androgen depletion and repletion in the rat ventral prostate: autoradiography and morphometric analysis. Prostate 1985;7:41–51.

231. Colombel MC, Buttyan R. Hormonal control of apoptosis: the rat prostate gland as a model system. Methods Cell Biol 1995;46:369–385.

232. Leger JG, Montpetit ML, Tenniswood MP. Characterization and cloning of androgen-repressed mRNAs from rat ventral prostate. Biochem Biophys Res Commun 1987;147:196–203.

233. Buttyan R, Zakeri Z, Lokshin R, Wolgemuth D. Cascade induction of *c-fos*, *c-myc*, and heat shock 70K transcripts during regression of the ventral prostate gland. Mol Endocrinol 1988;2:650–657.

234. Suzuki A, Matsuzawa A, Iguchi T. Down regulation of Bcl-2 is the first step on Fas-mediated apoptosis of male reproductive tract. Oncogene 1996;13:31–37.

235. Briehl MM, Miesfeld RL. Isolation and characterization of transcripts induced by androgen withdrawal and apoptotic cell death in the rat ventral prostate. Mol Endocrinol 1991;5:1381–1388.

236. Chang CS, Saltzman AG, Sorensen NS, et al. S. Identification of glutathione S-transferase Yb1 mRNA as the androgen- repressed mRNA by cDNA cloning and sequence analysis. J Biol Chem 1987;262:11901–11903.

237. Uemura H, Chang C. Antisense TR3 orphan receptor can increase prostate cancer cell viability with etoposide treatment. Endocrinology 1998;139:2329–2334.

238. Sensibar JA, Sutkowski DM, Raffo A, et al. Prevention of cell death induced by tumor necrosis factor alpha in LNCaP cells by overexpression of sulfated glycoprotein-2 (clusterin). Cancer Res 1995;55:2431–2437.

239. Nishi, N., Oya, H., Matsumoto, K, et al. Changes in gene expression of growth factors and their receptors during castration-induced involution and androgen-induced regrowth of rat prostates. Prostate 1996;28:139–152.

240. Wang Z, Tufts R, Haleem R, Cai X. Genes regulated by androgen in the rat ventral prostate. Proc Natl Acad Sci USA 1997;94:12999–13004.

241. Zhu N, Wang Z. Calreticulin expression is associated with androgen regulation of the sensitivity to calcium ionophore-induced apoptosis in LNCaP prostate cancer cells. Cancer Res 1999;59:1896–1902.

242. Martikainen P, Kyprianou N, Tucker RW, Isaacs JT. Programmed death of nonproliferating androgen-independent prostatic cancer cells. Cancer Res 1991;51:4693–700.

243. Furuya Y, Lundmo P, Short AD, et al. The role of calcium, pH, and cell proliferation in the programmed (apoptotic) death of androgen-independent prostatic cancer cells induced by thapsigargin. Cancer Res 1994;54:6167–6175.

244. Wertz IE, Dixit VM. Characterization of calcium release-activated apoptosis of LNCaP prostate cancer cells. J Biol Chem 2000;275:11470–11477.

245. Shabsigh A, Chang DT, Heitjan DF, et al. Rapid reduction in blood flow to the rat ventral prostate gland after castration: preliminary evidence that androgens influence prostate size by regulating blood flow to the prostate gland and prostatic endothelial cell survival. Prostate 1998;36: 201–206.

246. Buttyan R, Shabsigh A, Perlman H, Colombel M. Regulation of Apoptosis in the Prostate Gland by Androgenic Steroids. Trends Endocrinol Metab 1999;10:47–54.

247. Shabsigh A, Ghafar MA, de la Taille A, et al. Biomarker analysis demonstrates a hypoxic environment in the castrated rat ventral prostate gland. J Cell Biochem 2001;81:437–444.

248. Chang GT, Steenbeek M, Schippers E, et al. Characterization of a zinc-finger protein and its association with apoptosis in prostate cancer cells. J Natl Cancer Inst 2000;92:1414–1421.

249. Leuprolide versus diethylstilbestrol for metastatic prostate cancer. The Leuprolide Study Group. N Engl J Med 1984;311:1281–1286.

250. Prostate Cancer Trialists' Collaborative Group. Maximum androgen blockade in advanced prostate cancer: an overview of 22 randomised trials with 3283 deaths in 5710 patients. Lancet 1995;346:265–269.

251. Tyrrell CJ, Altwein JE, Klippel F, et al. Comparison of an LH-RH analogue (Goeserelin acetate, 'Zoladex') with combined androgen blockade in advanced prostate cancer: final survival results of an international multicentre randomized-trial. International Prostate Cancer Study Group. Eur Urol 2000;37:205–211.

252. Bayoumi AM, Brown AD, Garber AM. Cost-effectiveness of androgen suppression therapies in advanced prostate cancer. J Natl Cancer Inst 2000;92:1731–1739.

253. Wolff JM, Tunn UW. Intermittent androgen blockade in prostate cancer: rationale and clinical experience. Eur Urol 2000;38:365–371.

254. Bouchot O, Lenormand L, Karam G, et al. Intermittent androgen suppression in the treatment of metastatic prostate cancer. Eur Urol 2000;38:543–549.

255. Grossfeld GD, Chaudhary UB, Reese DM, et al. Intermittent androgen deprivation: update of cycling characteristics in patients without clinically apparent metastatic prostate cancer. Urology 2001;58:240–245.

256. Nejat RJ, Rashid HH, Bagiella E, et al. A prospective analysis of time to normalization of serum testosterone after withdrawal of androgen deprivation therapy. J Urol 2000;164:1891–1894.

257. Schulman CC, Debruyne FM, Forster G, et al. 4-Year follow-up results of a European prospective randomized study on neoadjuvant hormonal therapy prior to radical prostatectomy in T2-3N0M0 prostate cancer. European Study Group on Neoadjuvant Treatment of Prostate Cancer. Eur Urol 2000;38:706–713.

258. Scolieri MJ, Altman A, Resnick MI. Neoadjuvant hormonal ablative therapy before radical prostatectomy: a review. Is it indicated? J Urol 2000;164:1465–1472.

259. Gleave ME, La Bianca SE, Goldenberg SL, et al. Long-term neoadjuvant hormone therapy prior to radical prostatectomy: evaluation of risk for biochemical recurrence at 5-year follow-up. Urology 2000;56:289–294.

260. Messing EM, Manola J, Sarosdy M, et al. Immediate hormonal therapy compared with observation after radical prostatectomy and pelvic lymphadenectomy in men with node-positive prostate cancer. N Engl J Med 1999;341:1781–1788.

261. D'Amico AV, Schultz D, Loffredo M, et al. Biochemical outcome following external beam radiation therapy with or without androgen suppression therapy for clinically localized prostate cancer. JAMA 2000;284:1280–1283.

262. Gormley G, Stoner E, Bruskewitz R, et al. The effect of finasteride in men with benign prostatic hyperplasia. N Engl J Med 1992;327:1185–1191.

263. Stone NN, Clejan SJ. Response of prostate volume, prostate-specific antigen, and testosterone to flutamide in men with benign prostatic hyperplasia. J Androl 1991;12:376–380.

264. McConnell JD, Bruskewitz R, Walsh P, et al. The effect of finasteride on the risk of acute urinary retention and the need for surgical treatment among men with benign prostatic hyperplasia. Finasteride Long-Term Efficacy and Safety Study Group. [see comments]. N Engl J Med 1998;338:557–563.

265. Harman SM, Metter EJ, Tobin JD, et al. Longitudinal effects of aging on serum total and free testosterone levels in healthy men. Baltimore Longitudinal Study of Aging. J Clin Endocrinol Metab 2001;86:724–731.

266. Snyder PJ, Peachey H, Hannoush P, et al. Effect of testosterone treatment on body composition and muscle strength in men over 65 years of age. J Clin Endocrinol Metab 1999;84:2647–2653.

267. Kenny AM, Prestwood KM, Gruman CA, et al. Effects of transdermal testosterone on bone and muscle in older men with low bioavailable testosterone levels. J Gerontol A Biol Sci Med Sci 2001;56:M266–M272.

268. Zhao XY, Boyle B, Krishnan AV, et al. Two mutations identified in the androgen receptor of the new human prostate cancer cell line MDA PCa 2a. J Urol 1999;162:2192–2199.

269. Han G, Foster BA, Mistry S, et al. Hormone status selects for spontaneous somatic androgen receptor variants that demonstrate specific ligand and cofactor dependent activities in autochthonous prostate cancer. J Biol Chem 2000;276:11204–11213.

10 Androgens and Coronary Artery Disease

Fredrick C. W. Wu, MD
and Arnold von Eckardstein, MD

Contents

Introduction
Relationships Between Serum Levels of T and CAD: Observational Studies
Relationships Between Serum Levels of T and CAD: Interventional Clinical Studies
Relationships Between Serum Levels of T and CAD: Animal Studies
Effects of T on Cardiovascular Risk Factors
Effects of Androgens on Cells of the Arterial Wall and Vascular Function
DHEA-S and CAD in Men and Women
Estrogens and Cardiovascular Disease in Men
Summary and Conclusion
References

INTRODUCTION

Coronary artery disease (CAD) is one of the leading causes of mortality in men and women. Age-adjusted morbidity and mortality rates from CAD are 2.5-fold to 4.5-fold higher in men than in women *(1)*. This male preponderance is remarkably consistent across 52 countries with hugely divergent rates of CAD mortality and lifestyles *(2)*. Sex hormones can influence a multitude of factors implicated in the pathogenesis of atherosclerosis and coronary artery disease—the traditional view being that androgens are harmful and estrogens beneficial. However, the gender disparity in CAD may involve diverse mechanisms ranging from *in utero* sex hormone imprinting, gender-specific behavior, distribution of visceral body fat to vascular and myocardial structural/functional adaptation to aging, pressure overload, and disease *(3)*. As the therapeutic indications for androgen therapy widen to "non-classical" indications *(4)*, including male

From: *Contemporary Endocrinology: Androgens in Health and Disease*
Edited by: C. Bagatell and W. J. Bremner © Humana Press Inc., Totowa, NJ

contraception, physiological aging, chronic debilitating conditions, and hormone replacement in postmenopausal women *(5)*, it becomes increasingly pertinent to consider whether natural or induced changes in levels of testosterone (T) or dehydroepiandrosterone-S (DHEA-S) will impact on the risks of coronary artery disease in men and women. This review synthesizes data from a variety of disciplines into a global assessment of the relationship between androgens and CAD in men and women (*see* ref. *6* for more comprehensive coverage with a full bibliography).

RELATIONSHIPS BETWEEN SERUM LEVELS OF T AND CAD: OBSERVATIONAL STUDIES

T and CAD in Men

CROSS-SECTIONAL CLINICAL STUDIES

Of the 32 cross-sectional studies on the relationships between circulating T and CAD in men *(6,7)*, 16 found lower levels of T in cases compared to controls, whereas 16 showed no difference. As with all cross-sectional studies, the directionality of the relationship is indeterminate so that lower T levels may be either the consequence or a cause of CAD or may be associated with confounding variables such as insulin, lipids, changes in lifestyle, and medications. No study suggested that high levels of T were associated with CAD.

PROSPECTIVE COHORT OR CASE-CONTROL STUDIES

Of the seven non-cross-sectional studies *(8–14)*, none showed T to have any significant relationship or predictive value for incident CAD (*see* Table 1). The three prospective cohort studies followed 1009 Californian men aged 40–79 over 12 yr *(8)*, 2512 aged 45–59 in South Wales (Caerphilly) for 5 yr *(9)*, and 890 Baltimore men aged 53.8 ± 16 for up to 31 yr *(10)*. There was no correlation between baseline T levels and subsequent development of fatal or nonfatal CAD, stroke, or heart failure after adjusting for relevant confounders. These three cohort studies go a long way toward confirming that T is not an independent risk factor for CAD in men. In the four case-control studies, baseline T levels in cases of CAD and matched controls from the Honolulu Heart Programme *(11)*, Multiple Risk Factors Inverventional Trial *(12)*, Baltimore Longitudinal Study of Ageing *(13)*, and the Helsinki Heart Study *(14)* did not predict CAD events during observation periods of 6–8, 19–20, 9.5, and 5 yr respectively.

In summary, the 39 studies in the literature together provide a consistent dataset that shows the lack of a relationship between circulating T and incident or existing CAD in men. There is a suggestion, only from cross-sectional studies, that patients with CAD may have lower T levels; the nature of this relationship is unclear. None of the studies showed a positive relationship between T and CAD to suggest that high levels of this androgen may be a risk factor.

T and CAD in Women

Testosterone, bioavailable T, and androstendione did not differ significantly in 942 women with and without a history of heart disease at baseline and did not predict cardiovascular death or death from ischaemic heart disease *(18)*. In contrast, in a cross-sectional angiographic study of 109 postmenopausal women with chest pain, serum levels of free T were correlated with the extent of coronary artery narrowing *(19)*.

Table 1
Number of Studies Showing Negative (Favorable), Null, or Positive (Adverse)
Relationships Between T and DHEA
with Coronary/Cardiovascular Artery Disease in Males

Androgen	Study	n	Relationships Negative	Null	Positive
Testosterone	Cross-sectional	32	16	16	0
	Case control	4	0	4	0
	Prospective cohort	3	0	3	0
	Interventional[a]	6	6	0	0
	Animal[b]	9	4	3	2
DHEA and DHEA-S	Cross-sectional	10	6	3	1
	Case control	6	1	4	1
	Prospective cohort	6	1	5	0
	Animal[b]	5	5	0	0

[a] Including studies which used direct iv or intracoronary infusion of pharmacological doses of testosterone (15–17) but excluding 17 uncontrolled studies in the earlier literature from before 1950.
[b] Cardiovascular disease endpoints in experimental animal studies included aortic and coronary artery plaques or fatty streak lesions, myointimal proliferation.

However, free T and androstenedione were inversely correlated with carotid artery atherosclerosis in premenopausal and postmenopausal women (20).

POLYCYSTIC OVARIAN SYNDROME

Indirect evidence for the atherogenicity of androgens in women stems from cross-sectional data that consistently showed a strong obesity-independent cluster of cardiovascular risk factors, including insulin resistance, dyslipidemia, and impaired fibrinolysis in patients with polycystic ovarian syndrom (PCOS). Based on calculated-risk profiles, women with PCOS were predicted to have a relative risk for myocardial infarction of 7.4 : 1 (21).

In 102 consecutive women undergoing cardiac catheterization, Wild et al. (22) found a positive correlation between angiographic evidence of coronary artery disease and clinical evidence of hyperandrogenism. Similarly, in 143 women aged ≤60 yr referred because of chest pain or valvular heart disease, ultrasound evidence of polycystic ovaries (in 42% of patients) was associated with an increased number of stenosed coronary arteries (23). The prevalence of CAD was found to be significantly higher in 28 women (45–59 yr) who had undergone ovarian wedge resection over 18 yr ago compared to 752 aged-matched controls (24). In case-control studies using B-mode ultrasound, significantly increased carotid artery intima–media thickness was found in patients with PCOS compared to age-matched controls irrespective of body mass index (BMI), fat distribution, and other risk factors (25,26). This may be regarded as evidence in support of subclinical premature atherosclerosis in middle-aged (>45 yr) women independently related to the increased testosterone in PCOS. An increased prevalence of coronary artery calcification (which correlates with atherosclerosis) was found in 32 premenopausal (30–45 yr) women with PCOS compared with 52 controls using electron beam computed tomography *(27)*. However, in 18 healthy obese young women (32.7 ± 1.9 yr) with PCOS, endothelium-dependent and endothelium-independent vascular responses were normal compared to age-matched controls *(28)*.

Mortality and morbidity in over 786 women (over 45 yr of age) diagnosed to have PCOS on histopathological and hospital inpatient diagnostic records were compared retrospectively with 1060 age-matched controls. Despite significantly increased diabetes, hypertension, cholesterol and nonfatal cerebrovascular disease, standardized mortality ratio of 1.4 (95% confidence interval [CI]: 0.75–2.40) and the odds ratio of 1.5 (95% CI: 0.7–2.9) were not significantly increased *(29,30)*. In another cohort of 346 nonobese patients aged 30.3–55.7 yr diagnosed to have PCOS in a specialized clinic, the prevalence of cardiac complaints (serious heart disease or cardiac arrest) ascertained by telephone questionnaire was not significantly different from that in 8950 age-matched females in the general population *(31)*. However, both of these studies suffer from methological drawbacks such as underascertainment of PCOS *(29,30)* and the relative young age of the small cohort *(31)*.

In summary, although PCOS patients have an adverse-risk profile for CAD, whether this will lead to an increased and premature disease morbidity and mortality and, if so, whether this is causally related to chronic hyperandrogenemia *per se* as opposed to the associated risk factors remain unclear. Nevertheless, given the high prevalence of PCOS in the female population, this issue should remain a high priority target for future research.

RELATIONSHIPS BETWEEN SERUM LEVELS OF T
AND CAD: INTERVENTIONAL CLINICAL STUDIES

Endogenous Androgen Deprivation

A frequently cited but misquoted study *(32)* compared the life expectancy of 297 castrated inmates with 735 intact inmates (white males) in a single state institution for the mentally retarded. Castrated males lived an average of 13.6 yr longer than intact controls. However, the excess mortality in intact inmates was the result of infections with no difference in cardiovascular disease mortality between the two groups. The authors concluded that postpubertal castration did *not* decrease the frequency of deaths because of cardiovascular disease. In a historical review *(33)*, the life-span of 50 castrati singers (prepubertal castrates) born between 1581 and 1858 in Europe was 65.5 ± 13.8 yr compared to 64.3 ± 14.1 yr in 50 noncastrated singers. Prepubertal castration has no effect on longevity in men. The abolition of testicular androgens by prepubertal or postpubertal castration does not decrease cardiovascular mortality in men. This is supported by findings from cross-gender sex hormone treatment in 816 male-to-female transexuals aged 18–86 yr *(34)*. Administration of ethinylestradiol 100 µg/d and cyproterone acetate 100 mg/d for 7734 patient-years was not associated with any significant difference in cardiovascular mortality or morbidity compared to the general male population despite a 20-fold increase in venous thromboembolic complications.

Androgen Excess from Anabolic Steroid Abuse

Excessive androgen exposure in men is uncommon in clinical practice. However, anabolic–androgenic steroid (AAS) abuse in the general population is said to have reached epidemic proportion, with over 1 million current and former users in the United

States alone *(35–37)*. In two reviews of the literature covering a 12-yr period from 1987 to 1998 *(38,39)*, there was a total of 17 case reports of cardiovascular events in young male bodybuilders abusing pharmacological doses of AAS. Invariably, multiple preparations seldom prescribed in clinical practice, including oral 17α-alkylated androgens, were used simultaneously. There were 11 documented cases of acute myocardial infarction, 4 cardiomyopathy, and 2 strokes. It is not possible to draw firm scientific conclusions from these sporadic case reports, especially when the baseline denominator information on prevalence and extent of exposure is shrouded in uncertainty and secrecy. However, with the vast increase in abuse since the 1960s, there is no clear evidence for any rise in incidence of vascular events among likely users and ex-users of AAS. Nevertheless, it has been suggested that dose-dependent androgen-induced vasospasm, platelet aggregation, activation of coagulation cascade, atherogenic lipid profiles (decreased high-density lipoprotein [HDL] cholesterol and increased low-density lipoprotein [LDL] cholesterol and), and abnormal left-ventricular function and hypertrophy are relevant mechanisms precipitating sudden cardiac deaths in young power athletes and bodybuilders *(39)*. It must be emphasized that pathological data from men abusing exotic AASs in doses several orders of magnitude higher than those prescribed in the clinical setting should not be extrapolated to the legitimate therapeutic use of approved testosterone preparations or, indeed, to androgen physiology.

Exogenous T Treatment in Men with CAD

Studies (uncontrolled) from the 1940s suggested that T may improve symptomatic CAD in men *(6,7)*. More recent data are considered in this subsection.

Bolus intravenous or intracoronary injections of pharmacological doses of T acutely improved myocardial ischaemia or induced coronary artery dilatiation in a small number of men with CAD *(15–17)*. Whether this acute pharmacological action of T can be translated into a therapeutic effect remains to be determined.

In a randomized placebo-controlled double-blind study, T cypionate 200 mg im weekly for 8 wk decreased ST-segment depression during exercise testing in 25 men with positive tests *(40)*. In a placebo-controlled crossover (but not double blinded) study in 62 elderly men with CAD, oral T undecanoate for 4 wk improved subjective symptom scores and resting electrocardiograms (ECG) *(41)*. Transdermal testosterone 5 mg daily for 12 wk increased the time to 1-mm ST-segment depression in men with symptomatic CAD *(42)*.

These preliminary data suggest ECG changes can improve after (maximum of 12 wk) short-term T supplement in CAD patients with low T levels. It is unclear if the effects of T are based on specific cardiac actions or nonspecific improvements in skeletal muscle performance during exercise testing. Whether there are real symptomatic or functional benefits or decreased cardiovascular mortality from T treatment in the long term remain important but unanswered questions.

Exogenous T Treatment in Women

There is increasing interest in the use of T as part of postmenopausal hormone-replacement therapy (HRT) *(5,43,44)*. Whether the concurrent use of T will impact on the putative benefits of estrogen HRT on the cardiovascular system is currently unknown. In a 20-yr retrospective survey of 293 female-to-male transexuals aged 17–70 yr (mean: 34 yr) treated for 2 mo to 41 yr (total exposure of 2418 patient-years) with oral T undecanoate 160 mg daily or T (Sustanon) 250 mg im every 2 wk, there was no excess of cardiovascular (or all cause) mortality or morbidity compared with the general female population *(34)*.

In summary, interventional studies to decrease endogenous testosterone or administration of testosterone generally do not suggest a causal relationship between T exposure and the development of CAD. Although some preliminary information hints at possible beneficial effects on myocardial ischemia, prospective controlled data on cardiovascular disease endpoints (myocardial infarction, angina, mortality) from large-scale interventional studies using physiological doses of androgens are currently lacking.

RELATIONSHIPS BETWEEN SERUM LEVELS OF T
AND CAD: ANIMAL STUDIES

The influence of androgens on the development and progression of experimentally induced atherosclerosis has been investigated in six animal models with diet- or injury-induced atherosclerosis and two genetic atherosclerosis-susceptible mouse models *(see* ref. *6* for review) *(see* Tables 1 and 2). Larsen et al. *(45)* found no difference in the cholesterol content of abdominal aorta lesions before or after 17 wk of T treatment in male orchidectomized rabbits. A similar negative result was obtained with the anabolic steroid stanozolol *(46)*. Aortic arch atheroma formation was inhibited by estradiol in female but not male rabbits and T in male but not females rabbits and by combined estradiol and T administration in both sexes *(47)*. Interestingly, T treatment in female rabbits increased plaque sizes, but estradiol had no effect in male rabbits. The antiatherogenic effects of sex steroids appeared to involve gender-specific mechanisms. T did not have any effect on the myointimal proliferation response to balloon injury of the carotid artery in either male or female intact or gonadectomized rats, whereas estradiol inhibited this response in both sexes *(48)*. Castration of male rabbits resulted in increased aortic atherosclerosis, suggesting that endogenous T has an antiatherogenic effect *(49)*. The increase in aortic atherosclerosis can be reversed by of 80 mg daily oral T undecanoate or 500 mg daily of DHEA. In addition, 25 mg im T enanthate twice weekly, which raised circulating T levels by 10-fold, decreased aortic atherosclerosis. This suggests that androgens in pharmacological doses may have direct protective effects on the vasculature against atherosclerosis. In contrast, treatment of male chicks with T resulted in a dose-dependent increase in aortic atherosclerosis *(50)*. Similarly, T increased the extent of coronary atherosclerosis in female ovariectomized cynomolgus monkeys fed an atherogenic diet for 24 mo *(51)*. These effects were independent of various risk factors, including lipids. However, the acetylcholine-induced atherosclerosis-related coronary artery vasoconstriction was reversed by T treatment. Thus, despite the apparently adverse structural changes attributed to T, function of the coronary artery endothelium nevertheless improved *(51)*. With the same experimental model and design in female monkeys, coronary artery atherosclerosis was increased by the androgenic-anabolic steroid nandrolone treatment for 2 yr *(52)*. The coronary artery lumen area was significantly larger in the nandrolone-treated animals. Remodeling of the vessel wall and lumen could possibly counterbalance the increased plaque size.

Castration had no effect on atherosclerosis of either male or female Apo-E-deficient transgenic mice *(53)*. T decreased serum levels of cholesterol and inhibited the development of fatty streak lesions in the aorta *(53)*. Suppression of T by a gonadotropic-releasing hormone (GnRH) antagonist led to a decrease in atherosclerosis despite

Table 2
Number of Studies Showing Negative (Favorable), Null, or Positive (Adverse) Relationships
Between T and DHEA with Coronary/Cardiovascular Artery Disease in Females

Androgen	Subjects	Study	n	Negative	Null	Positive
				Relationships		
Testosterone	Females	Cross-sectional	3	1	1	1
		Prospective cohort	1	0	1	0
		Interventional	1	0	1	0
	PCOS females[a]	Cross-sectional	4	0	1	3
		Case control	6	0	3	3
	Female animals	Experimental[b]	6	2	1	3
DHEA and DHEA-S	Females	Cross-sectional	5	4	1	0
		Case control	1	0	1	0
		Prospective cohort	6	1	5	0
	Female animals	Experimental[b]	1	1	0	0

[a]Patients with PCOS with clinical and/or biochemical evidence of androgen excess is regarded as the independent variable.

[b]Cardiovascular disease endpoints in experimental animal studies included aortic and coronary artery plaques or fatty streak lesions, myointimal proliferation.

increases of cholesterol in male and decreases of HDL cholesterol in female Apo-E-deficient transgenic mice *(54)*. Exogenous T increased cholesterol levels and atherosclerotic lesions in intact male but decreased atherosclerotic lesions in female Apo-E-deficient mice *(55)*. In LDL-receptor-deficient male mice *(56)*, both castration and the aromatase inhibitor anastrazole increased the extent of fatty streak lesions in the aortic arch. Lesion formation was attenuated by treatment of orchidectomized animals with either T or estradiol. The atheroprotective effect of T was abolished by the simultaneous application of anastrazole. These results suggest that testosterone attenuates early atherogenesis by being aromatized to estrogens. The discrepancy between these three studies may partly be explained by the different dosages of T and gender-specific actions. The effects of T on early atherogenesis were not explained by changes in lipid levels in all three studies.

In summary, various animal models have highlighted the existence of different mechanisms in the evolution of atherosclerosis that can potentially be influenced by androgens. The inconsistent and conflicting results from these in vivo studies reflect the complexity of pathogenesis, the sexually dimorphic response to atherogenic triggers, as well as the gender-specific response to sex steroids. This serves as a timely caution to those holding oversimplistic views on the complex relationships between sex hormones and cardiovascular diseases.

EFFECTS OF T ON CARDIOVASCULAR RISK FACTORS

The effects of testosterone on cardiovascular risk factors are contradictory depending on whether associations with *endogenous* testosterone or effects of *exogenous* testosterone are being considered.

Endogenous T and Cardiovascular Risk Factors: Role of Adipose Tissue and Insulin

Correlations between plasma T and various cardiovascular risk factors are profoundly influenced by the interrelationships among T, adipose tissue, and insulin action. Furthermore, T shows opposite relationships with risk factors in men and women.

MEN

In men, plasma T levels are positively correlated with HDL cholesterol but inversely correlated with triglycerides, total cholesterol, LDL cholesterol, fibrinogen, and plasminogen-activator inhibitor-1 (PAI-1) (9,57–64). However, T shows even stronger inverse correlations with BMI, waist circumference, waist–hip ratio (WHR), visceral fat and circulating leptin, insulin, and free fatty acids. After adjustment for these measures of obesity and insulin resistance, the correlations between T and cardiovascular risk factors, but not with visceral fat or insulin, are no longer statistically significant (65–68). Low T in men is, therefore, a component of the metabolic syndrome, characterized by obesity, glucose intolerance or overt type 2 diabetes mellitus, arterial hypertension, hypertriglyceridemia, low HDL cholesterol, a procoagulatory state, and an antifibrinolytic state. What comes first in this apparently circular relationship between hypotestosteronemia, obesity, and insulin resistance is not clear. Hypogonadal men are frequently obese with increased levels of leptin and insulin (69–74). Body weight, leptin, and insulin levels decrease on T treatment in hypogonadal men (75–77) and eugonadal obese men (78–80), leading to a decrease of visceral fat, improved insulin sensitivity, and correction of dyslipidemia. Conversely, suppression of T by a GnRH antagonist increased serum levels of leptin and insulin (81). These data suggest that testosterone reduces visceral fat mass and improves insulin action. T stimulates lipolysis and reduces fat storage in adipocytes by upregulating androgen and β-adrenergic-receptor expression and activating adenylate cyclase, protein kinase A, and hormone-sensitive lipase (82,83). In cultured rat preadipocytes, androgens elicit an antiadipogenic effect, related to changes in the expression of the insulin-like growth factor (IGF-1) receptor (androgens and estrogens) and peroxisome proliferator-activated receptor (PPAR)-γ2 expression (estrogens) (84).

WOMEN

In women, serum T showed positive correlations with BMI and leptin levels (82,83,85,86). Low sex hormone-binding globulin (SHBG), which is an indirect measure of female hyperandrogenism, was associated with high BMI and WHR, as well as with high serum levels of leptin and insulin with low HDL cholesterol (87). In a prospective study, 20% of women with SHBG levels below the fifth percentile developed type 2 diabetes mellitus within 12 yr (88). Thus, hyperandrogenemia in women, in contrast to hypoandrogenemia in men, is a component of the metabolic syndrome.

POLYCYSTIC OVARIAN SYNDROME

Hyperandrogenic women with PCOS frequently have hypercholesterolemia, low HDL cholesterol, hypertriglyceridemia, elevated fibrinogen and PAI-1, and a family history of diabetes mellitus (89–98). Because many women with PCOS are overweight, it is unclear whether their dyslipidemic and procoagulatory states are secondary to insulin resistance (99,100) or whether hyperandrogenemia itself contributes to obesity and hyperinsulinemia (82,83,101–108).

Insulin action plays an important role in the pathogenesis of hyperandrogenemia in PCOS, where the ovaries remain insulin sensitive but tissues such as fat and muscle are resistant. Hyperinsulinemia therefore augments the luteinizing hormone (LH)- and ACTH-dependent hyperandrogenism via its cognate receptor and the inositolglycan pathway (109,110). Thus, metformin or the insulin sensitizer troglitazone significantly decreased serum levels of insulin as well as T in women with PCOS, independently of BMI or gonadotropins (111–114). Concomitantly, plasma levels of HDL cholesterol increased and plasma levels of PAI-1 decreased (110–112).

Although GnRH agonists (115) and androgen receptor blockade (116) in hyper-androgenic women improved insulin sensitivity and lipid profile (117), the magnitude of these changes was less than alterations in the opposite direction that usually encountered in PCOS. Short-term lowering of ovarian androgens by laparoscopic ovarian cautery did not alter insulin or lipid levels (118).

Supraphysiological doses of exogenous T administered to genetic females for gender reassignment therapy (119,120), nandrolone treatment in obese postmenopausal women (121), or T treatment of female cynomolgus monkeys (51) increased BMI, visceral fat, and muscle mass and decreased insulin sensitivity. Transient intrauterine or perinatal exposure to T predisposed female rats and marmoset monkeys to central adiposity and insulin resistance in adult life (54,122). Thus, there may be a vicious circle in which early androgen excess may contribute to insulin resistance in adult women with PCOS where hyperinsulinism aggravates the hyperandrogenism and associated clinical phenotype. A further hypothesis linking hyperandrogenism and insulin resistance is the concurrent dysregulation of ovarian/adrenal cytochrome P450c17α action (leading to excessive androgen synthesis) and insulin receptor function by excessive serine phosphorylation or decreased chironinositol (123–125). Deranged insulin action (independent of obesity) is very likely the root cause of the metabolic disarray in PCOS.

In summary, the role of T in determining cardiovascular risks is unclear. The associations between serum levels of T and cardiovascular risk factors are in opposite directions for men and women. These gender-specific correlations are further confounded by the bidirectional relationships among testosterone, adipose tissue, and insulin sensitivity. However, the weight of evidence would suggest that low endogenous T may be the driving factor for obesity, insulin resistance, and increased cardiovascular risk factors in men, whereas in women, in particular those with PCOS, altered insulin action appears to be critical for the development of the hyperandrogenaemia.

Effects of Exogenous T on Cardiovascular Risk Factors

In clinical studies, the effects of exogenous testosterone on cardiovascular risk factors differed considerably according to the dose, route of administration, duration of treatment, as well as the age, gender, and conditions of the recipients (see Table 3). The most consistent findings were decreases in plasma HDL cholesterol, lipoprotein(a) [Lp(a)], and fibrinogen.

HDL

Administration of AAS to either men or women were consistently found to cause substantial reductions of HDL cholesterol (35–38). Likewise, administration of supraphysiological dosages of testosterone to healthy eugonadal men in contraceptive studies (153–156,161), as well as androgen treatment of women with premenstrual

Table 3
Change in Lipids in Hypogonadal/Eugonadal Men Receving Testosterone Replacement

Study (ref.)	Patients	Mode of treatment	Duration	ΔLDL cholesterol	ΔHDL cholesterol	ΔTG	Δother risk factors
Hypogonadal Men							
Valdemarsson et al. 1987 (126)	10 Hypogonadal men	250 mg TE im/3 or 4 wk	9 mo	−6%	0	−14%	
Kirkland et al. 1987 (127)	14 Hypogonadal boys	100 or 200 mg TE im/mo	3 mo	n.d.	−14%	n.d.	
Sorva et al. 1988 (128)	13 Hypophy-sectomized men	100 mg TE im/2 wk	1 mo	−4%	−8%	−11%	ApoA-I: −11%
Jones et al. 1989 (129)	10 Klinefelter men	TE implant im	4 wk	+19%	−11%	−4%	ApoA-I: +8%
Hromadova et al. 1989 (130)	30 Sterile men	100 mg methyl-testosterone per day	30 d+??	−??%	+?? %		
Hana et al. 1991 (131)	9 Hypogonadal men	100 mg TI im/wk	24 mo	24%*	+19%	−30%	
Tenover et al. 1992 (132)	13 Hypogonadal elderly men	100 mg TE im/wk	3 mo	−15%*	−4%	−16%	ApoA-I: −11%
Bhasin et al. 1992 (133)	10 Hypogonadal men	Microcapsulated T im	12 wk	−7%	−16%	+14%	ApoA-I: −24% ApoB: −14%
Morley et al. 1993 (134)	8 Hypogonadal elderly men	200 mg TE im/2 wk	3 mo	n.d.	0	n.d.	
Salehian et al. 1995 (135)	63 Hypogonadal men or 2.5 mg T sublingual/d or 5 mg T sublingual/d	200 mg TE im/3 wk	2 mo	n.d.	−10% −8% −10%	n.d.	
Brodsky et al. 1996 (136)	5 Hypogonadal men	3 mg TC per kg body mass im every 2 wk	6 mo	+5%	−18%	+3%	
Katznelson et al. 1996 (137)	29 Hypogonadal men	100 mg TE or TC im/wk	6 mo	−6%	−10%	−20%	
Ozata et al. 1996 (138)	29 Hypogonadal men	250 mg TE im/3 wk	3 mo	+9%	+6%	0	

Reference	Subjects	Treatment	Duration				
Zglycienski et al. 1996 (139)	22 Hypogonadal men	200 mg TE im/2 wk	1 yr	-18%***	-9%*	-20%	
Arslanian et al. 1997 (140)	7 Boys with delayed puberty	50 mg TE im/2 wk	4 wk	-14%	-20%**	-9%	
Tripathy et al. 1998 (142)	10 Hypogonadal men	200 mg TE im/wk	12 wk	-41%	+5%	-25%	
Tan et al. 1998 (143)	11 Hypogonadal men	250 mg TE im/4 wk	12 wk	-2%	-1%	-12%	ApoA-I: -10%* Lp(a) -2%
Rabijekwski et al. 1998 (144)	30 Hypogonadal men	200 mg TE im/2 wk	12 mo	-16%	-4%	n.d.	
Jockenhövel et al. 1999 (145)	12 Hypogonadal men	100 mg mesterolone po/d	17 wk	-6%	-6%	-12%	
	13 Hypogonadal men	or 160 mg TU po/d		-8%	+9%-16%		
	15 Hypogonadal men	or 250 mg TE im/3 wk		+5%	+6%-8%		
	15 Hypogonadal men	or 1200 mg testosterone sc/d		0	-9%-11%		
Tan et al. 1999 (146)	10 Hypogonadal men	4 mg transdermal T/d	3 mo	-10%	-11%**	+3%	ApoA-I: -7%
Wang et al. 2000 (77)	227 Hypogonadal men	6 mg T/d scrotal patch vs gel with 50 mg or 100 mg T/d	180 d	n.s.	n.s.	n.s.	
Snyder et al. 2001 (147)	108 Hypogonadal elderly men	6 mg transdermal (scrotal) T/d	3 yr	0	-2%	-3%	ApoA-I: -3% ApoB: -5%
Howell et al. 2001 (141)	35 Hypogonadal men	2.5 mg transdermal T/d	1 yr	-11%*	0	+26%	
Dobs et al. 2001 (148)	20 Hypogonadal men	2-2.5 mg transdermal T/d	1 yr	-3%	-9%**	+16%*	
Ly et al. 2001 (149)	33 Hypogonadal men	70 mg transdermal DHT/d	3 mo	-11%*	0	-10%	
Eugonal Men							
Thompson et al. 1989 (150)	11 Eugonadal men	200 mg TE im/wk	6 wk	-16%*	-9%	+13%	
Friedl et al. 1990 (151)	18 Eugonadal men or with 250 mg testolactone/d or 20 mg methyl-testosterone/d	280 mg TE im/wk without	12 wk	n.d.	-4%	+10%	APOA-I: -12%
					-16%	+20%	0
					-33%	+40%	-40%

(continued)

Table 3 (continued)

Study (ref.)	Patients	Mode of treatment	Duration	ΔLDL cholesterol	ΔHDL cholesterol	ΔTG	Δother risk factors
Zmuda et al. 1993 (152)	14 Eugonadal men	200 mg TE im/wk, 250 mg testolactone/d, or both	3 wk	+2% −3% −1%	−15% −4% −20%	+17% −13% +3%	
Bagatell et al. 1994 (153)	19 Eugonadal men	200 mg TE im/wk	20 wk	−6%*	−15%*	+5%	ApoA-I: −8%
Meriggiola et al. 1995 (154)	36 Eugonadal men	200 mg TE im/wk	1 yr	−8%	−16%	n.d.	
Anderson et al., 1995 (155)	63 Eugonadal men	200 mg TE im/wk	1 yr	n.s.	−13%***	n.s.	Lp(a): −25%
Wu et al. 1995 (156)	189 Non-Chinese men 82 Chinese men	200 mg TE im/wk 200 mg TE im/wk	1 yr 1 yr	n.s.	−14% −2%	+10% (all)	
Marcovina et al. 1996 (157)	19 Eugonadal men	200 mg TE im/wk	20 wk	−8%	−14%*	+13%	Lp(a): −22%**
Grinspoon et al. 2000 (158)	54 Men with AIDS	200 mg TE im/wk	12 wk	−6%	−8%*	−25%	
Bhasin et al. 2001 (159)	61 Eugonadal men with suppressed T	25, 50, 125, 300, or 600 mg TE im/wk	20 wk	n.d.	Dose-dependent+ 10% to −20%***	n.d.	
Uyanik et al. 1997 (160)	37 Eugonadal men	120 mg TU po/d	2 mo	−25%**	+3%	−4%	APOA-I: −15% ApoB: +12%

ΔLDL, cholesterol change in plasma LDL cholesterol from pretreatment baseline; ΔHDL, cholesterol change in plasma HDL cholesterol from pretreatment baseline; ΔTG, change in plasma triglicerides from pretreatment baseline; T, testosterone; TE, testosterone enanthate; TC, testosterone cypionate; TU, testosterone undecanoate; TI, testosterone isobutyrate; DHT, dihydrotestosterone; n.s., not significant; n.d.: not done.

Changes were compared to follow-up, baseline (screening) are implausibly extreme and different from follow-up.

*$p < 0.05$, ** $p < 0.01$, *** $p < 0.001$ (as indicated by the authors of the original publications).

syndrome or menopause led to a decrease in HDL cholesterol *(162–164)*. Castration or suppression of endogenous testosterone with GnRH antagonists increased HDL cholesterol by about 20% *(81,165–172)*. The effect of GnRH antagonists can be prevented by coadministration of testosterone *(173)*. Taken together, these data indicate that testosterone exerts consistent effects on HDL metabolism. These effects are most marked on the large HDL subclass (i.e., HDL2) which is devoid of apolipoprotein A-II *(81,128,146,167)*.

Substitution of testosterone in hypogonadal men or in elderly men led to minor or no decrease in HDL cholesterol *(see* Table 3) *(77,126–129,143,145,150–174)*. A recent meta-analysis of 19 studies published between 1987 and 1999 *(175)* calculated that intramuscular administration of an average dosage of 179 ± 13 mg testosterone ester every 16 ± 1 d for 6 ± 1 mo was associated with an HDL cholesterol decrease of 2–5 mg/dL. This becomes less prominent with increasing age of treated men and duration of treatment. Testosterone substitution for up to 3 yr in men over the age of 50 yr did not produce any consistent changes in circulating lipid levels *(147,176)*. In a multicenter study of male contraception in younger men, a significant decrease in HDL cholesterol was found in non-Chinese subjects only *(156)*. Transdermal application of T or dihydrotestosterone (DHT) also exerted less effect on HDL cholesterol than intramuscular application *(148,149,141,174)*.

Lowering of HDL cholesterol by T is considered to increase cardiovascular risks because HDL cholesterol exerts several potentially antiatherogenic actions. However, in transgenic animal models, only increases of HDL cholesterol induced by ApoA-I overproduction but not by inhibition of HDL catabolism were consistently found to prevent atherosclerosis *(177)*. Therefore, using the mechanism of HDL modification and by inference, changes in metabolism rather than circulating levels of HDL cholesterol *per se* appear to determine the (anti-)atherogenicity of HDL *(177,178)*. T upregulates the scavenger receptor B1 (SR-B1) in the liver and stimulates selective cholesterol uptake. Hepatic lipase (HL) hydrolyzes phospholipids on the surface of HDL, thereby facilitating the selective uptake of HDL core lipids by SR-B1 *(177,179)*. The activity of HL in postheparin plasma is increased after the administration of exogenous T *(128,143,146,152,180)* and slightly decreased by suppression of T after GnRH antagonist treatment *(81)*. Increasing both SR-B1 and HL activities are consistent with the HDL-lowering effect of T, which reflects accelerated reverse cholesterol transport from the tissues to the liver. In accordance with this, transgenic mice overexpressing HL showed a dramatic fall in circulating HDL cholesterol levels, but atherosclerosis was inhibited rather than enhanced *(177,179,181)*. This highlights the pitfall of assuming that the HDL-lowering effect of exogenous T will increase cardiovascular risk. Paradoxically, the mechanism by which testosterone reduces circulating HDL cholesterol may actually confer protection from rather than promotion of atherosclerosis.

Lipoprotein(a)

Lipoprotein(a) [Lp(a)] has striking structural homology to plasminogen but no fibrinolytic activity. Lp(a) levels higher than 30 mg/dL are an independent risk factor for coronary, cerebrovascular, and peripheral atherosclerotic vessel diseases *(182)*. Administration of exogenous T to hypogonadal *(183)* or healthy men *(138,155,157,167,184)* decreased serum Lp(a) significantly by 22–59%. Lp(a) increased by 40–60% in men when endogenous T was suppressed by GnRH analogs *(168,183,185)*. The Lp(a)-lowering effect of T is independent of aromatization *(184)*. How T regulates Lp(a) is unknown. Whether changes in Lp(a) induced by T will affect cardiovascular risk is also unclear.

THE HEMOSTATIC SYSTEM

Administration of supraphysiological dosages of T to healthy men led to a sustained decrease of fibrinogen by 15–20% and significant decreases of PAI-1 *(186)*. Likewise, PAI-1 was decreased in men who received the anabolic androgen stanozolol *(187)*. In women, treatment of endometriosis with the weak androgen danazolol as well as post-menopausal HRT with tibolone, led to significant decreases of fibrinogen and PAI-1 levels *(188–190)*. These data indicate that T exerts anticoagulatory and profibrinolytic effects by lowering fibrinogen and PAI-1. However, high doses of androgens also decrease cyclooxygenase activity and increase platelet aggregability *(190,191)*.

In summary, exogenous T exerts significant dose-dependent effects on several cardio-vascular risk factors, most of which can be beneficial, namely lowering of Lp(a), insulin, fibrinogen, and PAI-1; the lowering of HDL cholesterol is considered harmful (but, in fact, can also be protective). These effects are most prominent at supraphysiological doses or if synthetic oral androgens are used, but they are minimal during hormone replacement of hypogonadal or elderly men. The nonlinear interactions of multiple risk factors and the confounding influence of obesity and insulin resistance make it impos-sible to predict the net effect of exogenous T on cardiovascular risks.

EFFECTS OF ANDROGENS ON CELLS OF THE ARTERIAL WALL AND VASCULAR FUNCTION

Vascular endothelial and smooth muscle cells, as well as macrophages and platelets, express androgen and estrogen receptors and the converting enzymes aromatase, 5α-reductase, and 17β-hydroxysteroid dehydrogenase *(see* ref. *6* for review). Androgens can therefore regulate vascular physiology and contribute to the pathogenesis of artherosclerosis both directly and via conversion to estradiol. Furthermore, the vascular effects of supraphysiological doses of T can also be mediated independently via mem-brane-receptor-associated ion channels.

Effects of Androgens on Vascular Reactivity

An early hallmark of atherosclerosis is decreased vascular responsiveness. This may be the result of impaired flow-mediated nitric oxide release from the endothelium (so-called endothelium-dependent mechanism) or an endothelium-independent disturbance in vascular smooth muscle relaxation in response to nitric oxide. Consequently, decreased vasodilation and enhanced vasoconstriction can lead to vasospasm and angina pectoris. Moreover, endothelial dysfunction also contributes to coronary events by promoting plaque rupture and thrombosis *(192–194)*.

Nitrate-induced dilation of the brachial arteries was significantly reduced in female-to-male transsexuals taking high-dose androgens *(195,198)* (*see* Table 4). Patients with prostate cancer and male-to-female transsexuals deprived of endogenous androgens had greater flow-induced but not in nitroglycerin-induced dilation of brachial arteries *(196,197)* (*see* Table 4).

In contrast, acute interventional studies with iv administration of T to male patients with CAD revealed apparently beneficial vasodilatory effects *(16,17,199)* (*see* Table 4). How-ever, the extremely high doses employed render the specificity and physiological relevance of these findings questionable. In postmenopausal women, T plus estradiol improved flow-mediated and nitrate-induced brachial artery vasodilatation in an uncontrolled study *(200)*.

Table 4
Effects of Testosterone on Vasoreactivity

Study (ref.)	Species	Artery	Study type	Dose[a]	Role of endothelium	Vasodilation
McCrohon et al. 1997 (197)	Human (M-to-F transsexual)	Brachial	Case control	0	Dependent	Increased
Herman et al. 1997 (196)	Human (M castrated)	Brachial	Case control	0	Dependent	Increased
New et al. 1997 (198)	Human (F-to-M transsexual)	Brachial	Case control	nmol	Dependent and independent	Decreased
McCredie et al. 1998 (195)	Human (F-to-M transsexual)	Brachial	Case control	nmol	Dependent and independent	Decreased
Webb et al. 1999 (16)	Human (M)	Coronary	Intervention	nmol	Independent	Increased
Rosano et al. 1999 (17)	Human (M)	Coronary	Intervention	μmol	?	Increased
				nmol	No effect	
Ong et al. 2000 (199)	Human (M)	Brachial	Intervention	μmol	Dependent	Increased
				nmol	No effect	
Warboys et al. 2001 (200)	Human (F)	Brachial	Intervention	nmol	Dependent and independent	Increased
Adams et al. 1995 (51)	Monkey (F)	Coronary	In vivo	nmol	Dependent	Increased
Chou et al. 1996 (201)	Dog (M and F)	Coronary	In vivo	μmol	Dependent	Increased
Farhat et al. 1995 (203)	Pig (M and F)	Coronary	Ex vivo	μmol	Dependent and independent	Increased
Quan et al. 1999 (206)	Pig (M and F)	Coronary	Ex vivo	μmol	Independent	Increased
Teoh et al. 2000 (205)				nmol	Decreased	
Yue et al. 1995 (204)	Rabbit (M and F)	Coronary	Ex vivo	μmol	Dependent and independent	Increased
Ceballos et al. 1999 (207)	Rat	Coronary	Ex vivo	nmol	Dependent	Decreased
Costarella et al. 1996 (202)	Rat (M)	Aorta	Ex vivo	μmol	Dependent and independent	Increased
Hutchison et al. 1997 (208)	Rabbit	Aorta	Ex vivo	nmol	Dependent	Decreased
Geary et al. 2000 (209)	Rat (M)	Cerebral	Ex vivo	μmol	Dependent	Increased

Note: M, male; F, female.
[a]Refers to change in serum levels: 0, castration; nmol, nanomolar; μmol, micromolar.

In vivo studies in monkeys and dogs of both sexes as well as most in vitro studies with animal vessels suggest that T exerts beneficial effects on vascular reactivity *(51,201)* *(see* Table 4). In vitro studies with isolated rings of coronary arteries and/or aortas from rats, rabbits, and pigs consistently found that T improved both endothelium-dependent and/or endothelium-independent vascular responsiveness *(202–209)* *(see* Table 4). Again, all of these studies employed supraphysiological to pharmacological doses of T, whereas physiological nanomolar dosages tended to inhibit vasodilatation *(205–208)*.

The cellular and molecular mechanisms by which T regulates vascular tone are not well understood. Evidence for and against endothelium-dependent or endothelium-independent mechanisms are summarized in Table 4. In vitro expression of nitric oxide synthase in human aortic endothelial cells was stimulated by estradiol but not by T *(210)*. T increased the response of coronary arteries to prostaglandin-F2α *(203,211)* whereas DHT increased the density of thromboxane receptors in smooth muscle cells *(212)*. However, pretreatment with the prostaglandin synthase inhibitor indomethacin had no effect on T-induced vasodilation; therefore the role of eicosanoids in the vascular actions of T is controversial *(201,204,205)*. Conversion to estradiol is not required because neither aromatase inhibitor nor the estrogen-receptor antagonist prevented the T-induced vasodilation *(201,204)*. Two observations also indicate that T, especially in supraphysiological doses, modulates vascular tone via nongenomic mechanisms. First, the androgen receptor antagonists flutamide and cyproterone acetate did not inhibit the effects of T on rabbit or pig coronary arteries *(204,205)*. Second, barium chloride attenuated the T-induced vasorelaxation of rabbit aortas and coronary arteries, indicating that T modulates the opening of potassium channels in vascular smooth muscle cells *(204)*.

In summary, T modulates vasoreactivity by both endothelium-dependent and endothelium-independent mechanisms, as well as by genomic and nongenomic modes of action. Physiological concentrations of T appear to inhibit vasodilatation by activation of the androgen receptor. In contrast, supraphysiological doses of testosterone can augment arterial vasodilatation through nongenomic actions.

Effects of T on Macrophage Functions

Increased uptake of oxidatively modified lipoproteins via type A scavenger receptors leads to the intracellular accumulation of cholesteryl esters in macrophages and thereby to foam cell formation *(213–216)*. T increases the oxidation of LDL by placental macrophages in vitro *(217)*. Dihydrotestosterone dose-dependently stimulates the uptake of acetylated LDL by scavenger receptor type A and intracellular cholesteryl ester accumulation in macrophages of male but not female donors *(218)*. The effect was blocked by the androgen receptor antagonist hydroxyflutamide *(218)*.

Nonhepatic and nonsteroidogenic cells such as macrophages cannot metabolize cholesterol and can only dispose of excess cholesterol by secretion. Cholesterol efflux from cells is therefore central to the regulation of the cellular cholesterol homeostasis. To date, two plasma membrane proteins are known to facilitate active cholesterol efflux *(see* Fig. 1). Interaction of the scavenger receptor B1 with mature lipid-containing HDL facilitates cholesterol efflux by reorganizing the distribution of cholesterol within the plasma membrane. The ATP-binding cassette transporter (ABC) A1 mediates phospholipid and cholesterol efflux to extracellular lipid-free apolipoproteins by translocating these lipids from intracellular compartments to the plasma membrane and/or by forming a pore within the plasma membrane, through which the lipids are secreted *(177)*.

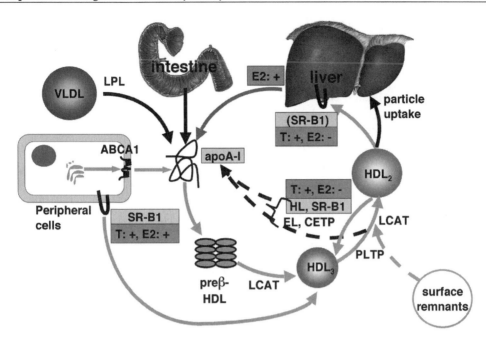

Fig. 1. Pathways of HDL metabolism and the influence of testosterone on reverse cholesterol transport. Mature HDL$_3$ and HDL$_2$ are generated from lipid-free ApoA-I (folded linear polypeptide) or lipid-poor pre-β_1-HDL as the precursors. These precursors are produced as nascent HDL by the liver or intestine or are released from lipolyzed VLDL and chlyomicrons (triglyceride-related lipoproteins [TGRL]) or by interconversion of HDL$_3$ and HDL$_2$ (broken black line). ABCA1-mediated lipid efflux from cells is important for initial lipidation; Lecithin cholesteryl acyl transferase (LCAT)-mediated esterification of cholesterol generates spherical particles that continue to grow upon ongoing cholesterol esterification, phospholipid transfer protein (PLTP)-mediated particle fusion, and surface remnant transfer. These mature HDL particles also continue to accept cellular cholesterol by processes that are facilitated by the scavenger receptor BI (SR-BI) and LCAT. Larger HDL$_2$ are converted into smaller HDL$_3$ on cholesteryl ester transfer protein (CETP)-mediated export of cholesteryl esters from HDL onto ApoB-containing lipoproteins, SR-B1-mediated selective uptake of cholesteryl esters into liver and steroidogenic organs, and hepatic lipase (HL)- and endothelial lipase (EL)-mediated hydrolysis of phospholipids. HDL lipids are catabolized either separately from HDL proteins (i.e., by selective uptake or via CETP-transfer) or together with HDL proteins (i.e., via uptake through as yet unknown HDL receptors or ApoE receptors). Both the conversion of HDL$_2$ into HDL$_3$ and the PLTP-mediated conversion of HDL$_3$ into HDL$_2$ liberate lipid-free or poorly lipidated ApoA-I (broken black line), which is either reused for the formation of mature HDL or is filtrated into the kidney. Gray arrows represent lipid transfer processes, black arrows represent protein transfer processes. The hepatic expression and activity of both HL and SR-B1 are upregulated by testosterone and downregulated by estradiol. Both testosterone and estradiol upregulate SR-BI expression in macrophages, thereby increasing cholesterol efflux from these cells onto lipidated HDL. In addition, estradiol upregulates the hepatic expression and secretion of ApoA-I. The actions of testosterone result in a lowering of circulating HDL cholesterol and an increase in reverse cholesterol transport. (Modified from ref. *177.*)

T upregulates the expression of the scavenger receptor B1 in human monocyte-derived macrophages, thereby stimulating HDL-induced cholesterol efflux. However, T does not affect expression of ABC A1 (von Eckardstein et al., unpublished). In summary, T modulates lipid transport mechanisms of macrophages which favour lipid accumulation (uptake of modified LDL via scavenger receptor type A) as well as lipid secretion (cholesterol efflux via scavenger receptor B1). The net effect is unclear.

Effects of T on Platelet Function

Aggregation of platelets is a prerequisite for thrombus formation and, hence, a critical step in acute coronary events. Administration of T cypionate to eugonadal men led to enhanced ex vivo platelet aggregation in response to the thromboxane analog I-BOP but not in response to thrombin *(219)*. T increases the expression of the androgen receptor in a megakaryocyte cell line, as well as in platelets *(220,221)*. Flutamide inhibited the stimulatory effect of testosterone on thromboxane receptor expression *(220,221)*, suggesting that the effect is mediated via the androgen receptor. Whether T exerts any effects on in vivo platelet aggregation and thrombus formation is currently not clear.

DHEA-S AND CAD IN MEN AND WOMEN

Dehydroepiandrosterone (DHEA) and its sulfate DHEA-S are weak but highly abundant adrenal androgens that show a marked progressive age-related decline in both men and women from the third decade onward *(222)*. There is a belief that the DHEA deficiency is associated with increased morbidity and mortality in the elderly *(223,224)*.

In men, an inverse *(225–232)*, null *(13,230,233–242)* or positive *(14,243)* relationship between DHEA-S levels and CAD have been reported (*see* Table 1). These observational studies are diminished by methodological shortcomings such as small sample size, cross-sectional analyses with no cause–effect differentiation, inadequate allowance for confounders (smoking and obesity), and the insensitivity of coronary angiography to detect early disease. Low DHEA-S levels appear to be associated with increased mortality from all causes in men over the age of 50 *(230,238)*, giving rise to the notion that this is a nonspecific marker of poor health *(240,244)*. Although a negative relationship between DHEA-S and CAD has been documented in cross-sectional studies in younger women *(17,229,231,245)*, all prospective and case-control studies *(16,238–242,246)* except one *(247)* in older or postmenopausal women showed that cardiovascular mortality was not associated with DHEA levels at baseline (*see* Table 2). Taken together, data from observational studies on DHEA-S are confounded, inconsistent, and do not support the hypothesis that DHEA-S "deficiency" is a risk factor for CAD.

In animal studies, DHEA consistently decreased atherosclerosis. Thus, all five studies *(48,248–251)* showed a significant reduction in spontaneous or balloon-injury-induced atherosclerotic lesions independently of lipids in rabbits. The use of animals with negligible physiological adrenal androgen production and pharmacological doses of DHEA render these data of doubtful relevance to man.

In summary, the epidemiological and experimental data on the relationship between DHEA and CAD are unconvincing.

ESTROGENS AND CARDIOVASCULAR DISEASE IN MEN

The importance of locally produced estrogens from aromatization of T in males for cardiovascular health is highlighted by recent human and transgenic mouse models of aromatase deficiency and estrogen resistance. In two men with undetectable circulating estradiol and estrone and high T as a result of P450 aromatase deficiency *(252,253)*, dyslipidaemia with elevated total and LDL cholesterol and triglyceride and decreased

HDL cholesterol was associated with insulin resistance. These metabolic abnormalities were correctable by low-dose oral or transdermal estrogen replacement. Insulin resistance, impaired glucose tolerance, and low HDL cholesterol were also apparent in a 28-yr-old male with a null mutation in estrogen-receptor (ER)α gene causing estrogen resistance *(254)*. Intact hepatic ERβ may have prevented full expression of dyslipdemia. Ultrafast electron beam computed tomgraphy imaging showed calcium deposition in the proximal left anterior descending coronary artery, indicating the presence of premature atherosclerosis *(255)*. Flow-mediated brachial artery vaosdilatation was absent, showing marked endothelial dysfunction *(256)*.

These rare experiments of nature suggest that estrogens are important in maintaining normal carbohydrate and lipid metabolism as well as normal endothelial-dependent nitric oxide-mediated vasodilatation in men. They are confirmed by data from transgenic knockout models *(257–259)*. The favorable effects of estrogens on HDL cholesterol demonstrated are also in accord with clinical studies using aromatase inhibitors in normal men (*see* the section Relationships Between Serum Levels of T and CAD; Interventional Clinical Studies).

SUMMARY AND CONCLUSION

Hypoandrogenemia in men and hyperandrogenemia in women are not only associated with increased risk of CAD but also with visceral obesity, insulin resistance, low HDL cholesterol, elevated triglycerides, LDL cholesterol, and PAI-1. These gender differences and confounders render the precise role of *endogenous* androgens in atherosclerosis unclear. *Exogenous* androgens, on the other hand, induce both apparently deleterious and beneficial effects on cardiovascular risk factors. Thus, T administration decreases HDL cholesterol, PAI-1 (apparently deleterious), Lp(a), fibrinogen, insulin, leptin and visceral fat mass (apparently beneficial) in men as well as women. However, androgen-induced declines in circulating HDL cholesterol are not necessarily proatherogenic, because it may reflect accelerated reverse cholesterol transport. Supraphysiological concentrations of T stimulate vasorelaxation; however, at physiological concentrations, inhibition of vasodilatation is observed in vitro. T increases macrophage uptake of modified lipoproteins ("proatherogenic") but it also stimulates the efflux of cellular cholesterol to HDL ("antiatherogenic"). The inconsistent data militate against a meaningful assessment of the net effect of T on the pathogenesis of atherosclerosis and global cardiovascular risk. However, current evidence does not support the concerns regarding cardiovascular risks from the therapeutic use of androgens in men. In contrast, the possibility that spontaneous or induced hyperandrogenaemia may increase the risks for CAD in women should be considered. The presentation of young women with PCOS therefore offers a valuable primary prevention opportunity against premature CAD.

REFERENCES

1. Lerner DJ, Kannel WB. Patterns of coronary heart disease morbidity and mortality in the sexes: a 26-year follow-up of the Framingham population. Am J Cardiol 1986;111:383–390.
2. Kalin MF, Zumoff B. Sex hormones and coronary disease: a review of the clinical studies. Steroids 1990;55:330–352.
3. Hayward CS, Kelly RP, Collins P. The roles of gender, the menopause and hormone replacement on cardiovascular function. Cardiovasc Res 2000;46:28–49.

4. Bhasin S, Bremner WJ. Clinical review 85: emerging issues in androgen replacement therapy. J Clin Endocrinol Metab 1997;82:3–7.

5. Davies SR. Androgens replacement in women: a commentary. J Clin Endocrinol Metab 1999;84:1886–1891.

6. Wu FCW, von Eckardstein A. Androgens and coronary artery disease. Endocr Rev, in press.

7. Alexandersen P, Haarbo J, Christiansen C. The relationship of natural androgens to coronary heart disease in males: a review. Atherosclerosis 1996;125:1–13.

8. Barrett-Connor E, Khaw KT. Endogenous sex hormones and cardiovascular disease in men. A prospective population based study. Circulation 1988;78:539–545.

9. Yarnell JWG, Beswick AD, Sweetnam PM, Riad-Fahmy D. Endogenous sex hormones and ischaemic heart disease in men. The Caerphilly Prospective Study. Arteriosclerosis Thromb 1993;13:467–471.

10. Harman SM, Metter EJ, Tobin JD, et al. Longitudinal effects of aging on serum total and free testosterone levels in healthy men. J Clin Endocrinol Metab 2001;86:724–731.

11. Cauley JA, Gutai JP, Kuller LH, Dai WS. Usefulness of sex steroid hormone levels in predicting coronary artery disease in men. Am J Cardiol 1987;60:771–777.

12. Phillips GB, Yano K, Stemmerman GN. Serum sex hormone levels and myocardial infarction in the Honolulu Heart Program. Pitfalls in prospective studies on sex hormones. J Clin Epidemiol 1988;41:1151–1156.

13. Contoreggi CS, Blackman MR, Andres R, et al. Plasma levels of estradiol, testosterone, and DHEAS do not predict risk of coronary artery disease in men. J Androl 1990;11:460–470.

14. Hautenen A, Manttari M, Manninen V, et al. Adrenal androgens and testosterone as coronary risk factors in the Helsinki Heart Study. Atherosclerosis 1994;105:191–200.

15. Webb CM, Adamson DL, de Zeigler D, Collins P. Effect of acute testosterone on myocardial ischemia in men with coronary artery disease. Am J Cardiol 1999;83:437–439.

16. Webb CM, McNeill JG, Hayward CS, et al. Effects of testosterone on coronary vasomotor regulation in men with coronary heart disease. Circulation 1999;100:1690–1696.

17. Rosano GM, Leonardo F, Pagnotta P, et al. Acute anti-ischemic effect of testosterone in men with coronary artery disease. Circulation 1999;99:1666–1670.

18. Barrett-Connor EL, Goodman-Gruen D. Prospective study of endogenous sex hormones and fatal cardiovascular disease in postmenipausal women. Br Med J 1995;311:1193–1196.

19. Phillips GB, Pinkernell BH, Jing TY. Relationship between serum sex hormones and coronary artery disease in postmenopausal women. Arteriosclerosis Thromb Vasc Biol 1997;17:695–701.

20. Bernini GP, Sgro' M, Moretti A, et al. Endogenous androgens and carotid intimal-medial thickness in women. J Clin Endocrinol Metab 1999;84:2008–2012.

21. Dahlgren E, Johannson S , Lindstedt G , et al. Woman with polycystic ovary syndrome wedge resected in 1956 to 1965: a long-term follow-up focussing on natural history and circulating hormones. Fertil Steril 1992;57:505–513.

22. Wild RA, Grubb B, Hartz van Nort JJ, et al. Clinical signs of androgen excess as risk factors for coronary artery disease. Fertil Steril 1990;54:255–259.

23. Birdsall M, Farquhar C, White H. Association between polycystic ovaries and extent of coronary artery disease in women having cardiac catheterization. Ann Intern Med 1997;126: 32–35.

24. Cibula D, Cifkova R, Fanta M, et al. Increased risk of non-insulin dependent diabetes mullitus, arterial hypertension and coronary artery disease in perimenopausal women with a history of the polycystic ovarian syndrome Human Reprod 2000;15:785–789.

25. Birdsall M, Farquhar C, White H. Association between polycystic ovaries and extent of coronary artery disease in women having cardiac catheterization. Ann Intern Med 1997;126:32–35.

26. Guzick DS, Talbott EO, Sutton-Tyrrell K, et al. Carotid atherosclerosis in women with polycystic ovary syndrome: initial results from a case-control study. Am J Obstet Gynecol 1996;174:1224–1229; discussion 1229–1232.

27. Christian RC, Dumesic DA, Yrtiska HJ, et al. Clinical hyperandrogenism and body mass index predict coronary calcification in perimenopausal women with polcystic ovarian syndrome. Endocrine Society Annual Meeting, 2000.

28. Mather KJ, Kwan F, Corenblum B. Hyperinsulinemia in polycystic ovary syndrome correlates with increased cardiovascular risk independent of obesity. Fertil Steril 2000;73:150–156.

29. Pierpoint T, McKeigue PM, Isaacs AJ, et al. Mortality of women with polycystic ovary syndrome at long-term follow-up. J Clin Epidemiol 1998;51:581–586.

30. Wild S, Pierpoint T, McKeigue P, Jacobs HS. Cardiovascular disease in women with polycystic ovary syndrome at long-term follow-up: a retrospective cohort study. Clin Endocrinol (Oxf) 2000;52:595–600.

31. Elting MW, Korsen TJM, Bezemer PD, Schoemaker J. Prevalence of diabetes, hypertension, and cardiac complaints in a follow-up study of a Dutch PCOS population. Human Reprod 2001;16: 556–560.

32. Hamilton JB, Mestler GE. Mortality and survival: comparison of eunuchs with intact men and women in a mentally retarded population. J Gerontol 1969;24:395–411.

33. Nieschlag E, Nieschlag S, Behre HM. Lifespan and testosterone. Nature 1993;366:215.

34. Van Kesteren PJ, Asscheman H, Megens JA, Gooren LJ. Mortality and morbidity in transsexual subjects treated with cross-sex hormones. Clin Endocrinol 1997;47:337–342.

35. Wilson JD. Androgen abuse by athletes. Endocr Rev 1988;9:181–199.

36. Council on Scientific Affairs. Medical and Non-medical uses of anabolic-androgenic steroids. JAMA 1990;264:2923–2937.

37. Yesalis CE, Kennedy NJ, Kopstein AN, Bahrke MS Anabolic-androgen steroid use in the United States. JAMA 1993;270:1217–1221.

38. Rockhold RW. Cardiovascular toxicity of anabolic steroids. Ann Rev Pharmacol Toxicol 1993;33:497–520.

39. Sullivan ML, Martinez CM, Gennis P, Gallagher EJ. The cardiac toxicity of anabolic steroids. Prog Cardiovas Dis 1998;41:1–15.

40. Jaffe MD. Effect of testosterone on on postexercise ST segment depression. Br Heart J 1977;39:1217–1222.

41. Wu SZ, Weng XZ. Therapeutic effects of an androgenic preparation on myocardial ischemia and cardiac function in 62 elderly male coronary heart disease patients. Chin Med J 1993;106:415–418.

42. English KM, Steed RP, Diver MJ, Jones TH, Channer KS. Low dose transdermal testosterone therapy improves angina threshold in men with chronic stable angina. Circulation 2000;102:1906–1911.

43. Snyder PJ. Editorial: the role of androgens in women. J Clin Endocrinol Metab 2001;86:1006–1007.

44. Miller KK, Sesmilo G, Schiller A, et al. androgen deficiency in women with hypopituitarism. J Clin Endocrinol Metab 2001;86:561–567.

45. Larsen BA, Nordestgaard BG, Stender S, Kjeldsen K. Effect of testosterone on atherogenesis in cholesterol-fed rabbits with similar plasma cholesterol levels. Atherosclerosis 1993;99:79–86.

46. Fogelberg M, Björkhem I, Diczfalusy U, Henriksson P. Stanozolol and experimental atherosclerosis: atherosclerosis development and blood lipids during anabolic steroid therapy of New Zealand white rabbits. Scand J Clin Lab Invest 1990;50:693–700.

47. Bruch B, Brehme U, Gugel N, et al. Gender-specific differences in the effects of testosterone and estrogen on thedevelopment of atherosclerosis in rabbits. Arteriosclerosis Thromb Vasc Biol 1997;17:2192–2199.

48. Chen SJ, Li HB, Durand J, Oparil S, Chen YF. Estrogen reduces myointimal proliferation after balloon injury of rat carotid artery. Circulation 1996;93:577–584.

49. Alexandersen P, Haarbo J, Byrjalsen I, et al. Natural androgens inhibit male atherosclerosis: a study in castrated, cholesterol-fed rabbits. Circ Res 1999;84:813–819.

50. Toda T, Toda Y, Cho BH, Kummerow FA. Ultrastructural changes in the comb and aorta of chicks fed excess testosterone. Atherosclerosis 1984;51:47–53.

51. Adams MR, Williams JK, Kaplan JR. Effects of androgens on coronary artery atherosclerosis and atherosclerosis-related impairment of vascular responsiveness. Arteriosclerosis Thromb Vasc Biol 1995;15:562–570.

52. Obasanjo IO, Clarkson TB, Weaver DS. Effects of the anabolic steroid nandrolone decanoate on plasma lipids and coronary arteries of female cynomolgus macaques. Metabolism 1996;45:463–468.

53. Elhage R, Arnal JF, Pieraggi M-T, et al.7 17β-estradiol prevents fatty streak formation in apolipoprotein E-deficient mice. Arteriosclerosis Thromb Vasc Biol 1997;17:2679–2684.

54. Eisner JR, Dumesic DA, Kemnitz JW, Abbott DH. Timing of prenatal androgen excess determines differential impairment in insulin secretion and action in adult female rhesus monkeys. J Clin Endocrinol Metab 2000;85:1206–1210.

55. von Dehn G, von Dehn O, Völker W, et al. Atherosclerosis in apolipoprotein E-deficient mice is decreased by the suppression of endogenous sex hormones. Horm Metab Res 2001;33:110–114.

56. Nathan L, Shi W, Dinh H, et al. Testosterone inhibits early atherogenesis by conversion to estradiol: Critical role of aromatase. Proc Natl Acad Sci USA 2001;98:3589–3593.

57. Barret-Connor EL. Testosterone and risk factors for cardiovascular disease in men. Diabetes Metab 1995;21:156–161.
58. De Pergola G. The adipose tissue metabolism: role of testosterone and dehydroepiandrosterone. Int J Obes Related Metab Disord 2000;24(Suppl 2):S59–S63.
59. Caron P, Bennet A, Camare R, et al. Plasminogen activator inhibitor in plasma is related to testosterone in men. Metabolism 1989;38:1010–1015.
60. Freedman DS, O 'Brien TR, Flanders WD. Relation of serum testosterone levels to high density lipoprotein cholesterol and other characteristics in men. Arterioscler Thromb 1991;11:307–315.
61. Glueck CJ, Glueck HI, Stroop D, et al. Endogenous testosterone, fibrinolysis, and coronary heart disease risk in hyperlipidemic men. J Lab Clin Med 1993;122:412–420.
62. Hämäläinen E, Adlercreutz H, Ehnholm C. Relationship of serum lipoproteins and apoproteins to the binding capacity of sex hormone binding globulin in healthy Finnish men. Metabolism 1986;35:535–541.
63. Kiel DP, Baron CA, Plymate SR. Sex hormones and lipoproteins in men. Am J Med 1989;87:35–39.
64. Yang XC, Jing TY, Gesnick LM, Phillips GB. Relation of hemostatic factors to other risk factors for coronary artery disease and to sex hormones in men Arteriosclerosis Thromb 1993;13:467–471.
65. Hergenc G, Schulte H, Assmann G, von Eckardstein A. Associations of obesity markers, insulin, and sex hormones with HDL-cholesterol levels in Turkish and German individuals. Atherosclerosis 1999;145:147–156.
66. Tchernof A, Labrie F, Belanger A, Despres JP. Obesity and metabolic complications: contribution of dehydroepiandrosterone and other steroid hormones. J Endocrinol 1996;150(Suppl):S155–S164.
67. Tsai EC, Boyko EJ, Leonetti DL, Fujimoto WY. Low serum testosterone level as a predictor of increased visceral fat in Japanese-American men. Int J Obes Relat Metab Disord 2000;24:485–491.
68. Simon D, Charles MA, Nahoul K, et al. Association between plasma total testosterone and cardiovascular risk factors in healthy adult men: The Telecom Study. J Clin Endocrinol Metab 1997;82:682–685
69. Pasquali R, Macor C, Vicennati V, et al. Effects of acute hyperinsulinemia on testosterone serum concentrations in adult obese and normal-weight men. Metabolism 1997;46:526–529.
70. Björntorp P. The regulation of adipose tissue distribution in humans Int J Obesity 1996;20:291–302.
71. Haffner SM, Valdez RA. Endogenous sex hormones: impact on lipds, lipoproteins, and insulin. Am J Med 1995;98(Suppl):S40–S47.
72. Marin P, Odén B, Björntorp P. Assimilation and mobilization of triglycerides in subcutaneous abdominal and femoral adipose tissue in vivo in men: effects of androgens. J Clin Endocrinol Metab 1995;80:239–243.
73. Vermeulen A. Decreased androgen levels and obesity in men. Ann Med 1996;28:13–15.
74. Couillard C, Gagnon J, Bergnon J, et al. Contribution of body fatness and adipose tissue distribution to the age variation in plasma steroids hormone concentration in men: the HERITAGE family study. J Clin Endocrinol Metab 2000;85:1026–1031.
75. Behre HM, Simoni M, Nieschlag E. Strong association between serum levels of leptin and testosterone in men. Clin Endocrinol 1997;47:237–240.
76. Sih R, Morley JE, Kaiser FE, et al. Testosterone replacement in older hypogonadal men: a 12 month randomized controlled trial. J Clin Endocinol Metab 1997;82:1661–1667.
77. Wang C, Swedloff RS, Iranmanesh A, et al. Transdermal testosterone gel improves sexual function, mood, muscle strength, and body composition parameters in hypogonadal men. Testosterone Gel Study Group. J Clin Endocrinol Metab 2000;85:2839–2853.
78. Marin P, Holmäng S, Jönsson L, et al. The effects of testosterone treatment on body composition and metabolism in middle aged men. Int J Obesity 1992;16:991–997.
79. Marin P, Holmäng S, Gustafsson C, et al. Androgen treatment of abdominally obese men. Obes Res 1993;1:245–251.
80. Rebuffé-Scrive M, Marin P, Bjorntorp P. Effect of testosterone on abdominal adipose tissue in men. Int J Obes 1991;15:791–795.
81. Büchter, D, Behre, HM, Kliesch, S, et al. Effects of testosterone suppression in young men by the gonadotropin releasing hormone antagonist cetrorelix on plasma lipids, lipolytic enzymes, lipid transfer proteins, insulin, and leptin. Exp Clin Endocrinol Diabet 1999;107:522–529.
82. Björntorp P. Hyperandrogenicity in women - a prediabetic condition? J Intern Med 1993;234:579–583.

83. Björntorp P. Fatty acids, hyperinsulinemia, and insulin resistance: which comes first? Curr Opin Lipidol 1994;5:166–174.

84. Dieudonne MN, Pecquery R, Leneveu MC, Giudicelli Y. Opposite effects of androgens and estrogens on adipogenesis in rat preadipocytes: evidence for sex and site-related specificities and possible involvement of insulin-like growth factor 1 receptor and peroxisome proliferator-activated receptor gamma2. Endocrinology 2000;141(2):649–656.

85. Mantzoros CS, Dunaif A, Flier JS. Leptin concentrations in the polycystic ovary syndrome. J Clin Endocrinol Metab 1997;82:1687–1691.

86. Rouru J, Anttila L, Koskinen P, et al. Serum leptin concentrations in women with polycystic ovary syndrome. J Clin Endocrinol Metab 1997;82:1697–1700.

87. Sherif K, Kushner H, Falkner BE. Sex hormone-binding globulin and insulin resistance in African-American women. Metabolism 1998;47:70–74.

88. Lindstedt G, Lundberg P, Lapidus L, et al. Low sex hormone binding globulin concentration as an independent risk factor for development of NIDDM: 12 yr follow up of population study of women in Gothenburg. Diabetes 1991;40:123–128.

89. Wortsman J, Soler NG. Abnormalities of fuel metabolism in the polycystic ovary syndrome. Obstet Gynecol 1982;60:342–345.

90. Mattson LA, Cullberg G, Hamberger L, et al. Lipid metabolism in women with polycystic ovary syndrome: possible implications for an increased risk for coronary heart disease. Fertil Steril 1984;42:579–584.

91. Wild RA, Palmer PC, Coulson PB, et al. Lipoprotein lipid concentrations and cardiovascular risk in women with polycystic ovarian syndrome. J Clin Endocrinol Metab 1985;61:946–951.

92. Conway GS, Agrawal R, Betteridge DJ, Jacobs HS. Risk factors for coronary artery disease in lean and obese women with the polycystic ovary syndrome. Clin Endocrinol 1992;37:119–125.

93. Dahlgren E, Janson PO, Johansson S, et al. Polycystic ovary syndrome and risk for myocardial infarction: evaluated from a risk factor model based on a prospective population study of women. Acta Obstet Gynecol Scand 1992;71:599–604.

94. Dahlgren E, Lapidus A, Janson P, et al. Hemostatic and metabolic variables in women with polycystic ovary syndrome. Fertil Steril 1994;61:455–460.

95. Talbott E, Guzick D, Clerici A, et al. Coronary heart disease risk factors in women with polycystic ovary syndrome. Arteriosclosis Thromb Vasc Biol 1995;15:821–826.

96. Sampson M, Kong C, Patel A, et al. Ambulatory blood pressure profiles and plasminogen activator inhibitor (PAI-1) activity in lean women with and without the polycystic ovary syndrome. Clin Endocrinol (Oxf) 1996;45:623–629.

97. von Eckardstein S, von Eckardstein A, et al. Elevated low density lipoprotein-cholesterol in women with polycystic ovary syndrome. J Gynecol Endocrin 1996;10:311–318.

98. Fox R. Prevalence of a positive family history of type 2 diabetes in women with polycystic ovarian disease. Gynecol Endocrinol 1999;13:390–393.

99. Penttila TL, Koskinen P, Penttila TA, et al. Obesity regulates bioavailable testosterone levels in women with or without polycystic ovary syndrome.Fertil Steril 1999;71:457–461.

100. Sozen I, Arici A. Hyperinsulinism and its interaction with hyperandrogenism in polycystic ovary syndrome. Obstet Gynecol Surv 2000;55:321–328.

101. Conway GS, Clark PM, Wong D. Hyperinsulinaemia in the polycystic ovary syndrome confirmed with a specific immunoradiometric assay for insulin. Clin Endocrinol 1993;38:219–222.

102. Chang RJ, Nakamura RM, Judd HL, Kaplan SA. Insulin resistance in nonobese patients with polycystic ovarian disease. J Clin Endocrinol Metabol 1983;57:356–359.

103. Dunaif A, Mandeli J, Fluhr H, Dobrjansky A. The impact of obesity on chronic hyperinsulinemia on gonadotropin release and gonadal steroid secretion in the polycystic ovary syndrome. J Clin Endocrinol Metabol 1988;66:131–139.

104. Graf MJ, Richards CJ, Brown V, et al. The independent effects of hyperandrogenaemia, hyperinsulinaemia, and obesity on lipid and lipoprotein profiles in women. Clin Endocrinol 1990;33:119–131.

105. Haffner SM. Sex hormone-binding protein, hyperinsulinemia, insulin resistance and noninsulin-dependent diabetes. Horm Res 1996;45:233–237.

106. Holte J, Bergh T , Berne C and Lithell H. Serum lipoprotein lipid profile in women with the polycystic ovary syndrome: relation to anthropometric, endocrine and metabolic variables. Clin Endocrinol 1994;41:463–471.

107. Franks S, Gilling-Smith C, Watson H, Willis D. Insulin action in the normal and polycystic ovary. Endocrinol Metab Clin North Am 1999;28(2):361–378.

108. Acién P, Quereda F, Matallin P, et al. Insulin, androgens, and obesity in women with and withoutpolycystic ovary syndrome: a heterogeneous group of disorders. Fertil Steril 1999;72:32–40.

109. Nestler JE, Jakubowicz DJ, de Vargas AF, et al. Insulin stimulates testosterone biosynthesis by human thecal cells from women with polycystic ovary syndrome by activating its own receptor and using inositolglycan mediators as the signal transduction system. J Clin Endocrinol Metab 1998;83:2001–2005.

110. Dunaif A, Thomas A. Current concepts in the polycystic ovarian syndrome. Ann Rev Med 2001;52:401–419.

111. Ehrmann DA, Cavaghan MK, Imperial J, et al. Effects of metformin on insulin secretion, insulin action, and ovarian steroidogenesis in women with polycystic ovary syndrome. J Clin Endocrinol Metab 1997;82:524–530.

112. Velazquez EM, Mendoza SG, Wang P, Glueck CJ. Metformin therapy is associated with a decrease in plasma plasminogen activator inhibitor 1, lipoprotein(a), and immunoreactive insulin levels in patients with the polycystic ovary syndrome. Metabolism 1997;46:454–457.

113. Pasquali R, Filicori M. Insulin sensitizing agents and polycystic ovary syndrome. Eur J Endocrinol 1998;138:253–254.

114. Kolodziejczyk B, Duleba AJ, Spaczynski RZ, Pawelczyk L. Metformin therapy decreases hyperandrogenism and hyperinsulinemia in women with polycystic ovary syndrome. Fertil Steril 2000;73:1149–1154.

115. Dahlgren E, Landin K, Krotkiewski M, et al. Effects of two antiandrogen treatments on hirsutism and insulin sensitivity in women with polycystic ovary syndrome. Hum Reprod 1998;13:2706–2711.

116. Morghetti P, Tosi F, Castello R et al. The insulin resistance in women with hyperandrogenism is partially reversed by antiandrogen treatment: evidence that androgens impair insulin action in women. J Clin endocrinol Metab 1997;81:952–960.

117. Diamanti-Kandarakis E, Mitrakou A, Raptis S, et al. The effect of a pure antiandrogen receptor blocker, flutamide, on the lipid profile in the polycystic ovary syndrome. J Clin Endocrinol Metab 1998;83:2699–2705.

118. Lemieux S, Lewis GF, Ben-Chetrit A, et al. Correction of hyperandrogenemia by laparoscopic ovarian cautery in women with polycystic ovarian syndrome is not accompanied by improved insulin sensitivity or lipid-lipoprotein levels. J Clin Endocrinol Metab 1999;84:4278–4282.

119. Polderman KH, Gooren LJ, Asschermann H et al. Induction of insulin resistance by androgens and estrogens. J Clin Endocrinol Metab 1994;79:265—271.

120. Elbers JM, de Jong S, Teerlink T, et al. Changes in fat cell size and in vitro lipolytic activity of abdominal and gluteal adipocytes after a one-year cross-sex hormone administration in transsexuals. Metabolism 1999;48(11):1371–1377.

121. Lovejoy JC, Bray GA, Bourgeois MO, et al. Exogenous androgens influence body composition and regional body fat distribution in obese postmenopausal women - a clinical research center study. J Clin Endocrinol Metab 1996;81(6):2198–2203.

122. Nilsson C, Niklasson M, Eriksson E, et al. Imprinting of female offspring with testosterone results in insulin resistance and changes in body fat distribution at adult age in rats. J Clin Invest 1998;101(1):74–78.

123. Dunaif A. Insulin resistance and the polycystic ovary syndrome: mechanism and implications for pathogenesis. Endocr Rev 1997;18:774–800.

124. Rosenfield RL. Ovarian and adrenal function in polycystic ovary syndrome. Endocrinol Metab Clin North Am 1999;28:265–293.

125. Nestler JE, Jakubowicz DJ, Reamer P, et al. Ovulatory and metabolic effects of d-chiro-inositol in the polycystic ovary syndrome. N Eng J Med 1999;340:1314–1320.

126. Valdemarsson S, Hedner P, Nilsson-Ehle P. Increase in hepatic lipase activity after testosterone substitution in men with hypogonadism of pituitary origin. Acta Med Scand 1987;221:363–366.

127. Kirkland RT, Keenan BS, Probstfield JL, et al. Decrease in plasma high density lipoprotein cholesterol levels at puberty in boys with delayed adolescence: Correlation with plasma testosterone levels JAMA 1987;257:502–507.

128. Sorva R, Kuusi T, Taskinene MR, et al. Testosterone substitution increases the activity of lipoprotein lipase and hepatic lipase in hypogonadal men. Atherosclerosis 1988;69:191–197.

129. Jones DB, Higgins B, Billet JS, et al. The effect of testosterone replacement on plasma lipids and apolipoproteins. Eur J Clin Invest 1989;19:438–441.
130. Hromadova M, Hacik T, Malatinsky E, et al. Some measures of lipid metabolism in young sterile men before and after testosterone treatment. Endoc Exp 1989;23:205–211.
131. Hana V, Marek J, Ceska R, et al. Influence of testosterone isobutyrate on serum lipoproteins during replacement therapy of hypogonadal men. Czech Med 1991;14:123–128.
132. Tenover JS. Effects of testosterone supplementation in the aging male. J Clin Endocrinol Metab 1992;75:1092–1098.
133. Bhasin S, Swerdloff RS, Steiner B, et al. A biodegradable testosterone microcapsule formulation provides uniform eugonadal levels of testosterone for 10-11 weeks in hypogonadal men. J Clin Endocrinol Metab 1992;74:75–83.
134. Morley JE, Perry HM 3rd, Kaiser FE, et al. Effects of testosterone replacement therapy in old hypogonadal males: a preliminary study. J Am Geriatr Soc 1993;41:149–152.
135. Salehian B, Wang C, Alexander G, et al. Pharmacokinetics, bioefficacy, and safety of sublingual testosterone cyclodextrin in hypogonadal men: comparison to testosterone enanthate—A Clinical Research Center Study. J Clin Endocrinol Metab 1995;80:3567–3575.
136. Brodsky IG, Balagopal P, Nair KS. Effects of testosterone replacement on muscle mass and muscle protein synthesis in hypogonadal men—a clinical research center study. J Clin Endocrinol Metab 1996;81:3469–3475.
137. Katznelson L, Finkelstein JS, Schoenfeld DA, et al. Increase in bone density and lean body mass during testosterone administration in men with acquired hypogonadism. J Clin Endocrinol Metab 1996;81:4358–4365.
138. Ozata M, Yildrimkaya M, Bulur M, et al. Effects of gonadotropin and testosterone treatment on lipoprotein(a), high density lipoprotein particles, and other lipoprotein levels in male hypogonadism. J Clin Endocrinol Metab 1996;81:3372–3378.
139. Zgliczynski S, Ossowski M, Slowinska-Srzednicka J, et al. Effect of testosterone replacement therapy on lipids and lipoproteins in hypogonadal and elderly men. Atherosclerosis 1996;121:35–43.
140. Arslanian S, Suprasongsin C. Testosterone treatment in adolescents with delayed puberty: changes in body composition, protein, fat, and glucose metabolism. J Clin Endocrinol Metab 1997;82:3213–3220.
141. Howell SJ, Radford JA, Adams JE, et al. Randomized placebo-controlled trial of testosterone replacement in men with mild Leydig cell insufficiency following cytotoxic chemotherapy. Clin Endocrinol (Oxf) 2001;55:315–324.
142. Tripathy D, Shah P, Lakshmy R, Reddy KS. Effect of testosterone replacement on whole body glucose utilisation and other cardiovascular risk factors in males with idiopathic hypogonadotrophic hypogonadism. Horm Metab Res 1998;30:642–645.
143. Tan KC, Shiu SW, Pang RW, Kung AW. Effects of testosterone replacement on HDL subfractions and apolipoprotein A-1 containing lipoproteins. Clin Endocrinol (Oxf) 1998;48:187–194.
144. Rabijewski M, Adamkiewicz M, Zgliczynski S. The influence of testosterone replacement therapy on well-being, bone mineral density and lipids in elderly men] Pol Arch Med Wewn 1998;100:212–221.
145. Jockenhövel F, Bullmann C, Schubert M, et al. Influence of various modes of androgen substitution on serum lipids and lipoproteins in hypogonadal men. Metabolism 1999;48:590–596.
146. Tan KC, Shiu SW, Kung AW. Alterations in hepatic lipase and lipoprotein subfractions with transdermal testosterone replacement therapy. Clin Endocrinol (Oxf) 1999;51:765–769.
147. Snyder PJ, Peachey H, Berlin JA, et al. Effect of transdermal testosterone treatment on serum lipid and apolipoprotein levels in men more than 65 years of age. Am J Med 2001;111:255–260.
148. Dobs AS, Bachorik PS, Arver S, et al. Interrelationships among lipoprotein levels, sex hormones, anthropometric parameters, and age in hypogonadal men treated for 1 year with a permeation-enhanced testosterone transdermal system. J Clin Endocrinol Metab 2001;86:1026–1033.
149. Ly LP, Jimenez M, Zhuang TN, et al. A double-blind, placebo-controlled, randomized clinical trial of transdermal dihydrotestosterone gel on muscular strength, mobility, and quality of life in older men with partial androgen deficiency. J Clin Endocrinol Metab 2001;86:4078–4088.
150. Thompson PD, Cullinane EM, Sady SP, et al. Contrasting effects of testosterone and stanozolol on serum lipoprotein levels JAMA 1989;261:1165–1168.
151. Friedl DKE, Hannan CJ, Jones RE, et al. High density lipoprotein cholesterol is not decreased if an aromatizable androgen is administered. Metabolism 1990;39:69–77.

152. Zmuda JM, Fahrenbach MC, Younkin BT. The effect of testosterone aromatization on high density lipoprotein cholesterol levels and post-heparin lipolytic activity. Metabolism 1993;39:69–77.

153. Bagatell CJ, Heiman JR, Matsumoto AM, et al. Metabolic and behavioural effects of high dose exogenous testosterone in healthy men. J Clin Endocrin Metab 1994;79:561–567.

155. Anderson RA, Wallace EM, Wu FCW. Effects of testosterone enanthate on serum lipoproteins in man. Contraception 1995;52:115–119.

154. Meriggiola MC, Bremner WJ, Paulsen CA. Testosterone enanthate at a dose of 200 mg/week decreases HDL-cholesterol levels in healthy men. Int J Androl 1995;18:237–242.

156. Wu FCW, Farley TMM, Peregoudov A, Waites GMH and World Health Organisation Task Force on Methods for the Regulation of Male Fertility Effects of exogenous testosterone in normal men: Experience from a multicentre contraceptive efficacy study using testosterone enanthate. Fertil Steril 1996;65:626–636.

157. Marcovina SM, Lippi G, Bagatell CJ, Bremner WJ. Testosterone-induced suppression of lipoprotein(a) in normal men: relation to basal lipoprotein(a) level. Atherosclerosis 1996;122: 89–95.

158. Grinspoon S, Corcoran C, Parlman K, et al. Effects of testosterone and progressive resistance training in eugonadal men with AIDS wasting. A randomized, controlled trial. Ann Intern Med 2000;133:348–355.

159. Bhasin S, Woodhouse L, Casaburi R, et al. Testosterone dose-response relationships in healthy young men. Am J Physiol Endocrinol Metab 2001;281:E1172–E1181.

160. Uyanik BS, Ari Z, Gumus B, et al. Beneficial effects of testosterone undecanoate on the lipoprotein profiles in healthy elderly men. A placebo controlled study. Jpn Heart J 1997;38:73–82.

161. Büchter D, von Eckardstein S, von Eckardstein A, et al. Clinical trial of a non-injectable male contraceptive: transdermal testosterone and oral levonorgestrel. J Clin Endocrinol Metab 1999;84:1244–1249.

162. Watts NB, Notelovitz M, Timmons MC, et al. Comparison of oral estrogens and estrogens plus androgen on bone mineral density, menopausal symptoms, and lipid-lipoprotein profiles in surgical menopause. Obstet Gynecol 1995;85:529–537.

163. Goh HH, Loke DF, Ratnam SS. The impact of long-term testosterone replacement therapy on lipid and lipoprotein profiles in women. Maturitas 1995;21:65–70.

164. Buckler HM, McElhone K, Durrington PN, et al. The effects of low-dose testosterone treatment on lipid metabolism, clotting factors and ultrasonographic ovarian morphology in women. Clin Endocrinol 1998;49:173–178.

165. Goldberg RB, Rabin D, Alexander AN, et al. Suppression of plasma testosterone leads to increase in serum total and high density lipoprotein cholesterol and apoproteins A-I and B. J Clin Endocrinol Metab 1985;60:203–207.

166. Bagatell CJ, Knopp RH, Vale WW, et al. Physiologic testosterone levels in normal men suppress high-density lipoprotein cholesterol levels. Ann Intern Med 1992;116:967–973.

167. Behre HM, Böckers A, Schlingheider A, Nieschlag E. Sustained suppression of serum LH, FSH, and testosterone and increase of high-density lipoprotein cholesterol by daily injections of the GnRH antagonist cetrorelix over 8 days in normal men. Clin Endocrinol (Oxf) 1994;40:241–248.

168. von Eckardstein A, Kliesch S, Nieschlag E, et al. Suppression of endogenous testosterone in young men increases serum levels of HDL-subclass LpA-I and lipoprotein(a). Clin Endocrinol Metab 1997;82:3367–3372.

169. Eri LM, Urdal P. Effects of the nonsteroidal androgen casodex on lipoproteins, fibrinogen and plasminogen activator inhibitor in patients with benign prostatic hyperplasia. Eur J Urol 1995;27:274–279.

170. Eri LM, Urdal P, Bechensteen AG. Effects of the luteinizing hormone-releasing hormone agonist leuprolide on lipoproteins, fibrinogen and plasminogen activator inhibitor in patients with benign prostatic hyperplasia. J Urol 1995;154:100–104.

171. Moorjani S, Dupont A, Labrie F, et al. Changes in plasma lipoproteins during various androgen suppression therapies in men with prostatic carcinoma: effects of orchiectomy, estrogen, and combination treatment with luteinizing hormone-releasing hormone agonist and flutamide. J Clin Endocrinol Metab 1988;66:314–322.

172. Denti L, Pasolini G, Cortellini P, et al. Changes in HDL-cholesterol and lipoprotein Lp(a) after 6-month treatment with finasteride in males affected by benign prostatic hyperplasia (BPH). Atherosclerosis 2000;152:159–166.

173. Bagatell CJ, Knopp RH, Bremner WJ. Physiological levels of estradiol stimulate plasma high density lipoprotein 2 cholesterol levels in normal men. J Clin Endocrinol Metab 1994;78:855–861.
174. Snyder PJ Peachey H, Berlin JA, et al. Effects of testosterone replacement in hypogonadal men. J Clin Endocrinol Metab 2000;85:2670–2677.
175. Whitsel EA, Boyko EJ, Matsumoto AM, et al. Intramuscular testosterone esters and plasma lipids in hypogonadal men: a meta-analysis. Am J Med 2001;111:261–269.
176. Tenover JS. Experience with testosterone replacement in the elderly. Mayo Clin Proc 2000;75(Suppl):S77–S82.
177. von Eckardstein, A, Nofer, JR, Assmann, G. HDL and coronary heart disease: Role of cholesterol efflux and reverse cholesterol transport. Arterioscler Thromb Vasc Biol 2001;20:13–27.
178. von Eckardstein A, Assmann G. Prevention of coronary heart disease by raising of HDL cholesterol? Curr Opin Lipidol 2000;11:627–637.
179. Santamarina-Fojo S, Haudenschild C. Role of hepatic and lipoprotein lipase in lipoprotein metabolism and atherosclerosis: studies in transgenic and knockout animal models and somatic gene transfer. Int J Tissue React 2000;22:39–47.
180. Glueck CJ, Gartside P, Fallat RW, Mendoza S. Effect of sex hormones on protamine inactivated and resistant postheparin plasma lipase. Metabolism 1976;25:625–630.
181. Krieger M. Charting the fate of the "good cholesterol": identification and characterization of the high-density lipoprotein receptor SR-BI. Annu Rev Biochem 1999;68:523–558.
182. von Eckardstein A, Schulte H, Cullen P, Assmann G. Lipoprotein(a) further increases the risk of coronary events in men with high global cardiovascular risk. J Am Coll Cardiol 2001;37: 2434–2439.
183. Berglund L, Carlström K, Stege R, et al. Hormonal regulation of serum lipoprotein(a) levels: effects of parenteral administration of estrogen or testosterone in males. J Clin Endocrinol Metab 1996;81:2633–2637.
184. Zmuda JM, Thompson PD, Dickenson R, Bausserman LL. Testosterone decreases lipoprotein(a) in men. Am J Cardiol 1996;77:1244–1247.
185. Arrer E, Jungwirth A, Mack D, Frick J, Patsch W. Treatment of prostate cancer with gonadotropin releasing hormone analogue: effect on lipoprotein(a). J Clin Endocrinol Metab 1996;81:2508–2511.
186. Anderson RA, Ludlam CA, Wu FCW. Haemostatic effects of supraphysiological levels of testosterone in normal men. Thromb Haemost 1995;74:693–697.
187. Verheijen JH, Rijken DC, Chang GT, Preston FE, Kluft C. Modulation of rapid plasminogen activator inhibitor in plasma by stanozolol. Thromb Haemost 1984;51:396–397.
188. Bjarnasson NH, Bjarnason K, Haarbo J, et al. Tibolone: Influence on markers of cardiovascular disease J Clin Endocrinol Metab 1997;82:1752–1756.
189. Crook D. Tibolone and the risk of arterial disease. J Br Menopause Soc 1999;S1:30–33.
190. Winkler UH. Effects of androgens on haemostasis Maturitas 1996;24:147–155.
191. Pilo R, Aharony D, Raz A. Testosterone potentiation of ionophere and ADP induced platelet aggregation: relationship to arachidonic acid metabolism. Thromb Haemost 1981;46:538–542.
192. De Caterina R. Endothelial dysfunctions: common denominators in vascular disease. Curr Opin Lipidol 2000;11:9–23.
193. Fuster V. Mechanisms lead to myocardial infarction: insights from studies in vascular biology. Circulation 1994;90:2126–2146.
194. Libby P. Molecular bases of the acute coronary syndromes. Circulation 1995;91:2844–2850.
195. McCredie RJ, McCrohon JA, Turner L, et al. Vascular reactivity is impaired in genetic females taking high-dose androgens. J Am Coll Cardiol 1998;32:1331–1335.
196. Herman SM, Robinson JTC, McCredie RJ, et al. Androgen deprivation is associated with enhanced endothelium-dependent dilatation in adult men. Arterioscler Thromb Vasc Biol 1997;17:2004–2009.
197. McCrohon JA, Walters WAW, Robinson JC, et al. Arterial reactivity is enhanced in genetic males taking high dose estrogens. J Am Coll Cardiol 1997;29:1432–1436.
198. New G, Timmins KL, Duffy SJ, et al. Long-term estrogen therapy improves vascular function in male to female transsexuals. J Am Coll Cardiol 1997;29:1437–1444.
199. Ong PJ, Patrizi G, Chong WC, et al. Testosterone enhances flow-mediated brachial artery reactivity in men with coronary artery disease. Am J Cardiol 2000;85:269–272.
200. Worboys S, Kotsopoulos, Teede H, et al. Evidence that parenteral testosterone therapy may improve endothelium-dependent and independent vasodilatation in postmenopausal women already receiving estrogen. J Clin Endocrinol Metab 2001;88:158–161.

201. Chou TM, Sudhir K, Hutchison SJ, et al. Testosterone induces dilatation of canine coronary conductance and resistance arteries in vivo. Circulation 1996;94:2614–2619.
202. Costarella CE, Stallone JN, Rutecki GW, Whittier FC. Testosterone causes direct relaxation of rat thoracic aorta. J Pharmacol Experiment Therap 1996;277:34–39.
203. Farhat MY, Wolfe R, Vargas R, et al. Effect of testosterone treatment on vasoconstrictor response of left anterior descend coronary artery in male and female pigs. J Cardiovasc Pharmacol 1995;25: 495–500.
204. Yue P, Chatterjee K, Beale C, et al. Testosterone relaxes rabbit coronary arteries and aorta. Circulation 1995;91:1154–1160.
205. Teoh H, Quan A, Leung SW, Man RY. Differential effects of 17beta-estradiol and testosterone on the contractile responses of porcine coronary arteries. Br J Pharmacol 2000;129:1301–1308.
206. Quan A, Teoh H, Man RY. Acute exposure to a low level of testosterone impairs relaxation in porcine coronary arteries. Clin Exp Pharmacol Physiol 1999;26:830–832.
207. Ceballos G, Figueroa L, Rubio I, et al. Acute and nongenomic effects of testosterone on isolated and perfused rat heart. J Cardiovasc Pharmacol 1999;33:691–697.
208. Hutchison SJ, Sudhir K, Chou TM, et al. Testosterone worsens endothelial dysfunction associated with hypercholesterolemia and environmental tobacco smoke exposure in male rabbit aorta. J Am Coll Cardiol 1997;29:800–807.
209. Geary GG, Krause DN, Duckles SP. Gonadal hormones affect diameter of male rat cerebral arteries through endothelium-dependent mechanisms. Am J Physiol Heart Circ Physiol 2000;279: H610–H618.
210. Hishikawa K, Nakaki T, Marumo T, et al. Up regulation of nitric oxide synthase by estradiol in human aortic endothelial cells. FEBS Lett 1995;360:291–295.
211. Murphy JG, Khalil RA. Decreased [Ca(2+)](i) during inhibition of coronary smooth muscle contraction by 17beta-estradiol, progesterone, and testosterone. J Pharmacol Exp Ther 1999;291:44–45.
212. Masuda A, Mathur A, Halushka PV. Testosterone increases thromboxane A2 receptors in cultured rat smooth muscle cells. Circ Res 1995;69:638–643.
213. Glass CK, Witztum JL. Atherosclerosis. the road ahead. Cell 2001;104:503–516.
214. de Winther MP, van Dijk KW, Havekes LM, Hofker MH. Macrophage scavenger receptor class A: A multifunctional receptor in atherosclerosis. Arterioscler Thromb Vasc Biol 2000;20:290–297.
215. Jessup W, Kritharides L. Metabolism of oxidized LDL by macrophages. Curr Opin Lipidol 2000;11:473–481.
216. Tabas I. Cholesterol and phospholipid metabolism in macrophages.Biochim Biophys Acta 2000;1529:164–174.
217. Zhu XD, Bonet B, Knopp RH. 17β-estradiol, progesterone, and testosterone inversely modulate low density lipoprotein oxidation and cytotoxicity in cultured placental trophoblast and macrophages. Am J Obstet Gynecol 1997;177:196–209.
218. McCrohon JA, Death AK, Nakhla S, et al. Androgen receptor expression is greater in macrophages from male than from female donors. A sex difference with implications for atherogenesis. Circulation 2000;101(3):224–226.
219. Ajayi AA, Mathur R, Halushka PV. Testosterone increases human platelet thromboxane A2 receptor density and aggregation responses. Circulation 1995;91:2742–2747.
220. Matsuda K, Mathur RS, Duzic E, Halushka PV. Androgen regulation of thromboxane A2/prostaglandin H2 receptor expression in human erythroleukemia cells. Am J Physiol 1993;265:E928–E934.
221. Matsuda K, Ruff A, Morinelli TA, et al. Testosterone increases thromboxane A2 receptor density and responsiveness in rat aortas and platelets. Am J Physiol 1994;267:H887–H893.
222. Vermeulen A. Dehydroepiandrosterone sulfate and ageing. Ann NY Acad Sci 1995;774:121–127.
223. Khaw KT. Dehydroepiandrosterone, dehydroepiandrosterone sulphate and cardiovascular disease. J Endocrinol 1996;150(Suppl):S149–S153.
224. Labrie F, Belanger A, Luu-The V, et al. DHEA and the intracrine formation of androgens and estrogens in peripheral target tissues: its role during aging. Steroids 1998;63:322–328.
225. Slowinska-Srzednicka J, Zgliczynski S, Ciswicka-Sznajderman M, et al. Decreased plasma dehydroepiandrosterone sulfate and dihydrotestosterone concentrations in young men after myocardial infarction. Atherosclerosis 1989;79:197–203.
226. Mitchell LE, Sprecher DL, Borecki IB, et al. Evidence for an association between dehydroepiandrosterone sulfate and non-fatal, premature myocardial infarction in males. Circulation 1994;89:89–93.

227. Feldman HA, Johannes CB, McKinlay JB, Longcope C. Low dehydroepiandrosterone sulfate and heart disease in middle-aged men: cross-sectional results from the Massachusetts Male Aging Study. Ann Epidemiol 1998;8:217–228.

228. Barrett-Connor E, Khaw KT, Yen SSC. A prospective study of dehydroepiandrosterone sulfate, mortality, and cardiovascular disease. N Engl J Med 1986;315:1519–1524.

229. Herrington DM, Gordon GB, Achuff SC, et al. Plasma dehydroepiandrosterone and dehydro-epiandrosterone sulfate in patients undergoing diagnostic coronary angiography. J Am Coll Cardiol 1990;16:862–870.

230. LaCroix AZ, Yano K, Reed DM. Dehydroepiandrosterone sulfate, incidence of myocardial infarction, and extent of atherosclerosis in men. Circulation 1992;86:1529–1535.

231. Ishihara F, Hiramatsu K, Shigematsu S, et al. Role of adrenal androgens in the development of arteriosclerosis as judged by pulse wave velocity and calcification of the aorta. Cardiology 1992;80:332–338.

232. Herrington DM. Dehydroepiandrosterone and coronary atherosclerosis. Ann NY Acad Sci 1995;774:271–280.

233. Phillips GB, Pinkernell BH, Jing TY. The association of hypotestosteronemia with coronary artery disease in men. Arterisclerosis Thromb 1994;14:701–706.

234. Hauner H, Stangl K, Burger K, et al. Sex hormone concentration in men with angiographically assessed coronary artery disease—relationship to obesity and body fat distribution. Klin Wochenschr 1991;69:664–668.

235. Schuler-Lüttmann S, Mönnig G, Enbergs A, et al. Insulin-like growth factor binding protein-3 is associated with the presence and extent of coronary arteriosclerosis. Arteriosclerosis Thromb Vasc Biol 2000;20:e10–e15.

236. Newcomer LM, Manson JE, Barbieri RL, et al. Dehydroepiandrosterone sulfate and the risk of myocardial infarction in US male physicians: a prospective study. Am J Epidemiol 1994;140:870–875.

237. Barrett-Connor E, Goodman-Gruen D. The epidemiology of DHEAS and cardiovascular disease. Ann N Y Acad Sci 1995;774:259–270.

238. Berr C, Lafon S, Debuire B, et al. Relationships of dehydroepiandrosterone sulfate in the elderly with functional, psychological and mental status and short-term mortality: a French community-based study. Proc Natl Acad Sci USA 1996;93:13,410–13,415.

239. Jansson JH, Nilsson TK, Johnson O. von Willebrand factor, tissue plasminogen activator, and dehydroepiandrosterone sulphate predict cardiovascular death in a 10 year follow up of survivors of acute myocardial infarction. Heart 1998;80:334–337.

240. Tilvis RS, Kahonen M, Harkonen M. Dehydroepiandrosterone sulfate, diseases and mortality in a general aged population. Aging (Milano) 1999;11:30–34.

241. Kiechl S, Willeit J, Bonora E, Schwarz S, Xu Q. No association between dehydroepiandrosterone sulfate and development of atherosclerosis in a prospective population study (Bruneck Study). Arteriosclerosis Thromb Vasc Biol 2000;20:1094–1100.

242. Trevedi DP, Khaw KT. Dehydroepiandrosterone sulfate and mortality in elderly men and women. J Clin Endocrinol Metab 2001;86:4171–4177.

243. Zumoff B, Troxler RG, O'Connor J, et al. Abnormal hormone levels in men with coronary artery disease. Arteriosclerosis 1982;2:58–67.

244. Moriyama Y, Yasue H, Yoshimura M, et al. The plasma levels of dehydroepiandrosterone sulfate are decreased in patients with chronic heart failure in proportion to the severity. J Clin Endocrinol Metab 2000;85:1834–1840.

245. Slowinska-Srzednicka J, Malczewska B, Srzednicki M, et al. Hyperinsulinaemia and decreased plasma levels of dehydroepiandrosterone sulfate in premenopausal women with coronary heart disease. J Intern Med 1995;237:465–472.

246. Barrett-Connor EL, Goodman-Gruen D. Prospective study of endogenous sex hormones and fatal cardiovascular disease in postmenipausal women. Br Med J 1995;311:1193–1196.

247. Barrett-Connor EL, Khaw KT. Absence of an inverse relation of dehydroepiandrosteroneysulfate with cardiovascular mortality in postmenopausal women. N Engl J Med 1987;317:711.

248. Gordon GB, Bush DE, Weisman HF. Reduction of atherosclerosis by administration of dehydro-epiandrosterone: a study in the hypercholesterolemic New Zealand white rabbit with aortic intimal injury. J Clin Invest 1988;82:58–64.

249. Arad Y, Badimon JJ, Badimon L, et al. Dehydroepiandrosterone feeding prevents aortic fatty streak formation and cholesterol accumulation in cholesterol-fed rabbits. Arteriosclerosis 1989;9:159–165.

250. Eich DM, Nestler JE, Johnson DE, et al. Inhibition of accelerated coronary atherosclerosis with dehydroepinadrosterone in the heterotopic rabbit model of cardiac transplantation. Circulation 1993;87:261–265.

251. Hayashi T, Esaki T, Muto E, et al. Dehydroepiandrosterone retards atherosclerosis formation through its conversion to estrogen: the possible role of nitric oxide. Arterioscler Thromb Vasc Biol 2000;20:782–792.

252. Morishima A, Grumbach MM, Simpson ER, et al. Aromatase deficiency in male and female siblings caused by a novel mutation and the physiological role of estrogens. J Clin Endocrinol Metab 1995;80:3689–3698.

253. Carani C, Qin K, Simoni M, et al. Effect of testosterone and oestradiol in a man with aromatase deficiency. New Eng J Med 1997;337:91–95.

254. Smith EP, Boyd J, Frank GR, et al. Estrogen resistance caused by a mutation in the estrogen-receptor gene in a man. N Engl J Med 1994;331:1056–1061.

255. Sudhir K, Chou TM, Chatterjee K, et al. Premature coronary artery disease associated with a disruptive mutation in the estrogen receptor gene in a man. Circulation 1997;96:3774–3777.

256. Sudhir K, Chou TM, Messina LM, et al. Endothelial dysfunction in a man with disruptive mutation in oestrogen-receptor gene. Lancet 1997;349:1146–1147.

257. Ohlsson C, Hellberg N, Parini P, et al. Obesity and disturbed lipoprotein profile in estrogen receptor-alpha-deficient male mice. Biochem Biophys Res Commun 2000;30:640–645.

258. Heine PA, Taylor JA, Iwamoto GA, et al. Increased adipose tissue in male and female estrogen receptor-alpha knockout mice. Proc Natl Acad Sci USA 2000;97:12729–12734.

259. Rubanyi GM, Frey AD, Kauser K, et al. Vascular estrogen receptors and endothelium-derived nitric oxide production in the mouse aorta. J Clin Invest 1997;99:2429–2437.

11 Androgens and Bone

Anne M. Kenny, MD and Lawrence G. Raisz, MD

CONTENTS

INTRODUCTION
OVERVIEW OF SKELETAL PHYSIOLOGY
ROLE OF SEX STEROIDS IN THE SKELETON
DIRECT EFFECTS OF ANDROGENS ON BONE CELLS
METABOLISM OF ANDROGEN IN BONE
ANDROGEN EFFECTS ON BONE IN VIVO: STUDIES IN ANIMAL MODELS
ROLE OF ANDROGENS IN THE SKELETON: HUMAN STUDIES
ROLE OF ANDROGENS IN THE PATHOGENESIS OF OSTEOPOROSIS
ANDROGEN THERAPY IN MEN
ANDROGEN THERAPY IN WOMEN
CONCLUSION
ACKNOWLEDGMENTS
REFERENCES

INTRODUCTION

Although it is clear that androgens play a critical role in the development and maintenance of the skeleton, there is great uncertainty about the mechanisms of their effects. Androgens can act directly on bone cells, but they can also act indirectly by altering mechanical forces through their effects on muscle or by conversion to estrogen through the action of aromatase. In this chapter, we provide a brief review of bone modeling and remodeling and its regulation as well as the mechanisms of bone loss in osteoporosis. We review the complex, conflicting data on the mechanism of direct androgen action on bone based largely in studies on cell and tissue cultures and animal models. Clinical studies on the role of sex hormones in skeletal development and age-related bone loss are summarized. We conclude by outlining some critical studies that might define the role of androgens in skeletal physiology and the pathogenesis and treatment of osteoporosis.

OVERVIEW OF SKELETAL PHYSIOLOGY

The skeleton is a metabolically active organ, constantly undergoing remodeling under the dual control of metabolic and structural needs. The formation of the skeleton begins

From: *Contemporary Endocrinology: Androgens in Health and Disease*
Edited by: C. Bagatell and W. J. Bremner © Humana Press Inc., Totowa, NJ

with a cartilage framework that then is converted to bone either through endochondral ossification in the long bones and vertebra or membranous bone formation adjacent to the cartilage in flat bones. During childhood, the skeleton grows by periosteal apposition and endosteal resorption, thus enlarging the marrow cavities *(1)*. This change in the form of bone is termed "modeling." At puberty, there is a rapid increase in bone mass *(2)*. There is both periosteal and endosteal apposition, particularly in males during puberty. After epiphyseal closure there is relatively little modeling of the skeleton. However, some increase in periosteal diameter can occur with aging, perhaps as a compensation for endosteal bone loss and weakening of skeletal structures *(3)*.

The continuous removal and replacement of packets of bone in the skeleton throughout life is termed "remodeling" *(4)*. The bone structural units (BSU) in remodeling are irregular platelike structures on the trabecular surfaces or cylindrical *osteons* in cortical bone. The remodeling cycle begins with *activation*. The activation process involves the effects of hormones and local factors on the previously inactive lining cells covering the bone surface and as well as stromal cells of the osteoblast lineage in the marrow or periosteum. These cells have a ligand for receptor activator of nuclear factor-$\kappa\beta$ (RANKL), which binds to a receptor on hematopoietic cells (RANK). This interaction results in replication, differentiation, and fusion of osteoclast precursors to form large multinucleated bone-resorbing cell *(5)*. There is a decoy receptor, osteoprotegerin (OPG), which can block this interaction and is an important local regulator *(6)*. In humans, the *resorption* phase lasts 2–3 wk and is followed by a *reversal* phase during which mononuclear cells are present on the bone surface. Osteoblast precursors then migrate to the bone surface and lay down successive layers of new bone. This *formation* phase replaces the removed tissue over a period of several months. Thus, the entire remodeling cycle may last 3–6 mo in humans *(7)*.

The regulation of bone remodeling is complex. Remodeling may be driven in part by the need to repair microdamage that results from repeated impact on the skeleton. Cortical and trabecular remodeling are clearly influenced by mechanical forces. Impact loading of the skeleton can stimulate new bone formation, and this process can also result in realignment of structure or modeling *(8)*.

Bone remodeling is also under the control of local factors and systemic hormones. Parathyroid hormone (PTH) stimulates bone remodeling, but depending on the dose and whether the increases in PTH are continuous or intermittent, there may be maintenance, loss, or gain of skeletal mass with PTH *(9,10)*. Vitamin D is critical for the supply of calcium and phosphorous for bone mineralization, but it can also stimulate bone resorption. Calcitonin is an inhibitor of bone resorption that appears to have relatively little role in regulation of bone remodeling in adult humans. The local regulators include cytokines, lipid mediators such as prostaglandins, and growth factors *(11–13)*. These factors may mediate the effects of systemic hormones and mechanical forces and are probably also responsible for the interactions between marrow and bone *(14)*. Physiological and pathological expansion of the marrow occurs at the expense of skeletal tissue, and marrow cells can produce factors that increase bone resorption.

Bone remodeling is normally tightly coupled; that is, the amount of bone removed by resorption is replaced by a similar amount of new bone through formation. However, during the pubertal growth spurt, bone mass is gained, partly because the new BSUs are larger and partly because new bone is added through modeling *(15)*. Menopausal and age-related bone loss are associated with an increase in both resorption and formation, but the bone formation response is insufficient *(16–18)*. Bone mass decreases because of complete loss of trabecular elements and endosteal bone by resorption and because the BSUs on trabecular surfaces are smaller because of impaired formation.

ROLE OF SEX STEROIDS IN THE SKELETON

Androgens and estrogens are critical in the development of the skeleton and in maintaining bone mass and strength throughout life *(19,20)*. The role of androgens in this process is complex *(19)*. Testosterone may act on androgen receptors in the skeleton directly or after conversion to dihydrotestosterone *(20,21)*. Androgens are the precursors for estrogens. Precursors such as androstenedione and dehydroepiandrosterone (DHEA) are presumed to act largely as sources of active androgen or estrogen but may also have direct effects *(22,23)*. There is some uncertainty about the bioavailability of circulating androgen to the skeleton. Both free androgen and androgen bound to albumin may be bioavailable, but it is also possible that testosterone bound to sex hormone-binding globulin (SHBG) can act on bone cells via SHBG receptors *(24–26)*. Because of these complexities, we can only describe the effects of sex steroids on bone in general terms. However, data from humans and experimental animals with androgen insensitivity, aromatase deficiency, or inactivating mutations of estrogen receptor-α (ERα) do help us identify the separate roles for androgen and estrogen.

DIRECT EFFECTS OF ANDROGENS ON BONE CELLS

Androgen receptors have been identified on bones cells of both the osteoblastic and osteoclastic lineages as well as chondrocytes *(27–29)*. The first description of androgen receptors in human osteoblasts *(30)* indicated that they were almost as abundant as estrogen receptors in both males and females. These receptors show similar binding affinity for testosterone and dihydrotestosterone (DHT) *(31)*. Androgen receptor levels can be upregulated by DHT *(32)*. There may also be a separate receptor for DHEA *(33)*, based on cell responses, but this has not been isolated. Androgens may also act on the cell membrane through a G-protein-coupled receptor, which can affect calcium entry and phospholipid turnover *(34,35)*. Androgen receptors have also been identified in isolated murine osteoclasts *(36)*.

Androgens have effects on proliferation, differentiation and apoptosis of osteoblastic cells *(37–40)*. However, widely different results have been reported, which probably depend on the types of cell studied as well as their stage of differentiation. For example, both positive and negative effects of androgens on proliferation have been reported *(41,42)*. Increased expression of transforming growth factor-β (TGF-β) appears to be a consistent response in many different cell culture systems *(33)*. Increase in expression of insulin-like growth factor (IGF-1) and its binding proteins has also been described *(43)*. These and other related effects are presumably responsible for the increase in osteoblast differentiation seen in androgen-treated cell cultures. Cell survival may also be prolonged by androgens, and this may be a nongenomic effect to prevent apoptosis *(13,44)*.

Androgens may alter the response of bone cells to other agonists. For example, PTH stimulation of cAMP *(45)* and prostaglandin production in response to interleukin-1 (IL-1) *(46)* and production of IL-6 *(47)* may be inhibited. These effects could result in inhibition of bone resorption by androgens.

METABOLISM OF ANDROGEN IN BONE

Bone cells have been shown to contain a number of enzymes that can metabolize androgens. Because these enzymes that can interconvert androgens and estrogens in bone cells, it is difficult to assess the specific roles of any single hormone *(48)*. Testosterone can be converted to DHT by 5α-reductase or to estradiol by aromatase. Bone cells can also form testosterone from androstenedione *(49,50)*. A genetic defect in aromatase results in marked skeletal abnormalities because of estrogen deficiency *(51,52)*, but the specific role of aromatase in bone has not been defined. It seems likely that 5α-reductase is of less importance for the maintenance of the skeleton, because deficiency of this enzyme does not result in any gross skeletal abnormalities *(53)*.

ANDROGEN EFFECTS ON BONE IN VIVO: STUDIES IN ANIMAL MODELS

The role of androgens in bone has been examined in rodent models, including ovariectomized and orchidectomized rats and mice, animals treated with inhibitors of aromatase or antiandrogens, and mice with defects in the androgen receptor or the aromatase enzyme. There are also limited studies in primates *(54,55)*. Orchidectomy in rats produces bone loss, associated with an increase in turnover similar to the effect of oophorectomy in females *(56,57)*. However, these changes could be the result of the loss of estrogen derived from testosterone rather than direct loss of testosterone. In oophorectomized rats, a high concentration of DHT appeared to decrease bone turnover *(58)*. Because DHT cannot be converted to estrogen, this indicates an androgen-receptor-mediated effect. Moreover, animals treated with either an antiestrogen or antiandrogen lose less bone than oophorectomized animals, whereas the combination of antiestrogen and antiandrogen treatment, or antihormonal treatment and oophorectomy results in equivalent bone loss but not as great an increase in bone turnover *(59)*. Inhibition of aromatase *(60)* or knockout of the enzyme *(61)* produces some bone loss in mice. However, the picture in male aromatase-deficient mice is somewhat different from that of orchidectomy, with a decrease in bone turnover and less bone loss *(62)*.

ROLE OF ANDROGENS IN THE SKELETON: HUMAN STUDIES

Both androgens and estrogens are critical for the growth and consolidation of the skeleton that occurs at puberty. There are sex differences; males show greater periosteal and endosteal apposition by modeling during puberty, supporting a specific role of androgen in this process. Studies of androgen insensitivity and estrogen deficiency, resulting from either defects in aromatase or loss of the estrogen receptor, have shed further light on the relative roles of these hormones in skeletal development *(51,52,63,64)*. One male with an inactivating mutation in ERα and two males with aromatase deficiency have been described as having a quite similar phenotype, with failure of epiphyseal closure, tall stature, high bone turnover, and decreased bone mineral density (BMD). With estrogen replacement, the patients with aromatase deficiency showed epiphyseal closure, decreased bone turnover, and, in one case, substantial increase in bone mass. These studies indicate that ERα is a critical receptor for regulation of bone turnover, but that androgen receptors may be sufficient to stimulate accelerated linear growth of the skeleton at puberty. Findings in androgen-insensitivity syndrome (AIS or testicular feminization) are somewhat contradictory. Patients with AIS are tall, phenotypic females with a male genotype and undescended testes. They are treated by castration and estrogen replacement. As adults, they do show a decrease in BMD *(65,66)*. When this is compared with normative *male* standards, there is substantial reduction with a Z-score of –1.8. Some of the difference in AIS patients may be the result of poor compliance with estrogen, but even in the estrogen-compliant group, the BMD is decreased *(67)*.

ROLE OF ANDROGENS IN THE PATHOGENESIS OF OSTEOPOROSIS

It is well established that men with severe hypogonadism lose bone *(68,69)*. This bone loss is associated with increased bone turnover and could result not only from the effects of decreased androgen but from the loss of estrogen, because the majority of endogenous estrogen in men is derived from gonadal testosterone. Osteopenia is also seen in men with delayed puberty, although it is less marked *(70–72)*. Hypogonadism acquired later in life can result in substantial bone loss in patients who have had surgical castration or been treated with gonadotrophin-releasing hormone (GnRH) analogs for prostate cancer *(73)*. These individuals may show increased skeletal sensitivity to PTH *(74)*.

The role of testosterone in the age-related decrease in bone density in men is not clear *(75–77)*. Bioavailable testosterone decreases with age, although total testosterone may show little or no decrease because SHBG increases with age *(24,78)*. Patients with hip fractures generally have lower testosterone levels than age-matched controls *(79,80)*. Studies relating testosterone levels to bone mass or rates of bone loss have yielded conflicting results *(81–85)*. One confounder is that SHBG is inversely related to body mass index so that heavier individuals are likely to have lower total testosterone, and these individuals are also likely to have higher BMDs. This may lead to a positive association between testosterone levels and BMD *(83)*. However, an inverse relationship between bioavailable testosterone and femoral neck BMD has been seen in the subpopulation of elderly men with low bioavailable testosterone levels *(84)*. Although there was no correlation with estradiol levels and BMD in these studies, this does not rule out a role for the estrogen produced from testosterone. Circulating estradiol levels may not fully reflect this production, because, as noted earlier, there is aromatase activity in bone and, therefore, local production of estrogen may be more important circulating levels *(86)*.

Studies of men presenting clinically with osteoporosis have shown that the estradiol level is more likely to be decreased than the testosterone level compared to non-osteoporotic age-matched controls *(87,88)*. In older men, increased vertebral fracture incidence, based on lateral spine radiographs, is associated with lower levels of estradiol but not lower levels total testosterone *(89)*. Morphometric studies of men with osteoporosis have also suggested that the pattern may be somewhat different from that seen in women. There is a greater component of decreased bone formation and less loss of trabeculae in the male patients *(17,90,91)*.

Androgen deficiency may also play a role in the pathogenesis of osteoporosis in women. Women who have had a hysterectomy and oophorectomy have relative androgen deficiency because the ovary is a major source of testosterone in postmenopausal women *(92)*. In addition, there is an age-related decline in adrenal androgens in women that is greater than that observed in men *(93)*.

The level of the major adrenal androgen DHEA was positively associated with BMD in women, but not in men *(94)*. Adrenal androgen may also play a role in skeletal development. Prepubertal girls with adrenal hyperplasia have increased bone density relative to bone age when compared either to normals or patients with central precocious puberty *(95)*. Despite the loss of androgen from oophorectomy, there appears to be no difference in bone density in estrogen-treated women whether or not their ovaries are present *(96)*. This may reflect the fact that exogenous estrogen also lowers androgen levels *(97)*.

There is evidence that androgens play a role in bone loss in women. In a study of androgen and estrogen dynamics, decreased testosterone and androstenedione production was found in women with vertebral crush fractures compared to age-matched controls, whereas there was no difference in estradiol or estrone production *(98)*. Moreover, height loss was associated with low testosterone levels in postmenopausal women *(99)*.

ANDROGEN THERAPY IN MEN

In men with severe testosterone deficiency hormone-replacement therapy can increase both bone density and lean body mass *(100–103)*. However, many patients continued to show low bone density despite apparently adequate replacement. This may have been a result of failure to achieve optimal peak bone mass, but an alternative might be inadequate conversion of testosterone to estrogen. In a recent short-term study, treatment of older men with an aromatase inhibitor resulted in a 40% decrease in estrogen and a significant increase in markers of bone resorption, as well as a decrease in markers of bone formation *(104)*. This occurred despite a 70% increase in testosterone, presumably as a result of a change in hypothalamic pituitary feedback. Thus it is possible that some estrogen should be added to testosterone in the treatment of hypogonadal men, but this hypothesis has not yet been tested.

The use of testosterone in older men who have normal or moderately reduced testosterone levels remains controversial *(105)*. In the past, androgen analogs such as nandrolone have been shown to increase bone density in this population. More recently, testosterone replacement in older men with relatively low but not severely hypogonadal levels was found to increase bone density in the spine *(106)* and the femur *(107)*. Testosterone therapy appeared to be relatively safe in these patients, with only small adverse changes in prostate-specific antigen, cholesterol profiles, or hematocrit. These studies were carried out in men who did not have symptomatic osteoporosis. In men with vertebral crush fractures, testosterone was shown to increase bone density, and this increase was associated with reductions in urinary deoxypyridinoline and *N*-telopeptide crosslinks. The treatment increased serum testosterone and estradiol and reduced SHBG *(108)*. Hence, the results could have been the result of increased bioavailable estradiol as well as testosterone. In short-term studies in men with low bioavailable testosterone, increasing bioavailable testosterone levels to normal range with testosterone replacement did not consistently alter biochemical markers *(109)*. Unfortunately, there are, as yet, no studies to indicate whether or not testosterone therapy can reduce the incidence of fractures in men with osteoporosis.

ANDROGEN THERAPY IN WOMEN

There are many clinical studies in which androgens have been administered to women with osteoporosis, largely as an adjunct to estrogen therapy *(110–112)*. These studies are difficult to interpret for a number of reasons. A wide variety of different compounds have been used, including compounds that have mixed androgen, estrogen, and progestin activity such as tibolone or norethindrone. An effective pure transdermal testosterone has only recently become available and used largely in women who have had an oophorectomy as replacement for effects on fatigue, lack of well-being, and diminished libido *(113)*. Interpretation of studies in which androgen is added to estrogen are confounded by the fact that estrogen increases and testosterone decreases SHBG. Thus, androgen treatment may simply increase bioavailability of estrogen. Studies showing that these combinations further decrease bone turnover, rather than increasing bone formation, support this possibility. Nevertheless, in short-term studies, adding methyltestosterone to estrogen appeared to have a separate and distinct effect because it reversed the reduction in markers of bone formation produced by estrogen alone *(111)*. The use of androgens in women is limited by side effects and safety concerns. These include increased hair growth, lowering of the voice, acne, and decreased high-density lipoprotein (HDL) cholesterol *(110)*.

Studies with androgen analogs such as stanozolol *(114)* and nandrolone *(115,116)* indicate that these compounds can increase bone mineral density, and histomorphometric studies suggest that they increase bone formation *(117)*. In most studies using combinations of estrogen and androgen, the combination therapy produces a greater increase in BMD than estrogen alone *(112,118–121)*. Here, again, there are no data on fracture prevention.

CONCLUSION

The data from cell and organ culture and animal studies clearly support a direct role for androgen in skeletal modeling and remodeling. There are both laboratory and clinical studies to indicate that the conversion of testosterone to estrogen is also critical in maintaining normal skeletal growth and turnover in men as well as women. However, the roles of androgen deficiency in the pathogenesis of osteoporosis and of androgen therapy and its treatment remain unresolved questions. It seems likely that testosterone, perhaps in relatively low doses, could benefit older men with low bioavailable testosterone levels. This could decrease fracture incidence not only by effects on bone but also by increasing muscle strength. With the current availability of long-acting injectable forms and transdermal patch preparations of testosterone, such studies are feasible. The use of supplemental androgen in women with osteoporosis is currently limited by side effects. This problem could be circumvented by the use of lower doses or the development of selective androgen-receptor modulators, parallel to the development of selective estrogen-receptor modulators, which have greater effects on the skeleton and lesser effects on classical androgenic targets. An important unresolved question is whether such androgen supplementation would be truly anabolic in this population or simply increase estrogen activity by its effects on SHBG or its conversion as a precursor. Only the former would represent a major therapeutic advance.

ACKNOWLEDGMENTS

This work has been supported by General Clinical Research Center (MO1-RR06192) and Claude Pepper OAIC (5P60-AG13631).

REFERENCES

1. Glastre C, Braillon P, Daid L, et al. Measurement of bone mineral density X-ray absorptiometry in normal children? Correlations with growth parameters. J Clin Endocrin Metab 1990;70:1330–1333.
2. Krabbe S, Christiansen C, Rodbro P, Transbol I. Effect of puberty on rates of bone growth and mineralization. Arch Dis Child 1979;54:950–953.
3. Mosekilde L. Sex differences in age-related loss of vertebral trabecular bone mass and structure—biomechanical consequences. Bone 1989;10:425–432.
4. Eriksen EF. Normal and pathological remodeling of human trabecular bone: three dimensional reconstruction of the remodeling sequences in normals and in metabolic bone disease. Endocr Rev 1986;7:379–408.
5. Yasuda H, Shima N, Nakagawa K, et al. Osteoclast differentiation factor is a ligand for osteoprotegerin/osteoclastogenesis-inhibitory factor and is identical to TRANCE/RANKL. Proc Natl Acad Sci USA 1998;95:3597–3602.
6. Kostenuik PJ, Shalhoub V. Osteoprotegerin: a physiologic and pharmacologic inhibitor of bone resorption. Curr Pharm Des 2001;7:613–635.
7. Parfitt AM. Osteonal and hemi-osteonal remodeling: thespatial and temporal framework for signal traffic in adult human bone. J Cell Biochem 1994;55:273–286.
8. Burger EH, Klein-Nulen J. Responses of bone cells to biomechanical forces in vitro. Adv Dent Res 1999;13:93–98.
9. Raisz L, Kream BE. Regulation of bone formation. Parts I and II. N Engl J Med 1983;309:29–35, 83–89.
10. Dempster DW, Cosman F, Parisien M, et al. Anabolic actions of parathyroid hormone on bone. Endocr Rev 1993;14:690–709.
11. Raisz LG. Local and systemic factors in the pathogenesis of osteoporosis. N Engl J Med 1988;318:818–28.
12. Raisz LG. Osteoporosis: current approaches and future prospects in diagnosis, pathogenesis, and management. J Bone Miner Metab 1999;17:79–89.
13. Manolagas SC. Birth and death of bone cells: basic regulatory mechanisms and implications for the pathogenesis and treatment of osteoporosis. Endocr Rev 2000;21:115–137.
14. Cheng MZ, Zaman G, Rawlison SC, et al. Enhancement by sex hormones of the osteoregulatory effects of mechanical loading and prostaglandins in explants of rat ulnae. J Bone Miner Res 1997;12:1424–1430.
15. Bonjour JP, Theintz G, Buchs B, et al. Critical years and stages of puberty for spinal and femoral bone mass accumulation durig adolescence. J Clin Endocrinol Metab 1991;73:555–563.
16. Parfitt AM, Matthews HE. Relationship between surface, volume, and thickness of iliac trabecular bone in aging and osteoporosis. J Clin Invest 1983;72:1396–1409.
17. Compston JE, Mellish RWE, Garrahan NJ. Age-related changes in iliac crest travecular bone loss in man. Bone Miner 1987;6:339–350.
18. Kim JG, Lee JY. Serum insulin-like growth factor binding protein profiles in postmenopausal women: their correlation with bone mineral density. Am J Obstet Gynecol 1996;174:1511–1517.
19. Vanderschuren D, Boonen S, Bouillon R. Action of androgens versus estrogens in male skeletal homeostasis. Bone 1998;23:391–394.
20. Compston JE. Sex steroids and bone. Physiol Rev 2001;81:419–447.
21. Davey RA, Hahn CN, May BK, Morris HA. Osteoblast gene expression in rat long bones: effects of ovariectomy and dihydrotestosterone on mRNA levels. Calcif Tissue Int 2000;67:75–79.
22. Baulieu EM, Thomas G, Legrain S, et al. Dehydroepiandrosterone (DHEA), DHEA sulfate, and aging: contribution of the DHEAge study to a sociobiomedical issue. Proc Natl Assoc Sci USA 2000;97:4279–4284.
23. Broeder CE, Quindry J, Brittingham K, et al. The Andro Project Physiological and hormonal influences of androstenedione supplementation in men 35 to 65 years old participating in a high-intensity resistance training program. Ann Int Med 2000;160:3093–3104.
24. Harman SM, Metter EJ, Tobin JD, et al. Longitudinal effects of aging on serum total and free testosterone levels in healthy men. Longitudinal Study of Aging. J Clin Endocrinol Metab 2001;86:724–731.
25. Nankin HR, Calkins JH. Decreased bioavailable testosterone in aging normal and impotent men. J Clin Endocrinol Metab 1986;63:1418–1420.

26. Rosner W, Hryb DJ, Khan MS, et al. Sex hormone-binding globulin mediates steroid hormone signal transduction at the plasma membrane. J Steroid Biochem Mol Biol 1999;69:481–485.

27. Abu EO, Horner A, Kusec V, et al. The localization of androgen receptors in human bone. J Clin Endocrinol Metab 1997;82:3493–3497.

28. Pederson L, Kremer M, Jodd J, et al. Androgens regulate bone resorption activity of isolated osteoclasts in vitro. Proc Natl Acad Sci USA 1999;6:505–510.

29. Bland R. Steroid hormone receptor expression and action in bone. Clin Sci 2000;98:217–240.

30. Colvard DS, Eriksen EF, Keeting PE, et al. Identification of androgen receptors in normal human osteoblast-like cells. Proc Natl Acad Sci USA 1989;86:854–857.

31. Benz DJ, Haussler MR, Thomas MA, et al. High-affinity androgen binding and androgenic regulation of alpha 1(I)-procollagen and transforming growth factor-beta steady state messenger ribonucleic acid levels in human osteoblast-like ostersarcoma cells. Endocrinol 1991;128: 2723–2730.

32. Wiren K, Keenan E, Zhang X, et al. Homologous androgen receptor up-regulation in osteoblastic cells may be associated with enhanced functional androgen responsiveness. Endocrinol 1999; 140:3114–3124.

33. Bodine PVN, Riggs BL, Spelsberg TC. Regulation of c-fos expression and TGF-β production by gonadal and adrenal androgens in normal human osteoblastic cells. J Steroid Biochem Mole Biol 1995;52:149–158.

34. Benten WP, Lieberherr M, Stamm O, et al. Testosterone signaling through internalizable surface receptors in androgen receptor-free macrophages. Mol Biol Cell 1999;10:3113–3123.

35. Lieberherr M, Grosse B. Androgens increase intracellular calcium concentration and inositol 1,4,5-trisphosphate and diacylglycerol formation via a pertussis toxin-sensitive G-protein. J Biol Chem 1994;269:7217–7223.

36. Mizuno Y, Hosoi T, Inoue S, et al. Immunocytochemical identification of androgen receptor in mouse osteoclast-like multinucleated cells. Calcif Tissue Int 1994;54:325–326.

37. Hofbauer LC, Khosla S. Androgen effects on bone metabolism: recent progress and controversies. Eur J Endocrinol 1999;140:271–286.

38. Kaspi CH, Wakley GK, Hierl T, Ziegler R. Gonadal and androgens are potent regulators of human bone cell metabolism in vitro. J Bone Miner Res 1997;12:464–471.

39. Kasperk CH, Wergedal JE, Farley JR, et al. Androgens directly stimulate proliferation of bone cells in vitro. Endocrinol 1989;124:1576–1578.

40. Kasperk CH, Wakley GK, Hierl T, Ziegler R. Gonadal and adrenal androgens are poten regulators of human bone cell metabolism in vitro. J Bone Miner Res 1997;12:464–471.

41. Takeuchi M, Kakushi H, Tohkin M. Androgens directly stimulate mineralization and increase androgen receptors in human osteoblast-like osteoscarcoma cells. Biochem Biophysi Res Commun 1994;204:905–911.

42. Czerwiec FS, Liaw JJ, Liu SB, et al. Absence of androgen-mediated transcriptional effects in osteoblastic cells despite presence of androgen receptors. Bone 1997;21:49–56.

43. Gori F, Hofbauer LC, Conover CA, Khosla S. Effects of androgens on the insulin-like growth factor system in an androgen-responsive human osteoblastic cell line. Endocrinol 1999;140:5579–5586.

44. Kousteni S, Bellido T, Plotkin LI, et al. Nongenetropic sex-nonspecific signaling through the estrogen or androgen receptors: dissociation from transcriptional activity. Cell 2001;104:719–730.

45. Fukayama S, Tashjian AH Jr. Direct modulation of androgens of the response of human bone cells (SaOS-2) to human parathyroid hormone (PTH) and PTH-related protein. Endocrinol 1989;125: 1789–1794.

46. Pilbeam CC, Raisz LG. Effects of androgens on parathyroid hormone and interleukin-1-stimulated prostaglandin production in cultured neonatal mouse calvariae. J Bone Miner Res 1990; 5:1183–1188.

47. Bellido T, Jilka RL, Boyce BF, et al. Regulation of interleukin-6 osteoclastogenesis and bone mass by androgens. J Clin Invest 1995;95:1886–1895.

48. Purohit A, Flanagan AM, Reed MJ. Estrogen synthesis by osteoblast cell lines. Endocrinol 1992;131:2027–2029.

49. Bruch HR, Wolf L, Budde R, et al. Androstenedione metabolism in cultured human osteoblast-like cells. J Clin Endocrinol Metab 1992;75:101–105.

50. Janssen JM, Bland R, Hewison M, et al. Estradiol formation by human osteoblasts via multiple pathways: relation with osteoblast function. J Cell Biochem 1999;75:528–537.

51. Morishima A, Grumbach MM, Simpson ER, et al. Aromatase deficiency in male and femal siblings caused by a novel mutation and the physiological role of estrogens. J Clin Endocrinol Metab 1995;80:3689–3698.

52. Bilezikian JP, Morishima A, Bell J, Grumbach MM. Increased bone mass as a result of estrogen therapy in a man with aromatase deficiency. N Eng J Med 1998;339:599–603.

53. Imperato-McGinley J. 5 Alpha-reductase-2 deficiency. Curr Ther Endocrinol Metab 1997;6:384–387.

54. Kasra M, Grynpas MD. The effects of androgens on the mechanical properties of primate bone. J Biomech Eng 1995;17:265–270.

55. Lundon K, Dumitriu M, Grynpas MD. Suprphysiologic levels of testosterone affect cancellous and cortical bone in the young female cynomolgus monkey. Calcif Tissue Int 1997;60:54–62.

56. Gunness M, Orwoll E. Early induction of alterations in cancellous and cortical bone histology after orchidectomy in mature rats. J Bone Miner Res 1995;10:1735–1744.

57. Vanderschueren D, Van Herck E, Suiker AM, et al. Bone and mineral metabolism in aged male rats: short and long term effects of androgen deficiency. Endocrinol 1992;130:2906–2916.

58. Mason RA, Morris HA. Effects of dihydrotestosterone on bone biochemical markers in sham and oophorectomized rats. J Bone Miner Res 1997;12:1431–1437.

59. Lea CK, Flanagan AM. Ovarian androgens protect against bone loss in rats made oestrogen deficient by treatment with ICI 182, 780. J Endocrin 1999;160:111–117.

60. Vanderschueren D, Van Herck E,, Nijs J, et al. Aromatase inhibition impairs skeletal modeling an decreases bone mineral density in growing male rats. Endocrinol 1997;138:23201–23207.

61. Oz OK, Zerwekh JE, Fisher C, et al. Bone has a sexually dimorphic response to aromatase deficiency. J Bone Miner Res 2000;15:507–514.

62. Miyaura C, Toda K, Inada M, et al. Sex and age-related response to aromatase deficiency in bone. Biochem Biophys Res Commun 2001;280:1062–1068.

63. Smith EP, Boyd J, Frank GR, et al. Estrogen resistance caused by a mutation in the estrogen-receptor gene in a man. N Engl J Med 1994;331:1056–1061.

64. Marcus R, Leary D, Schneider DL, et al. The contribution of testosterone to skeletal development and maintenance lessons from the androgen insensitivity syndrome. J Clin Endocrinol Metab 2000;85:1032–1037.

65. Soule SG, Conway G, Prelevic GM, et al. Osteopenia as a feature of the androgen insensitivity syndrome. Clin Endocrinol 1995;43:671–675.

66. Mauras N, O'Brien KO, Oerter Klein K, Hayes V. Estrogen suppression in males: metabolic effects. J Clin Endocrinol Metab 2000;85:2370–2377.

67. Munoz-Torres M, Jodar E, Quesada M, Escobar-Jiminez F. Bone mass in androgen-insensitivity syndrome: response to hormonal replacement therapy. Calcif Tissue Int 1995;57:94–96.

68. Stepan IJ, Lachman M, Zverina J, et al. Castrated men exhibit bone loss: Effect of calcitonin treatment on biochemical indices of bone remodeling. J Clin Endocrinol Metab 1989;69:523–527.

69. Finkelstein JS, Klibanski A, Neer RM, et al. Osteoporosis in men with idiopathic hypogonadotropic hypogonadism. Ann Intern Med 1987;106:354–361.

70. Finkelstein JS, Neer RM, Biller BM, et al. Osteopenia in men with a history of delayed puberty. N Engl J Med 1992;326:600–604.

71. Finklestein JS, Klibanski A, Neer RM. A longitudinal evaluation of bone mineral density in adult men with histories of delayed puberty. J Clin Endocrinol Metab 1996;81:1152–1155.

72. Finkelstein JS, Kilbanski A, Neer RM. Evaluation of lumber spine bone mineral density (BMD) using dual energy x-ray absorptiometry (DXA) in 21 young men with histories of constitutionally-delayed puberty. J Clin Endocrinol Metab 1998;83:4280–4283.

73. Kiratli BJ, Srinivas S, Perkash I, Terris MK. Progressive decrease in bone density over 10 years of androgen deprivation therapy in patients with prostate cancer. Urology 2001;57:127–132.

74. Leder BZ, Smith MR, Fallon MA, et al. Effects of gonadal steroid suppression on skeletal sensitivity to parathyroid hormone in men. J Clin Endocrinol Metab 2001;86:511–516.

75. Foresta C, Ruzza G, Mioni R, et al. Osteoporosis and decline of gonadal function in the elderly male. Horm Res 1984;19:18–22.

76. Francis RM, Peacock M, Aaron JE, et al. Osteoporosis in hypogonadal men: Role of decreased plasma 1,25-dihydroxyvitamin D, calcium malabsorption, and low bone formation. Bone 1986;7:261–268.

77. Tenover JS. Effects of testosterone supplementation in the aging male. J Clin Endocrinol Metab 1992;75(4):1092–1098.

78. Gray A, Berlin JA, McKinlay JB Longcope C. An examination of research design effects on the association of testosterone and male aging: results of a meta-analysis. J Clin Epidemiol 1991;44(7):671–684.

79. Stanley HL, Schmitt BP, Poses RM, Deiss WP. Does hypogonadism contribute to the occurrence of a minimal trauma hip fracture in elderly men? J Am Geriatr Soc 1991;39:766–771.

80. Jackson JA, Riggs MW, Spiekerman AM. Testosterone deficiency as a risk factor for hip fracture in men: a case control study. Am J Med Sci 1992;304:4–8.

81. Hannan MT, Felson DT, Anderson JJ. Bone mineral density in elderly men and women: results from the Framingham osteoporosis study. J Bone Min Res 1992;7(5):547–553.

82. Meier DE, Orwoll ES, Keenan EJ, Fagerstrom RM. Marked decline in trabecular bone mineral content in healthy men with age: Lack of association with sex steroid levels. J Am Geriatric Soc 1987;35:189–197.

83. Kenny AM, Gallagher JC, Prestwood KM, et al. Bone density, bone turnover, and hormone levels in men over age 75. J Gerontol Med Sci 1998;53A(6):M419–M425.

84. Kenny AM, Prestwood KM, Marcello KM, Raisz LG. Determinants of bone density in healthy older men with low testosterone levels. J Gerontol A: Biol Sci Med Sci 2000;55:M492–M497.

85. Slemenda CW, Christian JC, Reed T, et al. Long-term bone loss in men: effects of genetic and environmental factors. Ann Intern Med 1992;117(4):286–291.

86. Swerdloff RS, Wang C. Androgens, estrogens, and bone in men. Ann Intern Med 2000;133: 1002–1004.

87. Bernecker PM, Willvonseder R, Resch H. Decreased estrogen levels in male patients with primary osteoporosis. J Bone Miner Res 1995;10:S445 (abstract T364).

88. Resch H, Pietschmann P, Woloszczuk W, et al. Bone mass and biochemical parameters of bone metabolism in men with spinal osteoporosis. Eur J Clin Invest 1992;22:542–545.

89. Barrett-Connor E, Mueller JE, von Muhlen DG, et al. Low levels of estradiol are associated with vertebral fractures in older men, but not women: the Rancho Bernardo Study. J Clin Endocrinol Metab 2000;85:219–223.

90. Clarke BL, Ebeling PR, Jones JD, et al. Changes in quantitative bone histomorphometry in aging healthy men. J Clin Endocrin Metab 1996;81:2264–2270.

91. Jackson JA, Kleerekoper M, Parfitt AM, et al. Bone histomorphometry in hypogonadal and eugonadal men with spinal osteoporsis. J Clin Endocrinol Metab 1987;65:53–58.

92. Laughlin GA, Barrett-Connor E, Kritz-Jsilverstein D, von Muhlen D. Hysterectomy, oophorectomy, and endogenous sex hormone levels in older women: the Rancho Bernardo Study. J Clin Endocrinol Metab 2000;85:645–651.

93. Laughlin GA, Barrett-Connor E. Sexual dimorphism in the influence of advanced aging on adrenal hormone levels: the Rancho Bernardo Study. J Clin Endocrinol Metab 2000;85:3561–3568.

94. Greendale GA, Edelstein S, Barrett-Connor E. Endogenous sex steroids and bone mineral density in older women and men: the Rancho Bernardo Study. J Bone Miner Res 1997;12: 1833–1843.

95. Arisaka O, Hoshi M, Kanazawa S, et al. Effect of adrenal androgen and estrogen on bone maturation and bone mineral density. Metabolism 2001;50:377–379.

96. Kritz-Silverstein D, Barrett-Connor E. Oophorectomy status and bone density in older, hysterectomized women. Am J Prev Med 1996;12:424–429.

97. Tazuke S, Khaw KT, Barrett-Connor E. Exogenous estrogen and endogenous sex hormones. Medicine 1992;71:44–51.

98. Longcope C, Baker RS, Hui SL, Johnston CC Jr. Androgen and estrogen dynamics in women with vertebral crush fractures. Maturitas 1984;6:309–318.

99. Jassal SK, Barrett-Connor E, Edelstein SL. Low bioavailable testosterone levels predict future height loss in postmenopausal women. J Bone Miner Res 1995;10:650–654.

100. Katznelson L, Finkelstein JS, Schoenfeld DA, et al. Increase in bone density and lean body mass during testosterone administration in men with acquired hypogonadism. J Clin Endocrinol Metab 1996;81(12):4358–4365.

101. Katznelson L. Therapeutic role of androgens in the treatment of osteoporosis in men. Baillieres Clin Endocrinol Metab 1998;12:453–470.

102. Wang C, Swedloff RS, Iranmanesh A, et al. Transdermal testosterone gel improves sexual function, mood, muscle strength, and body composition parameters in hypogonadal men. J Clin Endocrinol Metab 2000;85:2839–2853.

103. Snyder PJ, Peachey H, Berlin JA, et al. Effects of testosterone replacement in hypogonadal men. J Clin Endocrinol Metab 2000;85:2670–2677.

104. Taxel P, Kennedy DG, Fall PM, et al. The effect of aromatase inhibition on sex steroids, gonadotropins, and markers of bone turnover in older men. J Clin Endocrinol Metab 2001;86:2869–2874.

105. Kaufman J, Johnell O, Abadie E, et al. Background for studies on the treatment of male osteoporosis: state of the art. Ann Rheum Dis 2000;59:765–772.

106. Snyder PJ, Peachey H, Hannoush P, et al. Effect of testosterone treatment on bone mineral density in men over 65 years of age. J Clin Endocrinol Metab 1999;85:1966–1972.

107. Kenny AM, Prestwood KM, Gruman CA, et al. Effects of transdermal testosterone on bone and muscle in older men with low bioavailable testosterone levels. J Gerontol A Biol Sci Med Sci 2001;56:M266–M272.

108. Anderson FH, Francis RM, Peaston RT, Wastell HJ. Androgen supplementation in eugonadal men with osteoporosis: effects of six months' treatment on markers of bone formation and resorption. J Bone Miner Res 1997;12(3):472–478.

109. Kenny AM, Prestwood KM, Raisz LG. Short-term effects of intramuscular and transdermal testosterone on bone turnover, prostate symptoms, cholesterol, and hematocrit in men over age 70 with low testosterone levels. Endocr Res 2000;26(2):153–168.

110. Watts NB, Notelovitz M, Timmons MC, et al. Comparison of oral estrogens and estrogens plus androgen on bone mineral density, menopausal symptoms, and lipid-lipoprotein profiles in surgical menopause. Obstet Gynecol 1995;85:529–537.

111. Raisz LG, Wiita B, Artis A, et al. Comparison of the effects of estrogen alone and estrogen plus androgen on biochemical markers of bone formation and resorption in postmenopausal women. J Clin Endocrinol Metab 1996;81:37–43.

112. Garnett T, Studd J, Watson N, Savvas M. A cross-sectional study of the effects of long-term percutaneous hormone replacement therapy on bone density. Obstet Gynecol 1991;78:1002–1007.

113. Shifren JL, Graunstein GD, Simon JA, et al. Transdermal testosterone treatment in women with impaired sexual function after oophorectomy. N Eng J Med 2000;343:682–688.

114. Chesnut CH, Ivey JL, Gruber HE, et al. Stanozolol in postmenopausal osteoporosis: therapeutic efficacy and possible mechanisms of action. Metabolism 1983;32:571–580.

115. Need AG, Morris HA, Hartley TF, et al. Effects of nadrolone decanoate on forearm mineral density and calcium metabolism in osteoporotic postmenopausal women. N Eng J Med 1987;41:7–10.

116. Hassager C, Riis BJ, Podenphant J, Christiansen C. Nandrolone decanoate treatment of post-menopausal osteoporosis for 2 years and effects of withdrawal. Maturitas 1989;11:305–317.

117. Beneton MN, Yates AJ, Rogers S, et al. Stanozolol stimulates remodeling of trabecular bone and net formation of bone at the endocortical surface. Clin Sci 1991;95:2886–2895.

118. Castelo-Branco C, Vicente JJ, Figueras F, et al. Comparative effects of estrongens plus androgens and tibolone on bone, lipid pattern and sexuality in postmenopausal women. Maturitas 2000;15:161–168.

119. Savvas M, Studd JW, Fogelman I, et al. Skeletal effects of oral oestrogen and testosterone in postmenopausal women. Br Med J 1988;297:331–333.

120. Savvas M, Studd JW, Norman S, et al. Increase in bone mass after one year of percutaneous oestradiol and testosterone implants in post-menopausal women who have previously received long-term oral oestrogens. Br J Obstet Gynaecol 1992;99:757–760.

121. Barrett-Connor E, Young R, Notelovitz M, et al. A two-year, double blind comparison of estrogen-androgen and conjugated estrogens in surgically menopausal women. Effects on bone mineral density, symptoms and lipid profiles. J Reprod Med 1999;44:1012–1020.

12 Androgens and the Hematopoietic System

Shehzad Basaria, MD
and Adrian S. Dobs, MD, MHS

CONTENTS

INTRODUCTION
HISTORICAL BACKGROUND
MECHANISM OF ACTION OF ANDROGENS
ERYTHROPOIETIC RESPONSE TO TESTOSTERONE IN NORMAL MEN
THERAPEUTIC USES OF ANDROGENS IN VARIOUS FORMS OF ANEMIAS
HEMATOCRIT AND CARDIOVASCULAR DISEASE
CONCLUSIONS
REFERENCES

INTRODUCTION

The role of androgens in the stimulation of erythropoiesis has been recognized for more than five decades. Men are known to have higher red cell mass than women, an observation that lead scientists to explore the role of androgens in various types of anemia. Of these, anemia secondary to renal insufficiency has been studied the most. Although recombinant human erythropoietin (rhEpo) has taken over the use of androgens in patients with renal failure, androgens may still have a role because of their efficacy and low cost. In this chapter, we will discuss the mechanism of action of androgens on the hematopoietic system, efficacy of androgens in the treatment of various anemias, and the erythropoietic side effects of androgens.

HISTORICAL BACKGROUND

Initial animal experiments showed an increase in hemoglobin level with androgen administration *(1)*. This was further confirmed by the observation that a significant decline in hematopoiesis occurs in rats after castration *(2)*. Administration of androgens to these animals resulted in an increase in the red blood cell counts *(3)*. Epidemiological studies have shown that men have higher hemoglobin and red cell mass than women *(4)*. This difference is apparent only after the pubertal spurt when males acquire an edge over females, likely the result of the secretion of androgens from their gonads *(5)*. This difference in red cell counts between the genders is not caused by the monthly menstrual

From: *Contemporary Endocrinology: Androgens in Health and Disease*
Edited by: C. Bagatell and W. J. Bremner © Humana Press Inc., Totowa, NJ

losses in women, because young women who have undergone hysterectomy still have lower hemoglobin levels compared to age-matched men *(5)*. Similar to animal studies, anemia develops in castrated and eunuchoid men *(1,2)*. This is reversed with androgen administration. The prevalence of anemia in both genders increases after age 60 and worsens with every decade thereafter *(6)*. This was further evaluated by Lipschitz et al., who found that elderly men with unexplained anemia had lower levels of erythroid precursors compared with nonanemic young men and elderly controls *(7)*.

MECHANISM OF ACTION OF ANDROGENS

Androgens stimulate erythropoiesis through a variety of direct and indirect ways. In this section we attempt to elucidate these mechanisms.

Stimulation of Erythropoietin Secretion

Animal studies have shown that androgen administration increases the synthesis and secretion of erythropoietin (Epo). Administration of androgens to female rats results in hypertrophy of renal tissue and an increase in Epo secretion *(8)*. Testosterone acts by binding to cytoplasmic receptors in the renal parenchymal cells. This hormone-receptor complex is transported to the nucleus where it results in transcription of certain proteins that increase cellular mass *(9)*, resulting in an increase in Epo synthesis and secretion. This observation is confirmed by animal studies showing that various doses of nandrolone decanoate when given to a mouse with renal failure results in an increase in Epo synthesis and hemoglobin concentration *(10)*. This increase in Epo secretion is blocked by injection of antierythropoietin antibody *(11)*, further proving that androgens act by increasing Epo levels.

Androgens also stimulate Epo synthesis in humans. Alexanian administered fluoxymesterone at a dose of 40 mg/m^2 to anemic men and control men and 10 mg/m^2 of fluoxymesterone to hypogonadal men and anemic women *(12)*. Two-thirds of the hypogonadal and/or anemic patients showed an elevation of red cell volume by at least 15%. All of the groups also showed an increase in the urinary levels of Epo. Humans (both genders) also have an extrarenal source of Epo and, therefore, even nephrectomized men respond to androgens *(13)*. The site of this extrarenal Epo synthesis remains unclear. Another study showed that the main mechanism by which androgens stimulate erythropoiesis is by stimulating secretion of Epo *(14)*. In this study, simultaneous administration to mice of cyproterone acetate (an antiandrogen) with testosterone propionate significantly decreased erythropoiesis. However, administration of synthetic Epo in the presence of cyproterone acetate did not inhibit erythropoiesis.

Action on Bone Marrow

Androgens stimulate erythroid colony-forming units in the bone marrow. Incubation of human bone marrow culture supplemented with variable testosterone concentrations results in stimulation of erythroid colony formation *(15)*. Androgens also convert the uncommitted bone marrow cells from Epo-nonreponsive to Epo-responsive cells. After these initial steps, Epo is mandatory for the maturation of these cells into the erythroid cell line. The combination of testosterone and Epo has a synergistic effect on erythropoiesis *(15)*. Testosterone makes the marrow cells Epo responsive and then Epo differentiates these uncommitted marrow cells into the erythroid cell line.

Iron Incorporation

Testosterone stimulates iron (Fe) incorporation into red blood cells (RBCs). Administration of androgens along with intravenous ^{59}Fe results in an increase in Fe uptake by the erythrocytes *(16)*. Administration of testosterone propionate three times a week to female mice increases RBC ^{59}Fe incorporation by 100% *(17)*. However, there is a delay of 96 h between the administration of testosterone and the maximal uptake of ^{59}Fe.

Red Cell Glycolysis

After entering the cells, androgens enhance the intracellular uptake of glucose. This leads to glycolysis *(18)*, resulting in the formation of high-energy phosphate bonds leading to DNA transcription and synthesis of mRNA in the erythroid cells. Erythropoiesis is seen after 6–12 h of glucose utilization *(18)*. This mechanism is believed to be independent of Epo.

ERYTHROPOIETIC RESPONSE
TO TESTOSTERONE IN NORMAL MEN

Before discussing the therapeutic efficacy of androgens in different disease states, it is important to study the erythropoietic response to androgens in a normal man. In one study, administration of 250 mg of testosterone enanthate for 5 mo to normal men failed to demonstrate any significant changes in blood parameters *(19)*. Palacios et al. conducted a study on 53 young men and administered testosterone with different dosing schedules *(20)*. Subjects were divided into two groups: The first group received 200 mg testosterone enanthate weekly and the second group received the same dose every 2 wk for 16 wk. Significant increase in RBC and white blood cell (WBC) counts were seen in the weekly group with no significant increase in the bimonthly group. Mild increases in hemoglobin and hematocrit were seen in both groups. This study showed that administration of twice the normal replacement dose to healthy young men results in a significant increase in red cell and white cell mass.

THERAPEUTIC USES OF ANDROGENS
IN VARIOUS FORMS OF ANEMIAS

Anemia of Renal Failure

Patients with renal failure are anemic because of decreased production of Epo *(21)*. Despite adequate hemodialysis, defective erythropoiesis does not normalize in this patient population *(22)*. Because humans have an extrarenal site for Epo synthesis, Epo levels have been detected in the plasma of anephric patients *(23)*. Androgens have been employed in the past for the treatment of anemia of end-stage renal disease (ESRD); however, with the introduction of rhEpo in the late 1980s, androgens have lost popularity. However, recent studies have shown that androgens may still have a role in erythropoiesis in these patients. In addition to their erythropoietic effect, androgens are cost-effective and have an anabolic effect. Initial studies reported that administration of 200 mg testosterone enanthate twice weekly in two ESRD patients resulted in an increase in Epo and hemoglobin levels and increased ^{59}Fe incorporation into erythrocytes *(24)*. In one of these patients, the transfusion requirements also significantly decreased. Richardson and Weinstein administered 400–600 mg testosterone enanthate weekly to

15 dialysis patients *(25)*. Thirteen of 15 patients showed a mean increase of hematocrit of 5.5% and red cell volume of 353 mL. Two patients who did not exhibit a satisfactory response initially were iron deficient and showed a satisfactory erythropoietic response after iron repletion *(25)*. This shows that adequate iron levels are mandatory for a satisfactory erythropoietic response to androgens. The majority of these patients also showed an increase in serum creatinine, suggesting an increase in muscle mass. In a recent study, eight male patients on peritoneal dialysis were given nandrolone decanoate 200 mg/wk for 6 mo *(26)*. Mean hemoglobin levels increased from 9.4 to 12.1 g/dL. This study showed that androgens can induce an erythropoietic response in patients undergoing both peritoneal and hemodialysis.

ESRD Patients: Anephric vs Intact Kidneys

Further studies were conducted to evaluate the efficacy of androgens in two groups of ESRD patients: those who were anephric and those with an intact kidney. In one study, testosterone administration resulted in a significant increase in packed-cell volume in three anephric patients *(27)*. Another study showed that fluoxymesterone increased packed-cell volume in two of three anephric patients *(22)*. Fried et al. attempted to differentiate the hematopoietic response in these two classes of patients by administering 150 mg testosterone propionate twice weekly to 11 patients with renal failure (5 were anephric and 6 with intact kidneys) *(28)*. The six patients with intact kidneys showed a significant rise in plasma Epo levels and packed-cell volume, whereas none of the anephric patients showed any response. This study suggested that androgens promote erythropoiesis in ESRD patients by releasing Epo even from the kidney remnants. Thus, the anemia of renal failure can become severe and refractory to androgen therapy when these patients undergo nephrectomy, suggesting that nephrectomy should be delayed as long as possible.

Dependency of Androgens on Epo in ESRD Patients

In one study, 25 anemic ESRD men on hemodialysis were treated with nandrolone decanoate 200 mg/wk intramuscularly for 6 mo *(29)*. Although there was an increase in mean hemoglobin levels in both groups, 15 patients showed an increase in Epo levels and 10 patients did not. There was no correlation between the degree of Epo elevation to the rise in hemoglobin levels. In 14 of these 25 patients, Epo and hemoglobin were measured after discontinuation of nandrolone. Although Epo levels returned to baseline 6 wk after the last dose of nandrolone, hemoglobin levels remained above the basal levels for 4 mo *(29)*. Furthermore, among these 14 patients, only 8 had initially shown an increase in Epo levels. These results suggest some additional unknown mechanisms by which androgens enhance erythropoiesis.

Androgen vs Epo in ESRD Patients

A comparison study to evaluate the efficacy of nandrolone decanoate 200 mg/wk and rhEpo 6000 IU/wk for 6 mo was conducted by Teruel et al. *(30)*. Androgens were given to men >50 yr of age and rhEpo was given to men <50 yr of age and to women. Although the increase in hemoglobin was similar in both groups, the androgen group experienced an increase in dry weight and serum albumin levels, signifying the anabolic effect of the androgen. Androgens were also more cost-effective. Furthermore, the patients in the rhEpo group experienced worsening of blood pressure.

ANDROGENS IN COMBINATION WITH RHEPO

Ballal et al. treated seven men with 2000 units rhEpo intravenously after each dialysis; eight other patients received the same dose of rhEpo in combination with nandrolone decanoate 100 mg/wk *(31)*. Patients receiving only rhEpo did not show any significant increase in hematocrit, whereas patients on combination therapy had a posttreatment hematocrit that was 9% higher compared to baseline. In another prospective study, one group of patients received 1500 U rhEpo thrice weekly for 26 wk and the other group received the same dose of rhEpo along with nandrolone decanoate 100 mg/wk *(32)*. The mean hematocrit increased in both groups; however, the increase in the rhEpo + nandrolone group was significantly greater than rhEpo alone. Contrary to the above-mentioned studies, one study failed to show any additional efficacy of nandrolone compared to rhEpo *(33)*.

Aplastic Anemia

Initial work to determine the efficacy of androgens in aplastic anemia was conducted on the pediatric population. Shahidi and Diamond initially suggested the effectiveness of testosterone and glucocorticoids in patients with aplastic anemia *(34)*. In 1969, Killander et al. conducted a trial of androgen plus prednisone in 19 children with aplastic anemia *(35)*. Patients were initially treated with high doses of prednisone (40–80 mg/d), and later the dose was reduced to 5–10 mg/d. Testosterone propionate was administered to seven patients at a dose of 3 mg/kg/d (six patients) and 1.7 mg/kg/d (one patient). The remaining 12 patients received methyltestosterone at 2 mg/kg/d. Eight children failed to show any response and died, whereas 2 initially responded but later relapsed and died. The remaining nine children responded favorably to androgens and corticosteroids and achieved good hemoglobin levels *(35)*. Severe bone marrow hypoplasia was the most unfavorable indicator of therapeutic response to androgens evident by the fact that among 11 responders, only 1 patient had severe marrow hypoplasia in contrast to 7 of 8 nonresponders. These data emphasize the importance of early diagnosis of patients with aplastic anemia (AA) before the marrow has become severely hypoplastic, because the response to androgens is poor once this stage is reached.

Recent studies have evaluated the treatment of AA only with androgens without any use of concomitant glucocorticoids. Duarte et al. used oxymetholone ($n = 32$) and methenolone ($n = 2$) orally in 34 patients *(36)*. Seven patients died within the first 2 mo of therapy and 10 had no response. The remaining 17 responded favorably, yielding a response rate of 50%. The median time to response was 3 mo. Among the responders, androgens resulted in normalization of all marrow cell lines and also decreased bleeding tendency. Patients with primary idiopathic AA (in contrast to secondary AA) and those with reticulocyte count >1% responded favorably. However, the strongest association was with neutrophil count of >500 mm³.

Palva and Wasastjerna treated 28 patients suffering from AA with oral methenolone at a dose of 1–2 mg/kg for 2–12 mo *(37)*. Methenolone normalized blood counts in 43% of the patients and the remission rate was 60% for patients with treatment period of at least 3 mo. These authors considered methenolone to be superior to testosterone in the treatment of AA with a remission rate of 50–70% compared to 5–40% *(37)*. Another study reported 50% survival rate after 4 yr of androgen treatment in patients with AA, a rate similar to bone marrow transplantation in those days *(38)*. Oxymetholone has also been reported to possess greater erythropoietic activity than testosterone and have produced remission rates of 70–100% *(39)*. In eight subjects with AA who were given oxymetholone for >2 mo, seven responded with an increase in hemoglobin (three of these patients had failed past testosterone treatment) *(39)*; six of them remained in remission for 22–33 mo. Oxymetholone also increases WBC and platelet count by 40% and 33%, respectively *(40)*.

Researchers have shown that the degree of hematopoietic response in patients with AA does not depend on the dose of androgens, but rather on the degree of marrow hypoplasia *(41)*. Fluoxymesterolone and norethandrolone were administered to 110 patients with AA at doses of 1 mg/kg/d and 0.2 mg/kg/d, respectively. Although the survival rate was higher among patients receiving high doses of androgens, however, further analysis showed that high-dose androgens improved survival only in those patients who had mild degree of AA.

Refractory Anemias

Myelodysplastic syndrome (MDS) is a state of ineffective erythropoiesis and is characterized by peripheral cytopenia in the presence of a normocellular or hypercellular bone marrow. Androgens have been used in the treatment of MDSs; however, the response has been less positive compared to AA. Kobaba et al. treated 27 patients with MDS with 5 different oral androgens *(42)*, with 11 patients responding favorably (efficacy 41%). The probability of survival was 75% for the responder group and 41% for the nonresponders. Six patients in the nonresponder group underwent transformation from refractory anemia to refractory anemia with excess blasts (worse form of MDS) compared to only one patient in the responder group. Oxymetholone has also been used in patients with myelofibrosis. Two patients in one study did not require transfusion for 9 and 14 mo, respectively, after oxymetholone treatment *(39)*.

Hemolytic Anemias

Androgens have been used in the management of sickle cell anemia and thalassemias with variable success. Earlier studies have reported a significant increase in red cell mass in patients with sickle cell anemia *(43)*. However, there is no effect of androgens on the sickling tendency or red cell survival. Craddock et al. have shown an improvement in hematological parameters in patients with thalassemia during oxymetholone therapy *(44)*. Androgens also increase hemoglobin levels in patients with paroxysmal nocturnal hemoglobinuria *(45)*. However, there is no increase in red cell life span.

Side Effects of Androgens

Androgen administration can result in adverse effects like virilization, acne, priapism, peliosis hepatis, and increased libido *(46)*. Teruel et al. recently reported that nandrolone decanoate given to hemodialysis patients for 6 mo resulted in a decline in HDL levels and an increase in triglyceride levels *(47)*. Although these side effects are commonly seen, we will focus our discussion on polycythemia, a major hematopoietic side effect of androgen therapy.

Polycythemia

A few studies have shown the development of polycythemia in patients treated with androgens. A study of hematopoietic parameters in 15 patients (52–78 yr) with primary hypogonadism treated with testosterone enanthate 300 mg/3 wk showed a significant increase in hematocrit (mean 49.4%) and RBC volume while on androgens (48). To further analyze the characteristics of the patients with different degrees of erythropoietic response, patients were divided into two groups: those who achieved hematocrit level of 48% or greater (n = 9) and those achieving <48% (n = 6). While off testosterone, both groups were similar in baseline demographic characteristics, hematocrit, red cell volume, and plasma volume. During androgen therapy, the <48% group had little change in these parameters; however, >48% group showed an increase in red cell volume along with a decrease in plasma volume, resulting in a higher hematocrit levels. Three of nine patients in the >48% group experienced cerebrovascular events while on testosterone therapy, achieving hematocrits of 53%, 58%, and 64%, respectively. The incidence of strokes in this group was 13%, much higher than in the general population (0.5–1.0%) (48). No patient in the <48% group had any cardiovascular events. The authors recommended that when there is an increase in hematocrit from baseline level of 15% or more or a hematocrit level of >48% is attained, a decision should be made regarding further continuation of androgen therapy.

Elderly men are particularly susceptible to develop polycythemia. Drinka et al. reported that two of eight hypogonadal elderly men developed polycythemia while receiving testosterone enanthate 150 mg/70 kg every 2 wk (49). These two men had the highest body mass index (BMI) in the group and their respective hematocrit levels were 53.4% and 57.3%. Both patients developed sleep apnea and one was documented to have nocturnal oxygen desaturation while on testosterone.

Androgens administered via different routes have a differential effect on hematopoietic parameters. Therapy with Androderm, the transdermal testosterone patch, results in a significantly lower rate of abnormal Hct elevations compared to intramuscular testosterone (15.4% vs 43.8%) (50). This may be the result of less total area under the curve in transdermal products. Similarly, in a recent study, none of the patients on transdermal testosterone gel became symptomatic, discontinued therapy, or withdrew from the study (51). These studies show that transdermal androgen preparations are less likely to result in polycythemia compared to intramuscular preparations.

These studies show that polycythemia can be a dangerous complication of androgen therapy. Although not studied prospectively, one should be cautious when giving androgens to patients with relative erythrocytosis, on diuretics, and smokers.

HEMATOCRIT AND CARDIOVASCULAR DISEASE

The relationship between hematocrit and coronary heart disease (CHD) has been known for a long time. An early autopsy study showed that patients with CHD had higher premortem hematocrits (52). The Puerto Rico Heart Health Program (53) showed that a higher hematocrit was associated with increased incidence of myocardial infarction and CHD-related death. The Honolulu Heart Program studied more than 8000 Japanese men prospectively for 10 yr (54) and found that subjects with hematocrit levels >45.4% had a higher rate of death resulting from CHD compared to any other cause.

Similar to CHD, elevated hematocrit is also a risk factor for stroke. A retrospective analysis of 500 patients found that men with hemoglobin of >15 g/dL or hematocrit of >44% were twice as likely to get cerebral infarctions than patients with lower values (55). For women, these values were >14 g/dL and >42%, respectively. Another study of 432 autopsy patients found that the risk of cerebral infarction increased steeply when the hematocrit level rose to >46% (56). The incidence of cerebral infarction was 18.3% with hematocrit values of 36–40%, 18.8% with hematocrit levels between 41% and 45%, 43.6% with a hematocrit level of 46–50%, and 50% with a hematocrit >50%. Interestingly, in elderly patients (>78 yr), the incidence of stroke increased when hematocrit levels rose >41%. The presence of hypertension did not influence the relationship between stroke and hematocrit levels. The infarctions were predominantly in the deep subcortical region, where the arterial caliber is smaller. The authors recommended that the optimum hematocrit in patients <78 yr should be kept between 41% and 45% and between 36% and 40% for those >78 yr. Another study showed that mortality resulting from acute stroke is higher in patients with a hematocrit value of >50% (57).

CONCLUSIONS

Androgens act on the hematopoietic system in a variety of ways. They induce release of Epo, increase bone marrow activity, and increase the incorporation of iron into the red cells. Androgens are useful agents in the treatment of anemia in patients with renal disease, aplastic marrow, hypogonadism, and hypopituitarism. They are as effective and less expensive than Epo. However, polycythemia remains a side effect of androgen therapy. Epidemiologic evidence suggests an increased risk of stroke with hematocrit in the top normal range (> 45%). Therefore, caution should be exercised during exogenous administration of androgens. The dose of testosterone should be reduced or the route of administration changed (from intramuscular to transdermal) if the level rises above 50% and discontinued if it rises above 52%. The risk–benefit ratio needs to be evaluated carefully in subjects who are at high risk for cardiovascular accident. In this population, the goal might be to maintain the hemtocrit level around 45%. Based on the available evidence, androgens should be strongly considered in the treatment of anemia related to renal disease, bone marrow depression, and hypogonadism.

REFERENCES

1. Vollmer EP, Gordon AS. Effect of sex and gonadotropic hormones upon the blood picture of the rat. Endocrinology 1941;29:828–837.
2. Steinglass P, Gordon AS, Charipper HA. Effect of castration and sex hormones on blood of the rat. Proc Soc Exp Biol Med 1941;48:169–177.
3. Crafts RC. Effects of hypophysectomy, castration and testosterone propionate on hemopoiesis in the adult male rat. Endocrinology 1946;39:401–413.
4. Hawkins WW, Speck E, Leonard VG. Variation of the hemoglobin level with age and sex. Blood 1954;9:999–1007.
5. Vahlquist B. The cause of the sexual differences in erythrocyte, hemoglobin and serum iron levels in human adults. Blood 1950;5:874–875.
6. McLennan WJ, Andrews GR, Macleod C, Caird FI. Anaemia in the elderly. Q J Med 1973;42:1–13.
7. Lipschitz DA, Mitchell CO, Thompson C. The anemia of senescence. Am J Hematol 1981;11:47–54.
8. Nathan DG, Gardner FH. Effects of large doses of androgen on rodent erythropoiesis and body composition. Blood 1965;26:411–420.
9. Paulo LG, Fink GD, Roh BL, Fisher JW. Effects of several androgens and steroid metabolites on erythropoietin production in the isolated perfused dog kidney. Blood 1974;43:39–47.
10. Yared K, Gagnon RF, Brox AG. Mechanisms of action of androgen treatment on the anemia of experimental chronic renal failure. J Am Soc Nephrol 1997;8:633A.
11. Schooley JC. Inhibition of erythropoietic stimulation by testosterone in polycythemic mice receiving anti-erythropoietin. Proc Soc Exp Biol Med 1966;122:402–403.
12. Alexanian R. Erythropoietin and erythropoiesis in anemic man following androgens. Blood 1969;33:564–572.

13. Shaldon S, Koch KM, Oppermann F, et al. Testosterone therapy for anaemia in maintenance dialysis. Br Med J 1971;3:212–215.
14. Medlinsky JT, Napier CD, Gurney CW. The use of an antiandrogen to further investigate the erythropoietic effects of androgens. J Lab Clin Med 1969;74:85–92.
15. Moriyama Y, Fisher JW. Effects of testosterone and erythropoietin on erythroid colony formation in human bone marrow cultures. Blood 1975;45:665–670.
16. Molinari PF, Rosenkrantz H. Erythropoietic activity and androgenic implications of 29 testosterone derivatives in orchiectomized rats. J Lab Clin Med 1971;78:399–410.
17. Naets JP, Wittek M. The mechanism of action of androgens on erythropoiesis. Ann NY Acad Sci 1968;149:366–376.
18. Molinari PF, Esber HJ, Snyder LM. Effect of androgens on maturation and metabolism of erythroid tissue. Exp Hematol 1976;4:301–309.
19. Mauss J, Borsch G, Bormacher K, et al. Effect of long-term testosterone oenanthate administration on male reproductive function: clinical evaluation, serum FSH, LH, testosterone, and seminal fluid analyses in normal men. Acta Endocrinol (Copenh) 1975;78:373–384.
20. Palacios A, Campfield LA, McClure RD, et al. Effect of testosterone enanthate on hematopoiesis in normal men. Fertil Steril 1983;40:100–104.
21. Gurney CW, Goldwasser E, Pan C. Studies on erythropoiesis VI. Erythropoietin in human plasma. J Lab Clin Med 1957;50:534–542.
22. Eschbach JW Jr, Funk D, Adamson J, et al. Erythropoiesis in patients with renal failure undergoing chronic dialysis. N Engl J Med 1967;276:653–658.
23. Naets JP, Wittek M. Erythropoiesis in anephric man. Lancet 1968;1:941–943.
24. DeGowin RL, Lavender AR, Forland M, et al. Erythropoiesis and erythropoietin in patients with chronic renal failure treated with hemodialysis and testosterone. Ann Intern Med 1970;72:913–918.
25. Richardson JR, Weinstein MB. Erythropoietic response of dialyzed patients to testosterone administration. Ann Intern Med 1970;73:403–407.
26. Navarro JF, Mora C, Rivero A, et al. Androgens as therapy for the treatment of anemia in peritoneal dialysis (PD) patients. Perit Dial Int 1998;18:S52.
27. Shaldon S, Patyna WD, Kaltwasser P, et al. The use of testosterone in bilateral nephrectomized dialysis patients. Trans Am Soc Artif Intern Organs 1971;17:104–107.
28. Fried W, Jonasson O, Lang G, Schwartz F. The hematologic effect of androgen in uremic patients. Study of packed cell volume and erythropoietin responses. Ann Intern Med 1973;79:823–827.
29. Teruel JL, Marcen R, Navarro JF, et al. Evolution of serum erythropoietin after androgen administration to hemodialysis patients: a prospective study. Nephron 1995;70:282–286.
30. Teruel JL, Marcen R, Navarro-Antolin J, et al. Androgen versus erythropoietin for the treatment of anemia in hemodialyzed patients: a prospective study. J Am Soc Nephrol 1996;7:140–144.
31. Ballal SH, Domoto DT, Polack DC, et al. Androgens potentiate the effects of erythropoietin in the treatment of anemia of end-stage renal disease. Am J Kidney Dis 1991;17:29–33.
32. Gaughan WJ, Liss KA, Dunn SR, et al. A 6-month study of low-dose recombinant human erythropoietin alone and in combination with androgens for the treatment of anemia in chronic hemodialysis patients. Am J Kidney Dis 1997;30:495–500.
33. Berns JS, Rudnick MR, Cohen RM. A controlled trial of recombinant human erythropoietin and nandrolone decanoate in the treatment of anemia in patients on chronic hemodialysis. Clin Nephrol 1992;37:264–267.
34. Shahidi NT, Diamond LK. Testosterone induced remission in aplastic anemia. Amer Dis Child 1959;98:293.
35. Killander A, Lundmark KM, Sjolin S. Idiopathic aplastic anaemia in children. Results of androgen treatment. Acta Paediatr Scand 1969;58:10–14.
36. Duarte L, Lopez Sandoval R, et al. Androstane therapy of aplastic anaemia. Acta Haematol 1972;47:140–145.
37. Palva IP, Wasastjerna C. Treatment of aplastic anemia with methenolone. Acta Haemat 1972;47:13–20.
38. Van Hengstum M, Steenbergen J, Haanen C. Clinical course in 28 unselected patients with aplastic anaemia treated with anabolic steroids. Br J Haematol 1979;41:323–333.
39. Sacks P, Gale D, Bothwell TH, Stevens K. Oxymetholone therapy in aplastic and other refractory anaemias. S Afr Med J 1972;46:1607–1615.

40. Sanchez-Medal L, Gomez-Leal A, Duarte L, Guadalupe Rico M. Anabolic androgenic steroids in the treatment of acquired aplastic anemia. Blood 1969;34:283–300.

41. French Cooperative Group for the Study of Aplastic and Refractory Anemias. Androgen therapy in aplastic anaemia: a comparative study of high and low-doses and of 4 different androgens. Scand J Haematol 1986;36:346–352.

42. Kobaba R, Kanamaru A, Takemoto Y, et al. Androgen in the treatment of refractory anemia. Int J Hematol 1991;54:103–107.

43. Lundh B, Gardner FH. The haematological response to androgens in sickle cell anaemia. Scand J Haematol 1970;7:389–397.

44. Craddock PR, Hunt FA, Rozenberg MC. The effective use of oxymetholone in the therapy of thalassaemia with anaemia. Med J Aust 1972;2:199–202.

45. Hartmann RC, Jenkins DE Jr, McKee LC, Heyssel RM. Paroxysmal nocturnal hemoglobinuria: clinical and laboratory studies relating to iron metabolism and therapy with androgen and iron. Medicine (Baltimore) 1966;45:331–363.

46. Watson AJ. Adverse effects of therapy for the correction of anemia in hemodialysis patients. Semin Nephrol 1989;9:30–34.

47. Teruel JL, Lasuncion MA, Rivera M, et al. Nandrolone decanoate reduces serum lipoprotein(a) concentrations in hemodialysis patients. Am J Kidney Dis 1997;29:569–575.

48. Krauss DJ, Taub HA, Lantinga LJ, et al. Risks of blood volume changes in hypogonadal men treated with testosterone enanthate for erectile impotence. J Urol 1991;146:1566–1570.

49. Drinka PJ, Jochen AL, Cuisinier M, et al. Polycythemia as a complication of testosterone replacement therapy in nursing home men with low testosterone levels. J Am Geriatr Soc 1995;43:899–901.

50. Dobs AS, Meikle WA, Arver S, et al. Pharmacokinetics, efficacy and safety of a permeation-enhanced testosterone transdermal system in comparison with bi-weekly injections of testosterone enanthate for the treatment of hypogonadal men. J Clin Endocrinol Metab 1999;84:3469–3478.

51. Wang C, Swerdloff RS, Iranmanesh A, et al. Transdermal testosterone gel improves sexual function, mood, muscle strength, and body composition parameters in hypogonadal men. J Clin Endocrinol Metab 2000;85:2839–2853.

52. Burch GE, DePasquale NP. The hematocrit in patients with myocardial infarction. JAMA 1962;180:63.

53. Sorlie PD, Garcia-Palmieri MR, Costas R Jr, Havlik RJ. Hematocrit and risk of coronary heart disease: the Puerto Rico Health Program. Am Heart J 1981;101:456–461.

54. Carter C, McGee D, Reed D, et al. Hematocrit and the risk of coronary heart disease: the Honolulu Heart Program. Am Heart J 1983;105:674–679.

55. Niazi GA, Awada A, al Rajeh S, Larbi E. Hematological values and their assessment as risk factor in Saudi patients with stroke. Acta Neurol Scand 1994;89:439–445.

56. Tohgi H, Yamanouchi H, Murakami M, Kameyama M. Importance of the hematocrit as a risk factor in cerebral infarction. Stroke 1978;9:369–374.

57. Lowe GD, Jaap AJ, Forbes CD. Relation of atrial fibrillation and high haematocrit to mortality in acute stroke. Lancet 1983;1:784–786.

13   Androgens and Body Composition

Laurence Katznelson, MD

CONTENTS

INTRODUCTION
TESTOSTERONE AND MALE HYPOGONADISM
TESTOSTERONE ADMINISTRATION IN HYPOGONADAL MEN
TESTOSTERONE ADMINISTRATION TO EUGONADAL MEN
ARE THERE APPLICATIONS OF TESTOSTERONE IN CHRONIC ILLNESS?
TESTOSTERONE AND WOMEN: ENDOGENOUS EFFECTS
    AND POTENTIAL USES
CONCLUSIONS
REFERENCES

INTRODUCTION

Ever since the clinical availability of androgens, it has been noted that androgens modulate body composition, leading to enhanced lean and diminished fat mass. Androgens have received particular attention with regard to improving body composition not only in normal populations but also in those with chronic illness with associated sarcopenia. For example, improvements in muscle mass following testosterone administration have been shown in sarcopenic states such as aging, cancer, and human immunodeficiency virus (HIV) wasting, although the implications of these changes with regard to function have not been well documented. The effects of androgens on fat mass have also generated much interest because of the potential effects of androgens in modulating cardiovascular risk. Additionally, there is excitement about the application of androgens to women because of the potential for beneficial effects on body composition in women with hypopituitarism and menopause. This chapter will provide an overview regarding both physiologic and supraphysiologic testosterone administration on body composition in eugonadal and hypogonadal individuals, including those with sarcopenia in the setting of chronic illness or aging. The potential applications of testosterone administration in these populations will be reviewed.

TESTOSTERONE AND MALE HYPOGONADISM

The rationale for investigating the effects of testosterone administration on body composition stems from cross-sectional studies that associate altered adipose deposition

From: *Contemporary Endocrinology: Androgens in Health and Disease*
Edited by: C. Bagatell and W. J. Bremner © Humana Press Inc., Totowa, NJ

in men with testosterone deficiency. Hypogonadal adult men have greater deposition of central fat compared to age and body mass index (BMI)-matched eugonadal men *(1)*. In a study utilizing computed tomography (CT) scans to quantify site-specific adiposity, we showed that hypogonadism was associated with more subcutaneous fat deposition, and there was a trend for more visceral fat compared to eugonadal men *(1)*. In a study of 23 healthy men, serum testosterone and free-testosterone levels correlated negatively both with visceral fat deposition and insulin levels *(2)*. These data indicate that lower testosterone levels correlate with increases in fat mass, with specific deposition in the central sites. In a cohort of 511 men aged 30–79 yr in 1972–1974, Khaw et al. *(3)* assessed the impact of androgens on central adiposity, estimated 12 yr later using the waist–hip circumference ratio. Levels of androstenedione, testosterone, and sex hormone-binding globulin (SHBG) measured at baseline were inversely related to accumulation of central adiposity. This suggests that lower testosterone levels have a contributory role in promoting central fat accumulation. Because central adiposity is associated with heightened cardiovascular risk, these data suggest that hypogonadism may have important implications with regard to health *(4,5)*. There have been no studies clearly demonstrating a link between testosterone deficiency and cardiac events.

TESTOSTERONE ADMINISTRATION IN HYPOGONADAL MEN

Investigations into the effects of testosterone on body composition are based on prior evidence of the nitrogen-retaining properties of testosterone in castrate animals *(6)* and historical evidence for behavioral effects of testosterone substitution in animals *(7)*. There are several models used to determine the effects of hypogonadism and testosterone administration in hypogonadism on body composition in men. One model utilizes biochemical castration to assess the effects of abrupt testosterone withdrawal on body composition. In a study by Mauras et al. *(8)*, Lupron depot was administered to six healthy young men (mean age: 23 yr) for 10 wk. Using dual-energy X-ray analysis (DEXA), there was a 2.1-kg reduction in fat-free mass and a 1.1-kg increase in fat mass, without a significant change in weight. There was a significant decrease in whole-body proteolysis and whole-body protein synthesis, a trend for a reduction in lipid oxidation rates, and a reduction in skeletal muscle insulin-like growth factor (IGF)-1 mRNA expression. These data show that a reduction in serum testosterone to castrate levels in young men is associated with a change in body composition, including an increase in fat mass, a decrease in lean mass, and a decline in protein synthesis and growth factor production in skeletal muscle. There were no changes in serum growth hormone (GH) and IGF-1 values during this study, suggesting that the observed effects on body composition and metabolism were the result of changes in testosterone alone. These changes in adiposity and fat-free mass are similar to trends seen in men with modest to moderate hypogonadism *(1)*.

The effects of androgen administration on body composition in adult men with hypogonadism have been investigated in multiple, nonplacebo-controlled studies. Katznelson et al. *(9)* administered intramuscular testosterone enanthate for 18 mo to 29 adult men with acquired hypogonadism (median age: 57 yr) who had never previously received testosterone therapy. At baseline, there was more percent body fat, measured by bioelectrical impedance, in hypogonadal compared to control men. Percent body fat decreased by 14% following testosterone-replacement therapy. Comparison of CT scans in 13 men showed that following treatment, there was a significant increase in lean mass (6%) in the erector spinae muscles, a 12% ($p < 0.01$) reduction in subcutaneous fat, and a 6% ($p = 0.08$) decrease in visceral fat. Other studies of the effects of androgens on body composition have included male subjects who were washed out from previous testosterone replacement. Wang et al. *(10)* administered testosterone via a sublingual cyclodextrin to 67 hypogonadal men for 6 mo, and, using DEXA, showed that fat-free mass increased by 0.9 kg and fat mass did not change. The increase in regional lean mass in the legs reached statistical significance. Leg press muscle strength, assessed by the one-repetition method, increased by 6%, whereas there was no change in arm strength. The changes in lean mass did not correlate with changes in leg strength. Wang et al. *(11)* administered two doses of transdermal testosterone gel (Androgel, 5 and 10 g) vs transdermal testosterone patch (Androderm) to 227 adult hypogonadal men for 180 d and showed an increase in fat-free mass and a corresponding reduction in fat mass (by DEXA). In this study, lean body mass increased in the testosterone gel group by an average of 1.6–3.3 kg, largely a function of dose of the testosterone gel. There was a corresponding modest incremental increase in lean body mass (1.0 kg) in the Androderm group. These findings paralleled the serum testosterone levels achieved by the different treatment modalities. The C_{avg} of serum testosterone in the treatment groups following 90 d of transdermal testosterone application was as follows: Androderm, 11.8 ± 0.8 nmol/L; Androgel 5 g, 17.2 ± 1.2 nmol; Androgel 10 g, 25.9 ± 1.4 nmol/L. These studies show that testosterone therapy of male hypogonadism consistently results in changes in body composition, with an enhancement of lean mass and a reduction in fat mass. Differences in body composition findings between these studies may be a function of the serum testosterone levels achieved. For example, the sublingual testosterone preparation resulted in briefer daily exposure to normal serum testosterone levels and less dramatic body composition changes than with either Androgel or Androderm *(12)*.

In assessing the effects of testosterone-replacement therapy on body composition, it is important to delineate the effects of testosterone on different body compartments using multiple modalities of body composition analysis. Bhasin et al. *(13)* administered testosterone enanthate injections for 12 wk to seven hypogonadal men (age: 21–47 yr). Total-body weight increased by 4.5 kg, fat-free mass (measured by underwater weighing) increased significantly by 5.0 kg, and percent body fat did not change (*see* Fig. 1). Using the deuterium water dilution method, fat-free mass increased by 6 kg. Total-body water increased by 5.1 kg, although the percent water did not change. Fat mass, derived by the deuterium water method, did not change. Whole-body leucine turnover did not change following testosterone administration, although the cross-sectional area of the arm and leg muscles increased significantly (by magnetic resonance imaging [MRI] scan). This study showed that increases in lean body mass following testosterone therapy may be demonstrated using multiple techniques and that changes in body compartments may vary depending on the instrument used for measurement. The apparent lack of change in whole-body leucine turnover, a surrogate for protein dynamics, may reflect the relatively low level of testosterone-induced change in muscle protein synthesis that may be difficult to detect using whole-body protein studies. In addition, this study did not examine the effects of testosterone on extracellular water: testosterone therapy has been associated with changes in water that may affect body composition interpretation with instruments such as bioelectrical impedance or DEXA. Of note, testosterone-replacement therapy was associated with a 22% increase in muscle strength in the bench press,

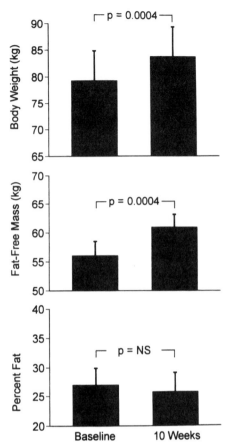

Fig. 1. Body weight, fat-free mass, and percent fat at baseline and after 10 wk of testosterone-replacement therapy in seven hypogonadal men. Data are presented as mean ± SEM. (From ref. *13*, reprinted with permission.)

assessed by the one-repetition method, and an increase in squat strength *(13)*. These data demonstrate that changes in body composition following testosterone-replacement therapy may be associated with enhanced strength.

To investigate the effects of testosterone administration on muscle protein synthesis and mass, Brodsky et al. *(14)* examined mixed skeletal muscle protein synthesis and substrate availability in five hypogonadal men aged 33–57 yr. Following 6 mo of biweekly testosterone cypionate injections (with dose adjustments based on serum levels), there was an 8.7-kg increase in fat-free mass and a 3.4-kg decrease in fat mass (by DEXA). The fractional synthesis rate of mixed skeletal muscle proteins increased significantly during testosterone treatment, as did the total muscle protein synthesis rate. There were no significant changes in levels of the major substrates for protein synthesis. These data show that the mechanism underlying the increase in muscle mass following testosterone-replacement therapy is, in part, the result of an increase in the synthesis of muscle proteins.

Differences in the absolute change in body composition measurements among the above studies probably reflect a combination of variability in the instruments used for measurements and levels of serum testosterone achieved. Changes in body water from testosterone substitution may affect fat-free mass analysis using bioelectrical impedance (a method that calculates fat and fat-free mass based on an estimated value for total-body water) and DEXA (a method that utilizes an estimated total-body-water value in fat-free mass calculations). Differential effects on water could lead to variability in measurements. Additionally, the largest changes in fat-free mass were observed in the study by Brodsky et al. *(14)*. The peak testosterone levels achieved by the biweekly testosterone intramuscular injections in this study were supraphysiologic. It is probable that a dose–response relationship between achieved testosterone levels and degree of change in fat and fat-free mass is responsible for these findings *(10–14)*.

With regard to the effects of testosterone administration on lipid profiles in hypogonadal men, most of the aforementioned studies have included measurement of plasma lipids before and after testosterone replacement. Modest reductions of high-density lipoprotein (HDL) cholesterol have been seen in some studies, although the clinical significance of these findings are unknown *(9,11)*. No other clear changes in lipid patterns have been described.

TESTOSTERONE ADMINISTRATION TO EUGONADAL MEN

Studies of the effects of testosterone on body composition in eugonadal men have led to important information with regard to changes in adiposity and lean body mass in the setting of pharmacologic testosterone administration. Effects of pharmacologic testosterone administration on body composition were shown by Forbes et al. *(15)* in an uncontrolled study of testosterone enanthate (3 mg/kg/wk) administration in seven healthy young men. Using ^{40}K (total-body potassium) measurements, the authors showed that there was a 12% increase in lean body mass and a 27% decline in body fat following 12 wk of testosterone treatment. Increments in urinary creatinine excretion suggested that the changes in muscle mass comprised most, if not all, of the increases in lean body mass. After discontinuation of testosterone, there was a decline in lean body mass, although after 5–6 mo, lean body mass remained higher than at baseline. These data suggest that pharmacologic testosterone administration may increase lean body mass and that these effects may be long lasting.

Welle et al. *(16)* administered testosterone enanthate at an approximate dose of 200 mg im every week for 3 mo to nine men (18–45 yr) with myotonic dystrophy. At baseline, subjects with myotonic dystrophy had approx 15 kg less lean body mass (measured by ^{40}K) compared to controls. Following 3 mo of testosterone administration, lean body mass increased by 4.9 kg (10%). These gains were maintained for 12 mo, although no further effects on lean body mass were observed. Basal metabolic rate increased by 10% during the 3 mo in the treated subjects. In this sarcopenic population, pharmacologic testosterone administration resulted in significant effects on lean body mass. Strength and performance were not measured in this study.

Administration of testosterone at pharmacologic doses to middle-aged men leads to changes in lean mass and selective alterations in site-specific adipose deposition. Marin et al. *(17)* randomized 25 men > 45 yr of age and the average BMI of 29 mg/kg^2 to either 80 mg testosterone undecanoate twice daily or placebo for 8 mo. Visceral fat (measured by abdominal CT scan) decreased by 0.4 kg ($p < 0.05$), whereas subcutaneous fat did not change following testosterone treatment. Lean body mass, measured by ^{40}K, did not change during treatment. The glucose disappearance rate increased by approx 20% in the treatment group only, suggesting that the reduction in visceral fat contributed to enhanced insulin sensitivity and that testosterone treatment may lead to improvements in cardio-vascular risk. Mean prostate volume increased by 12%, although serum prostate-specific antigen (PSA) and urine flow measurements did not change. Despite the increase in prostate volume, the PSA and functional assessments were reassuring with regard to prostate risks following pharmacologic testosterone treatment. To determine further whether testosterone may have selective effects on adipose metabolism, Marin et al. *(18)* administered 250 mg testosterone enanthate im 5 d prior to laparotomy for benign con-ditions in 17 middle-aged men. Lipid assimilation was measured with labeled oleic acid, administered 24 h prior to surgery, and adipose tissue biopsies of subcutaneous abdomi-nal, omental, and retroperitoneal tissues were collected during surgery. Compared to controls, there was a marked reduction in lipid uptake in the omental and retroperitoneal tissues, without change in lipid uptake in the subcutaneous fat. These data suggest that there may be differential androgen regulation of adipose tissue at different sites that may explain the above-described regional testosterone effects on adipose tissue *(17)*.

Because of these effects of testosterone on body composition, there has been wide-spread use of androgenic compounds by athletes based on the presumption that andro-gens will promote lean body mass *(19)*. Despite this intense use of androgens by athletes and bodybuilders, studies demonstrating beneficial androgen effects on body composi-tion have been controversial. Most of the earlier studies were neither blinded nor placebo controlled, were of insufficient treatment duration, or included interventions with exer-cise that were nonstandardized *(20)*. Additionally, athletes were often noncompliant with study procedures *(21,22)*. Therefore, although anabolic androgen use is pervasive, most studies either showed no effect or were controversial in interpretation.

To address this issue further, Bhasin et al. *(23)* investigated the effects of pharmacologic testosterone administration and resistance exercise on body composition and muscle strength in young healthy men. The men were randomized to four groups: placebo, no exercise; testosterone, no exercise; placebo plus exercise; testosterone plus exercise. Testosterone enanthate (600 mg im) vs placebo was administered weekly for 10 wk. Supervised strength training was performed 3 d/wk, and diets were standardized for protein and caloric intake. Testosterone administration alone resulted in increases in quadriceps area (measured by MRI) compared to placebo. The combination of testosterone and exercise produced greater gains in fat-free mass (9.5%, by DEXA) and muscle size (14.7% in triceps area and 14% in quadriceps area) than either placebo or exercise alone, and greater gains in muscle strength (24% in bench press strength and 39% in squat exercise capacity) than in either nonexercising group. Fat mass in the testosterone-treatment groups did not change. Safety studies showed no change in liver enzyme levels, serum PSA, prostate size, or morphology by digital rectal exam or hematocrit during the 10 wk. This study demonstrates that supraphysiologic test-osterone administration, especially when combined with strength training, increases fat-free mass, muscle size, and strength in normal men.

Griggs et al. *(24)* administered testosterone enanthate (3 mg/kg, im weekly) in a nonplacebo-controlled manner to nine healthy, eugonadal subjects aged 19–40 yr. Fol-lowing 12 wk of testosterone supplementation, lean body mass (measured by ^{40}K) increased by 12% and muscle mass (estimated by urinary creatinine excretion) increased by 20%. Muscle protein synthesis increased by 27%, suggesting that the increases in skeletal muscle were the result of anabolic effects on protein synthesis.

In summary, these studies, along with others *(25)*, show that administration of testosterone at supraphysiologic doses to normal men can lead to increases in lean body mass and reductions in fat mass. Supraphysiologic testosterone administration may result in some increases in strength, although more significant effects on strength are achieved in the setting of a combined exercise program *(23)*. Further studies are necessary to determine the potential adverse effects of supraphysiologic testosterone use on the prostate gland, hepatic function, lipids, and erythrocytosis.

The effects of testosterone on muscle mass are the result of increased muscle protein synthesis, as determined by infusion of stable leucine isotope infusions and muscle biopsies *(24)*. Effects of testosterone on whole-body protein synthesis using leucine flux experiments have been unremarkable, perhaps because of the relative low level of muscle protein synthesis vs total-body synthesis *(23,24)*.

ARE THERE APPLICATIONS OF TESTOSTERONE IN CHRONIC ILLNESS?

Because of the effects of testosterone in enhancing fat-free mass and muscle size, it has been suggested that there may be a role for testosterone in promoting lean body mass in catabolic states. In addition to aging, chronic illnesses such as HIV infection, chronic renal failure, and chronic obstructive lung disease are associated with testosterone deficiency, as are subjects receiving long-term supraphysiologic glucocorticoid administration *(26–28)*. These situations are also associated with muscle loss, suggesting a role for testosterone administration in promoting muscle mass and, potentially, muscle function in these situations.

Elderly Men and Sarcopenia: A Role for Testosterone?

Aging is associated with specific alterations in body composition. There is an approx 33% reduction in muscle mass between the ages of 30 and 80 yr, and this loss increases to 1% per year after the age of 70 yr *(29)*. This sarcopenia leads to diminished strength and function. Isometric and dynamic maximal voluntary strength of the quadriceps muscles decreases after the age of 50 yr and there is an approx 30% decrease in strength between 50 and 70 yr *(30)*. Muscle weakness is a common feature in elderly subjects who fall, a common cause of accidental injury and fracture in the elderly *(31,32)*. Aging is also associated with an increase in general adiposity, with specific deposition in the central, visceral area *(33,34)*. Because central adiposity is associated with hyperinsulinemia and enhanced cardiovascular risk, it is important to determine whether there are factors that may underlie these changes in body composition that may be reversible.

Multiple studies have demonstrated a decrease in serum testosterone levels in men with age *(35–37)*, although others have not *(38)*. Mean testosterone levels in men aged 80 yr are approx 60% of the level for men 25–50 yr *(39)*. The similarity of changes in muscle composition between castrate animals, hypogonadal men, and aging men suggests a role for relative hypogonadism in the decline of muscle composition/performance and the increase in adipose stores in the elderly *(40)*. In a community-based study of 775 older men, impaired glucose tolerance, assessed by oral glucose tolerance test (OGTT), and fasting plasma glucose were associated with lower total-testosterone levels *(41)*. These data suggest that relative testosterone insufficiency in elderly men may be associated with heightened cardiovascular risk.

There have been several studies evaluating the effects of testosterone replacement on body composition in elderly men. These studies have included subjects with serum testosterone or free-testosterone values below that of younger men, in order to address the hypothesis that raising levels into the midrange of younger men may have beneficial effects on body composition. Sih et al. *(42)* administered testosterone cypionate (200 mg) biweekly in a randomized, placebo-controlled study to 32 subjects for 12 mo. There were no differences in body fat (measured by bioelectrical impedance), but there was an increase in hand-grip strength. Tenover *(43)* administered testosterone enanthate (100 mg im, every week) vs placebo injections to 13 men > 56 yr of age in a crossover design study for 3 mo. In this study, testosterone treatment resulted in a 1.8-kg increase in lean mass (assessed by hydrostatic weighing) compared to placebo, and an increase in weight by 1.5 kg. In a randomized, double-blind placebo-controlled study of testosterone administration via scrotal patches in 108 men aged > 65 yr for 3 yr, testosterone treatment was associated with a 1.7-kg increase in lean mass (by DEXA) and a 2.3-kg reduction in fat mass *(44)* *(see* Fig. 2). In this study, there was no change in physical function and knee strength. These studies show that testosterone administration in elderly men leads to increases in lean body mass. Similar magnitudes of change in lean body mass were detected in the studies utilizing DEXA vs hydrostatic weighing for body composition measurement *(43)*. It is currently unknown whether these changes in lean body mass result in any clinical benefit with regard to physical function. In one study, testosterone administration (testosterone enanthate 100 mg im, every week) for 4 wk to six healthy elderly men resulted in an increase in muscle strength as assessed by isokinetic dynamometry and an increase in skeletal muscle protein synthesis *(45)*. It is not clear why increases in strength were noted in this study compared to the study by Snyder et al. *(44)*, but differences in study design, including study duration and lack of a placebo arm, may explain these findings. Although testosterone administration leads to a decrease in fat mass *(44)*, there are no studies in elderly men that assess the effects of testosterone on site-specific fat deposition. Additionally, there are no studies that demonstrate that testosterone administration leads to a reduction in cardiovascular risk in elderly men. Further studies are necessary to determine the potential benefits of testosterone repletion on physical function and cardiovascular risk in elderly men.

Despite the beneficial findings, there are potential long-term adverse consequences of testosterone that need to be considered with elderly men. The major concern regards prostate health. It has been reassuring that, in the longer-term studies, testosterone repletion has not been associated with an increase in prostate events, including bladder outlet obstruction, elevated PSA values, or detection of prostate cancer *(42,46)*. Erythrocytosis has also been detected *(42,46)*. Additionally, no consistent pattern of change in lipid profile has been demonstrated. Further long-term studies are critical for determining the long-term risks of testosterone administration to elderly men before consideration of widescale use in this population.

HIV-Infected Men: Use of Testosterone

The most common endocrine abnormality in HIV-infected individuals is testosterone deficiency, which is found in 25–60% of HIV-infected men *(47-49)*. Additionally, SHBG levels may be elevated by 39–51% in HIV-infected men, leading to further decreases in serum free-testosterone levels *(50)*. Testosterone deficiency is more prevalent among subjects who are more symptomatic from HIV, including men with a lower CD4 cell count, later stage of illness, and acquired immunodeficiency syndrome (AIDS) wasting syndrome (AWS) *(50)*. The AWS is characterized by progressive weight loss and a

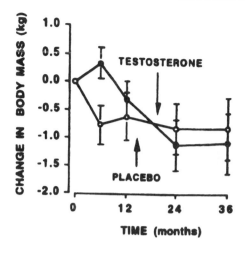

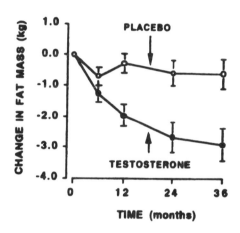

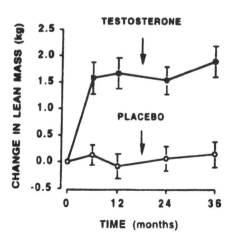

Fig. 2. Mean (±SE) change from baseline in total-body mass, fat mass, and lean mass as determined by DEXA in 108 elderly men treated with either testosterone or placebo. The decrease in fat mass and the increase in lean mass in the testosterone-treated subjects were different from those in the placebo treated subjects at 36 mo ($p < 0.05$). (From ref. *44*, reprinted with permission.)

disproportionate decline in lean body mass compared to fat mass, and it is associated with diminished survival *(52)*. Recent studies suggest a link between a decline in androgen levels in men with progressive AIDS and weight loss. Approximately half of HIV-infected men with AWS are hypogonadal *(53)*. In a nested case-control study of HIV-infected men, Dobs et al. *(54)* showed that weight loss was associated with a decline in bioavailable testosterone, and, once wasting was evident, there was a decline in total, free, and bioavailable testosterone. Furthermore, Grinspoon et al. *(55)* investigated androgen levels and body composition (using ^{40}K, DEXA, and 24-h urinary creatinine) in 20 hypogonadal men with AWS. In this study, lean body mass, muscle mass, and deterioration in exercise functional capacity correlated with serum testosterone levels. These data indicate that hypogonadism is common in HIV-infected men, and a decline in androgen levels correlate with weight loss, lean mass, and AWS. This suggests that testosterone insufficiency contributes to the sarcopenia of AWS and subsequent muscle dysfunction.

There have been several investigations into the effects of testosterone supplementation on body composition and muscle function in HIV-infected men *(56)*. Bhasin et al. *(57)* administered Androderm transdermal patches 10 mg/d in a randomized, double-blind, placebo-controlled study for 12 wk to hypogonadal (serum testosterone < 400 ng/dL) HIV-infected men without weight loss. Following testosterone administration, there was a significant increase in fat-free mass (using DEXA) by 1.4 kg, although the change in fat-free mass was not significantly different between the two treatment groups. There were no significant changes in total-body weight, strength (using 1-RM), or in Karnofsky performance scores. These data suggest that testosterone administration to hypogonadal HIV-infected men may result in an increase in lean body mass. In a study aimed at investigating the effects of testosterone administration on weight, quality of life, and muscle strength, Coodley and Coodley *(58)* administered testosterone cypionate (200 mg im, every 2 wk) for 12 wk to 39 HIV-infected men with >5% weight loss. The study subjects were not screened for serum androgen levels as inclusion criteria, although the authors state that, of those subjects with sera available at baseline for measurement, most of the patients were testosterone deficient. Following 3 mo, there was no difference in weight, although there was significant improvement in overall well-being and a tendency toward increased muscle strength. In another study involving open-label testosterone administration at a mildly pharmacologic dose followed by a 12-wk placebo-controlled phase, testosterone therapy (testosterone cypionate 400 mg im, every 2 wk) to HIV-infected men with serum testosterone <500 ng/dL resulted in an increase in weight by 3.7 lbs and mood *(59)*. Although these studies show that testosterone replacement may lead to an improvement in quality of life, there is still question as to whether testosterone supplementation may result in a significant reversal of weight loss seen with progressive HIV-infection associated with hypogonadism.

The effects of testosterone supplementation on body composition in subjects with overt AWS were investigated by Grinspoon et al. *(60)*. In this study, intramuscular testosterone enanthate (300 mg im, every 3 wk) was administered in a randomized double-blind placebo-controlled trial to 51 men with AWS and low serum free-testosterone values for 6 mo. Lean body mass (^{40}K), fat-free mass (DEXA), and muscle mass (24-h urinary creatinine excretion) were measured. Compared with placebo, testosterone-treated subjects significantly gained fat-free mass (1.8 kg), lean body mass (1.9 kg), and muscle mass (1.6 kg). There was no change in weight, exercise performance, viral load, or CD4 counts. These data suggest that, at least over 6 mo, testosterone-replacement therapy to men with AWS results in clear increases in lean and muscle mass, without a corresponding change in weight. In another study, testosterone administration increased muscle strength using the 1-RM method in 61 HIV-infected, hypogonadal men with weight loss randomized to testosterone enanthate (100 mg/wk) vs placebo for 16 wk (61). These studies show that testosterone-replacement therapy in HIV-infected, hypogonadal men with weight loss results in an increase in lean body mass and, depending on the strength outcome measure utilized, an increase in strength. No clear effects on physical function have been determined. In eugonadal, HIV-infected men with weight loss, pharmacologic testosterone therapy is more potent in increasing muscle mass, fat free mass, and strength (62,63). A potential concern of use of pharmacologic androgen administration in HIV-infected eugonadal men is the effect on lipid profile, as a decrease in HDL cholesterol levels may be seen (63). The long-term implications of these changes in body composition on function and survival need to be determined.

TESTOSTERONE AND WOMEN: ENDOGENOUS EFFECTS AND POTENTIAL USES

The relationship between testosterone and adipose distribution, including the correlation with endogenous testosterone levels and the effects of exogenous testosterone on visceral and subcutaneous fat depots, differs between men and women. As described earlier, abdominal obesity in men is associated with lower serum testosterone values, and testosterone administration to men may lead to reductions in both subcutaneous and visceral fat (1,9,17). In contrast, cross-sectional studies indicate that, in women, central fat accumulation, such as described by the waist-to-hip ratio, correlates with higher testosterone levels (64,65). There are several models in women that are useful in the consideration of the interaction of androgens and body composition.

1. In conditions of hyperandrogenism, such as polycystic ovarian syndrome (PCOS), there is a preponderance of central, visceral fat (65–67). The relative hyperandrogenism in PCOS is presumably the result of enhanced testosterone secretion by the ovaries and is associated with hyperinsulinemia. This association suggests that hyperandrogenism may contribute to visceral fat accumulation and subsequent hyperinsulinemia.
2. Another model useful in considering the effects of androgens on body composition in women is that of testosterone administration in female-to-male transsexuals. Elbers et al. (67) administered intramuscular testosterone esters every 2 wk to 10 nonobese, ovariectomized female to male transsexuals (mean age: 24 yr). Following 1 yr of testosterone administration, there was a significant reduction in subcutaneous fat, without change in visceral fat area, assessed by abdominal MRI scan. After 3 yr of testosterone treatment, there were no further effects on subcutaneous fat, but there was a 47% increase in visceral fat. Anabolic effects on skeletal muscle were detected, as evidenced by a 13% increase in muscle area at the level of the thigh within 1 yr. In a follow-up study, the same research group administered intramuscular testosterone esters every 2 wk to 20 female-to-male transsexuals for 12 mo (68). The findings in this study were similar, but a statistically significant increase in visceral fat (using MRI scan) was detected within 1 yr.
3. Menopause is associated with an approx 50% reduction in circulating testosterone levels (70). This decrement results from disruption of ovarian secretion of testosterone and ovarian and adrenal secretion of androstenedione, which is converted to testosterone. There has been much interest in investigating the utility of androgen replacement in postmenopausal women for improvement in quality of life and libido (71,72), but there

have been additional interesting findings with regard to effects on body composition. In a randomized trial, Lovejoy et al. *(40)* administered the anabolic androgen nandrolone (ND), spironolactone (SP), or placebo for 9 mo to 30 postmenopausal, obese women who underwent concurrent dietary management. All subjects lost weight during the study, and lean body mass (by DEXA) decreased in the SP and placebo groups. In contrast, lean body mass increased by approx 3 kg in the ND group. Additional body composition measurements were made with CT scans. There was a 10% increase in thigh muscle area in the ND group, without change in the other groups. The ND group also preferentially lost subcutaneous fat and gained visceral fat. In contrast, the SP and placebo groups lost visceral and subcutaneous fat, demonstrating the effects of androgens on visceral obesity in this population.

In another study, 33 postmenopausal women were randomized to receive implants of either estradiol (E) alone or estradiol combined with testosterone (E+T) *(73)*. Following 2 yr of treatment, there was no difference in total fat mass (by DEXA) between the groups *(73)*. However, there was an increase of 3.1 kg in fat free mass in the E+T group only. Additionally, there was an increase in intra-abdominal fat in the E+T group; the abdominal fat mass to fat free mass ratio declined in the E group but not the E+T group. Therefore, testosterone administration increased both fat-free mass and central adiposity.

These data indicate that endogenous testosterone or testosterone administration is associated with increased central fat accumulation, a situation in contrast to that of men. It is largely unknown whether these androgenic effects on body composition will enhance cardiovascular risk in women. The physiologic mechanisms underlying these findings are unclear. Differences between gender with regard to adipose distribution may stem from the importance of endogenous estrogens and the protective effect of estrogens on androgenic effects by downregulating androgen receptors *(74)*. The above-described findings in transsexuals and menopausal women were found largely in the setting of surgical or natural menopause, a situation without the potential protective effect of estrogen on androgen effects. There may also be differences in postreceptor regulatory effects of androgens in male and female adipose tissue *(75)*. Other reasons for the contrasting findings of the effects of androgens on adiposity between men and women may inclue variability in adipose tissue androgen-receptor density and the contribution of progesterone and cortisol to adipose tissue metabolism *(74)*.

There has been recent interest in the effects of androgens on body composition in HIV-infected women with AWS. Serum total and free-testosterone levels are lower in HIV-infected women compared to healthy women *(76)*. Androgen deficiency is highly prevalent among women with AWS and may result from undernutrition, illness, and/or HIV disease of the hypothalamic–pituitary–gonadal axis *(77)*. It has, therefore, been hypothesized that androgen administration may have beneficial effects on body composition in such women, although there are limited data in this regard *(78)*. In a randomized, double-blind, placebo-controlled trial in 53 women with AWS, Miller et al. *(79)* administered two doses of transdermal testosterone (to deliver 150 μg and 300 μg/d) vs placebo for 12 wk. The largest increase in body weight was in the 150-μg testosterone group (1.9 kg), and the largest increase in fat-free mass was in the 300-μg group. The discrepancy between the testosterone doses and the changes in body composition were unexplained. Clearly, further studies are necessary to determine the potential uses of androgens in modulating the body composition changes associated with AWS in women.

CONCLUSIONS

In men, testosterone deficiency is associated with a decrease in lean body mass and an increase in central fat stores. Testosterone-replacement therapy leads to an increase in lean body mass and a reduction in adiposity in hypogonadal men. These effects may be dosage related; hypogonadal or testosterone-sufficient subjects who receive supraphysiologic testosterone doses have more pronounced changes in lean and fat mass than men receiving physiologic testosterone replacement. Similarly, modest increases in certain measures of strength have been reported in studies of testosterone replacement therapy. Recent data suggest that higher doses of testosterone may lead to more profound changes in strength, particularly if coupled with a resistance exercise program. There may be a use for testosterone administration in subjects with sarcopenia resulting from catabolic states, although the long-term benefit-to-risk ratios need to be elucidated further.

REFERENCES

1. Katznelson L, Rosenthal DI, Rosol MS, et al. Using quantitative CT to assess adipose distribution in adult men with acquired hypogonadism. Am J Roentgenol 1998;170:423–427.
2. Seidell JC, Bjorntorp P, Sjostrom L, et al. Visceral fat accumulation in men is positively associated with insulin, glucose, and C-peptide levels, but negatively with testosterone levels. Metab: Clin Exp 1990;39:897–901.
3. Khaw KT, Barrett-Connor E. Lower endogenous androgens predict central adiposity in men. Ann Epidemiol 1992;2:675–682.
4. Simon D, Charles M, Nahoul K, et al. Association between plasma total testosterone and cardiovascular risk factors in healthy adult men: the Telecom study. J Clin Endocrinol Metab 1997;82:682–685.
5. Kissebah AH, Vydelingum N, Murray R, et al. Relation of body fat distribution to metabolic complications of obesity. J Clin Endocrinol Metab 1982;54:254–260.
6. Kochakian CD. Comparison of protein anabolic properties of various androgens in the castrated rat. Am J Physiol 1950;60:553–558.
7. Berthold AA. The transplantation of testes. Arch Anat Physiol Med 1849;42–46.
8. Mauras N, Hayes V, Welch S, et al. Testosterone deficiency in young men: marked alterations in whole body protein kinetics, strength, and adiposity. J Clin Endocrinol Metab 1998;83:1886–1892.
9. Katznelson L, Finkelstein JS, Schoenfeld DA, et al. Increase in bone density and lean body mass during testosterone administration in men with acquired hypogonadism. J Clin Endocrinol Metab 1996;81:4358–4365.
10. Wan, C, Eyre DR, Clark R, et al. Sublingual testosterone replacement improves muscle mass and strength, decreases bone resorption, and increases bone formation markers in hypogonadal men: a clinical research center study. J Clin Endocrinol Metab 1996;81:3654–3662.
11. Wang C, Swedloff RS, Iranmanesh A, et al. Transdermal testosterone gel improves sexual function, mood, muscle strength, and body composition parameters in hypogonadal men. Testosterone Gel Study Group. J Clin Endocrinol Metab 2000;85:2839–2853.
12. Salehian B, Wang C, Alexander G, et al. Pharmacokinetics, bioefficacy, and safety of sublingual testosterone cyclodextrin in hypogonadal men: comparison to testosterone enanthate—a clinical research center study. J Clin Endocrinol Metab 1995;80:3567–3575.
13. Bhasin S, Storer TW, Berman N, et al. Testosterone replacement increases fat-free mass and muscle size in hypogonadal men. J Clin Endocrinol Metab 1997;82:407–413.
14. Brodsky IG, Balagopal P, Nair KS. Effects of testosterone replacement on muscle mass and muscle protein synthesis in hypogonadal men-a clinical research center study. J Clin Endocrinol Metab 1996;81:3469–3475.
15. Forbes GB, Porta CR, Herr BE, Griggs, RC. Sequence of changes in body composition induced by testosterone and reversal of changes after drug is stopped (see comments). JAMA 1992;267:397–399.
16. Welle S, Jozefowicz R, Forbes G, Griggs RC. Effect of testosterone on metabolic rate and body composition in normal men and men with muscular dystrophy. J Clin Endocrinol Metab 1992;74:332–335.
17. Marin P, Holmang S, Jonsson L, et al. The effects of testosterone treatment on body composition and metabolism in middle-aged obese men. Int J Obes 1992;16:991–997.

18. Marin P, Lonn L, Andersson B, et al. Assimilation of triglycerides in subcutaneous and intra-abdominal adipose tissues in vivo in men: effects of testosterone. J Clin Endocrinol Metab 1996; 81:1018–1022.

19. Anonymous. American College of Sports Medicine. Position stand on the use of anabolic-androgenic steroids in sports. Sports Med Bull 1984;19:13–15.

20. Crist DM, Stackpole PJ, Peake GT. Effects of androgenic-anabolic steroids on neuromuscular power and body composition. J Appl Physiol 1983;54:366–370.

21. Freed DL, Banks AJ, Longson D, Burley DM. Anabolic steroids in athelics: crossover double-blind trial on weightlifters. Br Med J 1975;2:471–473.

22. Wilson JD. Androgen abuse by athletes. Endocr Rev 1988;9:181–199.

23. Bhasin S, Storer TW, Berman N, et al. The effects of supraphysiologic doses of testosterone on muscle size and strength in normal men (see comments). N Engl J Med 1996;335:1–7.

24. Griggs RC, Kingston W, Jozefowicz RF, et al. Effect of testosterone on muscle mass and muscle protein synthesis. J Appl Physiol 1989;66:498–503.

25. Young NR, Baker HW, Liu G, Seeman E. Body composition and muscle strength in healthy men receiving testosterone enanthate for contraception. J Clin Endocrinol Metab 1993;77:1028–1032.

26. Handelsman DJ, Dong Q. Hypothalamo-pituitary gonadal axis in chronic renal failure. Endocrinol Metab Clin North Am 1993;22:145–161.

27. Handelsman DJ. Hypothalamic-pituitary gonadal dysfunction in renal failure, dialysis and renal trans-plantation. Endocr Rev 1985;6:151–182.

28. Casaburi R. Rationale for anabolic therapy to facilitate rehabilitation in COPD. Baillieres Clin Endocrinol Metab 1998;12:407–418.

29. Tzankoff SP, Norris AH. Effect of muscle mass decrease on age-related BMR changes. J Appl Physiol: Respir Environ Exer Physiol 1977;43:1001–1006.

30. Larsson L, Grimby G, Karlsson J. Muscle strength and speed of movement in relation to age and muscle morphology. J Appl Physiol 1979;46:451–456.

31. Baker SP, Harvey AH. Fall injuries in the elderly. Clin Geriatr Med 1985;1:501–512.

32. Rubenstein LZ, Robbins AS, Josephson KR, et al. The value of assessing falls in an elderly population. A randomized clinical trial. Ann Intern Med 1990;113:308–316.

33. Borkan GA, Hults DE, Gerzof SG, et al. Age changes in body composition revealed by computed tomography. J Gerontol 1983;38:673–637.

34. Borkan GA, Hults DE, Gerzof SG, Robbins AH. Comparison of body composition in middle-aged and elderly males using computed tomography. Am J Phys Anthropol 1985;66:289–295.

35. Deslypere J, Vermeulen A. Leydig cell function in normal men: effect of age, life-style, residence, diet, and activity. J Clin Endocrinol Metab 1984;59:955–962.

36. Gray A, Feldman HA, McKinlay JB, Longcope C. Age, disease, and changing sex hormone levels in middle-aged men: results of the Massachusetts male aging study. J Clin Endocrinol Metab 1991;73:1016–1025.

37. Vermeulen A. Androgens in the aging male. J Clin Endocrinol Metab 1991;73:221–224.

38. Harman SM, Tsitouras PD. Reproductive hormones in aging men. I. Measurement of sex steroids, basal luteinizing hormone, and leydig cell response to human chorionic gonadotropin. J Clin Endocrinol Metab 1980;51:35–40.

39. Vermeulen A, Rubens R, Verdonck L. Testosterone secretion and metabolism in male senescense. J Clin Endocrinol Metab 1972;34:730–735.

40. Lovejoy JC, Bray GA, Bourgeois MO, et al. Exogenous androgens influence body composition and regional body fat distribution in obese postmenopausal women—a clinical research center study. pJ Clin Endocrinol Metab 1996;81:2198–2203.

41. Goodman-Gruen D, Barrett-Connor E. Sex differences in the association of endogenous sex hormone levels and glucose tolerance status in older men and women. Diabetes Care 2000;23:912–918.

42. Sih R, Morley JE, Kaiser FE, et al. Testosterone replacement in older hypogonadal men: a 12-month randomized controlled trial. J Clin Endocrinol Metab 1997;82:1661–1667.

43. Tenover JS. Effects of testosterone supplementation in the aging male. J Clin Endocrinol Metab 1992;75:1092–1098.

44. Snyder PJ, Peachey H, Hannoush P, et al. Effect of testosterone treatment on body composition and muscle strength in men over 65 years of age. J Clin Endocrinol Metab 1999;84:2647–2653.

45. Urban RJ, Bodenburg YH, Gilkison C, et al. Testosterone administration to elderly men increases skeletal muscle strength and protein synthesis. Am J Physiol 1995;269:E820–E826.

46. Snyder PJ, Peachey H, Hannoush P, et al. Effect of testosterone treatment on bone mineral density in men over 65 years of age. J Clin Endocrinol Metab 1999;84:1966–1972.

47. Croxson TS, Chapman WE, Miller LK, et al. Changes in the hypothalamic-pituitary-gonadal axis in human immunodeficiency virus-infected homosexual men. J Clin Endocrinol Metab 1989;68:317–321.

48. Coodley GO, Loveless MO, Nelson HD, Coodley MK. Endocrine function in the HIV wasting syndrome. J Acquired Immune Defic Syndrome 1994;7:46–51.

49. Raffi F, Brisseau JM, Planchon B, et al. Endocrine function in 98 HIV-infected patients: a prospective study. AIDS 1991;5:729–733.

50. Martin ME, Benassayag C, Amiel C, et al. Alterations in the concentrations and binding properties of sex steroid binding protein and corticosteroid-binding globulin in HIV+patients. J Endocrinol Invest 1992;15:597–603.

51. Wagner G, Rabkin JG, Rabkin R. Illness stage, concurrent medications, and other correlates of low testosterone in men with HIV illness. J Acquired Immune Defic Syndrome Hum Retrovirol 1995;8:204–207.

52. Kotler DP, Tierney AR, Wang J, Pierson RN Jr. Magnitude of body-cell-mass depletion and the timing of death from wasting in AIDS. Am J Clin Nutr 1989;50:444–447.

53. Dobs AS, Dempsey MA, Ladenson PW, Polk BF. Endocrine disorders in men infected with human immunodeficiency virus. Am J Med 1988;84:611–616.

54. Dobs AS, Few WL 3rd, Blackman MR, et al. Serum hormones in men with human immunodeficiency virus-associated wasting. J Clin Endocrinol Metab 1996;81:4108–4112.

55. Grinspoon S, Corcoran C, Lee K, et al. Loss of lean body and muscle mass correlates with androgen levels in hypogonadal men with acquired immunodeficiency syndrome and wasting. J Clin Endocrinol Metab 1996;81:4051–4058.

56. Cofrancesco J Jr, Whalen JJ, 3rd Dobs AS. Testosterone replacement treatment options for HIV-infected men. J Acquired Immune Defic Syndrome Hum Retrovirol 1997;16:254–265.

57. Bhasin S, Storer TW, Asbel-Sethi N, et al. Effects of testosterone replacement with a nongenital, transdermal system, Androderm, in human immunodeficiency virus-infected men with low testosterone levels. J Clin Endocrinol Metab 1998;83:3155–3162.

58. Coodley GO, Coodley MK. A trial of testosterone therapy for HIV-associated weight loss. AIDS 1997;11:1347–1352.

59. Rabkin JG, Wagner GJ, Rabkin R. Testosterone therapy for human immunodeficiency virus-positive men with and without hypogonadism. J Clin Psychopharmacol 1999;19:19–27.

60. Grinspoon S, Corcoran C, Askari H, et al. Effects of androgen administration in men with the AIDS wasting syndrome. A randomized, double-blind, placebo-controlled trial. Ann Intern Med 1998;129:18–26.

61. Bhasin S, Storer TW, Javanbakht M, et al. Testosterone replacement and resistance exercise in HIV-infected men with weight loss and low testosterone levels. JAMA 2000;283:763–770.

62. Strawford A, Barbieri T, Van Loan M, et al. Resistance exercise and supraphysiologic androgen therapy in eugonadal men with HIV-related weight loss: a randomized controlled trial. JAMA 1999;281:1282–1290.

63. Grinspoon S, Corcoran C, Parlman K, et al. Effects of testosterone and progressive resistance training in eugonadal men with AIDS wasting. A randomized, controlled trial. Ann Intern Med 2000;133:348–355.

64. Espeland MA, Stefanick ML, Kritz-Silverstein D, et al. Effect of postmenopausal hormone therapy on body weight and waist and hip girths. Postmenopausal Estrogen–Progestin Interventions Study Investigators. J Clin Endocrinol Metab 1997;82:1549–1556.

65. Evans DJ, Barth JH, Burke CW. Body fat topography in women with androgen excess. Int J Obes 1988;12:157–162.

66. Kirschner MA, Samojlik E, Drejka M, et al. Androgen-estrogen metabolism in women with upper body versus lower body obesity. J Clin Endocrinol Metab 1990;70:473–479.

67. Rebuffe-Scrive M, Cullberg G, Lundberg PA, et al. Anthropometric variables and metabolism in polycystic ovarian disease. Horm Metab Res 1989;21:391–397.

68. Elbers JMH, Asscheman H, Seidell JC, et al. Long-term testosterone administration increases visceral fat in female to male transsexuals. J Clin Endocrinol Metab 1997;82:2044–2047.

69. Elbers JM, Asscheman H, Seidell JC, Gooren LJ. Effects of sex steroid hormones on regional fat depots as assessed by magnetic resonance imaging in transsexuals. Am J Physiol 1999;276:E317–E325.

70. Judd HL. Hormonal dynamics associated with the menopause. Clin Obstet Gynecol 1976;19:775–788.

71. Davis SR, McCloud P, Strauss BJ, Burger H. Testosterone enhances estradiol's effects on postmeno-pausal bone density and sexuality. Maturitas 1995;21:227–236.
72. Barrett-Connor E, Young R, Notelovitz M, et al. A two-year, double-blind comparison of estrogen-androgen and conjugated estrogens in surgically menopausal women. Effects on bone mineral density, symptoms and lipid profiles. J Reprod Med 1999;44:1012–1020.
73. Davis SR, Walker KZ, Strauss BJ. Effects of estradiol with and without testosterone on body compo-sition and relationships with lipids in postmenopausal women. Menopause 2000;7:395–401.
74. Bjorntorp P. The regulation of adipose tissue distribution in humans. Int J Obes Relat Metab Disord 1996;20:291–302.
75. De Pergola G, Holmang A, Svedberg J, et al. Testosterone treatment of ovariectomized rats: effects on lipolysis regulation in adipocytes. Acta Endocrinol (Copenh) 1990;123:61–66.
76. Sinha-Hikim I, Arver S, Beall G, et al. The use of a sensitive equilibrium dialysis method for the measurement of free testosterone levels in healthy, cycling women and in human immunodeficiency virus-infected women. J Clin Endocrinol Metab 1998;83:1312–1318.
77. Grinspoon S, Corcoran C, Miller K, et al. Body composition and endocrine function in women with acquired immunodeficiency syndrome wasting. J Clin Endocrinol Metab 1997;82:1332–1337.
78. Javanbakht M, Singh AB, Mazer NA, et al. Pharmacokinetics of a novel testosterone matrix transdermal system in healthy, premenopausal women and women infected with the human immunodeficiency virus. J Clin Endocrinol Metab 2000;85:2395–2401.
79. Miller K, Corcoran C, Armstrong C, et al. Transdermal testosterone administration in women with acquired immunodeficiency syndrome wasting: a pilot study. J Clin Endocrinol Metab 1998;83:2717–2725.

14 Androgens and Sexual Function in Men and Women

John Bancroft, MD

CONTENTS

INTRODUCTION
ANDROGENS IN MEN
ANDROGENS IN WOMEN
COMPARISON OF ANDROGEN EFFECTS IN MEN AND WOMEN
REFERENCES

INTRODUCTION

The role of androgens in the sexual differentiation of male and female anatomical development is relatively clear. The evidence for a role for androgens in the masculinization of certain aspects of behavior is persuasive. Androgenic activation of sexual behavior, the subject of this chapter, is relatively clear for males, but much less clear for females. However, the idea that testosterone (T) is the "libido hormone" for women as well as men has been around for some time. There has been an upsurge of interest in the role of androgens in women's sexuality in the last 2–3 yr, particularly in the United States, fueled by the recent availability of new methods of testosterone administration to women. A careful, critical review of the literature is therefore timely. The male will be considered first, with some consideration of key issues at the end of that section. The evidence on the female will then be reviewed, together with a discussion of the key issues in that field. Finally, androgen effects in males and females will be compared and contrasted, and a number of theoretical and explanatory mechanisms proposed.

ANDROGENS IN MEN

Evidence that will be reviewed to evaluate the role of androgens in the sexuality of the human male includes studies of androgen deficiency and replacement, effects of aging, normal variations in androgen levels, androgens during sexual development, experimental studies of androgen manipulation, sexual effects of pharmacological agents that alter androgen levels, and clinical studies of men with low sexual desire. Because the most crucial and consistent evidence comes from studies of androgen deficiency and replacement, this will be considered first.

From: *Contemporary Endocrinology: Androgens in Health and Disease*
Edited by: C. Bagatell and W. J. Bremner © Humana Press Inc., Totowa, NJ

Androgen Deficiency and Replacement

There is now a modest but consistent literature on the effects of androgen deficiency, resulting from either hypogonadism or castration, and androgen replacement. The most informative and robust evidence comes from placebo-controlled evaluations of T replacement in hypogonadal men. In most such studies, subjects have been on hormone replacement and have had T withdrawn for a period of time before implementing placebo-controlled evaluation of reintroducing the T replacement. Although typically the number of men in such studies has been small, the results across studies have been gratifyingly consistent (1–6).

These studies have shown conclusively that within 3–4 wk of androgen withdrawal, there is a decline in sexual interest. In most men, there is eventually a reduction in the capacity for seminal emission. The effects on sexual activity with a partner are less predictable because of the varying influence of the partner. In men without partners, frequency of masturbation tends to follow the same pattern as sexual interest. These changes are reversed within 7–14 d of starting replacement. The time involved, which presumably depends on receptor upregulation, may depend on the length of time that the individual has been T deficient, but there have been no systematic studies of this issue in humans. The recent availability of transdermal delivery of T has allowed maintenance of more physiologically stable levels of T, and one study has shown that such replacement continues to maintain normal sexual function for at least 1 yr (7).

The relative importance of androgens in secondary hypogonadism (hypogonadotrophic hypogonadism, where testicular failure is secondary to deficient pituitary stimulation) compared to primary hypogonadism (i.e., hypergonadotrophic, with primary failure of the testes) has been questioned. Gooren (8) reported on two groups of six teenage males—one group hypogonadotrophic, the other hypergonadotrophic—all starting on androgen replacement for delayed onset of puberty between the ages of 14 and 18, and followed up 5–6 yr later. In spite of identical treatment regimes, the hypogonadotrophic group, although no different in erectile or ejaculatory capacity, showed less increase in the frequency and enjoyment of sexual activity and sexual interest and less positive change in mood and energy than the hypergonadotrophic group. In contrast, Skakkebaek et al. (3) found no differences in the patterns of response to T replacement in hypogonadotrophic and hypergonadotrophic subjects. Clopper et al. (9) found no difference between T replacement and gonadotrophin replacement in subjects with hypogonadotrophic hypogonadism. More recently, Finkelstein et al. (10) used a placebo-controlled design to evaluate varying levels of T administration in boys with delayed puberty. They found limited sexual effects of the T on sexuality, mainly on nocturnal emissions and some touching behaviors. In many cases of delayed puberty, the delay is followed by pubertal development. In other cases, the delay is the result of a lack of gonadotrophic stimulation that persists until treated. The hypogonadotrophic group in Skakkebaek et al. (3) study was a mixture of these two types. However, all of their cases had been on T replacement for from 6 mo to 17 yr before participation in the withdrawal/replacement study. More research is needed on this topic; presumably in many cases of delayed puberty, there are other delays apart from that of rising androgens. In all cases, there is likely to be delay in the necessary emotional, cognitive, and social learning that are necessary for "normal" manifestations of T on adult sexuality.

In general, the impact of T withdrawal and replacement on erectile function is more complex than that on sexual interest. One of the most predictable effects of T deficiency is a decline in spontaneous erections during sleep (nocturnal penile tumescence [NPT]). The frequency of such responses is not lessened, but the degree and duration of erection are substantially reduced. These deficits are normalized with T replacement *(5,6,11–13)*. Hypogonadal men may complain of problems with erectile response when awake, but it is not always clear whether this is a psychological problem associated with loss of sexual interest and consequent performance anxiety (e.g., refs. *5* and *14*) or whether it is a direct consequence of the T deficiency. Laboratory studies of erectile response of hypogonadal men to erotic stimuli indicate that they do not differ from eugonadal men in terms of maximum increase in circumference change *(5,12,15)* but they do differ in terms of latency and duration of erectile response and, possibly, in terms of rigidity *(13)*. The difference between the clear-cut impairment of NPT and the less obvious impairment of response to erotic stimuli is of interest and requires explanation. It may be that the NPT paradigm most clearly indicates the arousal aspect of sexual response, which appears to be T dependent *(16)*, whereas the response to erotic stimuli involves an information-processing component, which is relatively androgen independent, but where the accompanying androgen-dependent arousal determines the duration of the response and, in particular, the likelihood of the erectile response continuing beyond the duration of the external stimulus. The effects of T withdrawal on erectile response to erotic fantasy have been less studied and have been less consistent across studies and more research is required on this interesting aspect.

An interesting twist to this story resulted from a recent study of a new androgen, MENT *(17)*. To evaluate this compound, it was directly compared with a conventional testosterone ester in a withdrawal and replacement paradigm for hypogonadal men, of the kind described earlier. The study was carried out in two small groups of men: one in Scotland and the other in Hong Kong. This was the first study to involve hypogonadal men from outside Europe or North America. There were some interesting differences between the two groups of men. Although there were only minor differences between the two androgens, there were some interesting differences between the two groups of men. Although both showed the expected effects on waking erections, the effects on sexual interest were weak in the Hong Kong men, not reaching statistical significance, and the two groups clearly differed in terms of masturbation frequency. The Hong Kong men rarely masturbated and showed little increase, whereas the Scottish men showed a clear increase in masturbation frequency. This confronts us with the need to consider how biological effects are manifested under the influence of cultural factors, an aspect that had been ignored previously. The less culturally influenced the behavioral manifestation is, the more consistent we should expect to find androgen effects across cultures. The effect on NPT, for example, is unlikely to be culturally sensitive; the effect on frequency of masturbation is very likely to be. There is also a need to use measures of sexual effects that are appropriate for the cultural context. There may be some overlap here, in terms of mediating mechanisms, between the effects of culture and the effects of social and cognitive learning in relation to puberty, as discussed earlier.

The Effects of Aging

The relatively consistent results reported thus far have involved relatively young hypogonadal men. With the additional effects of aging, the picture becomes less clear. Schiavi *(18)* has reviewed the relevant literature well. First, the evidence is now clear that there is a variable but predictable decline in bioavailable T with increasing age. Earlier studies had presented a somewhat confusing picture of this issue, partly because of the failure to exclude the effects of poor physical health and partly because of a focus on total rather than free T. There is a change in the synchronicity of the hypothalamo–pituitary–gonadal axis, with altered sensitivity to negative feedback of T associated with reduced free-T levels and increases in luteinizing hormone (LH), which are not as great as they would be in younger men with the same T levels *(19)*. There is an increase in sex hormone-binding globulin (SHBG), possibly the result of an age-related increase in estradiol secretion by the Sertoli cells of the testis, resulting in relatively unaltered total T levels in spite of reduced free T.

Tsitouras et al. *(20)*, working with a group of healthy older men with relatively normal levels of T, divided their subjects into three groups according to the level of sexual activity; the high activity group had significantly higher levels of T than the low-activity group. In contrast, when they divided their subjects into those with and without erectile problems, they found no difference in T levels. In a careful study of healthy, medication-free men between the ages of 45 and 74, Schiavi *(18)* and his colleagues reported a clear decline in sexual interest, sexual arousability, and sexual activity with age. There was also a decline in frequency, duration, and degree of NPT with age. The relationship between the age-related declining free T and these other age-related changes was not straightforward, but could be explained by an age-related alteration in receptor responsiveness to T within the central nervous system (CNS). To support this hypothesis, they described three age-related patterns. In the younger age group (45–54 yr) no relationship was found between free-T levels and NPT, after age adjustment, consistent with the idea that at that age T levels are well above the threshold necessary for T effects. In the middle-age group (55–64 yr), a relationship was found between T and NPT, consistent with the idea that free-T levels are close to the threshold level in that age range; and in the older age group (65–74 yr), no relationship was found, suggestive of free-T levels falling below the threshold. This pattern could be partly explained by falling free T and partly by reduced receptor sensitivity to T effects.

Age-related changes in NPT also raise other interesting possibilities about age-related changes in T effects. As Schiavi et al. *(21)* have demonstrated, NPT is often reduced in older men who have no erectile problems to levels that in younger men would be suggestive of organic erectile dysfunction. The older man may maintain acceptable erectile function by means of increased direct tactile stimulation, and the reduced NPT may be a marker of his age-related decline in T-dependent central arousability.

In general, given the complexity of these various age-related processes we should not expect to find the same clear relationship between androgen withdrawal and replacement that have been found in younger hypogonadal men. In addition, there has still been no adequate placebo-controlled evaluation of testosterone replacement and its effects on sexuality in older men.

Adrenal androgens decline with age in both genders (*see* later subsection). In a placebo-controlled evaluation of dehydroepiandrosterone (DHEA) administration to men between 40 and 70 yr of age *(22)*, there was significant improvement in their somewhat crude measure of well-being, but no effect on "libido." In a more sophisticated study of 39 older men, aged 60–84, there were no differences between DHEA and placebo in the effects on measures of well-being and sexual function *(23)*.

Normal Variations in Androgen Levels

Although the normal range of plasma T is large, there is little predictable relationship between T levels within this range and measures of sexual interest or behavior *(24–26)*. Two studies in which erectile response to erotic stimuli was measured in the laboratory found a correlation between plasma T level and latency, but not degree of erectile response *(27,28)*. It is generally assumed that there is a level of plasma T above which increases in T will have little effect. This level is presumably within the normal range, may vary across individuals, and, as discussed earlier, could well increase with age. If such assumptions are correct, then the lack of correlations between circulating T and sexual parameters is not surprising, at least for younger men.

Testosterone shows a clear circadian pattern in younger men, with levels being at their highest during the latter part of the night and early morning and lowest in the evening. This pattern flattens out in older men *(29)*. The timing of this rhythm does vary somewhat on a seasonal basis, but the very limited evidence *(30)* suggests no relationship between the circadian rhythm and fluctuations in sexual interest or activity, but a possible relationship between the seasonal variation and seasonal peaks of sexual activity *(30–32)*.

Experimental Manipulations in Normal Men

LOWERING TESTOSTERONE

In a study of normal men, aged 20–40, Bagatell et al. *(33)* compared the effects of lowering T by means of a GnRH antagonist, NalGlu, on its own and in combination with different doses of T replacement. The design included a placebo group. This experimental manipulation lasted 6 wk, with 4-wk "pretreatment" and "posttreatment" phases. The medications were given on a weekly basis. The results clearly showed the reduction of sexual interest and activity when T levels were reduced with the NalGlu alone, consistent with the pattern of behavioral effects described earlier in the studies of hypogonadal men. In the lowest T-replacement regime (50 mg T enanthate weekly), the adverse behavioral changes were avoided even though blood levels of T were substantially lower than those pretreatment. However, blood samples were taken immediately before each weekly dose and, therefore, the T levels reported would be lower than those in the earlier part of the week. It is distinctly possible that if those end-of-week levels had been sustained for longer periods, a more negative picture would have appeared.

INCREASING TESTOSTERONE

The effects of increasing T in eugonadal men has become a topical issue because of the development of male contraceptives involving T administration. Anderson et al. *(34)* assessed the effects of supraphysiological levels of T in a single-blind, placebo-controlled study involving 31 healthy men who were part of an ongoing efficacy trial of hormonal male contraception. T enanthate injections 200 mg weekly were given for 8 wk in one group (T-only group), and placebo injections weekly were given for 4 wk, followed by 4 wk of the T enanthate injections in the other group (placebo/T group). Neither group showed any change in measures of sexual interactions with the partner or in frequency of masturbation. In both groups, however, there was an increase in scores on the Subscale 2 of the Sexual Experience Scale *(35)* during T administration, but not during placebo. This subscale measures the extent to which an individual seeks or allows (rather than avoids or rejects) sexual stimuli of an audiovisual or imaginary kind. It is, therefore, an index of sexual interest independent of interaction with a partner.

Bagatell et al. *(36)* gave T enanthate 200 mg im weekly for 20 wk. Ten of the 19 subjects also received the GnRH antagonist NalGlu to suppress endogenous T, the remaining nine received T only. Both groups achieved similarly elevated T levels during treatment. Behavioral measures showed no effects on frequency of sexual activities, including masturbation. There was however a nonsignificant increase in reports of spontaneous erections.

Su et al. *(37)* used a high and low dose of methyltestosterone in a placebo-controlled study of 20 healthy men. Each dose was taken for only 3 d, and there was just one measure relevant to sexuality, a visual analog rating of "sexual arousal." Precisely what this meant was not described, but this measure was significantly higher during the high dose than during placebo. On the other hand, Yates et al. *(38)* compared three dose levels of T in eugonadal men over a 14-wk period, in a single-blind, placebo-controlled design, and found no effect on frequency of orgasm or daily ratings of sexual interest. There is other limited evidence that athletes who take excessive amounts of anabolic steroids have higher coital and orgasmic frequency than athletes who do not use anabolic steroids, although, interestingly, they also reported a higher incidence of erectile problems *(39)*.

Carani et al. *(40)* evaluated the effects of T enanthate injections (150 mg) on NPT measured 2 d later, in a placebo-controlled study of eight normal young men. Supraphysiological levels of T did not affect frequency of rapid-eye-movement (REM) sleep episodes or the frequency, duration, or degree of NPT as measured by penile circumference change, but they did affect NPT measures of rigidity, resulting in greater and more prolonged rigidity. This was statistically significant, but a modest effect. The authors concluded that T was unlikely to have a differential effect on penile circumference and rigidity, but there may have been a ceiling effect for circumference and not for rigidity, allowing the additional enhancement of the latter.

Varying the Level Within the Normal Range

Buena et al. *(41)* took two groups of healthy men, aged 18–49 yr, and suppressed testicular function with a GnRH agonist (Lupron). One group was given a low-dose regime and the other was given a relatively high-dose regime of T replacement, producing serum T levels in the low and high parts of the normal range respectively. They were studied for 9 wk on this regime, and toward the end of this period, they were assessed for NPT in a sleep laboratory. The two groups did not differ in measures of sexual interest or activity or in NPT parameters, although rigidity of NPT was apparently not measured. These results are consistent with the idea that the normal "threshold" level of T is toward the lower part of the normal laboratory range and that increasing levels above that threshold has little effect on sexual variables. These results are also not inconsistent with those reported by Anderson et al. *(34)* and Carani et al. *(40)* because they did not include the same measures (i.e., SES2 and penile rigidity) that had shown the effects in the other two studies.

Developmental Aspects

The most substantial evidence relating to the role of androgens in early adolescent sexuality comes from a series of studies by Udry and his colleagues. Unfortunately, their results and the reported interpretations in relation to boys leave us with a somewhat confused picture. In a cross-sectional study of 102 boys in the ninth and tenth grades at school *(42)*, questionnaire assessment and blood sampling (on one occasion between 3 PM and 7 PM) were used. Questions covered the stage of pubertal developmental, though it is not clear whether spermarche was asked about. The Free-T Index (total T/SHBG) was found to be a strong predictor of "sexual motivation" and behavior, with stage of pubertal development not adding to the regression equation. They concluded that "free testosterone appears to affect sexual motivation directly... and not through the social interpretation of accompanying pubertal development." In a later, longitudinal study *(43)* over 3 yr, with six monthly questionnaires and hormonal assessments, they were unable to replicate the earlier cross-sectional findings: The stage of pubertal development was much more significant in predicting sexual interest and behavior than free T and, furthermore, no relationship between increasing levels of free T and measures of sexual interest and activity over the 3-yr period was found. They were unable to explain the differences between their two studies, but they concluded that hormones are not directly changing behavior, but that pubertal development is acting as a social signal, both to the boy himself and potential partners, that he is ready to engage in sexual activity. They did, however, find that both the level of testosterone and the stage of pubertal development at the initial assessment were predictors of coital status and sexual interest at later assessments. They focused on the initial free-T level and suggested that it was "a marker for an as-yet-unidentified motivational process."

These were difficult studies to carry out and not easily replicated and we should learn as much as we can from them. The authors' interpretations can be questioned on a number of levels. First, the predictive effect of both free-T and pubertal stage at time 1 is further evidence of the relationship between earlier age at puberty and higher levels of sexual interest and activity later, first reported by Kinsey et al. *(44)*. This is consistent with the idea that, in some way, boys with earlier puberty onset may be constitutionally more interested in sex (and possibly more responsive to T). Second, we should not assume, as these authors initially did, that the relatively simple relationship between high and low T levels and sexual interest demonstrated in replacement studies of hypogonadal men will also be evident in the rising levels of T around puberty. As discussed earlier, initial hormone replacement in men with delayed puberty shows a more complex and less predictable hormone–behavior relationship than is found with hypogonadal men who have gone through normal puberty and adolescent development prior to their hypogonadism (i.e., hypergonadotrophic hypogonadism). There is a fair amount of socially influenced learning relevant to sexual behavior at whatever age one goes through this pubertal process that impacts on the hormone–behavior effects. Third, it is quite possible that the central mechanisms involving T go through developmental stages as receptor regulation responds to rising hormone levels. It is also distinctly possible that rising T levels activate inhibitory mechanisms relevant to sexual response (e.g., the postejaculatory refractory period). Fourth, possibly the best direct behavioral marker of T effects, masturbation frequency, was not addressed in these studies; they found low reporting of masturbation. Halpern et al. *(45)* have recently followed up some of these males interviewed initially as young teenagers and asked them as young adults when they started masturbating. They found that masturbation during adolescence was more likely to be reported during this adult retrospective recall than during adolescence, by around 30%. Although we cannot be certain on this point, this is more likely to reflect underreporting during adolescence than overreporting during early adulthood.

A recent study at the Kinsey Institute has reported such retrospective data from two groups of men, one a group of undergraduates surveyed in 1998–1999, and the other, a much larger group of aged-matched college students from Kinsey's original study *(44)*. The onset of masturbation was reported to have occurred in the 2 yr either side of first ejaculation in 80%, the same proportion for both samples *(46)*. The temporal patterns were strikingly similar for these two samples 50 yr apart. Age at first ejaculation correlated highly with pubertal age derived from the wider range of pubertal markers in both samples. Here, we see a clear relationship between pubertal development and sexual behavior, which is less likely to be attributed to social signaling effects and is much more likely to be a behavioral manifestation of pubertal changes in hormone levels. In this study, the pubertal changes occurred in the developmentally normal age range.

Hormonal Manipulation to Control Deviant Sexual Behavior

The antiandrogen cyproterone acetate (CPA) has been used in Europe and Canada to control sexual behavior in sexual offenders. This compound combines a direct antiandrogenic action at the T receptor with an antigonadotrophic effect dependent on its progestational action. Bancroft et al. *(47)* compared the effects of CPA and ethinyl estradiol on 12 incarcerated sexual offenders. Both compounds reduced sexual interest and masturbatory activity and also erectile response to erotic fantasies and slides while having no effect on erectile response to erotic films. These results were very similar to those reported earlier for hypogonadal men. If this study had been carried out more recently and had involved measurement of both duration of erectile response and rigidity, then we may well have found subtle effects on the erectile responses to erotic films, as found by Carani et al. *(13)* in hypogonadal men. In this study, CPA substantially reduced total T, with no change in SHBG, whereas the estrogen substantially increased both total T and SHBG *(48)*. Presumably, there was a consequent reduction in free T with the estrogen, although it seems unlikely that this would have been as marked as with the CPA, raising the possibility that the estrogen as well as CPA may have had some direct antiandrogenic effects at the receptor level. Bradford and Pawlak *(49)* compared CPA with placebo in a 3 mo-treatment-period crossover design involving 19 sexual offenders. There was a significant treatment effect in reducing frequency of orgasms and sexual fantasies, but no effect on erectile response to erotic slides (although self-reported sexual arousal to the slides was reduced by CPA) or on measures of sexual interest. In a further study *(50)*, the effects of CPA on sexual arousal in response to a series of erotic audiotapes were evaluated in 20 pedophile offenders. Subjects were divided into high- and low-T groups according to baseline levels. CPA produced an overall reduction in sexual arousal compared to baseline and a weak interaction effect suggestive of a different pattern of response to the various erotic stimuli in the high- and low-T groups. These findings are difficult to interpret and there is no other data using auditory rather than visual stimuli for comparison.

Medroxyprogesterone acetate (MPA) is the drug most widely used in the United States for the control of deviant sexual behavior. Little in the way of controlled evaluation of its effects has been reported, and although there is ample evidence of its effects in reducing deviant sexual behavior (for review, *see* ref. *51*), its relevance to androgenic mechanisms is not clear. MPA certainly reduces circulating T and LH as a result of its antigonadotrophic effects *(52)*, but there may well be other direct negative progestational effects on central control of sexual behavior. There is also limited evidence of the use of GnRH agonists for controlling deviant sexual behavior *(53)*.

Sexual Side Effects of Medications

Several widely used anticonvulsants are associated with reduced sexual desire, probably because of their effect of increasing SHBG and lowering free T *(54)*. Fenwick et al. *(55)* showed that anticonvulsant-induced reduction in free T was associated with impairment of NPT. Newer anticonvulsants such as valproate, which do not alter androgen levels, do not have these sexual side effects.

Spironolactone, an aldosterone antagonist used in the treatment of hypertension, does not alter circulating levels of T or LH but is believed to have competitive binding effects at the T receptor. Side effects include loss of sexual interest, erectile problems, and gynecomastia *(56)*. Because of these assumed antiandrogenic effects, this drug is widely used by male-to-female transsexuals seeking demasculinization.

The treatment of prostatic cancer is of particular relevance. Because prostatic malignant cells are T sensitive, T levels are often lowered by surgical castration or by the use of antiandrogens is sometimes carried out. This results in a substantial impairment of sexual interest and erectile function, although, interestingly, there is a small minority of such patients who retain reasonably normal sexual function in spite of virtual elimination of androgen effects *(57)*.

Clinical Studies of Low Sexual Desire and Erectile Dysfunction

Although the experimental evidence reviewed earlier indicates a clear relationship between T levels and sexual desire and a much less certain relationship between T and erectile function, the clinical literature continues to be somewhat confused on these relationships. This is in part because sexual desire can be affected by factors other than T and in some men with erectile dysfunction, there is a secondary loss of sexual interest, presumably the result of psychological mechanisms. Conversely, men with low sexual desire may experience performance anxiety and associated erectile dysfunction. These relationships can sometimes be clarified by obtaining a clear history of one problem antedating the other *(58*, p. 97). The picture is further confounded by the fact that T levels may fall as a consequence of sexual problems. Jannini et al. *(59)* found that men with erectile dysfunction who responded to nonhormonal treatment showed a posttreatment increase in T levels, which was not found in those who did not respond.

There is, as yet, a serious lack of placebo-controlled evaluation of T therapy in men with low sexual desire or erectile dysfunction. In one small placebo-controlled study of eugonadal men, O'Carroll and Bancroft *(60)* found that in men with the primary complaint of low sexual desire, a modest but significant increase in sexual desire was produced by T treatment, but no improvement in erections was found in the men with erectile dysfunction. Similar studies are required in older men. Carani et al. *(61)* found, in a group of 14 "mildly hypogonadal" men with erectile dysfunction and a mean age of 37 yr, that some improvement in sexual response was produced by T replacement in those with the lowest levels of free T. Morales et al. *(22,62)* reported two uncontrolled studies of T treatment of "hypogonadal impotence." In the first study *(22)*, in which oral methyltestosterone was used, only 2 out of 22 subjects reported a "complete recovery of sexual function." In the second *(62)*, involving T undecanoate, 10 of the 23 subjects reported improvements in both sexual interest and erectile function, and 5 in sexual interest only. In neither of these reports was any information about age given, limiting the clinical relevance of this data.

In a report of a series of 1022 men presenting with erectile dysfunction *(63)*, low T levels were found in 4% of subjects less than 50 yr of age and in 9% of the older group. The authors commented that if they had restricted their estimation of T to men with low sexual desire, they would have missed 40% of the cases with low T and 37% of those who subsequently benefited from T replacement. They concluded by recommending that, to be cost-effective, measurement of serum T in cases of erectile dysfunction (ED) should only be carried out in patients aged less than 50 when there is low sexual desire or physical signs of T deficiency. However, serum T should be measured in all men with ED aged over 50.

Summary of Evidence in the Male

There is a consistency in the evidence showing a relationship between testosterone and both sexual interest and NPT in younger men. This is consistent with the main central effects of T being on central arousal associated with response to sexual stimuli *(16)*. As a consequence, thoughts about sex, accompanied by central arousal, are experienced as manifestations of "sexual interest." The association with NPT is suggestive of a testosterone-dependent "excitatory tone" dependent on central arousal mechanisms, which is allowed expression through penile erection when the inhibitory tone maintaining the normally flaccid penis is reduced or "switched off" during REM sleep (*see* ref. *64*, for further discussion).

The relevance of testosterone to erectile function is more subtle or complex. There may be testosterone-dependent mechanisms in the spinal cord and penis that are relevant, but we only have evidence of these in lower mammals. We can assume that T-dependent arousal mechanisms will augment erectile responses. However, other mechanisms, including cognitive processing of sexual stimuli, as well as age- and disease-related increases in erectile inhibitory tone, which are not T dependent, have an equal or greater influence on erectile response.

Whereas the picture is comparatively clear during young adulthood and midlife, developmental processes involved both around puberty and with aging are less well understood. It is conceivable that these two ends of the developmental spectrum involve complex changes in T receptor number and sensitivity, as well as other changes both centrally and peripherally, which makes physiological function of T more obscure at those times.

The concept of a threshold below which androgen deficiency occurs and above which increasing androgen levels has little effect is fairly consistently supported by the evidence. However, our ability to identify the "threshold level" remains crude. The level is likely to vary across individuals, and it may change with age and exposure to sustained and different levels of T. At present, we can only speculate on this issue. A number of studies have suggested that subtle effects may arise from increasing T to suprathreshold levels.

We have little systematic evidence on the timing of T effects on sexual responsiveness. The hormone-replacement studies discussed here suggest that, after a period of T withdrawal, it is several days or even 2–3 wk before replacement T has its maximum effects. On the other hand, short-term administration of T to eugonadal men has apparently produced effects, albeit subtle, within 3 d (e.g., refs. *37* and *40*). Further research is required on this fundamental issue.

ANDROGENS IN WOMEN

Developmental Aspects

Whereas androgens increase during the course of pubertal maturation in females, in comparison to males they start at a lower level and show a doubling of T through the stages of pubertal maturation compared to the 18-fold increase in T for boys *(65)*. There is an added complexity in the female; T production, which is predominantly from the ovary, shows a cyclical pattern accompanying ovulatory cycles. In an established and regular adult ovulatory cycle, T levels rise during the follicular phase and are at a maximum approximately for the middle third of the cycle, declining during the final third to reach the nadir during the first few days of the next follicular phase. Within the middle third, T levels may be relatively sustained or, as reported in some studies, show more discrete peri-ovulatory peaks. There is presumably some individual variability in this respect. There is a lack of evidence of what happens to T levels in adolescent postmenarcheal young women who have not yet established their regular adult pattern of ovarian cyclicity. Ankaberg and Norjavaara *(66)* studied T levels in a group of girls ranging from prepuberty to 2 yr postmenarche. Before puberty, they found T levels correlating with DHEA-S levels suggestive of the adrenals being the main prepubertal source of T. After the onset of puberty, T correlated more strongly with estradiol (E_2), suggestive of the ovary as the main source of T. However, although T levels were higher in mid and late puberty than in early puberty, the T-to-E_2 ratio was higher in early puberty than later.

When we consider peripubertal and early-adolescent T levels and their relationship to sexuality in females, we are again largely dependent on the work of Udry and his colleagues. Once again, their findings are somewhat confusing, comparable to their male studies. In their first cross-sectional study of white girls in the 8th, 9th, 10th grades, Udry et al. *(67)* found a relationship between T levels and measures of sexual interest and frequency or occurrence of masturbation, but not to whether they had experienced sexual intercourse. In their more recent longitudinal study of black and white postmenarcheal adolescent females *(68)*, T levels and increase in T were related to the transition to first intercourse, but not to measures of sexual interest or masturbation. As is the case for their male studies, this discrepancy is not easy to explain. However, given the greater complexity of the female ovarian cyclicity, particularly in early adolescence, there is greater scope for methodological confusion. In the first cross-sectional study, blood samples were collected between d 5 and 9 of the menstrual cycle, whereas in the later study, samples were collected between d 2 and 8. In neither case was the mid-third of the cycle, when T levels are maximum, sampled, and the 2- to 8-d sampling in the second study may have resulted in lower levels than would have been obtained using the 5- to 9-d sampling. The closer sampling is to the midcycle maximum, the more likely one is to find correlations with T-dependent behavior, as it is the maximum levels that are most likely to determine the behavior. The association between follicular T levels and transition to coitus may be reflecting some marker status of T level relevant to the ovarian cycle, rather than direct effects of the T.

As with males, one might expect T to be more directly related to sexual interest and self-directed behaviors, such as masturbation, than to sexual interaction with a partner. Therefore, it is of interest that in the report on age of onset of masturbation, cited earlier *(46)*, relating onset of masturbation in females to age at menarche, and in males ot age at spermarche, the picture is very different for females than for males, in whom age of onset was related to age at first ejaculation. In both the recent sample and the Kinsey sample collected 50 yr earlier, masturbation onset, for those who started to masturbate before first menarche or ejaculation, was, on average, 2 yr earlier in the females than the males in both samples, a significant difference in each case. In addition, the distribution of age of onset of masturbation was much wider in the females. Thus, whereas 80% of the males, in both samples, started masturbation in the period 2 yr either side of first ejaculation, the proportion of females, for the same time period either side of menarche, was 43% for the earlier sample and 36% for the recent sample. For the early and recent female samples respectively, 23% and 33% started 3 yr or more before menarche, and 34% and 31% started 3 yr or more after menarche. Although we had no hormonal data in these studies, we can reasonably conclude that the hormonal changes at puberty were much less influential in determining the age of onset of masturbation in the girls than in the boys. It is possible that the earlier onset of prepubertal masturbation in the girls may have been influenced by increases in adrenal androgens at adrenarche. However, one cannot escape the conclusion that females are much more variable in the extent to which this aspect of their emerging sexuality is influenced by androgens or other puberty-related hormones.

Normal Variations

THE MENSTRUAL CYCLE

Given that T varies in a predictable fashion during normal ovulatory cycles, we might expect to find any direct relationship between T level and behavior reflected in cyclical patterns of such behavior. There are, however, two caveats to using menstrual cycle data in this way. First, the midcycle rise in T is accompanied by a variety of other hormonal changes and it is not easy or even possible to distinguish between a cycle-related pattern resulting from T effects and those resulting from other effects. Second, what time relationship should we expect between midcycle rises in T and their behavioral consequences, if any? We have even less evidence on this issue than we have for the male (*see* ref. *69*, discussed in a later subsection).

Hedricks (*70*) described the major methodological inconsistencies in the literature that contribute to the variable picture. There was, however, a consistent finding of sexual activity being at its lowest during menstruation, although there are a number of explanations, in addition to low T levels, for this pattern. There was also a tendency, across studies, for indices of sexual interest or activity to be most marked during the follicular phase or around ovulation, although with considerable individual variability. This prevailing tendency is compatible with a T effect, but other explanations also have to be considered. If the cyclical variation in T influences the woman's sexuality, then we might expect to find correlations between the level of T reached during the cycle and patterns of behavior. Here, the evidence is again inconsistent. Persky et al. (*71*) and Morris et al. (*72*) found a correlation between midcycle levels of T and frequency of sexual activity with the partner across the cycle. Cutler et al. (*73*) found no relationship between luteal levels of T and frequency of sexual activity with a partner, although they did not include any measures of sexual interest. Bancroft et al. (*74*) found sexual interest and activity peaking in the midfollicular phase and decreasing in the middle third of the cycle when T was at its highest. In addition, they found a correlation ($r = 0.79$) between midcycle T and frequency of masturbation in those women who masturbated; correlations between T and aspects of sexual interaction with the partner were absent or in the opposite direction. Van Goozen et al. *(75)* found that FTI correlated with frequency of sexual intercourse through the cycle and with mean level of sexual interest. Masturbation frequency did not correlate significantly with FTI, but it did with total T and androstenedione levels. No adequate explanation for this discrepancy was offered. This pattern of correlations was basically the same whether peri-ovulatory or mean levels of androgen through the cycle were used. Schreiner-Engel et al. *(76)* found that women with higher midcycle T levels showed greater vaginal responses to erotic stimuli in the laboratory (particularly in the luteal phase), but reported less satisfactory sexual relationships with their partners than the low-T group.

PREGNANCY AND LACTATION

Pregnancy is a time of massive hormonal change, and whereas there are slight changes in T levels (a slight increase in T and a more substantial increase in SHBG, resulting in slightly reduced free T), they are modest compared with other hormonal changes and they have not been directly studied in relation to the pregnant woman's sexuality. Reduction in sexual interest and enjoyment is common during the postpartum period and is more marked in breastfeeding than bottle-feeding mothers *(77,78)*. Little attention has been paid, however, to the relationship between these postpartum behavioral changes and the woman's hormonal status. In one study *(79)*, 25 women were assessed prospectively for 6 mo postpartum, 19 of whom persisted with breastfeeding and 6 who changed to bottle-feeding within the first 6 wk. Not surprisingly, given the effects of lactation on ovarian function, the bottle feeders had higher T and androstenedione levels than the breastfeeding mothers. Of more relevance, five of the breast feeders reported reduced sexual interest, and their T and androstenedione levels were consistently and significantly lower than the breast feeders with no reduction in sexual interest. This is an important aspect of women's reproductive and sexual health that has received little attention.

The Effects of Aging and Menopause

Adrenal androgens decline with age over a relatively wide age span. This was most clearly shown in a study of oophorectomized women where the picture was not complicated by ovarian androgens *(80)*. However, this pattern has also been consistently found in other studies *(81–84)*. The situation with ovarian androgens is more complex, particularly with androstenedione, which is typically produced half by the adrenals and half by the ovaries in younger premenopausal women. Roger et al. *(85)* showed that T levels declined in women in the last few years before they reached menopause but not thereafter. This pattern has been replicated, as shown by the midcycle T peak *(86)* and by 24-h mean plasma total T measured on d 4–6 of the cycle *(87)*. Studies of postmenopausal women tend to show no relationship between T, androstenedione (A), and E_2, and either years past the menopause or actual age. The most important evidence comes from a longitudinal study of 172 women, all of whom changed from premenopausal to postmenopausal during the 7 yr of the study *(84)*. This study showed no change in total T but an *increase* in free T from premenopausal to postmenopausal. In a cross-sectional study of 141 women aged 40–60 yr, Bancroft and Cawood *(82)*, found T levels to be lower in postmenopausal than premenopausal women, a finding that has been reported in other studies. However, when other factors were taken into account, neither menopausal status nor age entered the multiple-regression equation accounting either for total testosterone or the free-androgen index (FAI).

Particularly confusing is the evidence relating to SHBG. Burger et al. *(84)* found a decrease in SHBG over their 7-yr study, the maximal decline occurring in the 2 yr before the final menstrual period. This was the explanation for the paradoxical increase in free T from premenopausal to postmenopausal. Bancroft and Cawood *(82)* found no difference in SHBG levels between premenopausal and postmenopausal women, whereas other reports suggestive of both reductions and increases have been published (*see* ref. *84*). This confounding of the relationship between age and ovarian androgen levels is partly the result of the complex role of the postmenopausal ovary. Ovarian interstitial cells can be stimulated by the postmenopausal rise in LH to produce T and A, sometimes excessively. In addition, factors such as body weight and insulin resistance influence this ovarian androgen production (*see* ref. *82* for a brief review of the evidence).

Given this somewhat complex picture, what might we reasonably expect to find from studies of androgen/sexual behavior relationships in women as they get older? A number of behavioral studies have reported a decline in sexual interest in women as they age (*see* ref. *68*, pp. 282–298). In contrast, Laumann et al. *(88)*, reporting on data from the National Health and Social Life Survey of men and women aged 18–59, found that the proportions of women indicating "a lack of desire for sex" during the past 12 mo did not vary significantly across the age groups and was, in fact, slightly lower in the oldest (50–59) age group. However, in a recent national telephone survey of 987 women in the United States carried out by the Kinsey Institute *(88a)*, women were asked how often they thought about sex during the past 4 wk. Frequency was lower in the older women, but low frequency was more likely to be associated with distress in the younger women. A potentially important difference between these two surveys, which might account for the discrepancy, is that Laumann et al. *(88)* asked the women to focus on "lack" of sexual interest, and their findings might reflect changing importance of sexual interest as women get older. In the Kinsey survey, simple frequency of sexual interest was assessed without any implication of whether the frequency was problematic or not. The Kinsey survey also included women up to the age of 65. The weight of evidence therefore points to an age-related decline in sexual interest in women, which may or may not be problematic for the older women.

If T levels are important for sexual interest in women, do they correlate with measures of sexual interest or activity as women get older? The earlier literature leaves us with a confused and inconsistent picture, partly because of the tendency to use univariate methods of analysis (*see* ref. *89*, for a brief review). Bachmann et al. *(90)* compared sexually active and sexually inactive naturally postmenopausal women and found no differences in estrogen or testosterone levels. In our study of 40- to 60-yr-old women *(89)*, roughly divided into premenopausal, perimenopausal, and postmenopausal groups, we found no relationship between frequency of sexual thoughts and either age, androgen levels, or menopausal status. However, also in this study, Subscale 2 of the Sexual Experience Scale *(35)*, which focuses on interest in noninteractional sexual stimuli, showed a negative correlation with age, but no relationship to androgen levels or menopausal status. Similar findings were reported by Dennerstein et al. *(91)*. In a group of women aged 48–58, no relationship was found between either menopausal status or androgen levels and any aspect of sexual functioning; age was negatively related to "sexual responsivity," a composite of ratings of arousal, orgasm, and enjoyment during sexual activities. Kirchengast et al. *(92)* studied 171 postmenopausal women and retrospectively assessed their decline in sexual interest since their last menstrual period.

Reported decline in sexual interest was associated positively with body weight but was unrelated to androgen levels. However, in each of these studies, the youngest women had presumably already reached the premenopausal T decline, and to adequately test the hormone–behavior relationship, the age range should include women before this developmental stage.

In the only longitudinal behavioral study of women in transition through the menopause so far published, McCoy and Davidson *(93)* found correlations between declining levels of T and coital frequency. However, only 16 women continued in this study (23 of the original 39 dropping out because they wanted hormone-replacement therapy [HRT]) and this number did not allow adequate multivariate analysis. The behavioral results of the much larger longitudinal study by the Melbourne group *(84)* are awaited with considerable interest.

Hormone Replacement and the Natural and Surgical Menopause

In spite of the above reviewed evidence, it is still often assumed that the menopause is associated with a decline in testosterone and that this fact is itself justification for using T in hormone replacement. It is of crucial importance to make the distinction between natural and surgical menopause. As already discussed, the evidence indicates that reduction of T in women occurs in the years before the natural menopause and that T levels, although variable across women, show no predictable change thereafter. With surgical removal of the ovaries, there is an immediate and substantial drop in circulating androgens. There are, however, other reasons for considering T replacement in HRT regimes for the natural menopause. The administration of exogenous estrogen in HRT increases SHBG and, consequently, reduces free T. Conversely, T administration will reduce SHBG levels and also, because of competitive binding with SHBG, increase the amount of free E_2. However, in evaluating the literature on T replacement with naturally or surgically menopausal women, a number of factors need to be taken into consideration.

1. Improvement in sexual interest or enjoyment may be secondary to more general improvement in well-being, mood, and energy. In a study of variations in mood and sexual interest through the menstrual cycle of young women, Sanders et al. *(94)* found that around one-third of the variability in sexual interest could be attributed to a more general variability in well-being. Cawood and Bancroft *(89)* found, in women aged 40–60 yr, that measures of mood and energy were the best predictors of sexual well-being, and this association has been strongly replicated in the recent Kinsey national survey of women, aged 20–65, referred to earlier *(88a)*.

2. Improvement in sexual interest and enjoyment may be secondary to improvement in vaginal dryness and associated dyspareunia, which can have negative repercussions on women's sexual enjoyment and, consequently, sexual interest.

3. Improvement in mood and well-being and, consequently, sexual interest associated with T administration may result from the effects of the exogenous T in increasing free E, rather than from direct T effects. Such an increase results from aromatization of T to E in the tissues, as well as preferential binding by T to SHBG. Although there is still uncertainty about the precise physiological role of steroid binding in influencing the relative impact of E and T *(95)*, this mechanism of using exogenous T to increase free E has been strongly advocated by Wallen and supported by experimental data from rhesus monkeys *(96)*. For these various reasons, it is not possible to establish whether improvement produced by a combined E + T regime is the result of the E, the T, or a combination of the two.

4. Studies using placebo control typically show a substantial placebo effect in improving well-being and sexual interest. Placebo control is, therefore, important.

With these caveats, what can we learn from studies of HRT in the natural or surgical menopause?

Natural Menopause. A number of studies, particularly earlier ones, included women with both natural menopause and surgical menopause, sometimes without even indicating the numbers of each. Where a study has a substantial majority of natural menopause subjects, it will be considered in this subsection. In those which have a substantial majority of surgical menopausal subjects, they will be considered in the next subsection.

Burger et al. *(97)* reported on 20 postmenopausal women whose lack of libido had persisted on "adequate oral estrogen replacement," but whose "other main symptoms, such as hot flushes and vaginal dryness," had been relieved. Fourteen of these women had gone through natural menopause. They were randomly assigned to either estrogen implant or estrogen plus testosterone implant. On average, the combined-implant group showed improvement in libido and sexual enjoyment within the first 6 wk, whereas the "estrogen-only" group did not. The latter group were, therefore, given an additional T implant and proceeded to show the same improvement as the combined group. It is noteworthy that no other symptoms were reported, and no indication was given of whether these women were suffering from tiredness, lack of concentration, or depression before starting the implants.

Myers et al. *(98)* studied 40 naturally postmenopausal women who were randomly assigned to 4 groups of 10 subjects each: P (Premarin only), PP (Premarin plus Provera), PT (Premarin plus methyltestosterone), and PL (placebo); they were assessed over a 10-wk period. Subjects were assessed with both self-ratings and laboratory measurement of vaginal pulse amplitude (VPA) response to erotic stimuli, a measure of genital response. There were no group differences in treatment effects on any of the sexuality variables, including VPA, except for masturbation. This showed a trend toward higher frequency and a significant increase in enjoyment of masturbation in the PT group. There was a trend ($p = 0.06$) toward group differences in mood, but, unfortunately, no further details were given of this measure. This study illustrates well the complex effects of exogenous hormone administration; in particular, an increase in SHBG in the P and PP groups and a significantly lower level of SHBG in the PT group. Given that the three treatment groups did not differ in their plasma E_2 levels, this demonstrates the likely increase of free E_2 as well as T in the PT group.

Davis et al. *(99)* studied 34 women, 2 of whom had had their ovaries removed. All had shown intolerance of or inadequate response to oral HRT. They were randomly assigned to either E implant or E+T implants, administered three times monthly for 2 yr. Women with specific complaints of low sexual desire were excluded. (It was considered unethical to randomly assign them to E only!). This exclusion is important and will be discussed further below. Women in both groups showed significant improvement in sexuality measures, and for most of the variables, the E+T group improved significantly more than the E group, except that toward the end of the 2-yr study period, there was a decline in the measures of sexuality that was attributed to a reduced frequency of implants because of continuing supraphysiological levels of T. This is a potentially interesting phenomenon that, as we will see, recurs in other studies using supraphysiological doses. This study is limited by having no measures of mood or well-being and behavioral measures only relating to sex.

Sherwin *(100)* randomly assigned "perimenopausal" women to four treatment regimes, involving either a low (0.625 mg) or high (1.25 mg) dose of Premarin for 25 d out of each month, and either Provera (5 mg) or placebo for d 15–25 of each month. Each woman took the assigned regime for 12 mo and was assessed with daily ratings during the 3rd, 6th, 9th and 12th mo. The main purpose of the study was to evaluate the effects of the progestogen on mood and sexuality. However, it incorporated a comparison of low and high estrogen (combined with placebo), which is of most relevance to this chapter. Results showed that the progestogen had a negative effect on mood, but not on sexuality. The mood effect was attenuated by the higher estrogen dose. Apparent from the graphed sexual interest data (Fig. 3 of ref. *100*), women in the high E + placebo group had substantially lower levels of sexual interest during the pretreatment month than the low E + placebo group, yet by the 6th mo and continuing through the 12th mo, they were showing noticeably higher levels of sexual interest. This was not commented on in the article.

Surgical Menopause. Because of the continuing role of the postmenopausal ovary in producing androgens, which also are available for conversion into estrogens, the woman with both ovaries removed is clearly in a state of gonadal steroid deficiency. Perhaps not surprisingly, the most persuasive evidence of an impact of testosterone on women's sexuality comes from controlled studies of hormone replacement in oophorectomized women. However, the evidence is not entirely straightforward.

Dennerstein et al. *(101)* studied 49 surgically menopausal women, all of whom had stable, satisfying sexual relationships, using a double-blind crossover design in which they spent 3 mo on each of four treatments: EE_2, l-norgestrel, combination of EE_2 and l-norgestrel, and placebo. The estrogen-only regime was significantly better than the others in improving sexual interest, enjoyment, and orgasmic frequency. This study, although not involving androgens, demonstrates that sexual measures can be improved by E administration. It also showed correlations between the measure of sexual desire and measures of mood, particularly "feelings of well-being." Dow et al. *(102)* studied 40 postmenopausal women, 34 of whom were surgically menopausal, and randomized them to estrogen-alone or estrogen-plus-testosterone implants. Women were only included if "loss of libido" was a problem in their relationship. The two treatment groups did not differ in the numbers who experienced dyspareunia. There was significant improvement in sexual interest and enjoyment as well as improvement in other symptoms in both treatment groups, and no differences between the treatments. Nathorst-Böös et al. *(103)* compared three age-matched groups of women, all of whom had undergone hysterectomy 2–6 yr previously. One group had had bilateral oophorectomy with no hormone replacement (Ovx), a second group had oophorectomy and received estrogen replacement (ERT), and the third group had their ovaries conserved (Hyx). Whereas the Ovx group was significantly more depressed and anxious than the other two, the two oophorectomized groups (Ovx and ERT) were both sexually impaired when compared to the Hyx group. Approximately 50% of women in these two groups complained of loss of libido. Thus whereas the estrogen replacement appeared to protect against mood change, it did not prevent impaired sexual function. Measures of free T, although lower in the ERT group than the other two groups, did not correlate with any of the sexuality measures.

Brincat et al. *(104)* studied 55 postmenopausal women already established on HRT. No details were given of the number of surgically menopausal women in this group, but the average age of 44.4 yr suggests that the majority were surgical. When the time came for further HRT (i.e., return of climacteric symptoms), they were randomly assigned to either E and T or placebo implants. Results showed significant symptom improvement across the board for the first 4 mo after active implant, but with some return of symptoms in the fifth and sixth months. There was no significant improvement in any symptom on the placebo implant, at any stage of the 6 mo. These results demonstrate the value of this combined regime, but do not evaluate the specific role of testosterone. The authors conclude that return of symptoms in the last 2 mo when E_2 and T levels were still within the normal range indicates that changing levels of E_2 and T are more important than absolute levels. Burger et al. *(105)* reported on 17 women, 11 of whom had undergone surgical menopause. They were selected because they complained of persistent symptoms, particularly loss of libido, in spite of treatment with Premarin 1.25 mg daily or Progynova 4 mg daily. They were given combined implants of E and T and assessed over 6 mo. Tiredness, lack of concentration and all measures of sexuality improved over the first 3 mo but relapsed over the last 3 mo. Once again, return of symptoms occurred in the presence of normal premenopausal levels of E_2 and T.

In the most sophisticated study in this field, Sherwin et al. *(106)* investigated women undergoing hysterectomy and bilateral oophorectomy. A 1-mo baseline assessment preceded the surgery. Postoperatively, women were assigned randomly to one of four treatment groups: estrogen only (E), testosterone only (T), estrogen plus testosterone (E+T), or placebo. These were given in monthly injections for 3 mo. All subjects then received 1 mo of placebo, following which they were crossed over to one of the other three treatment groups. A fifth group of younger women who had undergone hysterectomy only was assessed in the same way as a control for the effects of surgery. The E+T and T only conditions showed significantly higher levels of sexual interest, fantasy, and arousal than either the E only or placebo conditions. They did not differ in measures of sexual activity with partner or orgasm. Apart from its design, this study is also noteworthy because it focused on the immediate postoperative period in women who were not reporting significant sexual or mood problems preoperatively. In a separate article *(107)*, the effects on mood were reported, showing that mood was significantly better with all three hormone regimes compared with placebo. The T-only group also had significantly higher hostility scores than the other three groups. In a third article *(108)*, it was reported that energy level, well-being, and appetite were significantly higher in the two groups receiving T than in the E-only or placebo groups.

Sherwin and Gelfand *(109)* went on to study three groups of women, all of whom had been oophorectomized. One group had been established on a previous E+T regime; one group received monthly injections of E alone, and the third group had received no treatment (NT). Striking increases in sexual desire, fantasies, and arousal occurred in the E+T group 1 wk after the injection but by the second week, these variables were declining. By the fourth week, there were no differences between the E+T group and either the E or NT groups. In a separate article, Sherwin *(110)* reported on the mood changes in this study. The E+T group showed significantly less negative mood, in terms of anxiety, depression, hostility, tiredness, and clear headedness, than the NT group. The E+T group was also less anxious, depressed, and tired than the E group on d 8 postinjection (when improvement in the sexual variables was around maximal), "coincident with their higher levels of circulating T at that time." However, because mood correlated with E_2 levels and these levels remained within the physiological range and because T levels remained supraphysiological throughout, Sherwin concluded that the mood effects were the result of the E and not the T. It is not clear why E was clearly implicated for the mood changes and T for the sexual changes. There was also no attempt, in either this study or the earlier one, to examine possible relationships between sexuality and mood. A striking finding in the second study was the decline in behavioral response in the presence of continuing supraphysiological levels of T. Although the three groups in the Sherwin and Gelfand (109) study were selected to be comparable in terms of mental health and unproblematic sexual relationships, no explanation was given for why these three regimes had been selected for these particular women in the first place, and without such explanation, the question of whether there were relevant pretreatment differences between the groups remains.

Castelo-Branco et al. (111), in an open comparative study of hormone replacement in surgically menopausal women, assessed sexual functioning before HRT and after 12 mo on HRT. They compared estrogen alone (E), a combination of estrogen and a "weak" androgen (described as dihydroandrosterone enanthate, which is presumably meant to be dehydroepiandrosterone enanthate) (E+A), tibolone (Tb), a synthetic steroid with both estrogenic and androgenic properties, and no treatment (NT). All three treatments were associated with significant improvement in sexual functioning at the end of 1 yr. However, the E+A and Tb regimes produced more marked improvement than E alone.

Shifren et al. (112), making use of new developments in transdermal T administration, reported on 65 women who had undergone surgical menopause from 1 to 10 yr previously. Their average age was 47 yr (range: 31–56). All had impaired sexual function and all had been on Premarin, at least 0.625 mg daily for at least 2 mo when recruited for the study. All subjects continued on the same dose of oral estrogen through the study. After a 4-wk baseline assessment, they were all given daily transdermal patches with placebo (P), 150 μg T or 300 μg T as the daily dose, each for 12 wk with the order of presentation randomized. The principal methods of evaluation were the Brief Index of Sexual Functioning for Women (BISFW), expressed as percentage of mean score for "normal" women aged 20–55, and the Psychological General Well-Being Index (PGWI). These were administered at baseline and at the end of each of the 12-wk treatment periods. There was a substantial placebo response; however, taking the composite BISFW score, there was significantly more improvement with the high T dose than with placebo. Looking at the subscales, this effect was only significant for frequency of sexual activity and pleasure/orgasm, not for sexual desire or arousal [the opposite pattern reported by Sherwin et al. (106)]. For mood, there was a significantly greater improvement with the high dose for the composite score, and also for the depression and "positive well-being" subscales. The placebo response was more marked in the younger women; for those under 48 yr, there was no difference between placebo and active treatment on any variable; the overall significant effects depended on the older women. The explanation for this age effect is not clear. It may reflect that for younger women, loss of sexual interest or enjoyment is more problematic and, hence, the expectation of or need for improvement greater. It seems unlikely that T would be more effective in the older women, given that they had all had their ovaries removed. This study was also unusual in reporting levels of free T as well as total T, and these showed that whereas the total T levels were somewhat higher than normal on the higher T dose, the free T levels were closer to the upper part of the normal range. The transdermal route appears to have the advantage of delivering more physiological doses of T.

In a somewhat different type of study, Kaplan and Owett (113) reported on women who had been referred to them for sexual problems and who had either undergone cytotoxic therapy suppressing ovarian activity or had had both ovaries removed for the treatment of cancer. For the study, women were selected on the basis of their total-T levels, with 11 women having a T level less than 10 ng/dL and a comparison group of 11 women with T levels greater than 30 ng/dL. Although the authors concluded that T deficiency in women "produces a well-defined clinical syndrome," they also asserted that "the clinical features of Female Androgen Deficiency Syndrome and psychogenic hypoactive desire can be so similar as to be indistinguishable" on the basis of psychiatric or sexual history assessment. The crucial difference was the T level; the two groups differed significantly on two measures of sexual complaint: "decreased orgasm" and a "global symptom score."

   Summary of HRT Studies. As hormone replacement studies have had the greatest impact in influencing opinions of the role of T in women's sexuality, the main points from the studies reviewed, together with the four caveats listed earlier, will now be reconsidered. Only one study *(101)* directly examined the relationship between mood and sexuality, and the extent to which improvements in sexuality could be secondary to improvements in mood has not been addressed. Most studies did take the effect of vaginal dryness and its response to E into account. Even though several studies showed some improvement in sexuality variables using E alone, none considered the possibility that the effects of combining T with E could, at least, in part be the result of the resulting increase in free E_2, rather than simply the result of adding the direct effects of T. In only one study was there systematic evaluation of increasing the estrogen dose, although this was not the primary purpose of the study *(100)*, and whereas the benefits of higher E dose on mood was clearly indicated, apparent improvement in sexual interest received no comment.

   Only one study *(107)* evaluated the effects of T on its own. A few studies used a placebo control and the degree of placebo response varied considerably, possibly determined by whether or not subjects had already established sexual problems before entering the study and, hence, were more likely to be looking for a therapeutic response. Thus we see a substantial placebo response in the study of Shifrin et al. *(112)* in which women were selected on the basis of impaired sexual function, and no placebo response in Sherwin and Gelfand's *(107)* study in which women with satisfactory sexual lives were assessed immediately following surgery, before they had had time to establish any problems.

   Most of the studies using supraphysiological doses reported return of symptoms while T levels were still in the supraphysiological, or, at least, the normal physiological range. The only explanation offered for this striking phenomenon is that it is the changing rather than the absolute levels that are important. However, this is an unsatisfactory explanation and an alternative will be considered later.

Hormone Replacement of Adrenal Androgens

   As reviewed earlier, adrenal androgens decline with age in both men and women. Androstenedione has a substantial capacity for conversion to both E_2 and T; DHEA has a very limited capacity for conversion to T. There is little evidence, however, that DHEA is directly relevant to sexuality in either men or women. Cawood and Bancroft *(89)* in their study of 40–60-yr-old women found that levels of DHEA significantly predicted "positive affect and sensation seeking" and this mood measure was itself a predictor of sexual interest. Hence, DHEA may have indirect effects on sexual interest via its effect on general well-being. In a placebo-controlled evaluation of DHEA administration to women between 40 and 70 yr *(114)*, there was significant improvement in their somewhat crude measure of well-being, but no effect on "libido." Arlt et al. *(115)* evaluated DHEA replacement in women with adrenal insufficiency that was not age related and that had hitherto been treated with corticosteroids only. The addition of DHEA, compared to placebo, improved measures of depression, anxiety, general well-being, and sexual interest and responsiveness, although the greatest improvements were in the levels of depression and anxiety. These sexual effects could well have been secondary to improvements in general well-being and energy. Interestingly, these improvements were only clearly apparent after 4 mo of DHEA replacement.

Clinical Studies of Low Sexual Desire

Few studies have investigated T levels in women presenting specifically with problems of low sexual desire, rather than a more general set of menopause-related complaints. Stuart et al. *(116)* compared T levels in 11 women with the diagnosis of Inhibited Sexual Desire and 11 women with normal sexual desire and found no differences. Similarly, Schreiner-Engel et al. *(117)* compared 17 women, aged 27–39, who met DSM IV criteria for severe, persistent, and generalized loss of sexual desire, with 13 healthy sexually active women. They found no differences in T or other reproductive hormones. Riley and Riley *(118)* compared 15 women complaining of lifelong absence of sexual drive with a comparison group of 15 women. Testosterone was measured around midcycle. In the control group, FAI and total T correlated with sexual interest, whereas only total T correlated with coital frequency. In the patient group, the only significant correlation was between total T and coital frequency. The FAI index was significantly lower in the patient group, although neither total T nor SHBG differed, and none of the androgen levels were outside the normal laboratory range. Although the authors comment that this provides "further evidence that testosterone is involved in sexual drive," it is questionable to what extent T was determining the sexual drive. The differences in T between groups was subtle, whereas the measures of sexual interest and activity were markedly different.

Controlled studies of the treatment of sexual problems in women with testosterone have also been few. Carney et al. *(119)* studied 32 couples whose main problem was sexual unresponsiveness of the woman. Using a balanced factorial design, they compared the effects of either T or diazepam, given to the woman, each combined with sex therapy (on a weekly or monthly basis). The combination of T plus counseling was significantly superior to diazepam plus counseling on frequency of sexual thoughts, enjoyment of sex, and a number of other variables. Mathews et al. *(120)* attempted to replicate this study using placebo instead of diazepam and found no superiority of testosterone over placebo. To control for the possible confounding effect of the combined sex therapy, Dow and Gallagher *(121)* randomly allocated 30 couples, with the principal complaint of sexual unresponsiveness of the woman, to three treatment regimes, testosterone plus sex therapy, placebo plus sex therapy, and testosterone alone. The two combined therapy groups did not differ from each other, but both were superior to the testosterone alone treatment. The most likely explanation of the first study by Carney et al. *(119)* was that the apparent superiority of T was, in fact, the result of a negative impact of the diazepam on the effectiveness of the sex therapy.

Women with Endocrine Abnormalities

Hulter and Lundberg *(122)* reviewed 48 women with hypothalamo–pituitary disorders. Nearly all of these women had significant sexual problems, with 79% reporting loss of sexual interest. In comparing women with low and normal levels of T, no differences were found in level of sexual desire, vaginal lubrication, or orgasm. However, the women with low T were less likely to masturbate.

Effects of Steroidal Contraceptives

It has been know for some time that oral contraceptives (OCs), by both blocking ovulation and stimulating production of SHBG, are associated with reduced free-T levels. In spite of this, surprisingly little attention has been paid to possible effects of OCs on women's sexuality *(123)*. In a placebo-controlled study of women who had been sterilized, a combined OC (COC) was compared with a progestagen-only OC. The COC reduced sexual interest and, in some cases, induced negative mood in a proportion of women *(124)*. In another study, comparable effects were found to be relevant to discontinuation within the first 3 mo of OC use, both mood and sexual side effects being the strongest predictors of early discontinuation *(125)*. Whether these adverse sexual and mood effects are the result of lowered free T is a question waiting to be answered. An alternative explanation is a direct effect of the progestagen in the OC.

There is a limited amount of evidence on the relationship between T levels and sexuality in OC users. Bancroft et al. *(126)* compared two groups of students who were all sexually active, but one group was using COCs and the other was using nonsteroidal methods of contraception. As expected, the COC users had substantially lower free T than the nonusers, but in spite of this, their level of sexuality was higher, including a more positive attitude about their sexual partners. This underlines the fact that the personality of OC users, including their attitudes about premarital sexuality, is likely to be different than those who use other methods of contraception. In addition, the use of a safe contraceptive may have a sexually enhancing effect in the OC users. Furthermore, in any cross-sectional study such as this, those who experience negative sexual effects of the OC are likely to have selected themselves out. Of more interest is that levels of free T correlated with frequency of sexual intercourse as well as some aspects of enjoyment of sexual intercourse in the OC users but not the nonusers. Free T did not correlate with frequency of masturbation in either group. A subgroup of subjects from this study took part in a prospective study in which daily ratings of sexual interest and activity, well-being, and other variables were recorded over one cycle together with weekly blood samples *(127)*. This further confirmed that the non-OC users had higher free-T levels throughout the 4 wk of the cycle, but they also showed a significant fall in free T during menstruation. The OC users showed lower but more stable free-T levels. These two patterns of T were paralleled by daily ratings of sexual interest. Whereas free T and sexual interest remained fairly stable through the OC cycle, for nonusers there was a decline in both variables during the premenstrual and menstrual phases. In this study, this pattern could not be attributed to cyclical variation in mood, as both groups of subjects reported minimal cycle-related mood change.

In an earlier study *(128)*, 20 women with sexual problems that they attributed to OC use were compared with 20 women taking the same OCs but without sexual difficulties. Both groups showed similarly low T levels. The sexual-problem group then participated in a placebo-controlled, double-blind, crossover evaluation of oral androstenedione administration, which substantially increased circulating T levels. No sexual benefits were apparent from the increased T levels and this study failed to demonstrate that low T was causally related to the sexual difficulties. It was noteworthy that plasma T levels correlated significantly with measures of sexual interest in the no-problem group, but not in the problem group. This could be interpreted as evidence that once sexual problems become established in women, the complexity of psychosexual factors serves to obscure any hormone–behavior relationship. This same explanation could be used to account for the presence of correlations between free T and sexual activity in nonproblematic OC users, but no correlation in nonusers *(126)*. In that study, the nonusers showed various evidence that their sexual lives were more problematic than the OC users.

Clearly, this limited literature on free-T and OC use raises some fundamental questions that need further research. The substantial minority of OC users who discontinue because of negative sexual and mood effects could be demonstrating the effects of lowered free T. If so, that would suggest that lowering free T by OC use is of relevance to the sexuality and general well-being of some women but not all.

Effects of Antiandrogens in Women

Cyproterone acetate (CPA) is an antiandrogen that has been used for many years, at least in Europe, for treatment of androgen-dependent conditions such as acne and hirsutism in women. Little attention has been given to the possible sexual side effects of such treatment. Appelt and Strauss *(129)* reviewed seven studies from the 1970s reporting loss of libido in 1.2–33.3% of women. They commented that such side effects had not been systematically asked about in any of these studies and therefore depended on the women volunteering the information. Appelt and Strauss *(129)* studied 36 women who had not had sexual problems before starting on CPA, and of these, 16 (44%) reported negative effects on their sex life; this rises to 61% if women not in sexual relationships are excluded. They also cited two German studies from the 1960s showing that women with hirsutism and assumed high T did not have increased interest in sex. Instead, they tended to suffer from sexual problems that were attributed to the psychological impact of their hirsutism. The negative connotations of hirsutism in women are very culturally sensitive; in some cultures, increased body hair is regarded as sexually attractive. This is an issue that warrants cross-cultural study, although it should not be assumed that women with either hirsutism or acne have abnormally raised T levels; their problems may depend on increased target organ sensitivity to T in the skin.

Experimental Studies in Women

A recent study of eight healthy women with normal T levels, given sublingual doses of T in a placebo-controlled experiment, showed effects of increased T on genital response to erotic stimuli occurring 3–4 h after the peak increase in plasma T *(69)*. This seems surprisingly rapid for a genomic steroid effect.

This same group *(130)* studied eight young amenorrheic women with associated low weight, although none had the diagnosis of anorexia nervosa. They showed lower levels of sexual interest and activity and lower T levels than a comparison group of normally menstruating aged-matched women. The amenorrheic group was given testosterone undecanoate, 40 mg daily for 8 wk, and placebo for 8 wk in a double-blind crossover study. They were evaluated in a psychophysiology laboratory with measurement of vaginal pulse amplitude (VPA) in response to erotic fantasies and erotic films. Whereas response to fantasy did not differ between T and placebo, VPA was significantly greater in response to the film in the T condition. However, this effect was not reflected in subjective ratings of excitement or "lust." Nor did the two treatments differ in terms of daily ratings of sexuality or mood. This experiment therefore demonstrated an effect of increasing T on physiological response to erotic stimulation, which was not apparent in any subjective or mood measures.

Summary of Evidence in the Female

There are enough pointers in the literature reviewed to indicate that T has a role in the sexuality of women. However, the evidence is inconsistent and confusing, and, in a number of cases, contradictory. There are a number of possible explanations for this state of affairs.

1. Women may vary in the extent to which their sexuality is influenced by T. There is much indirect evidence to support this: the wide variation in age of onset of masturbation in women, suggestive of a variable impact of hormonal influences (46); the negative sexual effect that antiandrogens have in a proportion of women (129); the possibility that oral contraceptives reduce sexual interest by lowering free T but only in a proportion of women (124); the finding that sexual interest is lowered in many but not all women after oophorectomy (50% in ref. 103). Sherwin (131) commented that "considerable inter-subject variability in both plasma T levels and aspects of sexual behavior in oophorec-tomized women in response to a standard dose of E-A preparation has been observed in our studies." Yet, this possibility has received virtually no attention in the extensive literature on hormone replacement. If the responsiveness of women to the sexual effects of T does vary markedly across women, then we should expect to find considerable inconsistency across studies if this source of variability is not controlled.

2. Uncertainty about the extent to which observed behavioral effects of exogenous T are direct androgen effects or indirect effects resulting from increased availability of bioactive estrogen, resulting both from the conversion of T to E_2, and reduced binding of E_2 in the presence of increased T.

3. The sexuality of women is powerfully influenced by mood, energy, and well-being and these aspects are affected by a wide variety of factors. The possible relationship between T and mood will be considered in the final section. Although these aspects of affect have been assessed as well as sexuality in many of the studies considered, very few have directly considered the extent to which affect influences sexuality.

4. In addition to affect, the sexuality of women is powerfully influenced by other psychological mechanisms. This is implied by the finding in several studies of younger women, that the relationship between T and sexuality was most apparent in women whose sexuality was unproblematic (e.g., refs. 118, 128, and 130). Thus, whereas T may play a role in the sexuality of many women, its effects can easily be obscured by the coexistence of other psychological or affective factors.

COMPARISON OF ANDROGEN EFFECTS IN MEN AND WOMEN

What might we learn by directly comparing the effects of androgens in the two sexes?

1. The evidence is more consistent for the male than for the female, even though there are many more opportunities to study hormone–behavior relationships in women, and there is a much more substantial body of data. Apart from methodological considerations, which are more complex in women than men, potentially the most important factor accounting for this gender difference is a greater variability of behavioral responsiveness to androgens among women suggested earlier. There obviously is variability among men, but it appears to be of a much smaller magnitude.

2. Those women who are behaviorally responsive to T respond to levels of T that would be totally ineffective in men, This greater sensitivity to T in women is apparent in behavioral and other central nervous system (CNS) responses and is possibly less marked in the anabolic and skin effects of T.

3. Men and women may differ in the relationship between affect and sexuality. Although studies of androgen withdrawal and replacement in men show that mood, energy, and well-being are affected, the impact on these variables appears to be more influential and predictable in women than in men. The reasons for this are poorly understood. In general, the relationship between mood and sexuality has received very little attention. Conventional wisdom holds that sexual interest and, to some extent, responsiveness typically goes down in negative mood states. However, current research on this topic at the Kinsey Institute *(131a)* shows that a substantial minority of men experiences an increase in sexual interest when in negative mood states, to some extent with depression but more often with anxiety or stress. This paradoxical pattern is more likely in younger men. Our preliminary results with women suggest that whereas this paradoxical pattern does occur, it is less common than in men. The possible mechanisms involved in this relationship are beyond the scope of this chapter, but are, in any case, little understood. Whether the effects of T are involved remains uncertain.

4. A fundamental difference in male and female mechanisms of androgen production may be relevant. More than 90% of testosterone in the male is produced by the testes. By contrast, a substantial proportion of androgen production in women is from the adrenal glands and, hence, increased adrenal androgens can be expected in states associated with increased adrenal activity, such as anxiety, stress, or depression. There is limited evidence of androgen levels in such mood states, but they indicate that an increase in T is possible *(132–134)*. In the male, somewhat more attention has been paid to T levels in negative mood states; overall, the evidence is inconsistent, showing no change or a decrease, and with uncertainty in most studies whether the decrease is a cause or a consequence of the negative mood *(135)*. No evidence of an increased T in negative mood states in men has been found. Thus, it seems unlikely that the paradoxical increase in sexual interest in some men when in negative mood states could be caused by increased T, but this possibility needs to be ruled out. In women, it should be possible to establish whether those who report an increased sexual interest in negative mood states have a greater increase in their T levels than those who do not. In any case, this added complexity in women could be contributing to the overall confused picture.

5. The evidence is suggestive that testosterone–behavior relationships are more easily obscured by other psychological mechanisms in women than is the case for men, although this comparison warrants direct study. If so, this would imply that the hormone effects are more robust or predominant in the male.

6. In the male, the evidence supports the idea of a threshold above which increased T levels have little behavioral effect, and below which signs of androgen deficiency are likely to occur. The evidence does not support this same threshold concept in women. The most convincing behavioral effects of the administration of exogenous androgens involves supraphysiological levels; although in a number of studies, sensitivity to these levels appears to decrease over time. On the other hand, it remains possible that signs of androgen deficiency will occur if circulating levels of T fall too low, the critical level depending on a particular woman's sensitivity, although the effects of such deficiency on the woman's sexuality may be obscured by other psychological factors in the woman's life.

7. If the effects of T on genital response in males is comparatively subtle and complicated by other factors impacting on genital response, this would appear to be even more so in women.

Men are much more aware of their genital response, and perception of penile erection can have an enhancing effect on central arousal. Women are less aware of their genital responses, and as shown by Tuiten et al. *(130)*, effects that T may have on genital response are relatively easily dissociated from the woman's subjective experience of sexual interest or excitement. In comparison with men, women in general show much less agreement between their subjective reports of sexual arousal and genital measures of arousal *(136)*.

The Desensitization Hypothesis

The following is a theoretical attempt to explain some (but not all) of these gender differences in androgen effects on sexuality.

1. The greater variability in the sensitivity to androgens in women could result from a greater genetic variability in women, on the grounds that in women, behavioral responsiveness to gonadal steroids is less crucial to reproduction than is the case with men *(58,137,138)*. However, the mechanism by which a genetically determined sensitivity might be expressed differently in women and in men requires explanation.

2. One of the consequences of the far greater levels of T in men is that they show masculinizing effects, such as increased growth and muscle bulk, dependent on the peripheral anabolic effects of T. It has been postulated that if males were as sensitive to the CNS effects of T as females, then the behavioral effects of these masculinizing levels would be maladaptive. Hence, there is a need in the male to reduce responsiveness to androgen effects in the brain *(139)*.

3. Exposure to substantially higher levels of T during fetal development and also during the first few weeks postnatally could be responsible for desensitizing the CNS to T effects in the male. Such desensitization would presumably act at the genomic rather than the receptor stage of hormone action, as, at least in rodents and in the short term, both T and DHT exposure results in upregulation of T receptors *(140,141)*. A consequence of such desensitization in the male would be that genetically determined variations in CNS receptor responsiveness to T would be "flattened out," as well as allowing much higher levels of T from puberty onwards without hyperstimulation of CNS mechanisms.

4. With no such desensitization in females, the basic genetic variability would be more evident, at much lower levels of T, and manifested as greater variability in behavioral responsiveness, demonstrated from early adolescent development onward.

5. Evidence from studies of women with congenital adrenal hyperplasia (CAH), particularly the salt-losing variety associated with higher levels of T during fetal development, shows not only some degree of masculinization of behavior but also low levels of sexual interest and activity associated with low fertility *(142)*. Although in such cases there are a number of factors which could impair normal sexual development, this evidence is consistent with there being some degree of desensitization to the high fetal levels of T, which fall and remain low after birth when the CAH is treated.

6. An interesting question is whether this hypothetical desensitization mechanism is an "organizing effect" of high T that is only operative during early development or whether such suppression is possible if exposure to high levels occurs later in development. Evidence of "tolerance" to supraphysiological levels of T was reported in several of the HRT studies reviewed earlier. This suggests that such desensitization might occur later in life also, at least to some extent. If there is any validity in this "desensitization hypothesis," it is important that we know about it, as it could be highly relevant to long-term effects of sustained supraphysiological levels of T in older women. However, we should also keep in mind the possibility that there may be a decline in T-receptor sensitivity in women as they age comparable to that found in men.

Although by no means simple, this theoretical model is open to testing in both animal and clinical studies. In general, our understanding of the effects of androgens on human sexuality is far from complete, particularly in the female. Throughout this chapter, a number of issues warranting further research have been identified. With this renewed interest in androgen effects, it is to be hoped that we shall see many of these basic but unresolved questions answered in the near future.

REFERENCES

1. Davidson JM, Carmago CA, Smith ER. Effects of androgens on sexual behaviour of hypogonadal men. J Clin Endocrinol Metab 1979;48:955–958.
2. Luisi M, Franchi F. Double-blind group comparative study of testosterone undecanoate and mesterolone in hypogonadal male patients. J Endocrinol Invest 1980;3:305–308.
3. Skakkebaek NE, Bancroft J, Davidson DW, Warner P. Androgen replacement with oral testosterone undecanoate in hypogonadal men: a double blind controlled study. Clin Endocrinol 1981;14:49–61.
4. Salmimies P, Kockott G, Pirke KM, et al. Effects of testosterone replacement on sexual behavior in hypogonadal men. Arch Sex Behav 1982;11:345–353.
5. Kwan M, Greenleaf WJ, Mann J, et al. The nature of androgen action on male sexuality: a combined laboratory-self-report study on hypogonadal men. J Clin Endocrinol Metab 1983;57:557–562.
6. O'Carroll RE, Shapiro C, Bancroft J. Androgens, behaviour and nocturnal erection in hypogonadal men: the effects of varying the replacement dose. Clin Endocrinol 1985;23:527–538.
7. Arver S, Dobs AS, Meikle AW, et al. Improvement of sexual function in testosterone deficient men treated for 1 year with a permeation enhanced testosterone transdermal system. J Urol 1996;155(5): 1604–1608.
8. Gooren LJG. Hypogonadotropic hypogonadal men respond less well to androgen substitution treatment than hypergonadotropic hypogonadal men. Arch Sex Behav 1988;17:265–270.
9. Clopper RR, Voorhess ML, MacGillivray MH, et al. Psychosexual behavior in hypopituitary men: a controlled comparison of gonadotropin and testosterone replacement. Psychoneuroendocrinology 1993;18(2):149–161.
10. Finkelstein JW, Susman EJ, Chinchilli VM, et al. Effects of estrogen or testosterone on self-reported sexual responses and behaviors in hypogonadal adolescents. J Clin Endocrinol Metab 1998;83(7):2281–2285.
11. Cunningham GR, Hirshkowitz M, Korenman SG, Karacan I. Testosterone replacement therapy and sleep-related erections in hypogonadal men. J Clin Endocrinol Metab 1990;70:792–797.
12. Carani C, Bancroft J, Granata A, et al. Testosterone and erectile function: Nocturnal penile tumescence and rigidity, and erectile response to visual erotic stimuli in hypogonadal and eugonadal men. Psychoneuroendocrinology 1992;17(6):647–654.
13. Carani C, Granata ARM, Bancroft J, Marrama P. The effects of testosterone replacement on nocturnal penile tumescence and rigidity and erectile response to visual erotic stimuli in hypogonadal men. Psychoneuroendocrinology 1995;20(7):743–753.
14. Bancroft J, O'Carroll R, McNeilly A, Shaw R. The effects of bromocriptine on the sexual behaviour of a hyperprolactinaemic man. A controlled case study. Clin Endocrinol 1984;21:131–137.
15. Bancroft J, Wu FCW. Changes in erectile responsiveness during androgen therapy. Arch Sex Behav 1983;12(1):59–66.
16. Bancroft J. Are the effects of androgens on male sexuality noradrenergically mediated? Some consideration of the human. Neurosci Biobehav Rev 1995;19(2):325–330.
17. Anderson RA, Martin CW, Kung A, et al. 7α-Methyl-19-nortestosterone (MENT) maintains sexual behavior and mood in hypogonadal men. J Clin Endocrinol Metab 1999;84(10):3556–3562.
18. Schiavi RC. Aging and Male Sexuality. Cambridge University Press, Cambridge, 1999.
19. Veldhuis JD, Iranmanesh A, Mulligan T, Pincus SM. Disruption of the young-adult synchrony between luteinizing hormone release and oscillations in follicle-stimulating hormone, prolactin, and nocturnal penile tumescence (NPT) in healthy older men. J Clin Endocrinol Metab 1999;84(10): 3498–3505.
20. Tsitouras PD, Marti CE, Harman SM. Relationship of serum testosterone to sexual activity in healthy elderly men. J Gerontol 1982;37:288–293.
21. Schiavi RC, Schreiner-Engel P, Mandeli J, et al. Healthy aging and male sexual function. Am J Psychiatry 1990;147:766–771.

22. Morales A, Johnston B, Heaton JWP, Clark A. Oral androgens in the treatment of hypogonadal impotent men. J Urol 1994;152:1115–1118.

23. Flynn MA, Weaver-Osterholtz D, Sharpe-Timms KL, et al. Dehydroepiandrosterone replacement in aging humans. J Clin Endocrinol Metab 1999;84(5):1527–1533.

24. Raboch J, Starka L. Reported coital activity of men and levels of plasma testosterone. Arch Sex Behav 1973;2:309–315.

25. Kraemer HC, Becker HB, Brodie HTH, et al. Orgasmic frequency and plasma testosterone levels in normal human males. Arch Sex Behav 1976;5:125–132.

26. Brown WA, Monti PM, Corriveau DP. Serum testosterone and sexual activity and interest in men. Arch Sex Behav 1978;7:97–103.

27. Lange JD, Brown WA, Wincze JP, Zwick W. Serum testosterone concentration and penile tumescence changes in men. Horm Behav 1980;14:267–270.

28. Rubin H, Henson D, Falvo R, High R. The relationship between men's endogenous levels of testosterone and their penile responses to erotic stimuli. Behav Res Ther 1979;17:305–312.

29. Bremner WJ, Vitiello MV, Prinz PN. Loss of circadian rhythmicity in blood testosterone levels with aging in normal men. J Clin Endocrinol Metab 1983;56(6):1278–1281.

30. Reinberg A, Lagoguey M. Circadian and circannual rhythms in sexual activity and plasma hormones (FSH, LH and testosterone) of five human males. Arch Sex Behav 1978;7:13–30.

31. Udry JR, Morris NM. Seasonality of coitus and seasonality of birth. Demography 1967;4:673–680.

32. Smals AGH, Kloppenborg PWC, Benraad TJ. Circannual cycle in plasma testosterone levels in man. J Clin Endocrinol Metabol 1976;42:979–983.

33. Bagatell CJ, Heiman JR, Rivier JE, Bremner WJ. Effects of endogenous testosterone and estradiol on sexual behavior in normal young men. J Clin Endocrinol Metab 1994;78(3):711–716.

34. Anderson RA, Bancroft J, Wu FCW. The effects of exogenous testosterone on sexuality and mood of normal men. J Clin Endocrinol Metab 1992;75(6):1503–1507.

35. Frenken J, Vennix P. Sexuality Experience Scales Manual. Swets and Zeitlinger B.V., Zeist, The Netherlands, 1981.

36. Bagatell CJ, Heiman JR, Matsumoto AM, et al. Metabolic and behavioral effects of high-dose, exogenous testosterone in healthy men. J Clin Endocrinol Metab 1994;79(2):561–567.

37. Su T-P, Pagliaro M, Schmidt PJ, et al. Neuropsychiatric effects of anabolic steroids in male normal volunteers. JAMA 1993;269(21):2760–2764.

38. Yates WR, Perry PJ, MacIndoe J, et al. Psychosexual effects of three doses of testosterone cycling in normal men. Biol Psychiatry 1999;45:254–260.

39. Moss HB, Panzak GL, Tarter RE. Sexual functioning of male anabolic steroid abusers. Arch Sex Behav 1993;22(1):1–12.

40. Carani C, Scuteri A, Marrama P, Bancroft J. The effects of testosterone administration and visual erotic stimuli on nocturnal penile tumescence in normal men. Horm Behav 1990;24:435–441.

41. Buena F, Swerdloff RS, Steiner BS, et al. Sexual function does not change when serum testosterone levels are pharmacologically varied within the normal male range. Fertil Steril 1993;59(5):1118–1123.

42. Udry JR, Billy JOG, Morris NM, et al. Serum androgenic hormones motivate sexual behavior in adolescent boys. Fertil Steril 1985;43(1):90–94.

43. Halpern CT, Udry JR, Campbell B, Suchindran C. Testosterone and pubertal development as predictors of sexual activity: A panel analysis of adolescent males. Psychosom Med 1993;55:436–447.

44. Kinsey AC, Pomeroy WB, Martin CE. Sexual Behavior in the Human Male. WB Saunders, Philadelphia, 1948.

45. Halpern CJT, Udry JR, Suchindran C, Campbell B. Adolescent males' willingness to report masturbation. J Sex Res 2000;37(4):327–332.

46. Bancroft J, Herbenick D, Reynolds M. Masturbation as a marker of sexual development. In: Bancroft J, ed., Sexual Development. Indiana University Press, Bloomington, in press.

47. Bancroft J, Tennent G, Loucas K, Cass J. The control of deviant sexual behaviour by drugs: 1. Behavioural changes following oestrogens and anti-androgens. Br J Psychiatry 1974;125:310–315.

48. Murray MAF, Bancroft JHJ, Anderson DC, et al. Endocrine changes in male sexual deviants after treatment with anti-androgens, oestrogens or tranquillizers. J Endocrinol 1975;67:179–188.

49. Bradford JMW, Pawlak A. Double-blind placebo crossover study of cyproterone acetate in the treatment of the paraphilias. Arch Sex Behav 1993;22:383–402.

50. Bradford JMW, Pawlak A. Effects of cyproterone acetate on sexual arousal patterns of pedophiles. Arch Sex Behav 1993;22(6):629–641.

51. Bradford JMW, Greenberg DM. Pharmacological treatment of deviant sexual behaviour. Ann Rev Sex Res 1996;7:283–306.

52. Meyer WJ, Walker PA, Emory LE, Smith ER. Physical, metabolic, and hormonal effects on men of long-term therapy with medroxyprogesterone acetate. Fertil Steril 1985;43(1):102–109.

53. Thibaut F, Cordier B, Kuhn JM. Effect of a long-lasting gonadotrophin hormone-releasing hormone agonist in six cases of severe male paraphilia. Acta Psychiatr Scand 1993;87:445–450.

54. Toone BK, Wheeler M, Nanjee N, et al. Sex hormones, sexual activity and plasma anticonvulsant levels in male epileptics. J Neurol Neurosurg Psychiatry 1983;46:824–826.

55. Fenwick PBC, Mercer S, Grant R, et al. Nocturnal penile tumescence and serum testosterone levels. Arch Sex Behav 1986;15:13–22.

56. Sitsen JMA. Prescription drugs and sexual function. In: Sitsen JMA (ed.), Handbook of Sexology. Elsevier. 1988, pp. 425–461.

57. Rosseau L, Dupont A, Labrie F, Couture M. Sexuality changes in prostate cancer patients receiving antihormonal therapy combining the antiandrogen flutamide with medical (LHRH agonist) or surgical castration. Arch Sex Behav 1988;17(1):87–98.

58. Bancroft J. Human Sexuality and its Problems. Churchill Livingstone, Edinburgh, 1989.

59. Jannini EA, Screponi E, Carosa E, et al. Lack of sexual activity from erectile dysfunction is associated with a reversible reduction in serum testosterone. Int J Androl 1999;22:385–392.

60. O'Carroll R, Bancroft J. Testosterone therapy for low sexual interest and erectile dysfunction in men: a controlled study. Br J Psychiatry 1984;145:146–151.

61. Carani C, Zini D, Baldini A, et al. Effects of androgen treatment in impotent men with normal and low levels of free testosterone. Arch Sex Behav 1990;19(3):223–234.

62. Morales A, Johnston B, Heaton JPW, Lundie M. Testosterone supplementation for hypogonadal impotence: Assessment of biochemical measures and therapeutic outcomes. J Urol 1997;157(3): 849–854.

63. Buvat J, Lemaire A. Endocrine screening in 1,022 men with erectile dysfunction: Clinical significance and cost-effective strategy. J Urol 1997;158(5):1764–1767.

64. Bancroft J, Janssen E. The dual control model of male sexual response: a theoretical approach to centrally mediated erectile dysfunction. Neurosci Biobehav Rev 2000;24:571–579.

65. Nottelmann ED, Susman EJ, Dorn LD, et al. Developmental processes in early adolescence: relations among chronologic age, pubertal stage, height, weight, and serum levels of gonadotropins, sex steroids, and adrenal androgens. J Adolesc Health Care 1987;8:246–260.

66. Ankarberg C, Norjavaara E. Diurnal rhythm of testosterone secretion before and throughout puberty in healthy girls: correlation with 17β-estradiol and dehydroepiandrosterone sulfate. J Clin Endocrinol Metab 1999;84(3):975–984.

67. Udry JR, Talbert LM, Morris NM. Biosocial foundations of adolescent female sexuality. Demography 1986;23(2):217–229.

68. Halpern CJT, Udry JR, Suchindran C. Testosterone predicts initiation of coitus in adolescent females. Psychosom Med 1997;59:161–171.

69. Tuiten A, Van Honk J, Koppeschaar H, et al. Time course of effects of testosterone administration on sexual arousal in women. Arch Gen Psychiatry 2000;57:149–153.

70. Hedricks CA. Female sexual activity across the human menstrual cycle: a biopsychosocial approach. Ann Rev Sex Res 1994;5:122–172.

71. Persky H, Lief AI, Strauss D, et al. Plasma testosterone levels and sexual behavior of couples. Arch Sex Behav 1978;7:157–173.

72. Morris NM, Udry JR, Khan-Dawood F, Dawood MY. Marital sex frequency and midcycle female testosterone. Arch Sex Behav 1987;16:27–38.

73. Cutler WB, Garcia C-R, Huggins GR, Preti G. Sexual behavior and steroid levels among gynecologically premature premenopausal women. Fertil Steril 1986;48(4):496–502.

74. Bancroft J, Sanders D, Davidson D, Warner P. Mood, sexuality, hormones and the menstrual cycle III. Sexuality and the role of androgens. Psychosom Med 1983;45(6):509–516.

75. Van Goozen SHM, Wiegant VM, Endert E, et al. Psychoendocrinological assessment of the menstrual cycle: the relationship between hormones, sexuality, and mood. Arch Sex Behav 1997;26(4): 359–382.

76. Schreiner-Engel P, Schiavi RC, Smith H, White D. Sexual arousability and the menstrual cycle. Psychosom Med 1981;43:199–214.

77. Alder E, Bancroft J. The relationship between breastfeeding persistence, sexuality and mood in postpartum women. Psychol Med 1988;18:389–396.

78. Hyde JS, DeLamater J. Sexuality during pregnancy and the year postpartum. In: Travis CB, White JW, eds. Sexuality, Society, and Feminism. American Psychological Association 2000, pp. 167–180.

79. Alder E, Cook A, Davidson D, West C, Bancroft J. Hormones, mood and sexuality in lactating women. Br J Psychiatry 1986;148:74–79.

80. Crilly RG, Marshall DH, Nordin BE. The effect of age on plasma androstenedione concentration in oophorectomised women. Clin Endocrinol 1979;10:199–201.

81. Orentreich N, Brind JL, Rizer RL, Vogelman JH. Age changes and sex differences in serum dehydroepiandrosterone sulfate concentrations throughout adulthood. J Clin Endocrinol Metab 1984;59:551–555.

82. Bancroft J, Cawood EHH. Androgens and the menopause: A study of 40 to 60 year old women. Clin Endocrinol 1996;45:577–587.

83. Sulcová J, Hill M, Hampl R, Stárka L. Age and sex related differences in serum levels of unconjugated dehydroepiandrosterone and its sulphate in normal subjects. J Endocrinol 1997;154:57–62.

84. Burger HG, Dudley EC, Cui J, et al. A prospective longitudinal study of serum testosterone, dehydroepiandrosterone sulfate, and sex hormone-binding globulin levels through the menopause transition. J Clin Endocrinol Metab 2000;85(8):2832–2838.

85. Roger M, Nahoul K, Scholler R, Bagrel D. Evolution with ageing of four plasma androgens in postmenopausal women. Maturitas 1980;2:171–177.

86. Mushayandebvu T, Castracane VD, Gimpel T, et al. Evidence for diminished midcycle ovarian androgen production in older reproductive aged women. Fertil Steril 1996;65(4):721–723.

87. Zumoff B, Strain GW, Miller LK, Rosner W. Twenty-four-hour mean plasma testosterone concentration declines with age in normal premenopausal women. J Clin Endocrinol Metab 1995;80(4):1429–1430.

88. Laumann EO, Paik A, Rosen RC. Sexual dysfunction in the United States: Prevalence and predictors. JAMA 1999;281(6):537–544.

88a. Bancroft J, Loftus J, Long JS. Distress about sex: A national survey of women in heterosexual relationships. Arch Sex Behav 2003, in press.

89. Cawood EHH, Bancroft J. Steroid hormones, the menopause, sexuality and well-being of women. Psychol Med 1996;26:925–936

90. Bachmann GA, Leiblum SR, Kemmann E, et al. Sexual expression and its determinants in the postmenopausal woman. Maturitas 1984;6:19–29.

91. Dennerstein L, Dudley EC, Hooper JL, Burger H. Sexuality, hormones and the menopausal transition. Maturitas 1997;26:83–93.

92. Kirchengast S, Hartmann B, Gruber D, Huber J. Decreased sexual interest and its relationship to body build in postmenopausal women. Maturitas 1996;23:63–71.

93. McCoy NL, Davidson JM. A longitudinal study of the effects of menopause on sexuality. Maturitas 1985;7:203–210.

94. Sanders D, Warner P, Backström T, Bancroft J. Mood, sexuality, hormones and the menstrual cycle. I. Changes in mood and physical state: description of subjects and method. Psychosom Med 1983;45:487–501.

95. Mendel CC. The free hormone hypothesis: a physiologically based mathematical model. Endocr Rev 1989;10(3):232–274.

96. Wallen K, Parsons WA. Androgen may increase sexual motivation in estrogen-treated ovariectomized rhesus monkeys by increasing estrogen availability. Serono International Symposium on Biology of Menopause, 1998.

97. Burger H, Hailes J, Nelson J, Menelaus M. Effect of combined implants of oestradiol and testosterone on libido in postmenopausal women. Br Med J 1987;294:936–937.

98. Myers LS, Dixen J, Morrissette D, et al. Effects of estrogen, androgen, and progestin on sexual psychophysiology and behavior in postmenopausal women. J Clin Endocrinol Metab 1990;70:1124–1131.

99. Davis SR, McCloud P, Strauss BJG, Burger H. Testosterone enhances estradiol's effects on postmenopausal bone density and sexuality. Maturitas 1995;21:227–236.

100. Sherwin BB. The impact of different doses of estrogen and progestin on mood and sexual behavior in postmenopausal women. J Clin Endocrinol Metab 1991;72(2):336–343.

101. Dennerstein L, Burrows GD, Wood C, Hyman G. Hormones and sexuality: Effect of estrogen and progestogen. Obstet Gynecol 1980;56:316–322.

102. Dow MGT, Hart DM, Forrest CA. Hormonal treatments of sexual unresponsiveness in post-menopausal women: a comparative study. Br J Obstet Gynaecol 1983;90:361–366.
103. Nathorst-Böös J, von Schoultz B, Carlström K. Elective ovarian removal and estrogen replacement therapy—effects on sexual life, psychological well-being and androgen status. J Psychosom Obstet Gynaecol 1993;14:283–293.
104. Brincat M, Magos A, Studd JWW, et al. Subcutaneous hormone implants for the control of climacteric symptoms. Lancet 1984;1:16–18.
105. Burger HG, Hailes J, Menelaus M, et al. The management of persistent menopausal symptoms with oestradiol–testosterone implants: clinical, lipid and hormonal results. Maturitas 1984;6: 351–358.
106. Sherwin BB, Gelfand MM, Brender W. Androgen enhances sexual motivation in females: A prospective, crossover study of sex steroid administration in the surgical menopause. Psychosom Med 1985;47(4):339–351.
107. Sherwin BB, Gelfand MM. Sex steroids and affect in the surgical menopause: A double-blind, crossover study. Psychoneuroendocrinology 1985;10(3):325–335.
108. Sherwin BB, Gelfand MM. Differential symptom response to parenteral estrogen and/or androgen administration in the surgical menopause. Am J Obstet Gynecol 1985;151(2):153–160.
109. Sherwin BB, Gelfand MM. The role of androgen in the maintenance of sexual functioning in oophorectomized women. Psychosom Med 1987;49:397–409.
110. Sherwin BB. Affective changes with estrogen and androgen replacement therapy in surgically menopausal women. J Affect Disord 1988;14:177–187.
111. Castelo-Branco C, Vincente JJ, Figueras F, et al. Comparative effects of estrogens plus androgens and tibolone on bone, lipid pattern and sexuality in postmenopausal women. Maturitas 2000;34:161–168.
112. Shifren JL, Braunstein GD, Simon JA, et al. Transdermal testosterone treatment in women with impaired sexual function after oophorectomy. N Engl J Med 2000;343(10):682–688.
113. Kaplan HS, Owett T. The female androgen deficiency syndrome. J Sex Marital Ther 1993;19(1):3–24.
114. Morales AJ, Nolan JJ, Nelson JC, Yen SSC. Effects of replacement dose of dehydroepiandrosterone in men and women of advancing age. J Clin Endocrinol Metab 78(6):1360–1367.
115. Arlt, W., Callies, F., van Vlijmen, J.C., Koehler, I., et al. Dehydroepiandrosterone replacement in women with adrenal insufficiency. N Engl J Med 1999;341(14):1013–1020.
116. Stuart FM, Hammond DC, Pett MA. Inhibited sexual desire in women. Arch Sex Behav 1987;16(2):91–106.
117. Schreiner-Engel P, Schiavi RC, White D, Ghizzani A. Low sexual desire in women: the role of reproductive hormones. Horm Behav 1989;23:221–234.
118. Riley A, Riley E. Controlled studies on women presenting with sexual drive disorder: I. Endocrine status. J Sex Marital Ther 2000;;26:269–283.
119. Carney A, Bancroft J, Mathews A. Combination of hormonal and psychological treatment for female sexual unresponsiveness: a comparative study. Br J Psychiatry 1978;133:339–346.
120. Mathews A, Whitehead A, Kellett J. Psychological and hormonal factors in the treatment of female sexual dysfunction. Psychol Med 1983;13:83–92.
121. Dow MGT, Gallasher J. A controlled study of combined hormonal and psychological treatment for sexual unresponsiveness in women. Br J Clin Psychol 1989;28:201–212.
122. Hulter B, Lundberg PO. Sexual function in women with hypothalamo-pituitary disorders. Arch Sex Behav 1994;23(2):171–183.
123. Bancroft J, Sartorius N. The effects of oral contraceptives on well-being and sexuality. Oxford Rev Reprod Biol 1990;12:57–92.
124. Graham CA, Ramos R, Bancroft J, et al. The effects of steroidal contraceptives on the well-being and sexuality of women: a double blind, placebo-controlled, two centre study of combined and progestogen-only methods. Contraception 1995;52:363–369.
125. Sanders SA, Graham CM, Bass J, Bancroft J. A prospective study of the effects of oral contraceptives on sexuality and well-being and their relationship to discontinuation. Contraception 2001;64:51–58.
126. Bancroft J, Sherwin B, Alexander GM. Oral contraceptives, androgens, and the sexuality of young women. II. The role of androgens. Arch Sex Behav 1991;20(2):121–135.
127. Alexander GM, Sherwin BB, Bancroft J, Davidson DW. Testosterone and sexual behavior in oral contraceptive users and non-users: a prospective study. Horm Behav 1990;24:388–402.
128. Bancroft J, Davidson DW, Warner P, Tyrer G. Androgens and sexual behaviour in women using oral contraceptives. Clin Endocrinol 1980;12:327–340.

129. Appelt H, Strauss B. The psychoendocrinology of female sexuality: a research project. German J Psychol 1986;10(2):143–156.

130. Tuiten A, Laan E, Panhuysen G, et al. Discrepancies between genital responses and subjective sexual function during testosterone substitution in women with hypothalamic amenorrhea. Psychosom Med 1996;58:234–241.

131. Sherwin BB. A comparative analysis of the role of androgen in human male and female sexual behavior: Behavioral specificity, critical thresholds, and sensitivity. Psychobiology 1988;16:416–425.

131a. Bancroft J, Janssen E, Strong D, et al. The relationship between mood and sexuality in heterosexual men. Arch Sex Behav 2003, in press.

132. Baischer W, Koinig G, Hartmann B, Huber J, et al. Hypothalamic–pituitary–gonadal axis in depressed premenopausal women: elevated blood testosterone concentrations compared to normal controls. Psychoneuroendocrinology 1995;20:553–559.

133. Eriksson E, Sundblad C, Lisjoe P, et al. Serum levels of androgens are higher in women with premenstrual irritability and dysphoria than in controls. Psychoneuroendocrinology 1992;17(2-3):195–204.

134. Weber B, Lewicka S, Dueschle M, et al. Testosterone, androstenedione and dihydrotestosterone concentrations are elevated in female patients with major depression. Psychoneuroendocrinology 2000;25(8):765–771.

135. Seidman SN, Walsh BT. Testosterone and depression in aging men. Am J Geriatr Psychiatry 1999;7(1):18–33.

136. Everaerd W, Laan ETM, Both S, van der Velde J. Female sexuality. In L.T. Szuchman & F. Muscarella (eds.), Psychological perspectives on human sexuality New York: John Wiley & Sons, pp. 101–146.

137. Sanders D, Bancroft J. Hormones and the sexuality of women—the menstrual cycle. Clin Endocrinol Metab 1982;11:639–659.

138. Bancroft J. Hormones, sexuality and fertility in women. J Zool (Lond) 1987;213:445–454.

139. Bancroft J. Biological contributions to sexual orientation. In: McWhirter DP, Sanders SA, Reinisch JM, eds. Homosexuality/Heterosexuality. Oxford University Press, New York, 1990, pp. 101–111.

140. Menard CS, Harlan RE. Up-regulation of androgen receptor immunoreactivity in the rat brain by androgenic-anabolic steroids. Brain Res 1993;622:226–236.

141. Lu S, Simon NG, Wang Y, Hu S. Neural androgen receptor regulation: Effects of androgen and antiandrogen. J Neurobiol 1999;41:505–512.

142. Meyer-Bahlburg HFL. Commentary: What causes low rates of child-bearing in congenital adrenal hyperplasia? J Clin Endocrinol Metab 1999;84:1844–1847.

15 Androgens and Cognition

Monique M. Cherrier, PhD
and Suzanne Craft, PhD

CONTENTS

INTRODUCTION
EVIDENCE FROM ANIMAL STUDIES
EVIDENCE FROM HUMAN STUDIES
ENDOCRINE DISORDERS
SUMMARY
REFERENCES

INTRODUCTION

Androgens and their effects on behavior have been an area of study for over a century. In 1889, Brown-Sequard, using himself as case study, injected an extract from crushed animal testicles. He reported that this treatment gave him increased energy, muscular strength, stamina and mental agility *(1)*. Although crude, this approach led the way to the discovery of androgens. Since then, the focus of most androgen research has been in the area of reproductive function. More recently, the focus of attention has turned to hormone effects on the central nervous system (CNS) and aging, with particular emphasis on potential antiaging effects of hormone replacement therapy. This chapter will explore the complex relationship between androgens and cognition. We will first describe mechanisms by which hormones exert their effects in the CNS, including organizational and activational effects. Next, we will examine the relationship of androgens and cognition in humans, including endogenous levels and studies examining hormone manipulation in healthy young and older populations. Finally, we will examine the relationship between androgens and cognition as expressed through endocrine disorders that result in excessive or insufficient hormone levels. This chapter will feature cognition rather than mood, emotion, or other aspects of human behavior. Readers may refer to other chapters in this volume or Rubinow and Schmidt (1996) for a review of the relationship between androgens and mood or behavior *(2)*.

EVIDENCE FROM ANIMAL STUDIES
Hormonal Mechanisms of Action

Several CNS functions are regulated by gonadal steroids and, in particular, testosterone (T). Examples include prenatal sexual differentiation of the brain, adult sexual

From: *Contemporary Endocrinology: Androgens in Health and Disease*
Edited by: C. Bagatell and W. J. Bremner © Humana Press Inc., Totowa, NJ

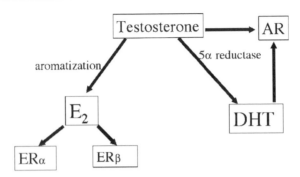

Fig. 1. Pathway of androgen metabolism and action in the CNS from T through dihydrotestosterone (DHT) via 5α-reductase and estradiol (E$_2$) via aromatase. Androgen receptor (AR), estrogen receptor-α (ERα) and -β (ERβ).

behavior, gonadotropin secretion, and cognition. The effects T are mediated through the androgen receptor (AR), which is widely, but selectively distributed throughout the brain *(3)*. Castration rapidly decreases AR expression and T upregulates neural AR in a dose-dependent manner in both male and female mice. T also acts via rapid, nongenomic methods of action through G-protein-coupled, agonist-sequestrable T membrane receptors that initiate a transcription-independent signaling pathway affecting calcium channels *(4–7)*. Thus, activational effects of androgens as discussed in a later subsection may occur through both genomic or nongenomic mechanisms.

Another important aspect of T action is its active metabolism in vivo. In the body, T is converted to E$_2$ by the enzyme cytochrome P450 aromatase, and to dihydrotestosterone (DHT) by the enzymes 5α-reductase (5α-R) types 1 and 2 *(see* Fig. 1). E$_2$ formed from T may then act on target organs via intracellular estrogen receptors α and β. DHT binds to androgen receptors with greater affinity than T and is a more potent androgen. Therefore, androgen effects may occur through T directly or via its active metabolites, E$_2$ and DHT.

Organizational Effects of Androgens

Organizational effects of androgens refer to permanent changes in brain structure and function as a result of exposure to androgens during a critical developmental window. For example, male rats castrated neonatally show a spatial ability pattern closer to the typical female rat pattern, whereas ovariectomized female rats treated with T neonatally demonstrate a typical male spatial ability pattern *(8)*. Intact female rats treated neonatally with T perform better on a maze task than male castrates and intact males *(9,10)*. These examples of permanent behavioral changes resulting from hormone manipulations during critical brain development periods are thought to be examples of organizational effects of hormones. Therefore, observed sex differences in healthy normal animals are thought to be the result of organizational effects of hormones.

Sexual dimorphisms have been shown to occur with regional concentrations of neuropeptides and neurotransmitters, brain physiology, and behavior *(11–13)*. For example, perinatal exposure of female rats to T eliminates the natural cyclic expression of gonadotropic secretion *(14)*. Previously identified sexually dimorphic brain regions include the hypothalamus, pituitary, corpus callosum, adrenal cortex, cerebellum, and prefrontal regions. With regard to cognitive tasks, a common finding is that males outperform females in many species on spatial tasks. This advantage on spatial tasks may be caused by a potential sexual dimorphism of the hippocampus and dentate gyrus, two structures that underlie spatial navigation and spatial memory. Female rats neonatally exposed to T demonstrate a more masculine or larger hippocampus, dentate gyrus, and corpus callosum *(15,16)*. Thus, the presence of androgens during critical developmental periods may produce sexual dimorphisms or sex differences for cognitive abilities.

Androgen Activational Effects

Androgens modulate cognition and behavior throughout the life-span. These modulation effects are termed "activational" effects of hormones. For example, postpubertal castrated male rats fail to demonstrate normal sexual behavior. However, sexual behavior can be restored to normal levels with T replacement *(17)*. Thus, certain behaviors are controlled to a large degree by androgens throughout the life-span. The mechanisms by which androgens exert these effects are likely complex. T replacement in castrated male rats results in decreased dopamine release, increased GABA turnover, and increased choline acetyltransferase (ChAT) levels *(2)*. These effects may occur rapidly, within hours or days, and can remain for years, affecting both brain structure, receptor sensitivity, and density *(18–20)*. The neuroregulatory effects of androgens occur in the frontal cortex, hypothalamus, amygdala, bed nucleus of stria terminalis, brainstem, and hippocampus *(2)*. Mice with age-related decreases in plasma T show a progressive impairment of spatial learning and memory related to T levels, which can be reversed with T administration *(21)*.

The activational effects of DHT on cognition are less well known. However, once formed, DHT is a potent steroid in the CNS. The affinity of DHT for the AR is four times that of T *(22)*. Like T, DHT upregulates neural AR following castration *(23)*. Although both T and DHT upregulate AR after castration, only DHT appears to sustain this effect for a prolonged period *(23)*.

The formation of E_2 results from aromatization of T. Brain aromatase activity (AA) in the male rat occurs primarily in the medial preoptic or anterior hypothalamus region *(24,25)*. Administration of the androgen-receptor antagonist flutamide with T or DHT in gonadectomized rats does not induce aromatase activity compared to T or DHT administered alone, suggesting that AA is androgen dependent *(24)*. E_2 treatment in the male rat partially upregulates AR after castration, although the effect is not nearly as strong as T or DHT *(26)*. E_2, like T, may act via nongenomic methods by binding to membrane receptors that are completely distinct from intracellular membrane receptors and can cause rapid signaling *(27)*. The functional role of E_2 in males is not well understood. E_2 appears to play an important and sometimes critical role in sexual behavior and social interaction behavior of male rats and other animals *(28,29)*. T and E_2 but not DHT modulate serotonin receptor mRNA and the density of serotonin receptors in the forebrain *(18,19)*. Thus, E_2 secondary to aromatization may be important with regard to mood.

EVIDENCE FROM HUMAN STUDIES

Endogenous Androgens

Measurable differences in certain cognitive abilities between men and women may be the result of the organizational effects of hormones. Hormones present during development of the CNS may produce structural changes resulting in behavioral differences. One area of cognitive abilities for which robust differences between men and women are typically observed is spatial abilities. The term "spatial" typically refers to tasks that have a geometric or three-dimensional aspect.

Studies in humans examining the relationship between endogenous androgen levels and cognitive performance have produced inconsistent results. Correlations between endogenous T levels and spatial abilities in men range from near zero to 0.53 *(30,31)*. In healthy young men, positive relationships have been found between circulating or endogenous T levels and visuospatial orientation *(30)*, spatial form comparison *(32)*, and composite visuospatial scores *(33)*. Positive relationships have also been found for tactual spatial tasks *(34,35)*. Other studies examining endogenous T levels have failed to find such a relationship between circulating androgen levels and visuospatial abilities *(36,37)*. Low T levels in men have also been found to be associated with better performance on spatial ability tasks, and high levels of estradiol have been associated with better visual memory in men *(36,38–40)*. In contrast, Gouchie and Kimura found that for male and female subjects divided into groups according to endogenous T levels (high vs low), the high-T women and low-T men demonstrated better spatial abilities compared to the low-T women and high-T men *(39)*. Finally, an examination of young men examined during periods of high vs low T levels from natural diurnal variation revealed a significant positive association with performance on a mental rotation test and average T levels but not with changes in T levels (i.e., high vs low), and there were no significant relationships between other tests (e.g., anagrams and an attention task) and T levels *(41)*. These findings have led some to suggest that the beneficial effects of T may be described by a curvilinear relationship such that low to moderate T levels improve cognitive abilities, but higher levels result in no further improvements or even decrements in some abilities (e.g., verbal) *(38,39)*.

In a comprehensive review of the literature, Kimura found large sex differences favoring males on spatial tasks sometimes approaching one standard deviation for targeting (e.g, throwing darts or catching a ball) and spatial orientation (e.g., imagined spatial rotation) *(42)*. Modest effect sizes were found for spatial visualization (e.g., imagining the result of folding paper in a precut shape), disembedding (finding a simple figure located in a more complex one), and spatial perception (e.g., determining the true vertical among distracting cues). Although some have suggested that experience with spatial tasks (e.g., driving, throwing, and catching) may account for these sex differences, studies controlling for experience continue to find sex differences and these differences may be present as early as 5 yr of age *(42–44)*.

Variability of results in the literature may be the result of wide variability in the selection of cognitive tests and their unique task demands. This includes use of the term "spatial" to describe numerous tests that may tap different cognitive processes or rely on different brain structures and networks. For example, men tend to outperform women on tasks that require spatial rotation or manipulation. Robust gender differences have been found for performance on the spatial rotation task (*see* Fig. 2), which requires imaginal rotation of an object *(45)*. It does not appear that this difference is the result of the three-dimensional aspect of the task, as these differences are also apparent on a test of two-dimensional rotation *(46)*. Interestingly, with a short training session and a virtual-reality adaptation of the mental rotation task, in which participants could manipulate a virtual-reality version of the complex design with their hands, these gender differences disap-

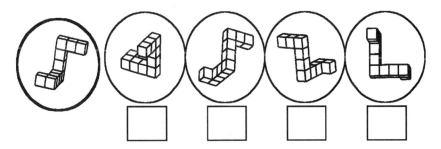

Fig. 2. Sample test item from the Mental Rotations Test. Three-dimensional item on the left is the stimulus item. Participants must choose two items on the right that match the stimulus item. Correct responses exactly match the stimulus item but have been rotated in three-dimensional space. Incorrect items do not match the stimulus item. (From ref. *45*.)

peared *(47)*. This latest result indicates a lack of gender differences on nonimagined spatial rotation tasks.

Memory for the location of objects is also considered a spatial task. Although recalling the location of objects clearly has a spatial component to it, several studies have demonstrated that women outperform men at recalling the location and spatial relationship between objects to be remembered in a spatial array *(48,49)*. Interestingly, this demonstrated difference between men and women on spatial tasks such as mental rotation and memory for spatial array is consistent with findings of gender differences on spatial navigation tasks. For example, men, on average, tend to use a Euclidean (distance) or cardinal direction (N, S, E, W) approach to spatial navigation, whereas women on average tend to use landmark references. Galea and Kimura (1993) found that when young men and women were required to learn a route on a tabletop map, men were able to learn the route in fewer trials, but women remembered more of the landmarks located along the route *(50)*. Studies comparing men and women on their ability to learn virtual-reality environments tend to support the findings of male advantage in landmark-free or landmark-limited environments *(51–53)*. Although there is some debate regarding the neural structures that underlie spatial navigation, most studies of humans and animals support a direct role for the hippocampus in spatial navigation or representation of large-scale space and the parahippocampal gyrus in recall of landmarks *(54–58)*. As noted previously, the hippocampus along with hypothalamus and other limbic structures are target areas for gonadal steroids. Male and female rats treated with T demonstrate a larger or more masculinelike hippocampus characterized by the size and assymetrical shape of the dentate gyrus *(16)*. Thus, these behavioral tendencies or cognitive styles may reflect differential effects of gonadal hormones on place and landmark systems in the hippocampus *(59)*.

Recent evidence from functional MRI (fMRI) studies provides further evidence that cognitive processing, in particular, processing of spatial information, activates specific brain regions and neural networks that are unique to the particular task demands. Shelton et al. (2001) found that healthy control participants activated right-sided hippocampus and parahippocampal regions when processing spatial information from a route or navigation perspective *(60)*. In contrast, when participants view the same information from a survey or ariel view, the cuneus, an area associated with processing complex visual information (objects or faces), demonstrated increased activation. Results indicate that specific cognitive task demands will activate unique corresponding brain regions or neural networks. In a similar fMRI experiment, men and women demonstrated activation of common brain regions associated with navigation (e.g., hippocampus, parahippocampus) while navigating through a virtual maze (61). However, a gender analysis revealed distinct activation of the left hippocampus in males, whereas females consistently recruited right parietal and right prefrontal cortex. In addition, men on average were significantly faster than women at finding their way out of the maze. Thus, evidence from human studies suggests that organizational and activational effects of hormones interact with the behavioral response to unique task demands and underlying neural networks associated with those task demands to produce the outcome of human behavioral performance.

Exogenous Androgens

Cognitive changes from exogenously manipulated androgen levels have been examined in healthy young men and women, transsexuals, and hypogonadal males (see following subsection). For example, Gordon and Lee (1986) examined cognitive performance in a group of healthy young men in response to administration of T enanthate (30). They administered a low dose of T enanthate (10 mg) to young men, followed by a battery of cognitive tests immediately after injection and 4 h later. They reported no appreciable effects from hormone administration, as participants demonstrated the same improvement from baseline to the second test session during the placebo condition as in the T condition. However, no hormone values were reported. Therefore, the relationship between cognition and hormone levels is unknown. In contrast, a group of female-to-male transsexuals (FMs) administered T, demonstrated improved spatial abilities, but with decreased verbal abilities (62). In a subsequent study by the same research group, beneficial effects of androgen treatment on spatial abilities were again confirmed in FMs and remained over a period of 1.5 yr (63). As expected, untreated male-to-female transsexuals (MFs) had higher scores on visuospatial tasks than untreated FMs, and after 3 mo of cross-sex hormone treatment, the group differences disappeared. Although findings of decreased verbal fluency from androgen treatment in FMs was not replicated, a pronounced effect on spatial abilities was replicated. This study shows that T had an enhancing, and not quickly reversible effect, on spatial ability performance, but no deleterious effect on verbal fluency in FMs. In contrast, antiandrogen treatment in combination with estrogen therapy had no observable effects on cognition in male-to-female transsexuals. However, Miles et al. (1998) (64) found male-to-female transsexuals demonstrated improved verbal memory in response to estrogen treatment with no differences between the treatment and control groups on tests of attention, mental rotation, or verbal fluency (64). Although it has been suggested that results from transsexual studies may be affected by comorbid psychiatric or mood conditions, there were no appreciable differences between the hormone-treated and wait-list groups in the Miles et al. (1998) study on mood measures (64). Further, in a population of healthy nontranssexual young women, Postma et al. (2000) found that short-term T admininstration (0.5 mg T cyclodextrine) resulted in improved spatial memory compared to placebo on some measures but not others (65).

Overall, the results from exogenous manipulation of androgens in healthy young men and women suggest that androgens may exert beneficial effects on spatial abilities. However, because of the study design and lack of documented change in hormone levels, findings to date remain inconclusive.

Aging Effects on Androgens

Serum levels of total T and bioavailable T (T that is not bound to sex hormone-binding globulin) decrease with age in men *(66,67)*. Although this decrease is gradual, it can result in decreased muscle mass, osteoporosis, decreased sexual activity, and changes in cognition *(66,68–71)*. Androgen-replacement therapy in normal older men has demonstrated benefits on bone mass, muscle strength, and sexual functioning *(72,73)*. However, these benefits may result from direct effects of T or from increased estradiol levels following aromatization of T. Recent evidence in the case of a patient with genetic aromatase deficiency suggests that bone mass changes and other physiological effects in men may, in fact, be attributable to changes in estradiol levels rather than to direct T effects *(74)*.

In addition to peripheral physiological effects, age-related declines in T levels may affect cognitive abilities. In healthy older men, endogenous T levels are significantly correlated with both visual and verbal memory and verbal fluency (0.53, 0.52 and 0.45, respectively) *(75)*. In a large, epidemiological cohort of healthy older males, the Ranch-Bernardo study, bioavailable T was significantly and positively correlated with verbal memory and a common cognitive screening test *(76)*. These associations were independent of age, education, body mass index, alcohol use, cigarette smoking, and depression. Thus, the association was not simply a reflection of health status.

Testosterone Replacement in Older Men

Although studies examining exogenous T administration in older men have produced mixed results, carefully designed prosposective studies with sensitive neuropsychological batteries tend to show significant effects. Sih et al. (1997), using a double-blind, placebo-controlled design, gave older, hypogonadal men biweekly injections of 200 mg T cypionate for 12 mo *(77)*. Fifteen men were randomly assigned to receive placebo and 17 men were randomly assigned to receive testosterone. The men were in good general health with a mean age of 68 yr. Tests of verbal and visual memory were administered prior to treatment and again after 6 mo. Although grip strength improved, memory measures remained unchanged. However, several reasons may account for lack of significant findings in this study. First, T levels did not change significantly from baseline levels during the course of T administration. Second, it is unclear when cognitive testing occurred relative to the T injection. Thus, cognitive testing may have occurred during times of trough T levels. In contrast, Janowsky et al. (1994) *(78)* found improvements in spatial abilities in a double-blind study using daily 15-mg T skin patches. In this study, 56 healthy older men (mean age: 67 yr) participated and were randomized to placebo or T for 3 mo of treatment. Participants were administered a battery of tests measuring semantic knowledge, constructional ability, verbal memory, fine motor coordination and divided attention prior to and after 3 mo of treatment. The treatment group demonstrated improvement on a measure of visuoconstructional ability (*see* Fig. 3).

More recently, Janowsky et al. (2000) found that T enanthate injections, 150 mg/weekly, improved spatial working memory in a group of healthy older males (*see* Fig. 4) *(79)*. These improvements were evident compared to an age-matched placebo group and exceeded practice effects demonstrated by young men (without T treatment). Working memory refers to one's ability to maintain information in mind while simultaneously manipulating or updating the information as needed. It is the mind's scratchpad; therefore, improvements in working memory can affect a number of cognitive and day-to-day tasks.

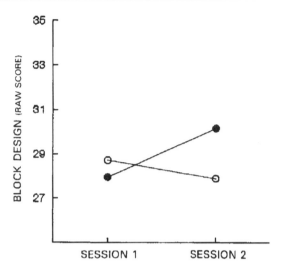

Fig. 3. Wechsler Adult Intelligence Scale—Revised Block Design subtest performance (total score) by a testosterone-supplemented group of healthy older eugonadal men (solid circles) and a placebo group (open circles) at Session 1 (baseline) and Session 2 (12 wk of daily 15-mg T skin patch use). The T-treated group demonstrated a significant improvement from baseline compared to placebo, as evidenced by a significant group by test session interaction $F(1,54) = 5.33$, $p = 0.025$. (From ref. *78*, reproduced with permission.)

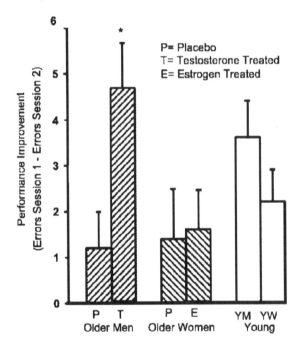

Fig. 4. Change in performance after 1 mo of placebo or hormone supplementation (150 mg intramuscular T enanthate weekly for men and 0.625 mg/d conjugated estrogen daily for women) in older subjects (stripped bars) or no treatment in the younger subjects (open bars). Older men on T supplementation showed an improvement in performance (fewer errors). Younger subjects showed the expected improvement on the task because of practice, whereas older subjects, without hormone supplementation or with estrogen supplementation did not. Brackets show standard error of the mean. (From ref. *79*, reproduced with permission.)

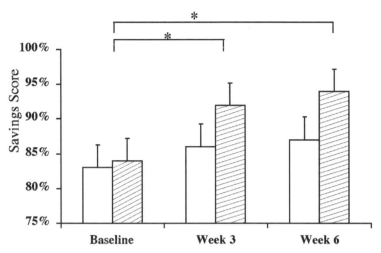

Fig. 5. Mean savings score on story recall (a measure of verbal memory) at baseline and wk 3 and 6 of treatment for placebo (open bars) and testosterone-treated (crosshatched bars) (100 mg im T enanthate weekly) healthy older men. The savings score is the number of exact words recalled from a short story after a 20-min delay divided by the number of words recalled immediately after hearing the story. Therefore, the savings score represents the percentage of information recalled. Standard error bars represent standard error of measurement. Asterisks and lines above the bars indicate significant changes from baseline in the T-treated group at wk 3 and 6, as indicated by the lines. (From ref. *80*, reproduced with permission.)

Consistent with these results, we have reported significant improvements in spatial and verbal memory in a group of healthy older men in response to short-term T administration *(80)*. Twenty-five healthy older men (mean age: 68 yr) were randomized to 100mg T enanthate or placebo and received treatment for 6 wk, followed by 6 wk of washout. Participants were administered a comprehensive battery of tests, including verbal and spatial memory, spatial abilities, verbal fluency, and selective attention. Testosterone-treated participants demonstrated significant improvements on spatial memory (recall of a walking route), spatial ability (block construction), and verbal memory (recall of a short story) *(see* Fig. 5). Improvements in spatial memory for a task that utilizes navigation in three-dimensional space and verbal memory have not been previously reported. Although improvements were not found for all cognitive measures, we did not expect changes on measures of verbal fluency or selective attention. Our results provide further evidence that T administration can result in beneficial, but selective, changes in cognition. This may be particularly important in a population of older adults who are at increased risk for memory deficits. In summary, these previous studies suggest that T administration may improve spatial and verbal memory, particularly for older males who have age-related decreases in endogenous testosterone levels.

ENDOCRINE DISORDERS

Congenital Adrenal Hyperplasia

Congenital adrenal hyperplasia (CAH) is a condition in which the developing fetus is exposed to excess levels of androgens during gestation. The most common cause of this androgen excess is 21-hydroxylase or 11β-hydroxylase deficiency *(81)*. The androgen excess results from loss of cortisol negative feedback regulation of ACTH secretion. About 75% of children with CAH have an associated deficiency in aldosterone production. The salt-wasting variety results in hyponatremia, hyperkalemia, and volume depletion that is usually present within the first 2 wk of life. The condition affects approx 1 in 5000 to 15,000 live births. The clinical presentation in genetic females includes pseudohermaphroditism, whereas affected males tend to have normal or early sexual development. Exposure to excess androgens during early development of the organism provides a unique opportunity to examine the organizational effects of hormones in humans.

There is some indication that individuals with CAH may demonstrate greater cerebral lateralization, as evidenced by a higher incidence of sinistrality (left-handedness) *(82,83)*. However, other studies have failed to support this *(84)*. MRI examination of CAH patients has revealed mixed findings with some evidence of atypical lateralization, abnormal white-matter distribution, or temporal lobe atrophy in about one-third of patients *(85–87)*. However, these abnormalities do not appear to be related to any detrimental neuropsychological performance or treatment status *(85,86)*. Increased incidence of learning disorders has been found in CAH patients, along with decrements in general intelligence quotient (IQ) level and verbal intelligence quotient (VIQ), suggesting that prenatal exposure to androgens may adversely affect the development of the left hemisphere or hemispheric lateralization, which would adversely affect verbal abilities *(85,87–91)*. For example, female CAH patients demonstrate significantly lower VIQ scores compared to unaffected sisters *(83,88,90)*. However, some evidence also supports a higher level of general intelligence in CAH patients *(85,92,93)*. In addition, studies of dichotic listening, a task that is sensitive to hemispheric lateralization, are not supportive of an atypical lateralization pattern in CAH patients *(84,94)*. In a dichotic listening task, different auditory inputs are simultaneously presented to each ear through headphones. In normal individuals with an intact corpus callosum, visual and auditory inputs sent to one hemisphere are quickly shared with the other. This task has been used to discover the typical pattern of left-hemisphere dominance for language.

One possible explanation for these findings may be that androgens specifically affect spatial abilities. In particular, if androgens are specific to spatial abilities, one would expect that CAH females would evidence superior spatial abilities compared to matched controls, whereas male CAH patients would evidence modest or no appreciable increase in spatial abilities compared to male controls. A study by Resnick et al. (1986) found CAH adolescent girls performed better than matched familial controls on tests of spatial ability (e.g., the Hidden Patterns Test, Card Rotations, and Mental Rotations) *(93)*. A more recent study by Hampson et al. (1998) also provides evidence that spatial abilities are specifically increased in CAH girls compared to controls *(95)*. This study examined a relatively young population of CAH patients (mean age 10 yr) matched for IQ level with controls. Participants were administered the Perceptual Speed Test, a task on which females typically outperform males, and the Spatial Relations Test, from the Primary Mental Abilities Test, a measure of spatial visualization on which males typically outperform females. CAH girls performed less well than controls on the perceptual speed task but outperformed the controls on the spatial test. This effect was large, nearly one standard deviation *(see* Fig. 6) and there was no difference between salt-wasters vs non-salt-wasters. Thus, the atypical advantage of CAH girls on the spatial task and a failure to find a typical advantage on the perceptual speed task represents a double-dissociation

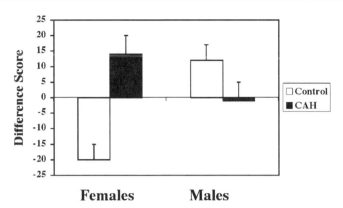

Fig. 6. Mean intraindividual difference scores in CAH and controls on the Primary Test of Mental Abilities reflecting the relative strength of spatial vs perceptual speed abilities in the four groups. Difference scores were calculated by subtracting the perceptual speed quotient from the spatial quotient for each child. A positive value indicates relatively greater proficiency in the spatial domain. Error bars represent the standard error of the mean. (From ref. 95, reproduced with permission.)

effect of androgens in this population. Although other studies have failed to find an advantage of spatial abilities in CAH girls (85,92), evidence of behavioral masculinization has also been reported in CAH girls (96–103). Thus, additional carefully designed studies may provide further information regarding the organizational effects of androgens on cognition in this population.

Isolated Hypogonadotropic Hypogonadism and Kallmann's Syndrome

Isolated hypogonadotropic hypogonadism (IHH) results from deficiency of gonadotropin-releasing hormone (GnRH) from the hypothalamus. When this type of hypo-gonadism is accompanied by anosmia from agenesis or malformation of the olfactory bulb, sulci, and tracts, this condition is termed Kallmann's syndrome (KS). It occurs in about 1 in 10,000 male births and males predominate in a ratio of 5 : 1. The syndrome can occur as an inherited or sporadic disorder. X-Linked, autosomal-dominant, and autosomal-recessive modes of inheritance have been described. For one-third or more of patients with KS, the defect is likely the result of an X-linked form of KS, caused by a defect in KAL. KAL encodes a protein, anosmin, that plays a key role in the migration of GnRH neurons and olfactory nerves to the hypothalamus (104). MRI studies have confirmed the absence or aplasia of the olfactory bulb in KS vs IHH patients (105). In IHH without anosmia, a defect in the GnRH receptor (GnRHR) has been reported to be responsible for reproductive function failure, and GnRHR mutations may be more common than previously appreciated in familial cases of normosmic IHH (106). Individuals are typically identified during adolescence when they evidence failure or a delay of puberty. It has been suggested that developmental anomalies arise in the CNS as a result of a chronic lack of T and estradiol. Reported neurologic abnormalities include anosmia, hyposmia, ocular motor abnormalities, pes cavus foot deformities, and impaired smooth pursuit eye movements and mirror movements (any synchronous movement of a corresponding muscle of another extremity occurring with the primary movement) *(107)*. Performance on mirror movements may be impaired because of a lack of inhibitory fibers in the corpus callosum. However, neuroradiology findings have failed to find defects in that area *(108)*.

Men with IHH demonstrate impairments in spatial abilities *(109,110)* and memory for both verbal and visual information *(111)*. Kertzman et al. (1990) found that IHH patients with abnormal mirror movements also demonstrated impairments on a measure of spatial attention *(112)*. This deficit was not the result of motor difficulties, as the IHH patients evidenced faster reaction times than controls. Alexander et al. (1998) examined 33 hypogonadal men receiving T-replacement therapy, 10 eugonadal men receiving T in a male contraceptive clinical trial and 19 eugonadal controls for changes in cognition in response to T treatment *(113)*. Cognitive tests included measures of visuospatial ability, verbal fluency, perceptual speed, and verbal memory. Group differences in testosterone levels were unrelated to performance on most cognitive measures, including visuospatial ability. However, hypogonadal men were impaired in their verbal fluency compared to eugonadal men at baseline, and they showed improved verbal fluency following T treatment.

We have also reported findings of changes in cognition from T treatment in a hypogonadal male with KS *(114)*. The patient was unusual, as he was first diagnosed with KS during a hospitalization for complaints of depression and weight loss at age 61. Clinical signs included an extremely low T level (essentially undetectable) along with low follicular-stimulating hormone (FSH) and leutinizing hormone (LH) levels. Upon further examination, the patient was found to have anosmia, fine auxiliary hair, fine pubic hair in a female distribution, and a long arm span. MRI revealed the absence of olfactory tracts and dual-energy X-ray analysis (DEXA) scan revealed markedly low bone density. After improvement in weight and stabilization of mood to the nondepressed range and prior to hormone-replacement therapy, the patient was administered a comprehensive neuropsychological battery. Following 6 wk of T enanthate (200 mg im q 2 k) treatment, the patient was retested. Measures included selected subtests from the Wechsler Adult Intelligence Scale—Revised (WAIS-R) (Digit Span & Arithmetic), Wechsler Memory Scale—Revised (WMS-R) Logical Memory subtest, Proactive Interference (PI) (a verbal list learning test), Stroop Test (a measure of selective attention), Visual Spatial Learning Test (VSLT), and a mental rotation task *(115–118)*. Following treatment, the patient demonstrated improvements in spatial memory and spatial ability measures (*see* Fig. 7) and modest declines in verbal memory (*see* Fig. 8). Attention (WAIS-R Digit Span), selective attention (Stroop), and reasoning (WAIS-R Arithmetic) did not change. Although the goal of hormonal treatment of male hypogonadism is typically to induce and maintain normal secondary sexual characteristics in adolescents, these studies indicate that changes in cognition may also occur with T treatment.

Klinefelter's Syndrome

Klinefelter's syndrome (XXY) or supernumary X is the result of the presence of surplus X chromosomes in phenotypic males *(119–121)*. Klinefelter's syndrome affects approximately 1 in 500 patients and is characterized by testicular failure, impaired spermatogenesis, elevated gonadotropin levels, and androgen deficiency *(119–121)*. Patients appear essentially normal until puberty and adulthood, when these symptoms become apparent. Distinguishing physical characteristics may include long legs and arm span, decreased facial and pubic hair, increased fat deposits in a female pattern, gynecomastia, and small testes and penis. Testosterone treatment during adolescence and adult-

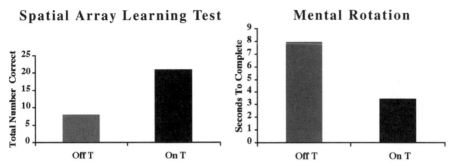

Fig. 7. Performance on the Spatial Array Learning Test—Revised and a mental rotation task in a 61-yr-old Kallman's patient before (light gray bars) and after 6 wk of T replacement (200 mg T enanthate biweekly) (black bars). For the Spatial Array Learning Test—Revised, the patient was required to learn seven abstract designs and their proper placement on a grid over several trials. The left side of graph represents the total number of correct responses summed across five trials. For the mental rotation task, the patient was asked to choose, between two possible choices, the correct response that represented the stimulus item rotated in space. The right graph represents choice reaction time; therefore, a decrease in response time represents an improvement.

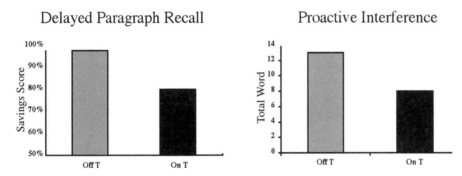

Fig. 8. Performance on the WMS-R Logical Memory Subtest and Proactive Interference (PI) measures of verbal memory in a 61-yr-old Kallman's patient before (light gray bars) and after 6 wk of T replacement (200 mg T enanthate biweekly) (black bars). For the WMS-R LM, the patient was required to listen to and recall two short narrative stories. The left side of graph represents the total number of story bits recalled after a 30-min delay. For PI, the patient was asked to listen to four successive word lists of semantically related words. The right graph represents the total number of words recalled from the four lists.

hood is the most common form of treatment with the goal of reducing long-term consequences of androgen deficiency such as osteoporosis.

Cognitive difficulties present during childhood and adolescence have been reported, and they include lower verbal IQ compared to performance IQ, developmental speech and language delays, learning disabilities (e.g., reading and written expression difficulties), and poor school performance *(122–125)*. However, because these difficulties have been reported prior to adolescence (when androgen deficiency develops), the connection between these difficulties and hormone imbalance is unclear. Recently, Patwardhan et al. (2000) found that Klinfelter's syndrome (XXY) men demonstrate a reduction in left temporal lobe gray-matter volumes on MRI compared with normal control subjects, suggesting that there may be brain structure changes related to previous findings of verbal learning disabilities in these patients *(126)*. In addition, patients who had never received T treatment evidenced significant reductions in left temporal lobe gray matter compared with those individuals who had received T supplementation. These findings suggest that in addition to organizing effects on brain structure during development, androgens can also affect neural structure and integrity throughout the human adult life-span.

SUMMARY

The studies reviewed in this chapter demonstrate a clear relationship between androgens and specific aspects of cognition. Observed effects of androgens on cognition may occur by several mechanisms, including direct effects of T or via T metabolites such as DHT or estradiol. Androgens act via both classic receptor-mediated genomic methods, as well as more recently characterized nongenomic methods. The temporal relationship of androgen effects was reviewed, including organizational effects that occur because of the presence of androgens during critical neural development periods that result in permanent changes in behavior and cognition, as observed with CAH and Klinefelter's patients. Considerable evidence also suggests that androgens exert modulating effects on cognition throughout the life-span, as demonstrated by observed cognitive changes in transsexual individuals undergoing hormone treatment and older adults receiving androgen supplementation. Taken together, there is strong support to indicate that androgens exert effects on cognition and in particular spatial abilities. Recent evidence from neuroimaging studies has extended our understanding of the complex interactions between androgens and cognition to suggest that organizational and activational effects of hormones interact with unique cognitive task demands and their associated neural networks. This recent neuroimaging evidence may help explain why androgens appear to have selective rather than widespread effects on cognition. Clearly, more research is needed in this area, and future research endeavors will likely further refine our understanding of these complex relationships.

REFERENCES

1. Brown-Sequard CE. The effects produced on man by subcutaneous injections of a liquid obtained from the testicles of animals. Lancet 1889;2:105.
2. Rubinow DR, Schmidt P. Androgens, brain, and behavior. Am J Psychiatry 1996;153:974.
3. Janne OA, Palvimo JJ, Kallio P, Mehto M. Androgen receptor and mechanism of androgen action. Ann Med 1993;25:83.
4. Lieberherr M, Grosse B. Androgens increase intracellular calcium concentration and inositol 1,4,5-trisphosphate and diacylglycerol formation via a pertussis toxin-sensitive G-protein. J Biol Chem 1994;269:7217.
5. Benten WP, Lieberherr M, Sekeris CE, Wunderlich F. Testosterone induces Ca2+ influx via nongenomic surface receptors in activated T cells. FEBS Lett 1997;407:211.
6. Benten WP, Lieberherr M, Stamm O, et al. Testosterone signaling through internalizable surface receptors in androgen receptor-free macrophages. Mol Biol Cell 1999;10:3113.
7. Benten WP, Lieberherr M, Giese G, et al. Functional testosterone receptors in plasma membranes of T cells. FASEB J 1999;13:123.
8. Dawson JLM, Cheung YM, Lau RTS. Developmental effects of neonatal skills in the white rat. Biol Psycol 1975;3:213.
9. Joseph R, Hess S, Birecree E. Effects of hormone manipulations and exploration on sex differences in maze learning. Behav Biol 1978;24:364.
10. Roof RL. Neonatal exogenous testosterone modifies sex difference in radial arm and Morris water maze performance in prepubescent and adult rats. Behav Brain Res 1993;53:1.

11. Stefanova N, Ovtscharoff W. Sexual dimorphism of the bed nucleus of the stria terminalis and the amygdala. Adv Anat Embryol Cell Biol 2000;158:1.
12. de Fougerolles Nunn E, Greenstein B, Khamashta M, Hughes GR. Evidence for sexual dimorphism of estrogen receptors in hypothalamus and thymus of neonatal and immature Wistar rats. Int J Immunopharmacol 1999;21:869.
13. Kirn J, Lombroso PJ. Development of the cerebral cortex: XI. Sexual dimorphism in the brain. J Am Acad Child Adolesc Psychiatry 1998;37:1228.
14. Gorski RA. Sexual dimorphisms of the brain. J Anim Sci 1985;61:38.
15. Nunez JL, Juraska JM. The size of the splenium of the rat corpus callosum: influence of hormones, sex ratio, and neonatal cryoanesthesia. Dev Psychobiol 1998;33:295.
16. Roof RL. The dentate gyrus is sexually dimorphic in prepubescent rats: testosterone plays a significant role. Brain Res 1993;610:148.
17. Hamburger-Bar R, Rigter H. Peripheral and central androgenic stimulation of sexual behaviour of castrated male rats. Acta Endocrinol (Copenh) 1977;84:813.
18. McQueen JK, Wilson H, Sumner BEH, Fink G. Serotonin transporter (SERT) mRNA and binding site densities in male rat brain affected by sex steroids. Brain Res Mol Brain Res 1999; 63:241.
19. Fink, G, Sumner, B, Rosie, R, et al. Androgen actions on central serotonin neurotransmission: relevance for mood, mental state and memory. Behav Brain Res 1999;105:53.
20. Sumner BE, Fink G. Testosterone as well as estrogen increases serotonin2A receptor mRNA and binding site densities in the male rat brain. Brain Res Mol Brain Res 1998;59:205.
21. Flood JF, Farr SA, Kaiser FE, et al. Age-related decrease of plasma testosterone in samp8 mice: replacement improves age-related impairment of learning and memory. Physiol Behav 1995;57:669.
22. Grino PB, Griffin JE, Wilson JD. Testosterone at high concentrations interacts with the human androgen receptor similarly to dihydrotestosterone. Endocrinology 1990;126:1165.
23. Lu S, Simon NG, Wang Y, Hu, S. Neural androgen receptor regulation: effects of androgen and antiandrogen. J Neurobiol 1999;41:505.
24. Roselli CE, Resko JA. Androgens regulate brain aromatase activity in adult male rats through a receptor mechanism. Endocrinology 1984;114:2183.
25. Resko JA, Pereyra-Martinez AC, Stadelman HL, Roselli CE. Region-specific regulation of cytochrome P450 aromatase messenger ribonucleic acid by androgen in brains of male rhesus monkeys. Biol Reprod 2000;62:1818.
26. Lynch CS, Story AJ. Dihydrotestosterone and estrogen regulation of rat brain androgen-receptor immunoreactivity. Physiol Behav 2000;69:445.
27. Schmidt BM, Gerdes D, Feuring M, et al. Rapid, nongenomic steroid actions: a new age? Front Neuroendocrinol 2000;21:57.
28. Roselli CE, Chambers K. Sex differences in male-typical copulatory behaviors in response to androgen and estrogen treatment in rats. Neuroendocrinology 1999;69:290.
29. Kellogg CK, Lundin A. Brain androgen-inducible aromatase is critical for adolescent organization of environment-specific social interaction in male rats. Horm Behav 1999;35:155.
30. Gordon HW, Lee PA. A relationship between gonadotropins and visuospatial function. Neuropsychologia 1986;24:563.
31. McKeever WF, Deyo RA. Testosterone, dihydrotestosterone, and spatial task performances of males. Bull Psychonom Soc 1990;28:305.
32. Christiansen K, Kussmann R. Androgen levels and components of aggressive behaviour in men. Horm Behav 1987;21:170.
33. Errico AL, Parsons OA, Kling OR, King AC. Investigation of the role of sex hormones in alcoholics' visuospatial deficits. Neuropsychologia 1992;30:417.
34. Tan U. The relationship between serum testosterone level and visuomotor learning in right handed young men. Int J Neurosci 1991;56:19.
35. Christiansen K. Sex hormone related variations of cognitive performance in !Kung San hunter-gathers of Namibia. Neuropsychobiology 1993;27:97.
36. Kampen DL, Sherwin BB. Estradiol is related to visual memory in healthy young men. Behav Neurosci 1996;110:613.
37. McKeever WF, Rich DA, Deyo RA, Conner RL. Androgens and spatial ability: failure to find a relationship between testosterone and ability measures. Bull Psychonom Soc 1987;25:438.
38. Moffat SD, Hampson E. A curvilinear relationship between testosterone and spatial cognition in humans: possible influence of hand preference. Psychoneuroendocrinology 1996;21:323.

39. Gouchie C, Kimura D. The relationship between testosterone levels and cognitive ability patterns. Psychoneuroendocrinology 1991;16:323.

40. Shute VJ, Pellegrino JW, Hubert L, Reynolds RW. The relationship between androgen levels and human spatial abilities. Bull Psychonom Soc 1983;21:465.

41. Silverman JM, Keefe RSE, Mohs RC, Davis KL. A study of the reliability of the family history method in genetic studies of Alzheimer disease. Alzheimer Dis Assoc Disord 1989;3:218.

42. Kimura D. Sex and Cognition, The MIT Press, Cambridge, MA 1999.

43. Vederhus L, Krekling S. Sex differences in visual spatial ability in 9-year-old children. Intelligence 1996;23:33.

44. Johnson E-S, Meade A-C. Developmental patterns of spatial ability: an early sex difference. Child Dev 1987;58:725.

45. Vandenberg SG, Kuse AR. Mental rotations, a group test of three-dimensional spatial visualization. Percept Motor Skills 1978;47:599.

46. Collins DW, Kimura D. A large sex difference on a two-dimensional mental rotation task. Behav Neurosci 1997;111:845.

47. Larson P, Rizzo A-A, Buckwalter J-G, et al. Gender issues in the use of virtual environments. Cyber Psychol Behav 1999;2:113.

48. McBurney D-H, Gaulin S-J-C, Devineni T, Adams C. Superior spatial memory of women: stronger evidence for the gathering. Evol Hum Behav 1997;18:165.

49. Eals M, Silverman I. The hunter-gatherer theory of spatial sex differences: proximate factors. Ethol Sociobiol 1994;15:95.

50. Galea LA, Kimura D. Sex differences in route learning. Pers Individ Diff 1993;14:53.

51. Sandstrom NJ, Kaufman J, Huettel SA. Males and females use different distal cues in a virtual environment navigation task. Cogn Brain Res 1998;6:351.

52. Moffat S-D, Hampson E, Hatzipantelis M. Navigation in a "virtual" maze: sex differences and correlation with. Evol Hum Behavior 1998;19:73.

53. Astur RS, Ortiz ML, Sutherland RJ. A characterization of performance by men and women in a virtual Morris water task: a large and reliable sex difference. Behav Brain Res 1998;93:185.

54. Maguire EA, Frackowiak RS, Frith CD. Recalling routes around London: activation of the right hippocampus in taxi drivers. J Neurosci 1997;17:7103.

55. Maguire EA, Frith CD, Burgess N, et al. Knowing where things are parahippocampal involvement in encoding object locations in virtual large-scale space. J Cogn Neurosci 1998;10:61.

56. Epstein R, Kanwisher N. A cortical representation of the local visual environment. Nature 1998;392:598.

57. Aguirre GK, D'Esposito M. Environmental knowledge is subserved by separable dorsal/ventral neural areas. J Neurosci 1997;17:2512.

58. Aguirre GK, Zarahn E, D'Esposito M. An area within human ventral cortex sensitive to "building" stimuli: evidence and implications. Neuron 1998;21:373.

59. Wilson FA, Riches IP, Brown MW. Hippocampus and medial temporal cortex. Neuronal activity related to behavioral responses during the performance of many tasks by primates. Behav Brain Res 1990;40:7.

60. Shelton AL, Gabrieli JD. Neural correlates of encoding space from route and survey perspectives. J Neurosci 2002;22:2711.

61. Gron G, Wunderlich AP, Spitzer M, et al. Brain activation during human navigation: gender-different neural networks as substrate of performance. Nat Neurosci 2000;3:404.

62. Van Goozen SHM, Cohen-Kettenis PT, Gooren LJG, et al. Activating effects of androgens on cognitive performance: causal evidence in a group of female-to-male transsexuals. Neuropsychologia 1994;32:1153.

63. Slabbekoorn D, van Goozen SH, Megens J, et al. Activating effects of cross-sex hormones on cognitive functioning: a study of short-term and long-term hormone effects in transsexuals. Psychoneuroendocrinology 1999;24:423.

64. Miles C, Green R, Sanders G, Hines, M. Estrogen and memory in a transsexual population. Horm Behav 1998;34:199.

65. Postma A, Meyer G, Tuiten A, et al. Effects of testosterone administration on selective aspects of object- location memory in healthy young women. Psychoneuroendocrinology 2000;25:563.

66. Tenover JS, Matsumoto AM, Plymate SR, Bremner WJ. The effects of aging in normal men on bioavailable testosterone and leuteinizing hormone secretion: response to clomiphene citrate. J Clin Endocrinol Metab 1987;65:1118.

67. Tenover J. Effects of testosterone supplementation in the aging male. J Clin Endocrinol 1992;75:1092.
68. Morley JE. Testosterone replacement and the physiologic aspects of aging in men. Mayo Clin Proc 2000;75(Suppl):S83.
69. Morley JE, Perry HM 3rd. Androgen deficiency in aging men: role of testosterone replacement therapy. [see comments]. J Lab Clin Med 2000;135:370.
70. Ravaglia G, Forti P, Maioli F, et al. Body composition, sex steroids, IGF-1, and bone mineral status in aging men. J Gerontol A: Biol Sci Med Sci 2000;55:M516.
71. Matsumoto AM. "Andropause"—are reduced androgen levels in aging men physiologically important? (editorial; comment). West J Med 1993;159:618.
72. Tenover JS. Androgen administration to aging men. Endocrinol Metab Clin N Am 1994;23:877.
73. Lund BC, Bever-Stille KA, Perry PJ. Testosterone and andropause: the feasibility of testosterone replacement therapy in elderly men. Pharmacotherapy 1999;19:951.
74. Carani C, Qin K, Simoni M, et al. Effect of testosterone and estradiol in a man with aromatase deficiency. N Engl J Med 1997;337:91.
75. Morely JE, Kaiser F, Raum WJ, et al. Potentially predictive and manipulable blood serum correlates of aging in the healthy human male: progessive decreases in bioavailable testosterone, dehydro-epiandrosterone sulfate, and the ratio of insulin-like growth factor to 1 growth hormone. Proc Natl Acad Sci USA 1997;94:7537.
76. Barrett-Connor E, Goodman-Gruen D, Patay B. Endogenous sex hormones and cognitive function in older men. J Clin Endocrinol Metab 1999;84:3681.
77. Sih R, Morley JE, Kaiser FE, et al. Testosterone replacement in older hypogonadal men: a 12 month randomized controlled trial. J Clin Endocrinol Metab 1997;82:1661.
78. Janowsky JS, Oviatt SK, Orwoll ES. Testosterone influences spatial cognition in older men. Behav Neurosci 1994;108:325.
79. Janowsky JS, Chavez B, Orowoll E. Sex steroids modify working memory. J Cogn Neurosci 2000;12:407.
80. Cherrier MM, Asthana S, Baker LD, et al. Testosterone supplementation improves spatial and verbal memory in healthy older men. Neurology 2001;57:80.
81. Orth DN, Kovacs WJ, Debold CR. The Adrenal cortex. In: Wilson JD, Foster DW, eds. Williams Textbook of Endocrinology, 8th ed. WB Saunders, Philadelphia, 1992 p. 489.
82. Nass R, Baker S, Speiser P, et al. Hormones and handedness: left-hand bias in female congenital adrenal hyperplasia patients. Neurology 1987;37:711.
83. Kelso WM, Nicholls MER, Warne GL. Effects of prenatal androgen exposure on cerebral lateralization in patients with congenital adrenal hyperplasia (CAH). Brain Cogn 1999;40:153.
84. Helleday J, Siwers B, Ritzen EM, Hugdahl K. Normal lateralization for handeness and ear advantage in a verbal dichotic listening task in women with congenital adrenal hyperplasia (CAH). Neuropsychologia 1994;32:875.
85. Sinforiani E, Livieri C, Mauri M, Bisio P. Cognitive and neuroradiological findings in congenital adrenal hyperplasia. Psychoneuroendocrinology 1994;19(1):55.
86. Nass R, Heier L, Moshang T, et al. Magnetic resonance imaging in the congenital adrenal hyperplasia population: increased frequency of white-matter abnormalities and temporal lobe atrophy. J Child Neurol 1997;12:181.
87. Plante E, Boliek C, Binkiewicz A, Erly WK. Elevated androgen, brain development and language/learning disabilities in children with congenital adrenal hyperplasia. Dev Med Child Neurol 1996;38:423.
88. Dittmann RW, Kappes MH, Kappes ME. Cognitive functioning in female patients with 21-hydroxylase deficiency. Eur Child Adolesc Psychiatry 1993;2:34.
89. Nass R, Baker S. Androgen effects on cognition: congenital adrenal hyperplasia. Psychoneuroendocrinology 1991;16:189.
90. Nass R, Baker S. Learning disabilities in children with congenital adrenal hyperplasia. J Child Neurol 1991;6:306.
91. Berenbaum SA, Korman K, Leveroni C. Early hormones and sex differences in cognitive abilities. Learning Individ Diff 1995;7:303.
92. Helleday J, Bartfai A, Ritzen EM, Forsman M. General intelligence and cognitive profile in women with congenital adrenal hyperplasia (CAH). Psychoneuroendocrinology 1994;19:343.
93. Resnick SM, Berenbaum SA, Gottesman II, Bouchard TJ. Early hormonal influences on cognitive functioning in congenital adrenal hyperplasia. Dev Psychology 1986;22:191.

94. Kelso WM, Nicholls MER, Warne GL, Zacharin M. Cerebral lateralization and cognitive functioning in patients with congenital adrenal hyperplasia. Neuropsychology 2000;14:370.
95. Hampson E, Rovet JF, Altmann D. Spatial reasoning in children with congenital adrenal hyperplasia due to 21-hydroxylase deficiency. Dev Neuropsychol 1998;14:299.
96. Berenbaum SA, Resnick SM. Early androgen effects on aggression in children and adults with congenital adrenal hyperplasia. Psychoneuroendocrinology 1997;22:505.
97. Berenbaum SA, Snyder E. Early hormonal influences on childhood sex-typed activity and playmate preferences: implications for the development of sexual orientation. Dev Psychol 1995;31:31.
98. Dittmann RW, Kappes MH, Kappes ME, Boerger D. Congenital adrenal hyperplasia: II. Gender-related behavior and attitudes in female salt-wasting and simple-virilizing patients. Psychoneuroendocrinology 1990;15:421.
99. Dittmann RW, Kappes MH, Kappes ME, Boerger D. Congenital adrenal hyperplasia: I. Gender-related behavior and attitudes in female patients and sisters. Psychoneuroendocrinology 1990;15:401.
100. Berenbaum SA, Hines M. Early androgens are related to childhood sex-typed toy preferences. Psychol Sci 1992;3(3):203.
101. Hines M, Kaufman FR. Androgen and the development of human sex-typical behavior: Rough-and-tumble play and sex of preferred playmates in children with congenital adrenal hyperplasia (CAH). Child Dev 1994;65:1042.
102. Zucker KJ, Bradley SJ, Oliver G, Blake J. Psychosexual development of women with congenital adrenal hyperplasia. Horm Behav 1996;30:300.
103. Dittmann RW, Kappes MH, Kappes ME, et al. Congenital adrenal hyperplasia I: Gender-related behaviors and attitudes in female patients and sisters. Psychoneuroendocrinology 1990;15:401–420.
104. Oliveira LM, Seminara SB, Beranova M, et al. The importance of autosomal genes in Kallmann syndrome: Genotype–phenotype correlations and neuroendocrine characteristics. J Clin Endocrinol Metab 2001;86:1532.
105. Vogel TJ, Stemmler J, Heye B, et al. Kallman syndrome versus idiopathic hypogonadotropic hypogonadism at MR imaging. Radiology 1994;191:53.
106. Beranova M, Oliveira LM, Bedecarrats GY, et al. Prevalence, phenotypic spectrum, and modes of inheritance of gonadotropin-releasing hormone receptor mutations in idiopathic hypogonadotropic hypogonadism. J Clin Endocrinol Metab 2001;86:1580.
107. Schwankhaus JD, Currie J, Jaffe M, et al. Neurologic findings in men with isolated hypogonadotropic hypogonadism. Neurology 1989;39:223.
108. Quintin R, Duke VM, De Zoysa PA, et al. The neuroradiology of Kallmann's syndrome: a genotypic and phenotypic analysis. J Clin Endocrinol Metab 1996;81:3010.
109. Hier DB, Crowley WF Jr. Spatial ability in androgen-deficient men. N Engl J Med 1982;306:1202.
110. Buchsbaum MS, Henkin RI. Perceptual abnormalities in patients with chromatin negative gonadal dysgenesis and hypogonadotropic hypogonadism. Int J Neurosci 1980;11:201.
111. Cappa, SF, Guariglia, C, Papagno, C, et al. Patterns of lateralization and performance levels for verbal and spatial tasks in congenital androgen deficiency. Behav Brain Res 1988;31:177.
112. Kertzman, C, Robinson, DL, Sherins, RJ, et al. Abnormalities in visual spatial attention in men with mirror movements associated with isolated hypogonadotropic hypogonadism. Neurology 1990;40:1057.
113. Alexander, GM, Swerdloff, RS, Wang, C, et al. Androgen–behavior correlations in hypogonadal men and eugonadal men. II. Cognitive abilities. Horm Behav 1998;33:85.
114. Cherrier, MM, Craft, S, Bremner, W, et al. Cognitive effects of exogenous testosterone administration in eugonadal and hypogonadal men. J Int Neuropsychol Soc 1998;4:16.
115. Wechsler, D. Weschler Adult Intelligence Scale—Revised, The Psychological Corporation, San Antonio, TX 1981.
116. Wechsler, D. Wechsler Memory Scale—Revised, The Psychological Corporation, San Antonio, TX 1987.
117. Malec JF, Ivnik RJ, Smith GE, et al. Visual Spatial Learning test: normative data and further validation. Psychol Assess 1992;4:433.
118. Lezak MD. Neuropsychologcial Assessment, 3rd Edition. Oxford University Press, New York, 1995.
119. Amory JK, Anawalt BD, Paulsen CA, Bremner WJ. Klinefelter's syndrome. Lancet 2000;356:333.
120. Smyth CM. Diagnosis and treatment of Klinefelter syndrome. Hosp Pract (Off Ed) 1999;34:111.
121. Smyth CM, Bremner WJ. Klinefelter syndrome. Arch Intern Med 1998;158:1309.

122. Ratcliffe S. Long-term outcome in children of sex chromosome abnormalities. Arch Dis Child 1999;80:192.
123. Money J. Specific neuro-cognitive impairments associated with Turner (45,X) and Klinefelter (47,XXY) syndromes: a review. Soc Biol 1993;40:147.
124. Mandoki MW, Sumner GS, Hoffman RP, Riconda DL. A review of Klinefelter's syndrome in children and adolescents. J Am Acad Child Adolesc Psychiatry 1991;30:167.
125. Walzer S, Bashir AS, Silbert AR. Cognitive and behavioral factors in the learning disabilities of 47,XXY and 47,XYY boys. Birth Defects Orig Artic Ser 1990;26:45.
126. Patwardhan AJ, Eliez S, Bender B, et al. Brain morphology in Klinefelter syndrome: extra X chromosome and testosterone supplementation. [see comments]. Neurology 2000;54:2218.

III APPLIED ANDROLOGY

16

Androgen Treatment
of the Hypogonadal Male

Alvin M. Matsumoto, MD

CONTENTS

INTRODUCTION
DIAGNOSTIC AND TREATMENT CONSIDERATIONS
   IN MALE HYPOGONADISM
THERAPEUTIC GOALS AND BENEFITS OF T TREATMENT
FORMULATIONS AVAILABLE FOR T-REPLACEMENT THERAPY
ANDROGEN FORMULATIONS UNDER DEVELOPMENT
POTENTIAL RISKS OF T TREATMENT AND MONITORING
SUMMARY AND CONCLUSIONS
REFERENCES

INTRODUCTION

Male hypogonadism is a common clinical condition that results in androgen deficiency and affects the health and well-being of boys and men of all ages. For example, androgen deficiency of varying degrees is a major manifestation of the Klinefelter syndrome, an XXY chromosomal disorder that affects approx 1 in 500 males *(1)*. Testosterone (T)-replacement therapy has proven beneficial effects in androgen-deficient hypogonadal men, and male hypogonadism is the main clinical indication for T treatment. Unfortunately, in a large proportion of hypogonadal men, androgen deficiency is undiagnosed, diagnosed long after its onset, or treated inappropriately.

The spectrum of clinical states associated with androgen deficiency is broad. Serum T levels are commonly low in men with chronic illness (e.g., chronic renal failure, obstructive pulmonary disease, and liver disease), acute illness (burns, surgery, critical medical illness), wasting syndromes (e.g., associated with human immunodeficiency virus [HIV] infection and cancer), the use of certain medications (e.g., glucocorticoids and central-nervous-system-acting medications, such as opiates), and in normal aging men (referred to as "andropause") *(2)*. These conditions are also associated with clinical manifestations of androgen deficiency, such as reduced muscle mass and strength, decreased bone mineral density, sexual dysfunction, diminished energy and well-being, and depressed mood. Preliminary studies suggest potential beneficial anabolic and behavioral effects of androgen therapy in men with these conditions *(3–8)*. Although the

From: *Contemporary Endocrinology: Androgens in Health and Disease*
Edited by: C. Bagatell and W. J. Bremner © Humana Press Inc., Totowa, NJ

long-term benefits and risks of T therapy in these disorders are not known, the potential for expanded uses of androgens has provided the impetus for the development of many new T formulations.

DIAGNOSTIC AND TREATMENT CONSIDERATIONS IN MALE HYPOGONADISM

The diagnosis of male hypogonadism is usually suspected when an individual presents with a clinical syndrome that is consistent with androgen deficiency and it is confirmed with measurements of serum T levels that demonstrate consistently low values *(2)*. It is important to consider the clinical manifestations of androgen deficiency in formulating the therapeutic goals of T-replacement therapy.

The clinical manifestations of androgen deficiency vary with the stage of sexual development of the individual *(2)*. Males with prepubertal androgen deficiency usually present as adolescents or young adults with delayed puberty. They manifest varying degrees of eunuchoidism, which is characterized by the following: lack of genitalia development (small penis); small testes (< 5 mL) and prostate; lack of male-pattern hair growth; long arms and legs relative to height, poorly developed muscle mass, and prepubertal fat distribution (eunuchoidal body habitus); low bone mineral density; high-pitched voice; poor libido and sexual function, energy, mood, motivation, and initiative; gynecomastia; failure to produce an ejaculate (aspermia) and initiate spermatogenesis; and a low hematocrit (in the female range).

Unless severe, androgen deficiency in adult males is usually more difficult to diagnose because the clinical manifestations are often subtle and/or attributed to other causes. Androgen-deficient men usually present with the following: poor sexual performance (diminished libido and erectile dysfunction); gynecomastia; infertility (because of impaired sperm production); decrease in the amount of pubic, chest, axillary, and facial hair; reduced muscle mass and strength; low bone mineral density (osteopenia or osteoporosis); diminished energy, motivation, and initiative; increased irritability and depressed mood; and mild hypoproliferative anemia. Testis size may be small (<15 mL) in men with a profound reduction in spermatogenesis, but it is often normal. Hot flushes may occur, mostly in men with a rapid onset of severe androgen deficiency.

If clinical manifestations suggest androgen deficiency, an initial measurement of serum total-T or free-T concentration is obtained, preferably in the morning (e.g., at approx 8 AM, the peak of the circadian variation in T levels) *(2,9)*. The use of an accurate and reliable T assay is crucial *(10–14)*. Most circulating T is bound to serum proteins, primarily sex hormone-binding globulin (SHBG) and albumin, and only 1–2% of T is free of protein binding. Therefore, in clinical situations that alter binding proteins, total-T assays that measure both free and protein-bound T may not accurately reflect biologically active T concentrations in blood.

In most local and many reference laboratories, both total-T and free-T levels are measured using automated platform-based, analog immunoassays that are highly variable and often of questionable accuracy *(10–14)*. Furthermore, both total-T and free-T levels measured using analog immunoassays vary directly with alterations in SHBG levels. Alterations in SHBG concentrations occur commonly and may affect total-T and free-T measurements by these analog methods. For example, moderate obesity, hypothyroidism, androgen or anabolic steroid administration, and nephrotic syndrome decrease SHBG concentrations and, therefore, lower total-T and free-T levels by analog methods, resulting potentially in a mistaken diagnosis of T deficiency. Conversely, aging, hyperthyroidism, hepatic cirrhosis, and androgen deficiency increase in SHBG and raise total-T and free-T levels by analog immunoassays, resulting potentially, in a mistaken impression of eugonadism.

It is for these reasons that in clinical situations where SHBG levels may be altered or serum total-T levels are in the low-normal or moderately low range (e.g., 200–350 ng/dL), free-T or bioavailable (free plus weakly albumin-bound or non-SHBG-bound) assays that are not affected by changes in SHBG concentrations should be used to confirm androgen deficiency. These assays include free T by equilibrium dialysis or centrifugation methods, bioavailable T by the ammonium sulfate precipitation method, or free and bioavailable T calculated from measurements of total-T and SHBG concentrations *(10–14)*. Unless SHBG levels are very low (e.g., nephrotic syndrome), total-T levels < 200 ng/dL in men with clinical manifestations consistent with T deficiency are usually diagnostic of androgen deficiency.

If the initial serum T level is low, patients should be evaluated for underlying acute or chronic illnesses, medications, or malnutrition to determine whether transient or reversible conditions associated with low T levels are present *(7)*. In these situations, a T level should be repeated after a recent illness is resolved completely, medications that may lower T are discontinued, and malnutrition is corrected. If these reversible causes of low T levels are not present or correctable, a serum T level should be repeated together with serum gonadotropin concentrations (i.e., luteinizing hormone [LH] and follicle-stimulating hormone [FSH] levels). Both because of significant biological and methodological variability in serum T concentrations, approx 15% of healthy young men may demonstrate a T level below the normal range in a 24-h period *(15)*. Therefore, before initiating T treatment, a repeat T level to confirm androgen deficiency is appropriate.

Serum gonadotropin levels should also be obtained prior to starting T therapy in order to differentiate androgen deficiency resulting from primary testicular disease (primary hypogonadism) from that resulting from hypothalamic–pituitary dysfunction or disease (secondary hypogonadism) *(2)*. Gonadotropin levels may be useful in the diagnosis of primary hypogonadism even in the presence of normal T concentrations. For example, approx 40% of men with Klinefelter's syndrome may have total T levels within the normal range, but all have elevated LH and/or FSH levels. Also, the diagnosis of secondary hypogonadism has important therapeutic implications. Secondary hypogonadism may be caused by hypothalamic–pituitary disease that may require therapeutic interventions other than T treatment alone (e.g., pituitary tumors that may cause local mass effects or be associated with deficiencies or hypersecretion of other anterior pituitary hormones). In some instances, treatment of the underlying etiology of hypothalamic–pituitary dysfunction may correct androgen deficiency (e.g., treatment of Cushing's syndrome or hyperprolactinemia). Finally, in men with gonadotropin deficiency, but otherwise normal testis function, who are interested in fathering children, induction of both androgen and sperm production and restoration of fertility may be achieved using gonadotropin therapy or, in men with hypothalamic hypogonadism, pulsatile gonadotropin-releasing hormone (GnRH) treatment. Therefore, a careful investigation of the etiology of secondary hypogonadism is needed prior to initiation of T-replacement therapy.

For optimal clinical management of patients, it is important to consider etiological factors other than androgen deficiency that may contribute as much or more to clinical manifestations *(7)*. For example, in middle-aged to older men who present primarily with sexual dysfunction, androgen deficiency may contribute to loss of libido and failure of erections, but underlying neurovascular disease and/or medications are usually the major causes of erectile dysfunction. In these men, T treatment does not fully correct erectile failure, and additional therapy (e.g., sildenafil or alprostadil) is usually necessary for a satisfactory clinical outcome in these men. In men with osteoporosis and androgen deficiency, it is essential to perform a comprehensive evaluation for other common causes of bone loss (e.g., vitamin D deficiency, medications, immobility or inactivity, alcohol abuse, hyperparathyroidism) and to undertake measures to prevent falls in order to decrease the risk of fractures.

THERAPEUTIC GOALS AND BENEFITS OF T TREATMENT

The therapeutic goals of androgen-replacement therapy in male hypogonadism are to correct or improve the clinical consequences of T deficiency (outlined in the previous section); therefore, they depend on whether hypogonadism occurs in prepubertal boys or adults *(16)*.

In boys with hypogonadism causing delayed puberty, the therapeutic goals of T treatment are the following: induce secondary sexual characteristics (growth of the penis and scrotum and male hair pattern); stimulate long bone growth, acquisition of peak bone mass, and, eventually, closure of epiphyses without compromising adult height potential; increase muscle mass and strength and cause a redistribution of fat mass; enlarge the larynx and deepen the voice; stimulate male sexual behavior and function (libido and erections); induce other behavioral changes (improve energy, mood, motivation and initiative); and increase red blood cell production (into the normal adult male range).

The goals of androgen treatment in adult hypogonadal men are the following: improve or restore normal sexual function (libido and erectile function); stimulate growth and restore normal male hair pattern; improve muscle mass and strength; increase bone mineral density and reduce the risk of fractures; improve energy, motivation, initiative and mood, and reduce irritability; and increase hematocrit (into the normal adult male range). Because spermatogenesis requires high local T concentrations that are not achievable by exogenous androgen administration, T therapy does not stimulate spermatogenesis and testis size, nor does it restore fertility in hypogonadal men. Treatment of infertility in hypogonadal men is usually only possible in those with secondary hypogonadism using gonadotropin or GnRH therapy.

Beneficial clinical effects are usually produced with androgen-replacement therapy in hypogonadal men when serum T concentrations are increased into the broad normal range of T levels. The dose–response effects of T differ in different target organs and have not been characterized fully *(17–20)*. However, recent studies suggest some T actions exhibit threshold effects (e.g., libido that is stimulated maximally at relatively low T levels) *(19)*. In contrast, other actions of T demonstrate continuous dose–response effects within the physiological range of T levels and above (e.g., muscle mass) *(17,18)*. In some patients (e.g., elderly men with severe prostate disease), low-dose T supplementation rather than full androgen replacement may be necessary and sufficient to induce some desired clinical effects such as anabolic actions on muscle and bone, while minimizing stimulation of prostate growth.

FORMULATIONS AVAILABLE FOR T-REPLACEMENT THERAPY

Testosterone formulations that are available in the United States for treatment of male hypogonadism include parenteral 17β-hydroxyl T esters and transdermal T patches or gel (*see* Table 1) *(16)*. Although oral 17α-alkylated androgen preparations (e.g., methyltestosterone and fluoxymesterone) are available, they have low biopotency and bioavailability, and it is difficult to achieve full androgen replacement with these weak androgens *(16)*. Also, they significantly lower high-density lipoprotein (HDL) and raise low-density lipoprotein (LDL) cholesterol, are expensive, and have the potential to cause hepatotoxicity (cholestasis, jaundice, peliosis hepatis, and benign and malignant hepatic tumors). Because oral 17α-alkylated androgens have fewer therapeutic benefits and are associated with potentially greater risks compared to T esters or transdermal T formulations, they should not be used for androgen-replacement therapy of hypogonadal men.

Parenteral T Esters

Prior to the availability of transdermal T formulations, the long-acting, clinically equivalent, parenteral 17β-hydroxyl T esters T enanthate (Delatestryl®; Bio-Technology General, Iselin, NJ) and cypionate (Dep-Testosterone®, Pharmacia &Upjohn, Kalamazoo, MI) were the most effective, practical inexpensive, and safe preparations for androgen replacement in hypogonadal men *(16,21,22)*. Although transdermal T formulations provide a more physiological T replacement and are effective and practical alternatives to T injections, 17β-hydroxyl T esters continue to be used for androgen-replacement therapy, primarily because they are the least expensive method of T treatment. Also, some subjects who have been treated both with parenteral and transdermal T prefer T ester injections. Hydrophobic 17β-hydroxyl T esters are formulated in an oil vehicle (sesame oil for T enanthate and cottonseed oil for T cypionate). Following intramuscular injection, T esters are released slowly and hydrolyzed rapidly to T following release, resulting in an extended duration of T release and action into the circulation.

In adult hypogonadal men, the usual starting dose of T enanthate or cypionate is 150–200 mg im every 2 wk. Following injection of 200 mg of a T ester, serum T levels increase to the upper normal range or above for a few days and then gradually decline over 2 wk to the lower normal range or sometimes below, prior to the next injection (*see* Fig. 1A) *(21,22)*. This wide excursion of serum T levels between T ester injections may be associated with disturbing fluctuations in sexual desire and function, energy, and mood. In men who experience reduced libido, energy, and mood prior to their next injection, shortening the dosing interval to every 10 d may alleviate these symptoms. Some men prefer being treated with 75–100 mg T enanthate or cypionate im weekly in order to minimize fluctuations in serum T levels and symptoms. Administration of larger doses of T esters less frequently than every 2 wk (e.g., 300 mg im every 3 wk or 400 mg im every 4 wk) is not recommended. These higher doses usually produce very large fluctuations in blood T levels, characterized by more prolonged markedly supraphysiologic concentrations for several days following an injection and levels below the normal range after 3 wk *(22)*. Most patients are able to learn and perform self-administration of intramuscular T ester injections or have a family member administer the injections.

In men with severe, long-standing androgen deficiency, the profound alterations in sexuality, behavior, and physical appearance induced by full androgen-replacement

Table 1
T-Replacement Formulations Available in the United States

Formulation	Usual adult dosage	Cost[a]	Advantages	Disadvantages
Parenteral T esters				
T enanthate* (Delatestryl®) or T cypionate** (Depo-Testosterone®)	Adult T-replacement therapy 150–200 mg im every 2 wk or 75–100 mg im every wk Low-dose T supplementation 50–100 mg im every 2 wk T treatment of prepubertal boys 50–100 mg im monthly, increasing to every 2 wk and then to adult replacement dosages	$30/mo* (200 mg/2 wk) $15/mo** (200 mg/2 wk)	Long clinical experience Inexpensive Some dose flexibility Approved for use in boys	im injections, discomfort High to low T levels → fluctuations in libido, energy, mood Erythrocytosis > with transdermal formulations
T propionate	25–50 mg im 3 times/wk	$10/mo (50 mg tiw)	Short half-life Rapid ↓ T levels after stopped	Frequent im injections, discomfort High to low T levels → fluctuations in libido, energy, mood Rarely used
Transdermal T patches				
Testoderm® (matrix, scrotal patch with adhesive strips)	4 or 6 mg every AM	$100/mo (6 mg/d)	Physiological T levels, circadian variation No injections	Adequate size, clean and shaven scrotum, briefs needed Poor adhesion to skin High DHT levels More expensive than T esters Limited dose flexibility Scrotal location unacceptable to some

318

Formulation	Dose	Cost[a]	Advantages	Disadvantages
Androderm® (permeation-enhanced, reservoir, nonscrotal patch)	5–7.5 mg every PM	$120/mo (5 mg/d)	Physiological T levels, circadian variation; No injections; Good adhesion; Normal DHT levels	Frequent skin irritation, occasionally severe (↓ by coapplication of corticosteroid cream); More expensive than Testoderm; Higher dose requires 2 patches; Limited dose flexibility
Testoderm TTS® (non-permeation-enhanc reservoir, nonscrotal patch)	5–10 mg every AM	$110/mo (5 mg/d)	Physiological T levels, circadian variation; No injections; Less skin irritation than Androderm	Poor adhesion to skin; More expensive than Androderm; Larger patch than others; Higher dose requires 2 patches; Limited dose flexibility
Transdermal T gel AndroGel® T in hydroalcoholic gel	50–100 mg every AM	$165/mo (50 mg/d)	Steady-state T levels	Potential transfer of T to women and children by contact (prevented by clothing and washing after 2 h); No injections; Little skin irritation
Subcutaneous T pellets Tesopel® Pellets	225–450 mg (3–6 pellets) implanted sc every 3–4 mo	$30/mo (450 mg/3 mo)	Long-term, steady-state T levels	Minor surgical procedure; Extrusion, bleeding, and infection, although uncommon; Pellets not easily removable; Very seldom used

[a]Approximate average wholesale price (AWP) from 2001 Drug Topics Redbook, Medical Economics Thomson Health Care, Montvale, NJ, 2001.
Note: DHT = dehydrotestosterone.

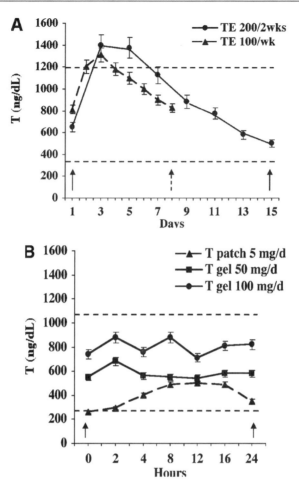

Fig. 1. Mean serum T concentrations during T-replacement therapy in hypogonadal men. **(A)** Serum T levels after the last injection of 100 mg T enanthate im every week (triangles) or 200 mg im every 2 wk (circles), at the end of 12 wk of treatment. Arrows represent the times of T enanthate injections, and dashed lines represent the normal range for T (adapted from ref. *22*). **(B)** Serum T levels before and after applications of T gel (AndroGel) 5 g (50 mg of T, squares) or 10 g (100 mg of T, circles) daily, or a T patch (Androderm) 5 mg (triangles) daily, after 90 d of treatment. Arrows represent the times of transdermal T application (time 0 was 0800 h), and dashed lines represent the normal range for T (adapted from ref. *23*).

therapy may be quite distressing both to the patients and their sexual partners. Counseling of hypogonadal men and their partners prior to and during T treatment plays an important role in reducing the likelihood of serious adjustment problems associated with androgen therapy. In some men, initiating therapy with a low dosage of T (e.g., 100 mg T enanthate or T cypionate every 2 wk) for several months, followed by a gradual escalation to a full androgen-replacement dosage may be the most prudent approach.

In some clinical situations, a full androgen-replacement dosage may not be necessary (e.g., elderly men with severe prostate disease in whom the anabolic actions of T on muscle and bone are the primary therapeutic goals). In these instances, low-dose T supplementation (e.g., 50–100 mg T enanthate or cypionate im every 2 wk or less) may be sufficient to induce the desired clinical effects, such as anabolic actions on muscle and bone, while minimizing potential adverse effects, such as stimulation of prostate growth. There is some evidence that low-dose T treatment may produce anabolic effects, even though serum T levels are not sustained within the normal range *(24–26)*. In this regard, low-dose androgen supplementation may be similar to glucocorticoid-replacement therapy with hydrocortisone, in which the duration of its biological action in tissues is not reflected by the serum concentrations of this steroid hormone. However, the clinical effects of low-dose T supplementation have not been evaluated fully in controlled trials.

An alternative to low-dose androgen supplementation with T enanthate or T cypionate is the use of the shorter-acting 17β-hydroxyl T ester T propionate, 25–50 mg im three times weekly *(16)*. Because of its short half-life, discontinuation of this preparation results in a more rapid fall in serum T levels and shorter duration of action compared to T enanthate and T cypionate. Therefore, an advantage of this preparation is rapid withdrawal of androgen replacement if adverse effects should develop. However, the frequent im injections needed to maintain normal T levels make this T ester a less desirable option to most patients, and T propionate is rarely used except perhaps in short-term therapeutic trials.

The clinical response to androgen replacement and occasionally serum T levels are used to monitor the adequacy T-replacement therapy in hypogonadal men *(16)*. Most hypogonadal men experience increases in libido, sexual function and activity, energy, well-being, motivation, and mood, and decreases in irritability within the first few months of T treatment. Anabolic effects such as increases in muscle mass and strength, body hair growth, and bone mineral density occur throughout the subsequent several months to years of androgen therapy. If the clinical response to androgen therapy is not adequate or wanes toward the end of the injection interval, measurements of blood T concentrations may be useful. Serum T levels measured either at the expected peak or midpoint (1–2 d and 5–7 d after an injection, respectively) or nadir (just before the next injection) between T ester injections may help to document an inadequate dose or absorption (e.g., in a very obese man) or dosing interval, respectively *(16,27)*. Some practitioners routinely monitor T levels after initiating of androgen therapy in order to determine the adequacy of replacement and to avoid over replacement.

In boys with prepubertal androgen deficiency and delayed puberty, T treatment is usually withheld until approx 14 yr of age (bone age at least 10.5 yr) *(28–30)*. Occasionally, therapy is initiated at a younger age if delayed sexual development and growth causes severe psychological distress in affected boys and their families. In order to avoid premature closure of long bone epiphyses and compromise of adult height potential, therapy is initiated with a very low dose of T enanthate or T cypionate (e.g., 50–100 mg im monthly). This dosage of T ester is sufficient to stimulate long-bone growth and induce some virilization without interfering with the spontaneous pubertal onset that occurs eventually in boys with constitutional delayed puberty. The latter is clinically and biochemically indistinguishable from delayed puberty caused by permanent hypogonadotropic hypogonadism (e.g., Kallmann's syndrome). Therefore, T treatment in boys with delayed puberty is intermittent. T therapy is continued for 3–6 mo and then stopped for 3–6 mo to determine whether spontaneous pubertal onset or progression occurs, as evidenced initially by an increase in testes size to > 8 mL. If spontaneous pubertal development does not occur, intermittent T treatment is continued, and the T ester dosage is increased gradually to 50–100 mg im every 2 wk, and then to full adult replacement doses, over the next several years. By avoiding intramuscular injections, transdermal T patches or gels would provide potentially very useful alternatives for the treatment of prepubertal androgen deficiency. However, these T formulations have not been tested and are not approved for use in prepubertal boys.

Transdermal T Formulations

Three transdermal T patches and a transdermal T gel are available as safe and effective alternatives to T esters for T-replacement therapy in hypogonadal men (*see* Table 1) *(16,31)*. They are useful in men who prefer to avoid or are unable to tolerate or administer intramuscular T ester injections. In contrast to T ester injections, T patches produce physiological T levels that exhibit a normal circadian variation, and T gel produces steady-state physiological T concentrations. However, all of these transdermal T delivery systems require daily application, are more expensive than androgen-replacement therapy using T ester injections, and possess some limitations (e.g., scrotal application site, skin irritation, poor skin adherence or absorption, limited dose flexibility, and potential for contact transfer). Many of these limitations are a consequence of the need to deliver relatively large amounts (5–10 mg) of T through skin that requires a thin, vascular area of skin (e.g., scrotal skin), a large patch or skin surface area of application, or solvents (e.g., alcohol) and permeation-enhancing agents. In some men, inherent skin sensitivity is also factor that may limit the use of some transdermal T formulations.

A scrotal T patch (Testoderm; Alza, Palo Alto, CA) was the first transdermal T delivery system available for T replacement in hypogonadal men *(32–34)*. This system contains T within the matrix of the patch, and because it is applied to the thin, highly vascular skin of the scrotum, it does not require permeation-enhancing agents. Scrotal T patches are available in two sizes that deliver either 6 mg (60 cm^2) or 4 mg (40 cm^2) of T daily. Long-term daily morning application of the Testoderm patch maintains normal physiological T levels that mimic the circadian variation of endogenous T and improves clinical manifestations of androgen deficiency *(35–37)*. After 3–4 wk of daily use, serum T levels are measured 2–4 h after application of the patch in order to assess the adequacy of T delivery. This patch requires application on an adequate size, clean, dry, and, preferably, shaven scrotum and the use of brief-type underwear for optimal adhesion. These requirements may not be acceptable to some hypogonadal men. Because of poor adherence to scrotal skin, thin adhesive strips were added to a subsequent version of this patch. Some men may experience skin irritation and itching. Serum levels of dihydrotestosterone (DHT), a more potent androgen than T, increase to above the normal range as a result of the high 5α-reductase activity in scrotal skin. The clinical significance of chronic exposure to high circulating DHT levels in androgen-responsive organs such as the prostate is unclear, but careful monitoring for the development of adverse androgenic effects should be performed. No increase in prostate disease was observed in small, short-term controlled studies of older men treated with the Testoderm patch *(35–37)* or DHT gel formulations *(38–40)*, but these studies do not address potential long-term risks. The subsequent availability of nonscrotal T patches (*see* the following paragraph) has supplanted the use of the scrotal T patch for androgen-replacement therapy.

A permeation-enhanced, nonscrotal T patch (Androderm, Watson, Corona, CA) that is composed of a central reservoir containing T and permeation enhancers in an alcohol-based gel within an adhesive patch was developed an alternative to scrotal T patches for androgen replacement-therapy *(41,42)*. It is applied daily to nonscrotal skin (e.g., back, abdomen, upper arms or thigh), avoiding areas over a bony prominence. Long-term nightly application of this patch in hypogonadal men also maintains serum T levels in the physiological range with a normal circadian variation, and it improves the clinical manifestations of androgen deficiency *(43–45)*. Androderm patches are available in two sizes that deliver 2.5 mg (37 cm^2) or 5 mg (44 cm^2) of T daily. Application of a single 5-mg Androderm patch usually produces serum T levels in the low- to mid-normal range. Production of T concentrations that are consistently in the mid- to high-normal range usually requires application of two Androderm patches (e.g., one 2.5-mg patch plus one 5-mg patch *(46)*. After 3–4 wk of daily use, morning serum T levels are measured 8–10 h after application of the patch on the previous evening in order to assess the adequacy of T delivery. The major limitation to use of this patch is skin irritation that occurs in at least approx 30% of patients *(43,47–49)*. The degree of skin irritation is highly variable—commonly minor redness and rarely severe burnlike reactions. Pretreatment of skin under the reservoir with triamcinolone acetonide 0.1% cream reduces the incidence and severity of skin irritation produced by the Androderm patch *(50)*. In contrast to the scrotal T patch, serum DHT levels remain within the normal range with this nonscrotal patch. However, it is more expensive than the scrotal T delivery system.

A non-permeation-enhanced, reservoir, nonscrotal T patch (Testoderm TTS; Alza, Palo Alto, CA) is also available for T-replacement therapy in hypogonadal men *(51–53)*. It is composed of a relatively large reservoir containing T in an alcohol-based gel (without permeation enhancers) within a lightly adhesive patch. It is applied daily to nonscrotal skin (e.g., back, abdomen, or upper buttocks) and pressed firmly in place. Daily morning application of this patch in hypogonadal men maintains physiological serum T levels that mimic the normal circadian variation of endogenous T. The Testoderm TTS patch delivers approx 5 mg (60 cm^2) of T daily. Application of a single 5-mg patch usually produces serum T levels in the low- to mid-normal range. Production of T concentrations that are consistently in the mid- to high-normal range usually requires application of two 5-mg patches *(51)*. After 3–4 wk of daily use, serum T levels are measured 2–4 h after application of the patch in order to assess the adequacy of T delivery. Because it does not use permeation-enhancing agents and has less adhesive, the Testoderm TTS patch causes much less skin irritation than the Androderm patch *(54)*. However, the major limitation to use of this patch is its poor adherence to skin, especially with sweating. Serum DHT levels also remain within the normal range with this nonscrotal T patch. The Testoderm TTS patch is slightly less expensive than the Androderm patch. Recently, this patch was withdrawn from the market by its manufacturers.

Most recently, a transdermal formulation of T in a 1% hydroalcoholic gel (AndroGel; Unimed/Solvay, Buffalo Grove, IL) became available for androgen replacement in hypogonadal men *(23)*. It is applied daily in the morning to clean, dry skin of the shoulders and upper arms and/or abdomen and flanks, and allowed to dry. Hands should be washed with soap and water after application of the gel. The application sites should be covered with clothing and contact with water (e.g., showering or swimming) should be avoided for 5–6 h. Long-term daily application of AndroGel in hypogonadal men maintains steady-state physiological serum T levels and improves the clinical manifestations of androgen deficiency *(56,57)*. AndroGel is packaged in packets of two sizes that deliver 25 mg (2.5-g packet) or 50 mg (5-g packet) of T daily. After 90 d treatment,

Androgel 5 g (50 mg of T) and 10 g (100 mg of T) daily produced serum T concentrations in the mid- and high-normal range, respectively, compared to Androderm 5 mg daily that produced serum T levels in the low- to mid-normal range (Fig. 1B) *(23)*. After 2 wk of daily use, morning serum T levels are measured in order to assess the adequacy of T delivery. AndroGel may also produce serum DHT levels above the normal range, probably as a result of the large surface area of skin covered. However, local skin irritation occurs in ≤ 5% of patients. The major limiting factor to the use of AndroGel for androgen-replacement therapy is cost. It is the most expensive T formulation that is available, and if more than one packet (e.g., 5 g) of AndroGel is required for adequate replacement, the cost is prohibitive for most patients. There is also concern with this formulation regarding transfer of T from application sites on the skin of patients to women (especially pregnant women) and children. Precautions to minimize potential transfer of T to others include thorough washing of hands immediately after application of AndroGel, covering application sites with clothing, and thorough washing of areas that come into contact with application sites. Also, 5–6 h (and occasionally as soon as 1–2 h) after application, showering is permitted that washes off residual T on the surface of the skin with minimal effect on the absorption of T from subcutaneous sites.

Subcutaneous T Pellets

Testosterone pellets (Testopel Pellets, Bartor Pharmacal, Rye, NY), 225—450 mg, (three to six 75-mg pellets) implanted subcutaneously every 3–4 mo are available for long-term androgen-replacement therapy in hypogonadal men, but is very seldom used in the United States. Outside of the United States, subcutaneous implantation of T pellets has been used more commonly for androgen replacement. Using a different formulation, subcutaneous implantation of 600–1200 mg (three to six 200-mg pellets) is accomplished using a trocar that is introduced through a small skin incision *(57–59)*. These T implants produce sustained, nearly zero-order release of T into circulation, and maintain steady-state physiological serum T levels for 4–6 mo. Because a minor surgical procedure is required two to three times yearly to implant a large number pellets and there is a potential for extrusion and other local side effects and difficulty in removing pellets if necessary, this method of T replacement is not acceptable to many hypogonadal men.

ANDROGEN FORMULATIONS UNDER DEVELOPMENT

Recently, there has been an eruption of interest by pharmaceutical companies in developing new and possibly more selective androgen formulations or compounds. This interest has been ignited in part by the realization that male hypogonadism is a common clinical disorder, but also by the potential for expanded indications for androgen treatments (e.g., chronic illnesses and wasting syndromes, age-related androgen deficiency [andropause] and hormonal male contraception).

There is considerable interest in developing new short-acting T formulations—in particular, orally active preparations—both for androgen-replacement therapy of hypogonadal men and low-dose androgen supplementation. In countries outside the United States, an oral, 17β-hydroxyl ester, T undecanoate has been available for many years and used to provide safe and effective androgen replacement in hypogonadal men *(24,60)*. Unlike oral 17α-alkylated androgens, T undecanoate formulated in oleic acid is absorbed from the gastrointestinal tract directly into the lymphatic system, bypassing initial hepatic inactivation, and is not associated with hepatotoxicity. Androgen replacement usually requires high doses (80–240 mg daily) and administration in divided doses (two to three times daily). Absorption of T undecanoate is quite variable and is dependent on concomitant ingestion of a meal. Thus, serum T levels and clinical responses produced are highly variable.

A new formulation of T undecanoate and a bioadhesive buccal T tablet, both administered twice daily, are being tested for androgen replacement in hypogonadal men and registration in the United States. In previous studies, T complexed to 2.5–5 mg hydroxypropyl-β-cyclodextrin administered sublingually to hypogonadal men resulted in a rapid increase in serum T levels that peaked in 20–40 min and lasted for only 2–4 h (25,26,61). Despite these unfavorably pharmacokinetics, T cyclodextrin improved sexual function, mood, and muscle strength and reduced markers of bone resorption, supporting the notion that the biological actions of T may not be reflected by its serum levels and that sustained physiological concentrations may not be necessary for some clinical effects of T.

In some countries in Europe, a 2% hydroalcoholic DHT gel formulation is used for androgen replacement therapy of young hypogonadal men (38). Recently, DHT gel formulations have also been tested in older hypogonadal men (39,40,62). A rationale that is proposed for the its use in treatment of hypogonadal men is that DHT administration may suppress endogenous gonadotropins and T secretion, thereby lowering intraprostatic T and DHT concentrations and preventing prostatic stimulation (63). Also, because it is not aromatizable, DHT may not induce or worsen gynecomastia in hypogonadal men. However, evidence for these potential advantages of DHT over T for androgen-replacement therapy is lacking. As with T gel, there is concern regarding transfer of this more potent androgen to females and children who come in contact with skin sites of application. Furthermore, because DHT is not aromatizable and endogenous gonadotropin and estrogen (E_2) secretion are suppressed, there is concern regarding the potential consequences of estrogen deficiency produce in hypogonadal men treated with DHT (e.g., on bone, brain, and lipids). Finally, other transdermal T-gel formulations and patches are being developed for androgen-replacement therapy in hypogonadal men.

In addition to these short-acting androgen preparations, a number of long-acting formulations are being developed that produce prolonged release of T and sustained serum T levels in the normal range, both for use in androgen replacement in young hypogonadal men and other potential uses such as hormonal male contraception. In hypogonadal men, the 17β-hydroxyl esters, [T undecanoate formulated in castor or tea seed oil (64,65) and T buciclate (66)] were administered im every 6–12 wk to maintain serum T levels within the eugonadal range (the latter in the low-normal range). Also, intramuscular or subcutaneous injections of T incorporated into biodegradable microcapsules produce serum T concentrations in the eugonadal range for 10–11 wk (67,68). Although these long-acting T preparations show promise, major limitations of these formulations include the large (4 mL) injection volumes, which require two separate injection sites and are often uncomfortable, and their highly variable bioavailability.

Finally, there is expanding interest in developing "designer" androgens that will maintain the beneficial effects of T on muscle, bone, sexual function, behavior, mood, cognition, and cardiovascular function but will have reduced adverse actions or protective effects on the prostate gland, lipid profile, and cardiovascular risk. Based on the knowledge that tissue-specific androgen action involves interactions among the androgen receptor and tissue-specific coactivator and corepressor proteins, an approach that is being used to develop such compounds is to identify nonsteroidal, orally active selective androgen-receptor modulators (SARMs), analogous to selective estrogen receptor modulators (SERMs), such as raloxifene *(69,70)*. Although SARMs may have selective androgen actions on different target organs, they will probably not have intrinsic estrogen activity. Unless specific SARMs do not suppress endogenous gonadotropin and E_2 secretion, administration of these compounds will probably produce a state of relative estrogen deficiency, similar to that which occurs with the administration of non-aromatizable androgens, such as DHT. Therefore, specific clinical indications (e.g., muscle-wasting syndromes) that take advantage of a SARMs unique tissue-selective properties will need to be identified. Carefully performed studies of their clinical benefits and risks will need to be performed, with attention to effects on target organs (e.g., bone) that are normally mediated, in part, by aromatization of T to E_2.

Another approach used to develop a "designer" androgen is to identify an androgen that undergoes aromatization to an estrogen but, unlike T, not does not undergo 5α-reduction to a more potent androgen. One such androgen that was synthesized over 20 yr ago is 7α-methyl-19-nortestosterone, also known as MENT *(71)*. In orchidectomized monkeys, compared to T, MENT is 10 times more potent in stimulating body weight gain and suppressing gonadotropins but only twice as potent in stimulating prostate growth *(72)*. In hypogonadal men, two subcutaneous MENT acetate implants maintain stable MENT concentrations, sexual function, and mood for 6 wk *(73)*. However, longer-term effects on body composition (muscle and fat mass and bone mineral density) relative to its effects on prostate size have not been evaluated fully.

POTENTIAL RISKS OF T TREATMENT AND MONITORING

Androgen treatment is absolutely contraindicated in men with prostate cancer and breast cancer *(16)*. Because these are androgen-dependent malignancies, T treatment may stimulate tumor growth. This has been demonstrated most definitively in men with metastatic prostate cancer in whom rapid growth and expansion of metastatic tumors may cause worsening of severe bone pain or spinal cord compression. Prior to initiating T-replacement therapy, a careful breast examination for masses should be performed in all hypogonadal men, and digital rectal examination (DRE) for a prostate nodule or induration should be performed in middle-aged and older men with androgen deficiency. Measurement of serum prostate-specific antigen (PSA) is useful in men at higher risk for prostate carcinoma (e.g., older men) and those with an abnormal DRE or family history of prostate cancer.

Relative contraindications to androgen therapy include patients with untreated obstructive sleep apnea in whom T treatment may worsen sleep-disordered breathing and associated oxygen desaturation, men with significant erythrocytosois at baseline in whom further stimulation of erythropoiesis may result in hyperviscosity and vascular complications, and patients with severe edematous states (e.g., severe congestive heart failure, nephrotic syndrome, or hepatic cirrhosis) in whom fluid retention associated with T treatment may worsen edema.

In general, androgen-replacement therapy using either T ester injections or transdermal T formulations are tolerated very well and serious adverse effects are rare *(16)*. Acne and increased oiliness of the skin is relatively common in patients receiving T therapy for induction of puberty and responds to local skin measures (e.g., retinoic acid), antibiotics, and/or reduction in T dosage. Frontal balding or androgenic alopecia may develop in genetically predisposed hypogonadal men during T treatment. Mild to moderate weight gain usually occurs as a result of both the anabolic actions of T and sodium and water retention. Clinically significant edema does not usually occur except in men with underlying edematous conditions (*see* previous paragraph). Excessive stimulation of libido and erections are rare and occur mostly in boys and men with severe, long-standing androgen deficiency treated with higher doses of T. In these patients, symptoms usually resolve spontaneously or with a reduction in the dosage of T. Contrary to popular belief, T replacement in physiological or moderately supraphysiological dosages does not cause excessive aggressiveness or anger *(18,25,55,74,75)*. Although social aggressiveness, motivation, and initiative are increased, irritability and anger are reduced with androgen-replacement therapy. As mentioned earlier, the stimulation of normal libido and more aggressive behavior and physical changes induced by T in men with long-standing androgen deficiency may be distressing to patients and their sexual partners. Therefore, careful counseling regarding behavioral and physical changes that are expected should be instituted prior to and during T treatment.

In hypogonadal men, T-replacement therapy stimulates erythropoiesis and increases hematocrit from the female range into the normal adult male range *(76)*. Occasionally, T administration causes excessive erythrocytosis that may require reduction or, if severe, temporary discontinuation of therapy and/or therapeutic phlebotomy. Although adverse effects associated with T-induced erythrocytosis are poorly documented in the literature, there is concern that a severe increase in red cell volume and associated blood viscosity may predispose some patients, especially older men, to vascular thrombosis. Therefore, measurement of a hematocrit should be performed prior to starting T treatment, shortly after initiation of T (e.g., 3–6 mo) and then yearly during therapy. Of note is that some hypogonadal men who develop erythrocytosis on androgen therapy have underlying predisposing conditions, such as hypoxia resulting from chronic lung disease or obstructive sleep apnea. Compared to hypogonadal men treated with T ester injections that produce slightly supraphysiological T levels for a few days after administration, excessive erythrocytosis occurs less commonly in men with transdermal T patches that produce more physiological T levels *(77)*.

Testosterone-replacement therapy in hypogonadal men may induce or worsen obstructive sleep apnea *(78,79)*. The prevalence of clinically significant obstructive apnea during T treatment is not known, but it is probably low. However, significant apnea is associated with significant morbidity and mortality, and sleep apnea is also associated with low T levels. Therefore, hypogonadal men (especially those at increased risk [e.g., obese men]) should be questioned about symptoms of obstructive sleep apnea (e.g., apnea or loud snoring during sleep, sleep disturbance, or daytime somnolence), both prior to and during T replacement. If symptoms are present prior to or develop during T therapy, a formal sleep study should be performed, and if obstructive sleep apnea is confirmed, treatment should be instituted (e.g., continuous positive airway pressure) before T is started or continued. If the patient is unresponsive or cannot tolerate treatment, T should not be instituted or discontinued.

Occasionally, gynecomastia develops in patients receiving T treatment, especially in boys or young men receiving androgens for induction of puberty and severely hypogonadal men receiving relatively high doses of T who have a predisposing condition, such as hepatic cirrhosis *(16)*. Careful examination usually reveals some gynecomastia and increased amounts subcutaneous fat tissue of the chest in hypogonadal men prior to initiation of androgen therapy. Furthermore, small amounts of palpable breast tissue (usually ≤ 2 cm) are commonly detectable in eugonadal men. Therefore, it is important to do a careful breast examination prior to and during T therapy.

Testosterone-replacement therapy in hypogonadal men increases prostate size to volumes that are similar to those of age-matched eugonadal men, but it does not cause excessive stimulation of prostate growth and enlargement *(80,81)*. There is no evidence that androgen-replacement therapy worsens symptoms, urine flow, or urinary retention associated with benign prostatic hyperplasia (BPH) that may require invasive intervention, such as transurethral resection of the prostate (TURP). However, long-term controlled studies have not been performed to evaluate these issues in the population of men over age 45 yr who are at increased risk for developing clinically significant BPH. Therefore, caution should be exercised when treating middle-aged to older men, especially those with moderate to severe symptoms of BPH prior to T treatment, and monitoring of symptoms should be performed *(82)*. Symptoms of BPH should be assessed (e.g., using the American Urological Association Symptom Index or International Prostate Symptom Score) prior to and during T replacement in these men. Low-dose T supplementation and/ or concomitant therapy for BPH (e.g., α-adrenergic receptor antagonists, 5α-reductase inhibitors, or bladder outlet procedures) should be considered in patients with moderate to severe symptoms.

There is no evidence that T treatment causes prostate cancer. However, in middle-aged to older hypogonadal men, the most concerning potential long-term risk of T-replacement therapy is stimulation of growth of previously unrecognized localized or metastatic prostate cancer or, in older men particularly, growth of pre-existing subclinical (microscopic) prostate cancer into clinically apparent and significant disease *(7)*. Although there is evidence that T treatment will stimulate the growth of metastatic and locally invasive prostate cancer, the effect of T on subclinical prostate cancer is not known. Long-term, prospective, controlled trials are needed to determine whether T therapy will stimulate growth and progression of subclinical microscopic prostate cancer into clinically evident and significant disease.

Serum PSA levels are reduced in hypogonadal men and increased to levels observed in age-matched eugonadal men with androgen replacement *(80)*. Whether an individual physician monitors PSA levels before and during T replacement therapy in an older hypogondal men depends, to some extent, on whether they feel PSA screening in eugonadal men is justified *(7,83)*. The practice of yearly PSA screening in eugonadal men over the age of 45 yr is controversial and its utility has not been demonstrated convincingly. Increasingly however, it is becoming a standard of care in many communities, and many patients are demanding PSA screening. An argument raised for more intensive PSA monitoring during T treatment in older hypogonadal men is that a potentially disease-modifying therapeutic intervention is being initiated, often with a T formulation that produces transient supraphysiological T levels (T esters). Therefore, for clinical and medical legal reasons, more careful monitoring of PSA levels is prudent. An argument against more intensive PSA monitoring is that abnormal PSA levels that trigger a prostate biopsy are more likely to occur in older hypogonadal men on T treatment and, therefore, there is an increased likelihood of detecting subclinical prostate cancer for which treatment is unclear. Even if subclinical prostate cancer discovered on biopsy does not affect overall mortality, the potential medical, surgical, psychological, socioeconomic, legal, and ethical consequences of this diagnosis may be great. Taking these considerations into account, a recent consensus recommendation is that in older hypogonadal men, a DRE and PSA level be monitored prior to starting therapy, shortly after starting therapy (e.g., at 3–6 mo), and then yearly (7,84).

Because men have a higher risk of coronary artery disease than women and T administration may suppress HDL cholesterol, leading to a more atherogenic lipid profile, there is concern that T replacement in hypogonadal men will increase the risk of heart disease. In severely androgen-deficient young men, T-replacement therapy decreases HDL cholesterol concentration (85–88). In general, the degree of reduction in HDL cholesterol is greater in more severely androgen-deficient men and with higher physiological or supraphysiological T dosages, and it is much greater with nonaromatizable, oral 17α-alkylated androgens (16). In contrast, T treatment of older mildly hypogonadal men does not suppress HDL cholesterol, and total and LDL cholesterol are either not affected or decreased (7). The clinical significance of these T-induced lipoprotein changes on cardiovascular risk is not known. Furthermore, most cross-sectional epidemiological studies suggest that low T levels are associated with an increase in the risk and severity of coronary artery disease, and longitudinal studies fail to find a relationship between T levels and development of coronary heart disease (7,83,89,90). Also, intervention studies suggest that T treatment may improve exercise-induced coronary ischemia and angina (91–97). However, long-term controlled studies are needed to determine the effects of T treatment on major cardiovascular outcomes, such as the incidence of coronary death, myocardial infarction, and stroke. At present, cardiovascular health and plasma lipids should be evaluated as dictated by general practices, and more intensive monitoring is not justified.

Potentially serious hepatotoxicity occurs predominantly with the use of oral 17α-alkylated androgens, and rarely, if ever, occurs with the use of injectable T esters or transdermal T formulations (16). Routine testing of liver enzymes is not necessary with the use of the latter preparations for androgen replacement in hypogonadal men.

By suppressing endogenous gonadotropin production, T treatment reversibly suppresses spermatogenesis to varying degrees, depending on the T formulation, dosage, and duration of treatment, underlying etiology of hypogonadism, and baseline spermatogenesis (2). The suppression of sperm production may further impair fertility in hypogonadal men receiving androgen therapy. This effect of T therapy is usually only clinically relevant in men with hypogonadotropic hypogonadism with otherwise normal testes. In gonadotropin-deficient men, if fertility is desired, androgen therapy should be discontinued and gonadotropin treatment should be started initially with human chorionic gonadotropin (hCG) and then, if necessary, with combined hCG and human menopausal gonadotropin (hMG) or hFSH administration (2). In the absence of concomitant testicular disease (e.g., cryptorchidism), previous T-replacement therapy does not impair the subsequent induction of spermatogenesis with gonadotropin therapy.

Occasionally, local discomfort or bleeding may occur at the site of T ester injections. Using proper intramuscular injection techniques may minimize these side effects. Administration of T esters subcutaneously usually causes severe local irritation and pain. Rarely, patients may experience an allergic reaction to the injection vehicle, sesame oil (T enanthate), or cottonseed oil (T cypionate). As discussed previously, transdermal T patches may cause local skin irritation, itching, contact dermatitis, and, occasionally, more severe reactions. Skin reactions occur more commonly with the Androderm patch than with the Testoderm and Testoderm TTS patches and AndroGel.

SUMMARY AND CONCLUSIONS

Male hypogonadism is a common clinical condition that affects the health and well-being of boys and men of all ages. T-replacement therapy has proven beneficial effects on body composition (muscle, bone, and fat mass), sexual development and function, and behavior and mood. Unfortunately, androgen deficiency is often not diagnosed or treated inappropriately. The diagnosis of male hypogonadism is suspected when individuals present with a clinical syndrome that is consistent with androgen deficiency, and it is confirmed by the presence of repeatedly low serum T levels. The clinical manifestations of androgen deficiency vary with the stage of sexual development and are subtler in men compared to prepubertal boys with hypogonadism. T levels should be measured using an accurate and reliable assay that is preferably not affected by alterations in SHBG concentrations and should be repeated to confirm the diagnosis of androgen deficiency. Other important management considerations include the evaluation of potentially reversible causes of androgen deficiency, concomitant gonadotropin and T measurements to diagnosis secondary hypogonadism that has important therapeutic implications, and consideration of other etiological factors that may contribute clinical manifestations.

The goals of androgen-replacement therapy in male hypogonadism are to correct or improve the clinical consequences of T deficiency and, therefore, depend on whether hypogonadism occurs in prepubertal boys or adults. Currently, T formulations that are available for androgen replacement are T esters injections and transdermal T patches or gel. T esters are effective and safe and provide the least expensive method of T replacement, but they usually require intramuscular injections every 1–2 wk, and are associated with wide excursions in T levels that may cause fluctuations in symptoms. Transdermal T patches or gel provide more physiological T levels but require daily application, may cause skin irritation, and are more expensive than T esters. A number of new short- and long-acting androgen formulations and designer androgens and SARMs are currently being developed that should greatly expand the methods available for androgen treatment in the future.

Prostate cancer and breast cancer are absolute contraindications, and untreated obstructive sleep apnea, erythrocytosis, and severe edematous states are relative contraindications to T treatment. In general, androgen-replacement therapy is tolerated very well and serious adverse effects are rare. Occasionally, T treatment may cause excessive erythrocytosis and, rarely, it may induce or worsen obstructive sleep apnea. Therefore, hematocrit and symptoms of sleep apnea should be assessed prior to and during T therapy. In middle-aged to older hypogonadal men, monitoring of DRE and PSA for prostate cancer and BPH symptoms are also recommended. However, the long-term risks of T treatment in older hypogonadal men on incidence of clinical prostate cancer, severity and need for invasive intervention for BPH, and cardiovascular outcomes, such as cardiac death, myocardial infarction, and stroke, are unknown. A large, long-term, prospective, randomized, placebo-controlled trial is needed to determine both the potential risks and benefits of chronic T treatment in older hypogonadal men.

REFERENCES

1. Amory JK, Anawalt BD, Paulsen CA, Bremner WJ. Klinefelter's syndrome. Lancet 2000;356:333–335.
2. Matsumoto AM. The testis. In: Felig P, Frohman LA, eds. Endocrinology and Metabolism, 4th Edition. McGraw-Hill, New York, 2001, pp. 635–705.
3. Bhasin S, Storer TW, Asbel-Sethi N, et al. Effects of testosterone replacement with a nongenital, transdermal system, Androderm, in human immunodeficiency virus-infected men with low testosterone levels. J Clin Endocrinol Metab 1998;83:3155–3162.
4. Grinspoon S, Corcoran C, Askari H, et al. Effects of androgen administration in men with the AIDS wasting syndrome. A randomized, double-blind, placebo-controlled trial. Ann Intern Med 1998; 129:18–26.
5. Grinspoon S, Corcoran C, Stanley T, et al. Effects of hypogonadism and testosterone administration on depression indices in HIV-infected men. J Clin Endocrinol Metab 2000;85:60–65.
6. Handelsman DJ, Liu PY. Androgen therapy in chronic renal failure. Baillieres Clin Endocrinol Metab 1998;12:485–500.
7. Matsumoto AM. Andropause: clinical implications of the decline in serum testosterone levels with aging in men. J Gerontol A: Biol Sci Med Sci 2002;57:M76–M99.
8. Reid IR, Wattie DJ, Evans MC, Stapleton JP. Testosterone therapy in glucocorticoid-treated men. Arch Intern Med 1996;156:1173–1177.
9. Bremner WJ, Vitiello MV, Prinz PN. Loss of circadian rhythmicity in blood testosterone levels with aging in normal men. J Clin Endocrinol Metab 1983;56:1278–1281.
10. Giraudi G, Cenderelli G, Migliardi M. Effect of tracer binding to serum proteins on the reliability of a direct free testosterone assay. Steroids 1988;52:423–424.
11. Rosner W. Errors in the measurement of plasma free testosterone. J Clin Endocrinol Metab 1997;82:2014–2015.
12. Rosner W. An extraordinarily inaccurate assay for free testosterone is still with us. J Clin Endocrinol Metab 2001;86:2903.
13. Vermeulen A, Verdonck L, Kaufman JM. A critical evaluation of simple methods for the estimation of free testosterone in serum. J Clin Endocrinol Metab 1999;84:3666–3672.
14. Winters SJ, Kelley DE, Goodpaster B. The analog free testosterone assay: are the results in men clinically useful? Clin Chem 1998;44:2178–2182.
15. Spratt DI, O'Dea LS, Schoenfeld D, et al. Neuroendocrine-gonadal axis in men: frequent sampling of LH, FSH, and testosterone. Am J Physiol 1988;254:E658–E666.
16. Matsumoto AM. Clinical use and abuse of androgens and antiandrogens. In: Becker KL, ed. Principles and Practice of Endocrinology and Metabolism, 3rd Edition. Lippincott Williams & Wilkins, Philadelphia, PA, 2001, pp. 1181–1200.
17. Bhasin S, Storer TW, Berman N, et al. The effects of supraphysiologic doses of testosterone on muscle size and strength in normal men. N Engl J Med 1996;335:1–7.
18. Bhasin S, Woodhouse L, Casaburi R, et al. Testosterone dose–response relationships in healthy young men. Am J Physiol Endocrinol Metab 2001;281:E1172–E1181.
19. Buena F, Swerdloff RS, Steiner BS, et al. Sexual function does not change when serum testosterone levels are pharmacologically varied within the normal male range. Fertil Steril 1993;59:1118–1123.
20. Singh AB, Hsia S, Alaupovic P, et al. The effects of varying doses of T on insulin sensitivity, plasma lipids, apolipoproteins, and C-reactive protein in healthy young men. J Clin Endocrinol Metab 2002;87:136–143.
21. Nankin HR. Hormone kinetics after intramuscular testosterone cypionate. Fertil Steril 1987;47:1004–1009.
22. Snyder PJ, Lawrence DA. Treatment of male hypogonadism with testosterone enanthate. J Clin Endocrinol Metab 1980;51:1335–1339.
23. Swerdloff RS, Wang C, Cunningham G, et al. Long-term pharmacokinetics of transdermal testosterone gel in hypogonadal men. J Clin Endocrinol Metab 2000;85:4500–4510.
24. Gooren LJ. A ten-year safety study of the oral androgen testosterone undecanoate. J Androl 1994;15: 212–215.
25. Wang C, Alexander G, Berman N, et al. Testosterone replacement therapy improves mood in hypogonadal men—a clinical research center study. J Clin Endocrinol Metab 1996;81:3578–3583.
26. Wang C, Eyre DR, Clark R, et al. Sublingual testosterone replacement improves muscle mass and strength, decreases bone resorption, and increases bone formation markers in hypogonadal men—a clinical research center study. J Clin Endocrinol Metab 1996;81:3654–3662.

27. Bhasin S, Bremner WJ. Clinical review 85: Emerging issues in androgen replacement therapy. J Clin Endocrinol Metab 1997;82:3–8.
28. De Luca F, Argente J, Cavallo L, et al. Management of puberty in constitutional delay of growth and puberty. J Pediatr Endocrinol Metab 2001;14:953–957.
29. Houchin LD, Rogol AD. Androgen replacement in children with constitutional delay of puberty: the case for aggressive therapy. Baillieres Clin Endocrinol Metab 1998;12:427–440.
30. Soliman AT, Khadir MM, Asfour M. Testosterone treatment in adolescent boys with constitutional delay of growth and development. Metabolism 1995;44:1013–1015.
31. Amory JK, Matsumoto AM. The therapeutic potential of testosterone patches. Expert Opin Invest Drugs 1998;7:1977–1988.
32. Cunningham GR, Cordero E, Thornby JI. Testosterone replacement with transdermal therapeutic systems. Physiological serum testosterone and elevated dihydrotestosterone levels. JAMA 1989;261:2525–2530.
33. Findlay JC, Place V, Snyder PJ. Treatment of primary hypogonadism in men by the transdermal administration of testosterone. J Clin Endocrinol Metab 1989;68:369–373.
34. Findlay JC, Place VA, Snyder PJ. Transdermal delivery of testosterone. J Clin Endocrinol Metab 1987;64:266–268.
35. Behre HM, von Eckardstein S, Kliesch S, Nieschlag E. Long-term substitution therapy of hypogonadal men with transscrotal testosterone over 7–10 years. Clin Endocrinol (Oxf) 1999;50:629–635.
36. Snyder PJ, Peachey H, Hannoush P, et al. Effect of testosterone treatment on bone mineral density in men over 65 years of age. J Clin Endocrinol Metab 1999;84:1966–1972.
37. Snyder PJ, Peachey H, Hannoush P, et al. Effect of testosterone treatment on body composition and muscle strength in men over 65 years of age. J Clin Endocrinol Metab 1999;84:2647–2653.
38. de Lignieres B. Transdermal dihydrotestosterone treatment of "andropause." Ann Med 1993;25:235–241.
39. Kunelius P, Lukkarinen O, Hannuksela ML, et al. The effects of transdermal dihydrotestosterone in the aging male: a prospective, randomized, double blind study. J Clin Endocrinol Metab 2002;87:1467–1472.
40. Ly LP, Jimenez M, Zhuang TN, et al. A double-blind, placebo-controlled, randomized clinical trial of transdermal dihydrotestosterone gel on muscular strength, mobility, and quality of life in older men with partial androgen deficiency. J Clin Endocrinol Metab 2001;86:4078–4088.
41. Meikle AW, Arver S, Dobs AS, et al. Pharmacokinetics and metabolism of a permeation-enhanced testosterone transdermal system in hypogonadal men: influence of application site-a clinical research center study. J Clin Endocrinol Metab 1996;81:1832–1840.
42. Meikle AW, Mazer NA, Moellmer JF, et al. Enhanced transdermal delivery of testosterone across nonscrotal skin produces physiological concentrations of testosterone and its metabolites in hypogonadal men. J Clin Endocrinol Metab 1992;74:623–628.
43. Arver S, Dobs AS, Meikle AW, et al. Long-term efficacy and safety of a permeation-enhanced testosterone transdermal system in hypogonadal men. Clin Endocrinol (Oxf) 1997;47:727–737.
44. Kenny AM, Bellantonio S, Gruman CA, et al. Effects of transdermal testosterone on cognitive function and health perception in older men with low bioavailable testosterone levels. J Gerontol A: Biol Sci Med Sci 2002;57:M321–M325.
45. Kenny AM, Prestwood KM, Gruman CA, et al. Effects of transdermal testosterone on bone and muscle in older men with low bioavailable testosterone levels. J Gerontol A: Biol Sci Med Sci 2001;56:M266–M272.
46. Brocks DR, Meikle AW, Boike SC, et al. Pharmacokinetics of testosterone in hypogonadal men after transdermal delivery: influence of dose. J Clin Pharmacol 1996;36:732–739.
47. Bennett NJ. A burn-like lesion caused by a testosterone transdermal system. Burns 1998;24:478–480.
48. Jordan WP Jr. Allergy and topical irritation associated with transdermal testosterone administration: a comparison of scrotal and nonscrotal transdermal systems. Am J Contact Dermatitis 1997;8:108–113.
49. Parker S, Armitage M. Experience with transdermal testosterone replacement therapy for hypogonadal men. Clin Endocrinol (Oxf) 1999;50:57–62.
50. Wilson DE, Kaidbey K, Boike SC, Jorkasky DK. Use of topical corticosteroid pretreatment to reduce the incidence and severity of skin reactions associated with testosterone transdermal therapy. Clin Ther 1998;20:299–306.
51. Singh AB, Norris K, Modi N, et al. Pharmacokinetics of a transdermal testosterone system in men with end stage renal disease receiving maintenance hemodialysis and healthy hypogonadal men. J Clin Endocrinol Metab 2001;86:2437–2445.

52. Yu Z, Gupta SK, Hwang SS, et al. Transdermal testosterone administration in hypogonadal men: comparison of pharmacokinetics at different sites of application and at the first and fifth days of application. J Clin Pharmacol 1997;37:1129–1138.

53. Yu Z, Gupta SK, Hwang SS, et al. Testosterone pharmacokinetics after application of an investigational transdermal system in hypogonadal men. J Clin Pharmacol 1997;37:1139–1145.

54. Jordan WP Jr, Atkinson LE, Lai C. Comparison of the skin irritation potential of two testosterone transdermal systems: an investigational system and a marketed product. Clin Ther 1998;20:80–87.

55. Wang C, Swerdloff RS, Iranmanesh A, et al. Transdermal testosterone gel improves sexual function, mood, muscle strength, and body composition parameters in hypogonadal men. Testosterone Gel Study Group. J Clin Endocrinol Metab 2000;85:2839–2853.

56. Wang C, Swerdloff RS, Iranmanesh A, et al. Effects of transdermal testosterone gel on bone turnover markers and bone mineral density in hypogonadal men. Clin Endocrinol (Oxf) 2001;54:739–750.

57. Handelsman DJ, Conway AJ, Boylan LM. Pharmacokinetics and pharmacodynamics of testosterone pellets in man. J Clin Endocrinol Metab 1990;71:216–222.

58. Handelsman DJ, Mackey MA, Howe C, et al. An analysis of testosterone implants for androgen replacement therapy. Clin Endocrinol (Oxf) 1997;47:311–316.

59. Jockenhovel F, Vogel E, Kreutzer M, et al. Pharmacokinetics and pharmacodynamics of subcutaneous testosterone implants in hypogonadal men. Clin Endocrinol (Oxf) 1996;45:61–71.

60. Skakkebaek NE, Bancroft J, Davidson DW, Warner P. Androgen replacement with oral testosterone undecanoate in hypogonadal men: a double blind controlled study. Clin Endocrinol (Oxf) 1981;14:49–61.

61. Salehian B, Wang C, Alexander G, et al. Pharmacokinetics, bioefficacy, and safety of sublingual testosterone cyclodextrin in hypogonadal men: comparison to testosterone enanthate—a clinical research center study. J Clin Endocrinol Metab 1995;80:3567–3575.

62. Wang C, Iranmanesh A, Berman N, et al. Comparative pharmacokinetics of three doses of percutaneous dihydrotestosterone gel in healthy elderly men—a clinical research center study. J Clin Endocrinol Metab 1998;83:2749–2757.

63. Swerdloff RS, Wang C. Dihydrotestosterone: a rationale for its use as a non-aromatizable androgen replacement therapeutic agent. Baillieres Clin Endocrinol Metab 1998;12:501–506.

64. Nieschlag E, Buchter D, Von Eckardstein S, et al. Repeated intramuscular injections of testosterone undecanoate for substitution therapy in hypogonadal men. Clin Endocrinol (Oxf) 1999;51:757–763.

65. Zhang GY, Gu YQ, Wang XH, et al. A pharmacokinetic study of injectable testosterone undecanoate in hypogonadal men. J Androl 1998;19:761–768.

66. Behre HM, Nieschlag E. Testosterone buciclate (20 Aet-1) in hypogonadal men: pharmacokinetics and pharmacodynamics of the new long-acting androgen ester. J Clin Endocrinol Metab 1992;75:1204–1210.

67. Amory JK, Anawalt BD, Blaskovich PD, et al. Testosterone release from a subcutaneous, biodegradable microcapsule formulation (Viatrel) in hypogonadal men. J Androl 2002;23:84–91.

68. Bhasin S, Swerdloff RS, Steiner B, et al. A biodegradable testosterone microcapsule formulation provides uniform eugonadal levels of testosterone for 10–11 weeks in hypogonadal men. J Clin Endocrinol Metab 1992;74:75–83.

69. Negro-Vilar A, Jordan WP Jr. Selective androgen receptor modulators (SARMs): a novel approach to androgen therapy for the new millennium. J Clin Endocrinol Metab 1999;84:3459–3462.

70. Roy AK, Tyagi RK, Song CS, et al. Androgen receptor: structural domains and functional dynamics after ligand-receptor interaction. Ann NY Acad Sci 2001;949:44–57.

71. Sundaram K, Kumar N. 7Alpha-methyl-19-nortestosterone (MENT): the optimal androgen for male contraception and replacement therapy. Int J Androl 2000;23:13–15.

72. Cummings DE, Kumar N, Bardin CW, et al. Prostate-sparing effects in primates of the potent androgen 7alpha-methyl-19-nortestosterone: a potential alternative to testosterone for androgen replacement and male contraception. J Clin Endocrinol Metab 1998;83:4212–4219.

73. Anderson RA, Martin CW, Kung AW, et al. 7Alpha-methyl-19-nortestosterone maintains sexual behavior and mood in hypogonadal men. J Clin Endocrinol Metab 1999;84:3556–3562.

74. Anderson RA, Bancroft J, Wu FC. The effects of exogenous testosterone on sexuality and mood of normal men. J Clin Endocrinol Metab 1992;75:1503–1507.

75. Tricker R, Casaburi R, Storer TW, et al. The effects of supraphysiological doses of testosterone on angry behavior in healthy eugonadal men—a clinical research center study. J Clin Endocrinol Metab 1996;81:3754–3758.

76. Shahidi NT. Androgens and erythropoiesis. N Engl J Med 1973;289:72–80.

77. Dobs AS, Meikle AW, Arver S, et al. Pharmacokinetics, efficacy, and safety of a permeation-enhanced testosterone transdermal system in comparison with bi-weekly injections of testosterone enanthate for the treatment of hypogonadal men. J Clin Endocrinol Metab 1999;84:3469–3478.
78. Matsumoto AM, Sandblom RE, Schoene RB, et al. Testosterone replacement in hypogonadal men: effects on obstructive sleep apnoea, respiratory drives, and sleep. Clin Endocrinol (Oxf) 1985;22:713–721.
79. Schneider BK, Pickett CK, Zwillich CW, et al. Influence of testosterone on breathing during sleep. J Appl Physiol 1986;61:618–623.
80. Behre HM, Bohmeyer J, Nieschlag E. Prostate volume in testosterone-treated and untreated hypogonadal men in comparison to age-matched normal controls. Clin Endocrinol (Oxf) 1994;40:341–349.
81. Jin B, Conway AJ, Handelsman DJ. Effects of androgen deficiency and replacement on prostate zonal volumes. Clin Endocrinol (Oxf) 2001;54:437–445.
82. Jackson JA, Waxman J, Spiekerman AM, et al. Prostatic complications of testosterone replacement therapy. Arch Intern Med 1989;149:2365–2366.
83. Bhasin S, Buckwalter JG. Testosterone supplementation in older men: a rational idea whose time has not yet come. J Androl 2001;22:718–731.
84. Swerdloff RS, Blackman MR, Cunningham GR, et al. Summary of the Consensus Session from the 1st Annual Andropause Consensus 2000 Meeting. The Endocrine Society, Bethesda, MD, 2000, pp. 1–6.
85. Bagatell CJ, Bremner WJ. Androgen and progestagen effects on plasma lipids. Prog Cardiovasc Dis 1995;38:255–271.
86. Bagatell CJ, Knopp RH, Vale WW, et al. Physiologic testosterone levels in normal men suppress high-density lipoprotein cholesterol levels. Ann Intern Med 1992;116:967–973.
87. Jockenhovel F, Bullmann C, Schubert M, et al. Influence of various modes of androgen substitution on serum lipids and lipoproteins in hypogonadal men. Metabolism 1999;48:590–596.
88. Whitsel EA, Boyko EJ, Matsumoto AM, et al. Intramuscular testosterone esters and plasma lipids in hypogonadal men: a meta-analysis. Am J Med 2001;111:261–269.
89. Alexandersen P, Haarbo J, Christiansen C. The relationship of natural androgens to coronary heart disease in males: a review. Atherosclerosis 1996;125:1–13.
90. Phillips GB, Pinkernell BH, Jing TY. The association of hypotestosteronemia with coronary artery disease in men. Arteriosclerosis Thromb 1994;14:701–706.
91. English KM, Steeds RP, Jones TH, et al. Low-dose transdermal testosterone therapy improves angina threshold in men with chronic stable angina: a randomized, double-blind, placebo-controlled study. Circulation 2000;102:1906–1911.
92. Jaffe MD. Effect of testosterone cypionate on postexercise ST segment depression. Br Heart J 1977;39:1217–1222.
93. Rosano GM, Leonardo F, Pagnotta P, et al. Acute anti-ischemic effect of testosterone in men with coronary artery disease. Circulation 1999;99:1666–1670.
94. Sigler LH, Tulgan J. Treatment of angina pectoris by testosterone propionate. NY State J Med 1943;43:1424–1428.
95. Webb CM, Adamson DL, de Zeigler D, Collins P. Effect of acute testosterone on myocardial ischemia in men with coronary artery disease. Am J Cardiol 1999;83:437–439.
96. Webb CM, McNeill JG, Hayward CS, et al. Effects of testosterone on coronary vasomotor regulation in men with coronary heart disease. Circulation 1999;100:1690–1696.
97. Wu SZ, Weng XZ. Therapeutic effects of an androgenic preparation on myocardial ischemia and cardiac function in 62 elderly male coronary heart disease patients. Chin Med J (Engl) 1993;106:415–418.

17   Androgens and Puberty

Erick J. Richmond, MD
and Alan D. Rogol, MD, PhD

CONTENTS

DEFINITION OF PUBERTY
PHYSIOLOGY OF NORMAL PUBERTY
GROWTH HORMONE AND SEX STEROID HORMONE INTERACTIONS
   DURING PUBERTY
THE ROLE OF ANDROGENS VS ESTROGENS DURING PUBERTY
COMMON USES OF EXOGENOUS TESTOSTERONE IN CHILDREN
SUMMARY
REFERENCES

DEFINITION OF PUBERTY

Puberty is the process of physical maturation manifested by an impressive acceleration of linear growth in mid- to late adolescence and the appearance of secondary sexual characteristics. The secondary sexual characteristics are a result of androgen production from the adrenals in both sexes (adrenarche)—testosterone from the testes in the male and estrogens from the ovaries in females (gonadarche). Although the rapid growth spurt had previously been attributed directly to the rising concentrations of gonadal steroid hormones, an indirect effect mediated through altered growth hormone release and insulin-like growth factor I (IGF-1) predominates *(1)*.

The traditional definition of precocious puberty is the appearance of any sign of secondary sexual maturation before the age of 8 yr in girls and 9 yr in boys. A large study sponsored by the American Academy of Pediatrics in young healthy girls suggests that puberty begins at an earlier age today than previously *(2)*. Consequently a change in the age of the lower limit of normal puberty in girls was proposed recently by the Lawson Wilkins Pediatric Endocrine Society *(3)*. On the other hand, two recent studies in boys *(4,5)* did not show a distinct trend toward earlier maturation, and in one of them *(5)*, the investigators did not find a significant difference in the timing of puberty based on race. Thus, puberty is considered normal in boys, if it starts after age 9 yr and before 13.5 yr.

From: *Contemporary Endocrinology: Androgens in Health and Disease*
Edited by: C. Bagatell and W. J. Bremner © Humana Press Inc., Totowa, NJ

PHYSIOLOGY OF NORMAL PUBERTY

Secondary Sexual Characteristics

The method described by Tanner (stages 1–5) *(6)* is the most widely utilized throughout the world for assessing sexual maturation. Although pubic hair is usually the first evidence of puberty, reddening and thinning of the scrotum and increased testicular size are the first physical findings of puberty among boys. In general, pubertal testicular enlargement has begun when the longitudinal measurement of a testis is greater than 2.5 cm (excluding the epididymis) or the volume is equal to or greater than 4 mL *(7)*. The right testis is usually larger than the left, and the left is located lower in the scrotum than the right.

The phallus is more accurately measured in the stretched, flaccid state. The length of the erectile tissue (excluding the foreskin) increases from an average of 6.2 cm in the prepubertal stage to 12.4 ± 2.7 cm in the white adult; in black men, the mean length is 14.6 cm, and in Asians, it is 10.6 cm *(8)*.

During puberty the male larynx, cricothyroid cartilage, and laryngeal muscles enlarge; the voice breaks at approx 13.9 yr and the adult voice is achieved by 15 yr of age *(9)*.

Pubertal Growth Spurt

The pubertal growth spurt can be divided into three stages: the stage of minimal growth velocity just before the spurt (takeoff velocity); the stage of most rapid growth, or peak height velocity (PHV); and the stage of decreased velocity and cessation of growth at epiphyseal fusion. Boys reach PHV approx 2 yr later than girls and are taller at takeoff; PHV occurs at stages 3 to 4 of puberty in most boys and is completed by stage 5 in more than 95% of boys *(10,11)*. The mean takeoff age is 11 yr and the PHV occurs at a mean age of 13.5 yr in boys.

The total height gain in boys between takeoff and cessation of growth is approx of 31 cm *(12)*. The mean height difference between adult men and women is 12.5 cm.

Bone Age and Body Composition

Skeletal maturation is assessed by comparing radiographs of the hand, the knee, or the elbow with standards of maturation in a normal population *(13)*. In normal children, bone age, an index of physiological maturation, does not have a well-defined relationship to the onset of puberty and is as variable as the chronologic age. However, in boys with delayed puberty, bone age correlates better with the onset of secondary sexual characteristics than does chronologic age.

There are dramatic changes during puberty in males, including increases in lean body mass, skeletal mass, bone mineral density (BMD), and body water and decrease in percentage fat mass *(14)*. In boys, bone mineral density reaches a peak at 17.5 yr, after the PHV, a factor that may result in a period of increased fragility and susceptibility to fracture following trauma *(15)*.

Gonadotropins

Pulsatile gonadotropin secretion has been documented at all ages, especially since the more sensitive third-generation immuno-chemiluminometric assays have become available. Puberty is heralded by an increase in the amplitude of luteinizing hormone (LH) and follicle-stimulating hormone (FSH) secretion which is detectable before the external signs of puberty are evident. Initially, biologically relevant surges of LH release occur during sleep, resulting in elevations of early-morning gonadal steroid hormone levels, which then wane throughout the day. With maturity, this release occurs regularly throughout the day *(16)*. The intermittent release of gonadotropins is reflective of the episodic release of gonadotropin-releasing hormone (GnRH) *(17)*. The increased sex hormone production by the testes results from increased LH stimulation; FSH stimulates primarily maturation of the tubules and spermatogonia.

Testosterone, Estrogen, and Adrenal Steroids

In human neonates, the levels of circulating growth hormone (GH) are higher in the male. This is most likely related to higher levels of gonadal steroid hormones in the male during the first months of life. Female neonates have circulating testosterone levels that fall to childhood values by the second week of life. In contrast, male infants have a rise in testosterone concentrations to midpubertal levels beginning at about 2 wk of age, which peak at 1–2 mo and then slowly decline to prepubertal values by 6 mo of age *(18)*.

Nighttime elevations of serum testosterone are detectable in the male before the onset of physical signs of puberty and during early puberty after the development of sleep-entrained secretion of LH *(19)*. In the daytime, testosterone levels begin to increase at approx 11 yr when the testis volume is at least 4 mL, and continue to rise throughout puberty *(20)*. The steepest increment in testosterone levels occurs between pubertal stages 2 and 3; mean testosterone levels can rise from 0.7 to 8 nmol/L (from 0.2 to 2.4 ng/mL) within 10 mo *(21)*.

Although the measurement of the ratio of testosterone to its metabolites has been advocated as a means of detecting the use of illicit androgen preparations by athletes, the ratio of testosterone to epitestosterone in the urine may be elevated normally during the progression through puberty. Consequently, the validity of this procedure during puberty is questionable *(22)*. Testosterone and other steroids can be measured in saliva for screening purposes and for monitoring therapy *(23)*.

Several recent studies have evaluated the effects of testosterone on body composition and strength. Bhasin and colleagues *(24)* administered 100 mg testosterone enanthate weekly for 10 wk to seven hypogonadal men with very low serum testosterone levels. Serum testosterone increased sevenfold, body weight increased by 4.5 kg (mean), fat-free mass increased by 5.0 kg (mean), and body fat did not change. Thus, almost all of the weight gain was explained by the increase in fat-free mass. Arm and leg muscle cross-sectional areas, assessed by magnetic resonance imaging (MRI), increased significantly. Substantial increases in muscle strength were also noted after testosterone treatment.

The mechanisms underlying the effects of androgens on bone are probably multifactorial. Androgen receptors have been found on the osteoblast, suggesting that androgens have direct, local effects on bone metabolism *(25)*. In addition, in vitro studies have shown that androgens may stimulate osteoblast differentiation, suggesting that testosterone stimulates osteoblast function and bone formation directly *(26)*. Testosterone may affect bone resorption by modulating either the local production of osteoclast-regulatory interleukins and other cytokines, or the osteoclast response to circulating calcium-regulatory hormones. In testosterone deficiency, an enhanced production of interleukin-6 (IL-6) by osteoblasts leads to osteoclastogenesis and increased bone resorption *(27)*. Accelerated bone resorption may contribute to the osteopenia in hypogonadal men. The administration of gonadal steroids, including androgens, leads to a decreased production of IL-6 by osteoblasts and, consequently, reduced osteoclast activity *(28)*. These studies suggest that androgens may dampen bone resorption through an inhibition of osteoclast action. Also, it has been postulated that androgens may regulate bone metabolism through a modulation of the response of bone cells to parathyroid hormone (PTH) and IGF-1 *(29,30)*.

In the male, approx 75% or more of estradiol is derived from extraglandular aromatization of testosterone and (indirectly) androstenedione; the remainder is secreted by the testes *(31)*. Many actions of testosterone on growth, skeletal maturation, and accrual of bone mass are the result of its aromatization to estrogen *(32)*. Aromatase is absent or barely detectable in prepubertal testes, but is easily measurable in late puberty; in normal testes, aromatase is predominantly present in Leydig cells, but tumors of either Sertoli or Leydig cells may have increased aromatase activity *(33)*.

In boys, low levels of estradiol are present before puberty and rise throughout maturation until the adolescent growth spurt occurs, and decrease thereafter *(34)*.

There is a progressive increase in plasma levels of dehydroepiandrosterone (DHEA) and its sulfated form (DHEA-S) in both boys and girls beginning by the age of 7 or 8 and continuing throughout early adulthood. The increase in the secretion of adrenal androgens and their precursors is known as adrenarche.

Plasma DHEA has a diurnal rhythm similar to that of cortisol, but levels of plasma DHEA-S show less variation and serve as a useful biochemical marker of adrenarche.

Dissociation of adrenarche and gonadarche occurs in several disorders of sexual maturation, including premature adrenarche (onset of pubic or axillary hair before age 8) and central precocious puberty *(35)*.

GROWTH HORMONE AND SEX STEROID HORMONE INTERACTIONS DURING PUBERTY

During adolescence, the interactions between GH and the sex steroid hormones are striking. Several studies of adolescent boys have demonstrated that the rising level of testosterone during puberty has a central role in augmenting spontaneous GH secretion and IGF-1 production *(1)*.

The ability of testosterone to stimulate pituitary GH secretion is transient, perhaps secondary to a fundamental, but transitory, change in the GH autonegative feedback during puberty. GH and IGF-1 levels fall significantly during late puberty and adulthood despite continuous high concentrations of gonadal steroid hormones.

Studies of adolescents with panhypopituitarism or selective deficiencies of GH or the gonadal steroid hormones have been instrumental in verifying the synergism between GH and the sex steroid hormones at puberty. In males with panhypopituitarism, full-replacement doses of GH and testosterone are required to normalize plasma IGF-1 levels and to achieve maximal growth potential *(36)*. In a study of men with hypogonadotropic hypogonadism, Liu and colleagues found that GH secretion and IGF-1 levels did not rise to normal until appropriate testosterone replacement was given *(37)*. Similarly, Aynsley-Green and colleagues demonstrated that gonadal steroid hormones alone are not enough to sustain normal pubertal growth in these patients *(38)*. Moreover, untreated individuals with idiopathic GH deficiency undergo a greatly attenuated adolescent growth spurt despite adequate levels of sex steroid hormones.

Studies in adolescents with constitutional delay of growth and puberty (CDGP) have demonstrated the vital interaction between GH and sex steroid hormones. In these subjects, administration of exogenous testosterone alone leads to a dramatic increase in GH secretion, plasma IGF-1 concentrations, and growth velocity (*see* the subsection Constitutional Delay of Growth and Puberty). Central precocious puberty is characterized by a significant rise in gonadal steroid hormone levels, GH secretion, and growth velocity. Following suppression of the hypothalamic–pituitary–gonadal axis with GnRH analogs, a significant decline in growth velocity, rate of skeletal maturation, GH secretion, and plasma IGF-1 concentrations are noted (39,40). Girls with Turner syndrome, who lack endogenous estrogen production, display a twofold to threefold increase in GH secretion following the administration of very small doses of estrogen (41). Based on the previous clinical observations, it is clear that the *interaction* between GH and the sex steroid hormones is necessary to achieve physiologic growth and sexual development during the pubertal years (42).

THE ROLE OF ANDROGENS VS ESTROGENS DURING PUBERTY

Individuals with complete androgen insensitivity (formerly termed "testicular feminization") demonstrate that androgens are not necessary to support normal adolescent growth or to achieve pubertal levels of GH and IGF-1, if sufficient levels of estrogens are present (43). Affected individuals have a normally timed pubertal growth spurt and attain adult height intermediate between mean heights for men and women. Aromatization of the high levels of testosterone produces elevated concentrations of estradiol which correlate positively with plasma IGF-1 levels. Gonadectomy results in a rapid decline in sex steroid hormone levels as well as GH secretion and IGF-1 levels.

Estrogen plays a pivotal role in skeletal maturation during puberty. Adolescent girls with Turner syndrome before estrogen therapy and boys with CDGA before testosterone therapy have a significant delay in skeletal maturation. A 28-yr-old man with an estrogen-receptor gene mutation who was fully virilized, had a bone age of only 15 yr and continued to grow in length (44). Similar clinical presentations are described in individuals with mutations of the aromatase gene. Despite elevated androgen concentrations in these subjects, levels of estradiol and estrone are very low, resulting in tall stature and delayed skeletal maturation. Males have eunuchoid skeletal proportions. Taken together, these observations confirm that estrogens are vital for physiologic bone maturation and proportions (but not linear growth) in both men and women.

Nonaromatizable Androgens

Unlike testosterone, oxandrolone and dihydrotestosterone (DHT) cannot be converted to estrogens by the aromatase enzyme system. Studies utilizing these compounds have helped delineate the differential effects of androgens and estrogens on GH secretion. The response of DHT and testosterone on GH secretion and IGF-1 levels were compared in boys with CDGP (45). A significant decrease in the integrated serum GH concentrations, but no changes in plasma IGF-1 concentrations were found after DHT administration compared with a significant increase in both parameters following testosterone therapy. This study suggests that the marked increase in mean and pulsatile GH levels at puberty is not the result of a direct androgen effect, but perhaps, it results from an estrogen-receptor-dependent mechanism.

There have been a number of investigations to show the growth-augmenting effects of oxandrolone. Oxandrolone has been used in the treatment of boys with CDGA to increase linear growth velocity without a disproportionate advancement of skeletal maturation, decrease in adult height, or excessive virilization (46). Rosenfeld and co-workers (47) have the longest and most extensive study of oxandrolone and GH treatment in girls with Turner syndrome. They demonstrated the benefits of this combination therapy on growth velocity and adult height. More recently, Nilsson and colleagues (48) treated a group of 17 girls with Turner syndrome with oxandrolone and GH. The mean adult height was 154.2 cm, which is equivalent to a mean net gain of 8.5 cm over the projected adult height. Fewer studies have been done to evaluate the effect of this synthetic androgen on GH release. Results of GH secretory activity and IGF-1 levels, however, are conflicting, but most of the evidence indicates that there is no stimulatory effect of oxandrolone on GH secretion despite its ability to increase the growth rate.

Androgen and Estrogen Receptor Blockade

Studies utilizing selective androgen-receptor or estrogen-receptor blockade have been more helpful in elucidating the differential effects of androgens and estrogens on the GH/IGF-1 axis. Flutamide, a nonsteroidal antagonist of the androgen receptor, administered to normal, late pubertal boys in an amount large enough to increase serum LH, free-testosterone, and estradiol level, has been associated with an increase in GH secretion (49). The increase in GH secretion was the result of an increase of both the maximal GH secretory rate and the mass of GH secreted per burst. A smaller increase in the frequency of GH secretory episodes was noted, but no changes in GH half-life were detected. Interruption of the negative feedback loop as a result of androgen blockade resulted in the above-noted elevations in LH, total estradiol, and free-testosterone concentrations. The observed rise in GH secretion and estradiol concentrations secondary to flutamide-induced blockade of the androgen receptor may reflect either enhanced estrogen-mediated effects or a reduced effect of androgen-mediated inhibition of the GH/IGF-1 axis.

Tamoxifen is a nonsteroidal antagonist of the estrogen receptor. When administered to adolescent boys, it has been associated with a significant decrease in GH secretion and IGF-1 levels (50). Diminished GH secretion results from the decrease in the maximal secretory rate and number of secretory bursts, with a trend toward a lower GH mass secreted per burst. No changes in the GH half-life or metabolic clearance rate or in the concentrations of testosterone, estradiol, or LH were observed.

These observations indicate that endogenous estrogens have a facilitatory role in the neuroendocrine control of the GH/IGF-1 axis in adolescent boys. It is possible that any stimulatory role of androgens on GH secretion is exerted through the estrogen receptor.

Effects of Sex Steroids on Bone Mineralization During Puberty

Puberty is a critical period to increase the rate of bone formation and to maximize bone mineral content and bone strength. More than 90% of peak skeletal mass is present by age 18 yr. It is the bone mass at this time that accounts for at least one-half of the variability in bone mass in the elderly (51).

Increases in height and weight are the strongest correlates of skeletal mineralization during childhood and adolescence (52). There are gender differences in bone density during childhood and adolescence because of differences in the timing of growth and puberty, resulting in females reaching peak bone mass earlier than males, although bone density values at peak bone mass are similar between the sexes.

Recent investigations have suggested that peak bone mass may be attained as early as late adolescence in the hip and spine *(53)*. In healthy adolescents, bone mass increases throughout childhood, with maximal bone mass accrual occurring in early to midpuberty and slowing in late puberty. Longitudinal data from healthy girls demonstrate that the rate of accrual in bone mass is most pronounced between 11 and 14 yr of age and falls significantly after 16 yr of age and/or 2 yr after menarche *(54)*. These data suggest that there is a critical window in time to maximize bone mass in early and midpuberty; the majority of bone mass will have accumulated by late puberty.

The presence of osteopenia in subjects with abnormal pubertal development demonstrates the critical impact of pubertal hormone changes on normal bone mineral acquisition. Adult patients with hypogonadotropic hypogonadism commonly have osteopenia, resulting from inadequate bone mineral accrual during puberty and/or abnormal bone remodeling after puberty *(55)*. Some adult men with a history of CDGP have decreased bone mass *(56)*. Androgen receptors are located in growth-plate osteoblasts in males and females and are thought to mediate the anabolic effects of testosterone on bone *(57)*. However, estrogen appears to be the more important sex steroid involved in skeletal maturation and mineralization, although it is unknown whether estradiol acts directly on bone or indirectly by stimulating other mediators of bone growth.

Patients with aromatase deficiency or estrogen-receptor defects have a phenotype that includes tall stature and normal secondary sexual characteristics, however, they have osteopenia and skeletal immaturity in adulthood, despite normal androgen levels *(58)*. Treatment of a male with aromatase deficiency with estrogen resulted in dramatic increase in bone density and completion of skeletal maturation, indicating the critical role of estrogen in skeletal mineralization and maturation *(59)*.

COMMON USES OF EXOGENOUS TESTOSTERONE IN CHILDREN

The most common conditions in children where treatment with testosterone may be beneficial are those associated with permanent hypogonadism (hypergonadotropic and hypogonadotropic hypogonadism) and CDGP, a physiologic form of hypogonadotropic hypogonadism.

Constitutional Delay of Growth and Puberty

Constitutional delay of growth and puberty is a frequent variant of normal pubertal maturation. It is characterized by a slowing of the growth rate as well as by a delay in the timing and tempo (rate of progression of the various stages) of puberty *(60)*. Typically, these boys seek medical evaluation in the early teens as they become aware of the discrepancy in sexual development and height between themselves and their peers. Clinically, they have a height age (the age corresponding to the height at which the patient's height is at the 50% percentile) that is delayed with respect to the chronological age, but it is concordant with their bone age. Sexual development is prepubertal or early pubertal and is again appropriate for the bone age, but delayed for chronological age. There is often a family history of one parent or a sibling of either sex having also been a "late bloomer."

Height velocity continues at a prepubertal rate or slows slightly as a prepubertal *dip*, in contrast to peers of the same chronological age, whose height velocity begins to accelerate at the age of 12–13 yr. When the height is plotted on the standard growth curve, the height gain of these boys appears to be decelerating because the standard growth curve incorporates the pubertal growth spurt at an "average" age. This further accentuates the difference between the delayed boys and their normally developing counterparts. The apparent deceleration in growth compared with chronologically matched peers is usually a compelling concern of the patient and/or his family and brings the adolescent to medical attention. Biochemically, boys with CDGP resemble normal boys with comparable bone ages. Serum levels of GH, IGF-1, IGF-BP3, LH, FSH, and testosterone may be dimished for chronological age, but they are normal when compared with levels in boys of the same stage of sexual development (61,62). The suppressed hypothalamic–pituitary–gonadal axis found in CDGP represents an extension of the physiological hypogonadotropic hypogonadism present since infancy. Without intervention, most boys with constitutional delay of growth and adolescence will undergo normal pubertal development spontaneously and will reach their target height as predicted from parental stature (63). Development may, however, occur several years after that of their peers, and many adolescents suffer significant emotional distress because they differ in their appearance from their peers during these years.

Androgen therapy was initially proposed to alleviate this psychological stress. Recent data have emerged supporting androgen therapy in these boys for its beneficial effects on bone mass and body composition, in addition to the psychological benefits (64).

In our practice, we use testosterone enanthate or cypionate 50–100 mg im every 4 wk for 3 mo. At the next visit, almost all boys will report some increase in appetite, body weight, and height, and many show early testicular enlargement. An early-morning testosterone level measured at least 3 wk after the last injection usually represents the boy's endogenous testosterone production. If no physiologic changes are apparent after 3 mo, the dose may be increased by 25–50 mg administered every 4 wk. Treatment is continued for another 3 mo, and the boys are then re-evaluated. An increase in testicular size indicates gonadotropin release despite the negative feedback effects of the exogenous testosterone. (Boys with permanent hypogonadotropic hypogonadism will not have testicular growth.) If growth and development cannot be sustained without therapy after 1 yr of testosterone treatment, the presence of permanent hypogonadotropic hypogonadism is more likely and further investigation is required.

Permanent Hypogonadism

In hypogonadotropic hypogonadism, insufficient pulsatile secretion of GnRH and the resulting LH and FSH deficiency lead to sexual infantilism. The degree of this deficit varies and, hence, the phenotype can vary from complete sexual infantilism to conditions that are difficult to differentiate from CDGP (see Table 1).

The GnRH deficiency may be secondary to a genetic or developmental defect not detected until the age of the expected puberty, or it may be the result of a tumor, an inflammatory process, a vascular lesion, or trauma. The use of pulsatile GnRH administration is not practical for the routine induction of puberty in adolescent boys; therefore, long-term testosterone replacement is the treatment of choice for hypothalamic or pituitary gonadotropin deficiency.

Congenital or acquired gonadotropin deficiency resulting from central nervous system lesions requires testosterone-replacement therapy at the normal age of onset of puberty. An exception may occur when GH deficiency coexists; in this condition it is generally advisable to initiate testosterone replacement by age 14 yr to maximize linear growth.

Table 1
Causes of Hypogonadotropic Hypogonadism

1. CNS disorders
   a. Genetic disorders
   b. Tumors
   c. Infiltrative diseases including Langerhans cell histiocytosis
   d. Trauma
2. Isolated gonadotropin deficiency
   a. Idiopathic
   b. Kallmann's syndrome
   c. X-Linked adrenal hypoplasia congenita
   d. Isolated LH deficiency
3. Miscellaneous disorders
   a. Prader–Willi syndrome
   b. Laurence–Moon syndrome
   c. Bardet–Biedl syndrome
   d. Chronic diseases
   e. Other genetic syndromes

Patients with hypergonadotropic hypogonadism have impaired secretion of gonadal steroids, which results in decreased negative feedback upon the hypothalamus and elevated FSH and LH levels. Klinefelter's syndrome and its variants and primary or secondary testicular failure are included in this category. Plasma testosterone and LH levels should be monitored every 6 mo during puberty and yearly thereafter in patients with Klinefelter's syndrome. If the LH level rises more than 2.5 standard deviations above the mean value or if the testosterone level decreases below the normal range for age, testosterone-replacement therapy is strongly recommended.

Gonadal steroid treatment regimens are the same in both hypogonadotropic hypogonadism and hypergonadotropic hypogonadism. Boys are given testosterone enanthate, 50–100 mg im every 4 wk at the start and increased gradually to adult replacement doses of 200 mg every 2–3 wk (65). Skin patches of testosterone (2.5 and 5 mg) and the recently approved gel formulation may be useful in motivated teenagers, although experience with these forms is minimal in the adolescent male.

SUMMARY

Puberty describes the complex physiological transition between childhood and adulthood. Dramatic physical changes occur, most notably the development of secondary sexual characteristics and the pubertal growth spurt, in which gonadal steroids play a pivotal role. Accompanying the increase in gonadal steroids is an increase in growth hormone secretion. Evidence suggests that adequate growth hormone and gonadal steroids are *both* necessary for the attainment of a normal pubertal growth velocity. The complex interplay between these two hormonal axes has been under intensive basic and clinical research. Recent studies have enhanced the understanding of the relevant role of gonadal steroids in body composition, skeletal maturation, and bone mass accrual during puberty. Most boys with constitutional delay of growth and puberty will undergo normal puberty without intervention; however, androgen therapy may have beneficial effects on bone mass and body composition, in addition to its psychological benefits.

Permanent hypogonadism may be secondary to insufficient pulsatile secretion of GnRH (hypogonadotropic hypogonadism) or testicular failure despite high levels of gonadotropins (hypergonadotropic hypogonadism). In both conditions, testosterone treatment is indicated to induce and/or maintain sexual maturation and to maximize linear growth.

REFERENCES

1. Veldhuis JD, Roemmich JN, Rogol AD. Gender and sexual maturation-dependent contrasts in the neuroregulation of growth hormone secretion in prepubertal and late adolescent males and females-a general clinical research center-based study. J Clin Endocrinol Metab 2000;85:2385–2394.
2. Herman-Giddens ME, Slora EJ, Wasserman RC, et al. Secondary sexual characteristics and menses in young girls seen in office practice: a study from the Pediatric Research in Office Settings network. Pediatrics 1997;99:505–512.
3. Kaplowitz PB, Oberfield SE. Reexamination of the age limit for defining when puberty is precocious in girls in the United States: implications for evaluation and treatment. Drug and Therapeutics and Executive Committees of the Lawson Wilkins Pediatric Endocrine Society. Pediatrics 1999; 104:936–941.
4. Sonis WA, Comite F, Blue J, et al. Behavior problems and social competence in girls with true precocious puberty. J Pediatr 1985;106:156–160.
5. Biro FM, Lucky AW, Huster GA, Morrison JA. Pubertal staging in boys. J Pediatr 1995;127:100–102.
6. Tanner JM. Growth at adolescence. Charles C Thomas, Springfield, IL, 1962.
7. Zachmann M, Prader A, Kind HP. Testicular volume during adolescence: cross-sectional and longitudinal studies. Helv Paediatr Acta 1974;29:61–72.
8. Sutherland RS, Kogan BA, Baskin LS, et al. The effect of prepubertal androgen exposure on adult penile length. J Urol 1996;156:783-787.
9. Karlberg P, Taranger J. The somatic development of children in a Swedish urban community. Acta Paediatr Scand 1976;258(Suppl):1–48.
10. Tanner JM, Whitehouse RH, Marubini E, Resele LF. The adolescent growth spurt of boys and girls of the Harpenden growth study. Ann Hum Biol 1976;3:109–126.
11. Largo RH, Gasser T, Prader A, et al. Analysis of the adolescent growth spurt using smoothing spline functions. Ann Hum Biol 1978;5:421–434.
12. Abbassi V. Growth and normal puberty. Pediatrics 1998;102:507–511.
13. Greulich WS, Pyle SI. Radiograph Atlas of Skeletal Development of the Hand and Wrist. Stanford University Press, Stanford, CA, 1959.
14. Roemmich JN, Clark PA, Mai V, et al. Alterations in growth and body composition during puberty: III. Influence of maturation, gender, body composition, fat distribution, aerobic fitness, and energy expenditure on nocturnal growth hormone release. J Clin Endocrinol Metab 1998;83:1440–1447.
15. Bonjour JP, Theintz G, Law F, et al. Peak bone mass. Osteoporos Int 1994;4(Suppl 1):7–13.
16. Delemarre-Van De Waal HA, Wennink JM, Odink RJ. Gonadotrophin and growth hormone secretion throughout puberty. Acta Paediatr Scand 1991;372(Suppl):26–31.
17. Knobil E. The neuroendocrine control of the menstrual cycle. Recent Prog Horm Res 1980;36: 53–88.
18. Winter JS, Hughes IA, Reyes FI, Faiman C. Pituitary–gonadal relations in infancy: 2. Patterns of serum gonadal steroid concentrations in man from birth to two years of age. J Clin Endocrinol Metab 1976;42:679–686.
19. Boyar RM, Rosenfeld RS, Kapen S, et al. Human puberty. Simultaneous augmented secretion of luteinizing hormone and testosterone during sleep. J Clin Invest 1974;54:609–618.
20. August GP, Grumbach MM, Kaplan SL. Hormonal changes in puberty. 3. Correlation of plasma testosterone, LH, FSH, testicular size, and bone age with male pubertal development. J Clin Endocrinol Metab 1972;34:319–326.
21. Knorr D, Bidlingmaier F, Butenandt O, Fendel H. Plasma testosterone in male puberty. I. Physiology of plasma testosterone. Acta Endocrinol (Copenh) 1974;75:181–194.
22. Dehennin L, Delgado A, Peres G. Urinary profile of androgen metabolites at different stages of pubertal development in a population of sporting male subjects. Eur J Endocrinol 1994;130:53–59.

23. Boas SR, Cleary DA, Lee PA, Orenstein DM. Salivary testosterone levels in male adolescents with cystic fibrosis. Pediatrics 1996;97:361–363.
24. Bhasin S, Storer TW, Berman N, et al. Testosterone replacement increases fat-free mass and muscle size in hypogonadal men. J Clin Endocrinol Metab 1997;82:407–413.
25. Abu EO, Horner A, Kusec V, et al. The localization of androgen receptors in human bone. J Clin Endocrinol Metab 1997;82:3493–3497.
26. Kasperk CH, Wergedal JE, Farley JR, et al. Androgens directly stimulate proliferation of bone cells in vitro. Endocrinology 1989;124:1576–1578.
27. Manolagas SC, Jilka RL. Bone marrow, cytokines, and bone remodeling. Emerging insights into the pathophysiology of osteoporosis. N Engl J Med 1995;332:305–311.
28. Bellido T, Jilka RL, Boyce BF, et al. Regulation of interleukin-6, osteoclastogenesis, and bone mass by androgens. The role of the androgen receptor. J Clin Invest 1995;95:2886–2895.
29. Fukayama S, Tashjian AH Jr. Direct modulation by androgens of the response of human bone cells (SaOS-2) to human parathyroid hormone (PTH) and PTH-related protein. Endocrinology 1989;125: 1789–1794.
30. Itagane Y, Inada H, Fujita K, Isshiki G. Interactions between steroid hormones and insulin-like growth factor-I in rabbit chondrocytes. Endocrinology 1991;128:1419–1424.
31. Weinstein RL, Kelch RP, Jenner MR, et al. Secretion of unconjugated androgens and estrogens by the normal and abnormal human testis before and after human chorionic gonadotropin. J Clin Invest 1974;53:1–6.
32. Mauras N, O'Brien KO, Welch S, et al. Insulin-like growth factor I and growth hormone (GH) treatment in GH-deficient humans: differential effects on protein, glucose, lipid, and calcium metabolism. J Clin Endocrinol Metab 2000;85:1686–1694.
33. Inkster S, Yue W, Brodie A. Human testicular aromatase: immunocytochemical and biochemical studies. J Clin Endocrinol Metab 1995;80:1941–1947.
34. Klein KO, Martha PM Jr, Blizzard RM, et al. A longitudinal assessment of hormonal and physical alterations during normal puberty in boys. II. Estrogen levels as determined by an ultrasensitive bioassay. J Clin Endocrinol Metab 1996;81:3203–3207.
35. Sklar CA, Kaplan SL, Grumbach MM. Evidence for dissociation between adrenarche and gonadarche: studies in patients with idiopathic precocious puberty, gonadal dysgenesis, isolated gonadotropin deficiency, and constitutionally delayed growth and adolescence. J Clin Endocrinol Metab 1980;51:548–556.
36. Metzger DL, Kerrigan JR, Rogol AD. Gonadal steroid hormone regulation of the somatotrophic axis during puberty in humans: mechanisms of androgen and estrogen action. Trends Endocrinol Metab 1994;5:290–294.
37. Liu L, Merriam GR, Sherins RJ. Chronic sex steroid exposure increases mean plasma growth hormone concentration and pulse amplitude in men with isolated hypogonadotropic hypogonadism. J Clin Endocrinol Metab 1987;64:651–656.
38. Aynsley-Green A, Zachmann M, Prader A. Interrelation of the therapeutic effects of growth hormone and testosterone on growth in hypopituitarism. J Pediatr 1976;89:992–999.
39. Mansfield MJ, Rudlin CR, Crigler JF Jr, et al. Changes in growth and serum growth hormone and plasma somatomedin-C levels suppression of gonadal sex steroid secretion in girls with central precocious puberty. J Clin Endocrinol Metab 1988;66:3–9.
40. Conn PM, Crowley WF Jr. Gonadotropin-releasing hormone and its analogs. Annu Rev Med 1994;45: 391–405.
41. Mauras N, Rogol AD, Veldhuis JD. Increased hGH production rate after low-dose estrogen therapy in prepubertal girls with Turner's syndrome. Pediatr Res 1990;28:626–630.
42. Zhang J, Peddada SD, Malina RM, Rogol AD. Longitudinal assessment of hormonal and physical alterations during normal puberty in boys: VI. Modeling of growth velocity, mean growth hormone (mean GH) and serum testosterone (T) concentrations. Am J Hum Biol 2000;12:814–824.
43. Zachmann M, Prader A, Sobel EH, et al. Pubertal growth in patients with androgen insensitivity: indirect evidence for the importance of estrogens in pubertal growth of girls. J Pediatr 1986;108:694–697.
44. Smith EP, Boyd J, Frank GR, et al. Estrogen resistance caused by a mutation in the estrogen-receptor gene in a man. N Engl J Med 1994;331:1056–1061.
45. Keenan BS, Richards GE, Ponder SW, et al. Androgen-stimulated pubertal growth: the effects of testosterone and dihydrotestosterone on growth hormone and insulin-like growth factor-I in the treatment of short stature and delayed puberty. J Clin Endocrinol Metab 1993;76:996–1001.

46. Stanhope R, Buchanan CR, Fenn GC, Preece MA. Double blind placebo controlled trial of low dose oxandrolone in the treatment of boys with constitutional delay of growth and puberty. Arch Dis Child 1988;63:501–505.

47. Rosenfeld RG, Frane J, Attie KM, et al. Six-year results of a randomized, prospective trial of human growth hormone and oxandrolone in Turner syndrome. J Pediatr 1992;121:49–55.

48. Nilsson KO, Albertsson-Wikland K, Alm J, et al. Improved final height in girls with Turner's syndrome treated with growth hormone and oxandrolone. J Clin Endocrinol Metab 1996;81:635–640.

49. Metzger DL, Kerrigan JR. Androgen receptor blockade with flutamide enhances growth hormone secretion in late pubertal males: evidence for independent actions of estrogen and androgen. J Clin Endocrinol Metab 1993;76:1147–1152.

50. Metzger DL, Kerrigan JR. Estrogen receptor blockade with tamoxifen diminishes growth hormone secretion in boys: evidence for a stimulatory role of endogenous estrogens during male adolescence. J Clin Endocrinol Metab 1994;79:513–518.

51. Louis O, Demeirleir K, Kalender W, et al. Low vertebral bone density values in young non-elite female runners. Int J Sports Med 1991;12:214–217.

52. Slemenda CW, Reister TK, Hui SL, et al. Influences on skeletal mineralization in children and adolescents: evidence for varying effects of sexual maturation and physical activity. J Pediatr 1994;125:201–207.

53. Matkovic V, Jelic T, Wardlaw GM, et al. Timing of peak bone mass in Caucasian females and its implication for the prevention of osteoporosis. Inference from a cross-sectional model. J Clin Invest 1994;93:799–808.

54. Bass S, Delmas PD, Pearce G, Hendrich E, et al. The differing tempo of growth in bone size, mass, and density in girls is region-specific. J Clin Invest 1999;104:795–804.

55. Finkelstein JS, Klibanski A, Neer RM, et al. Osteoporosis in men with idiopathic hypogonadotropic hypogonadism. Ann Intern Med 1987;106:354–361.

56. Finkelstein JS, Neer RM, Biller BM, et al. Osteopenia in men with a history of delayed puberty. N Engl J Med 1992;326:600–604.

57. Abu EO, Horner A, Kusec V, et al. The localization of androgen receptors in human bone. J Clin Endocrinol Metab 1997;82:3493–3497.

58. Morishima A, Grumbach MM, Simpson ER, et al. Aromatase deficiency in male and female siblings caused by a novel mutation and the physiological role of estrogens. J Clin Endocrinol Metab 1995;80(12):3689–3698.

59. Bilezikian JP, Morishima A, Bell J, Grumbach MM. Increased bone mass as a result of estrogen therapy in a man with aromatase deficiency. N Engl J Med 1998;339:599–603.

60. Houchin LD, Rogol AD. Androgen replacement in children with constitutional delay of puberty: the case for aggressive therapy. Baillieres Clin Endocrinol Metab 1998;12:427–440.

61. Sanayama K, Noda H, Konda S, et al. Spontaneous growth hormone secretion and plasma somatomedin-C in children of short stature. Endocrinol Jpn 1987;34:627–633.

62. Kerrigan JR, Martha PM Jr, Blizzard RM, Christie CM, Rogol AD. Variations of pulsatile growth hormone release in healthy short prepubertal boys. Pediatr Res 1990;28:11–14.

63. Crowne EC, Shalet SM, Wallace WH, et al. Final height in boys with untreated constitutional delay in growth and puberty. Arch Dis Child 1990;65:1109–1112.

64. Bertelloni S, Baroncelli GI, Battini R, et al. Short-term effect of testosterone treatment on reduced bone density in boys with constitutional delay of puberty. J Bone Miner Res 1995;10:1488–1495.

65. Bourguignon JP. Linear growth as a function of age at onset of puberty and sex steroid dosage: therapeutic implications. Endocr Rev 1988;9:467–488.

18   Androgens in Older Men

J. Lisa Tenover, MD, PhD

CONTENTS

INTRODUCTION
ANDROGEN CHANGES WITH NORMAL AGING
AGE-RELATED CHANGES IN ANDROGEN TARGET ORGANS
CLINICAL STUDIES OF ART
ANDROGEN REPLACEMENT METHODS
CONCLUSION
REFERENCES

INTRODUCTION

The 2000 US census data has demonstrated that the number of older men is growing faster than the number of older women. In comparison to the 1990 census, the number of men over the age of 65 yr has increased by 15%, whereas the number of women over that age has increased 10%. In absolute numbers, older women still outnumber older men, but the gap between the genders in closing. This has many potential implications in regards to aging men's health issues and surely will add impetus to trying to bring more clarity to the topic of male hormone replacement for older men (male HRT, or androgen replacement therapy [ART]).

The practice of giving androgens to older men in an attempt to retrieve or maintain youthful characteristics is based on two major factors: (1) there is a decline in serum testosterone levels as men age and (2) there are concomitant changes in androgen target organs that are similar to what is seen in hypogonadal young adult men prior to receiving testosterone replacement. Thus, ART can be approached from either a therapeutic or a preventive viewpoint: One is trying either to restore or improve some physical entity or function in an androgen target organ or to prevent the decline in the same. Rigorous scientific investigation of the benefits and risks of ART, however, is now only in about its second decade and there have not yet been any large multicenter controlled clinical trials of this therapy. In addition, there currently is no consensus on what hormonal or clinical criteria to use to decide which older men should receive ART. Despite this lack of clinical information on ART, the public and media interest in this topic is abundant, and testosterone sales, at least in the United States, continue to increase.

From: *Contemporary Endocrinology: Androgens in Health and Disease*
Edited by: C. Bagatell and W. J. Bremner © Humana Press Inc., Totowa, NJ

In aging men, the combination of declining levels of androgen (predominantly testosterone) levels and the development of potentially related symptoms and physiological changes is known as "andropause" or (partial) androgen deficiency of the aging male, or (P)ADAM. This chapter will review what currently is known about PADAM and the data on the beneficial and adverse effects of ART.

ANDROGEN CHANGES WITH NORMAL AGING

The levels of all components of serum testosterone (T) decline as adult men age. Early data regarding this were often suspect, because studies often did not control for overall health, smoking, obesity, or time of day of the sampling, all factors that can influence T levels (for review, see ref. 1). However, more recent cross-sectional studies have borne out this age-related change (2–5), and there are now at least three longitudinal studies that also have demonstrated this decline in serum T (6–8). Most of the data on T levels and age are derived from studies in which the vast majority of men enrolled were Caucasian. Some smaller cross-sectional evaluations of men of African-American (9) or Asian (10) descent suggest that these ethnic groups also may demonstrate this age-related testosterone decline. Serum dihydrotestosterone (DHT) levels, in general, do not change appreciably with age (5), but circulating DHT is probably less important than that which is formed within a given tissue (11). Serum estradiol levels either are unchanged or may rise slightly in men as they age (12–14).

The age-related decline in serum T is largely the result of decreased production by the testis, which demonstrates blunted T production even when maximally stimulated with luteinizing hormone (LH) (12,14). The hypothalamus also plays a role, demonstrating chaotic secretion and increased sensitivity to sex steroid negative feedback (15). Serum gonadotropin levels increase somewhat with age, but in most older men, even those with quite low testosterone, gonadotropin levels are still within the normal adult male range (5). The ratio of bioactive to immunoreactive LH also may decline slightly with age (16,17), but this is only a minor contributor to the decline in T production. Testosterone metabolism slows with normal aging, but not enough to offset the decline in production.

Although age alone has a strong predictive value for lower serum T levels, concomitant disease such as diabetes mellitus (5), liver disease (18), hemochromatosis (19), and others (20) also can contribute. There are a number of medications that have been associated with lower androgen levels, including ketoconazole (21), cimetidine (22), and glucocorticoids (23). Significant obesity, especially abdominal obesity, can be associated with lower T levels (24). The descriptor PADAM usually applies to healthy older men, but the issue of ART should be relevant to those men who have reasons other than just age for low T production.

Although there is agreement that T levels decline as men age, defining which older men are androgen deficient and might warrant ART has not been codified. One of the impediments to establishing a consensus is the lack of a practical, clinically useful biochemical parameter of androgen action. The physiological changes and symptoms that can be attributed to PADAM have complicated pathogenesis and could be affected by a variety of factors, low testosterone being only one of them. In addition, it is still not clear which component of serum T is the best measure of assessing androgen availability to the androgen receptor in the various target tissues.

Serum total T is composed of several components: free (unbound) T, T loosely bound to albumin, and T more tightly bound to sex hormone-binding globulin (SHBG; see Fig. 1).

$$
\text{Total T} \quad = \quad
\left.
\begin{array}{l}
\left[\text{Free T} \quad\underline{\quad\quad}\right] \\
+ \\
\text{Albumin-T} \underline{\quad}\rfloor \\
+ \\
\left\lfloor \text{SHBG-T} \right.
\end{array}
\right\} \quad \underline{\quad} \text{Bioavailable T}
$$

Fig. 1. The three components that comprise human serum total testosterone.

The combination of free T and albumin-bound T is called "bioavailable" T. Epidemiological studies have shown that it is the bioavailable T that best correlates with parameters such as bone mineral density *(25)* and sexual function *(26)* in older men and is predictive for the development of frailty in inner-city African-American males *(9)*. It is not known, however, whether non-SHBG-bound T is the T component that is bioavailable to every androgen target organ. In addition, not all target-organ effects of testosterone are the result of the steroid directly, but they also can be the result of one of its metabolites, such as estradiol in bone *(27)* and DHT in the prostate *(11)*. Because gonadotropin levels are not usually outside the normal adult male range in older men, their measurement generally is not helpful in defining "androgen deficiency" in this age group.

The selection of a particular component of serum T to use in defining an older man as being androgen deficient has several implications. One is that it will have an ultimate effect on the "prevalence" of PADAM in the older male population. Because SHBG levels tend to rise with age in men *(5,8,13)*, the level of bioavailable T declines more profoundly with age than does the level for total T *(17,28)*. If androgen deficiency is defined in older men by a serum total T below the normal range (two standard deviations below the mean value) for young adult men, then about one-quarter to one-third of Caucasian men over the age of 65 yr might meet this criterion, whereas if non-SHBG-bound T is used, then 50% of older men may well meet this criterion *(29,30)*. The other area of impact relates to the accuracy, availability, and cost of the assays used to measure the T components. The assay for total T is straightforward, is widely available, and is the least expensive of the T assays. Analog free-T assays have been shown to be inaccurate *(31)*, but doing the assay by equilibrium dialysis is tedious and expensive. Bioavailable T also is more difficult to assay, not available except in a few select centers, and the most costly. There is some movement toward using measurements of total T and SHBG, and then calculating bioavailable T or free T *(31,32)*, but there is no unanimity as yet on the formulas to use or the value range that defines "testosterone deficiency" in older men.

Adding to the lack of clarity is that fact that there are no specific androgen target-organ dose–response data for older men. Based on data from young hypogonadal men replaced with T, one would expect that target organs will vary in their threshold response. For example, it may take much lower T levels to restore libido than is needed to restore muscle mass. Given the uncertainties of the T assays vis-à-vis biological importance of the measured value, along with the insufficient clinical study data to help in defining PADAM, at this time it may be more important to select men for ART based on those who have one or more specific androgen target-organ deficiencies and who also have T levels that are low enough that meaningful changes in T can be made with physiological replacement.

Table 1
Changes in Androgen Target Organs with Normal Aging
and with T Replacement in Young Hypogonadal Men

| Target organ | Changes seen with aging | Young adult hypogonadal men | |
		Pre-T[a]	With T treatment
Muscle mass	↓	↓	↑
Muscle strength	↓	↓	↑
Fat mass	↑	↑	↓
Bone mineral density	↓	↓	↑
Libido	↓	↓	↑
Erectile function	↓	↓	↑
Sense of well-being or mood	↔/↓	↓	↑

[a]Compared to age-matched eugonadal men; ↓: decreased; ↑: increased; ↔: no change.

AGE-RELATED CHANGES IN ANDROGEN TARGET ORGANS

Androgens are known to have a variety of important physiologic actions, including effects on muscle, bone, mood, prostate, bone marrow, cognitive function, and sexual function. In hypogonadal young men who are replaced with T, changes in these various areas have been reported (*see* Table 1). Declining lean body mass and strength, increased fat mass, declining bone mineral density (BMD), decreased libido and potency, a decline in general sense of well-being, and increased irritability are associated in variable degrees with male aging (*see* Table 1).

Muscle and Fat

Sarcopenia, the loss of muscle mass, is an important finding with aging. The cumulative decline in lean body mass, predominantly muscle mass, with age is about 35–40% between the ages of 20 and 80 yr *(33,34)*. This loss of muscle mass results predominantly from a decrease in the number of type II, fast twitch fibers important for production of power *(35)*. In healthy older people, there is a strong correlation between muscle mass and muscle strength *(36)*, but the causes of the decline in muscle mass and strength with age are probably multifactorial. Decreased muscle strength can lead to decreased physical function *(37)*. Androgens have long been known for their anabolic effects, and physiological replacement of T in hypogonadal young men *(38)* or supraphysiological treatment of eugonadal young men *(39)* has been shown to result in increases in lean body mass, muscle size, and strength.

As muscle mass declines with age, body weight remains relatively constant, because fat mass increases *(40)*. Much of this is intra-abdominal fat, which has metabolic and clinical implications *(41)*. Independent of age, abdominal fat mass has been shown to correlate inversely with serum free-T levels *(42,43)*.

Bone

Male osteoporosis is becoming an important clinical entity as the life-span of men increases *(44)*. After age 60 yr, hip fracture rates in men increase dramatically, doubling each decade *(45)*. Mortality after hip fracture is higher in men than in women *(46)*. Both cross-sectional and longitudinal studies have shown that even healthy older men lose bone mass with age (44). Hypogonadism is one cause of male osteoporosis, and low T levels are a risk factor for minimal trauma hip fracture in older men (47). Men who are physically or chemically castrated in adult life demonstrate a significant decline in BMD (48,49). Young adult men with acquired androgen deficiency have lower BMD than age-matched controls (50), and T replacement in this group is associated with significant increases in both vertebral and hip BMD (51). Bioavailable T levels have been shown to correlate positively with BMD in older men (25), as have bioavailable estradiol levels (27).

Sexual Function

Numerous measures of sexual function change as men age, including a decline in orgasmic frequency, an increase in erectile dysfunction (ED), and a decline in quality and quantity of sexual thoughts and enjoyment (52). Data to support a relationship between T levels and the decline in many aspects of sexual function with age are scarce, however. Especially with ED, the correlation data would suggest low T levels have only a minimal role in the etiology of this condition in the older man. Although T may have some effect on optimal penile rigidity, through its effect in regulating nitric oxide synthase activity in the smooth muscle of the corpora cavernosa, the prevalence of low T is not significantly different between older men with and without impotence (53). In young hypogonadal men, T replacement improves a variety of sexual behaviors, including sexual thoughts, sexual desire, spontaneous erections, and frequency of sexual activity (54). The threshold level of serum T needed for optimal sexual function, however, has not been determined, but it may be relatively low. T administration does not seem to improve ED in men with normal T levels (55).

Mood and Cognitive Function

Androgens may improve aspects of mood, such as irritability and depressive affect, when given to hypogonadal young adult men (56). Compared to nondepressed men, elderly men who are depressed have been reported to have lower total T levels (57) and, similarly, lower bioavailable T levels have been associated with depressed mood in a large cross-sectional study of older men (58).

The relationship between T and cognitive function in men is not clear because of a lack of data, the many different cognitive processes that can and have been assessed, and the timing of the androgen exposure in relation to the subject age. The effects of androgens seem to be specific to certain domains, with some studies showing a positive correlation with spatial performance and others reporting improvement in verbal fluency (59). One epidemiological study of older men reported a positive association between total and bioavailable T levels and better performance on tests of verbal memory and mental control (60).

Erythropoiesis

Androgens are known to stimulate red blood stem cells and the production of erythropoietin (61); androgen receptors are found in cultured erythroblasts (62). Adult men have higher hemoglobin levels, hematocrits, and red blood cell mass than do adult women, and these sex differences are not present before puberty (63). Young hypogonadal men have lower red blood cells counts and hemoglobin levels than do their age-matched controls, and these parameters increase when T is replaced (64). Likewise, studies in which eugonadal men have been supplemented with androgens have shown an increase in hematocrit with therapy (65). Healthy older men tend to have similar or slightly lower hematocrits compared with normal young adult men (61,66).

Cardiovascular Disease

Androgens often have been categorized as having a negative impact on cardiovascular health. This has been based on the higher incidence of cardiovascular disease (CVD) in men compared to women of the same age, the decrease of high-density lipoprotein (HDL) cholesterol levels at puberty in boys (67), the worsening of the atherogenic lipid profile in young adult men who are taking nonaromatizable androgens (68), and the increase in HDL cholesterol seen when either young or old men are made hypogonadal (69). On the other hand, epidemiological studies have reported a positive correlation between free T and HDL cholesterol levels (70) and a negative correlation with fibrinogen and plasminogen activator inhibitor levels (71). Short-term infusion studies with T have shown a direct arterial vasodilatory effect (72) and prolongation of time until ischemia during exercise testing in men with known CVD (73).

Prostate

Androgens have a role in promoting both benign prostate hyperplasia (BPH) and prostate adenocarcinoma, two independently distributed, but common, diseases in older men. Although epidemiological studies have not demonstrated that circulating levels of androgens are implicated in the etiology of either disease, androgen deprivation therapy has been used for the treatment of both. Serum prostate-specific antigen (PSA) levels and prostate volumes are lower in hypogonadal nonelderly adult men, and both these parameters increase to normal, but not above normal, following T replacement (74). Older men with prostate cancer may have low T levels (75).

CLINICAL STUDIES OF ART

As with any therapy, knowledge of the possible benefits and potential adverse effects of treatment, characteristics of the persons for whom those benefits and risks are most likely to occur, the dose–response profile of the target organ(s) of interest, and the relative benefit–to–risk ratio for the hormone doses to be utilized are all important information. Unfortunately, these data for ART are limited at this time, and therapeutic decisions are being made, by necessity, without complete information. Limitations in using the data from currently available trials to assist with making decisions about utilization of ART in a clinical practice include (1) the lack of uniformity in the hormonal values used as study entrance criterion, (2) the variety of treatment modalities utilized and the androgen levels obtained with therapy, (3) the diversity in outcome parameters measured, (4) the relatively small number of participants who have been studied, (5) the short periods of treatment that have been evaluated (most studies are 12 mo or less in duration), and (6) the lack of experience with the use of ART in men other than those with robust health and who are less than 75 yr of age. Direct extrapolation of the current clinical ART data obtained from generally healthy men to what might be expected to occur in more frail populations should be done with caution; although the benefits of ART may be more pronounced in this latter group, the risks may also increase.

Table 2
Possible Benefits and Risks of ART

Benefits	Risks
Preserve/improve bone mass and prevent fractures	Promote fluid retention
Increase muscle mass and strength	Precipitate or worsen sleep apnea
Increase stamina and physical function	Cause gynecomastia
Decrease cardiovascular disease risk	Increase cardiovascular disease risk
Improve libido	Produce polycythemia
Improve aspects of cognition	
Improve well-being and mood	Hasten development of benign or malignant prostate disease

Table 2 lists the possible benefits and risks of ART. Many of these have been evaluated in some form in the various ART trials, although there are very little data in some areas.

ART and Bone

Studies of ART in older men that have dealt with some aspect of the effect on bone have all utilized T as the treatment androgen. This may be important, because T is converted to estradiol in vivo and older men receiving ART often show a substantial increase in serum estradiol levels. Because bioavailable estradiol has been shown to be a better predictor of BMD in older men than any component of T, it is possible that the effects of ART on bone in older men could be mediated through its conversion to estradiol.

The published ART studies to date have lasted from 3 to 36 mo, with the shorter studies measuring biochemical parameters of bone turnover and the longer studies evaluating bone mineral density. Some, but not all, of the studies enrolled older men who were osteoporotic at baseline. There are, as yet, no data on the effect of ART on fracture rates in older men.

As shown in Table 3, these studies have generally shown an increase in BMD and a slowing of bone degradation with ART *(76–81)*. One other study in older men taking chronic glucocorticoids reported an increase in vertebral BMD with T treatment *(82)*. The studies of ART have varied considerably in the baseline T levels of participants, in the T levels achieved with therapy, and in the length of treatment. These differences, along with the lack of knowledge about the serum T levels or length of treatment needed to achieve optimal effects on BMD, may explain some of the discrepancy between the findings of the various studies.

ART and Body Composition and Strength

There have been a number of published studies in which body composition and/or muscle strength were evaluated during androgen therapy in older men *(76,77,80,83–88)*. In general, these studies have demonstrated a decline in fat mass and an increase in lean body mass (LBM) with ART *(see* Table 4). The decline in fat mass that is seen in some of the studies might be expected to lead to an improvement in insulin sensitivity, as was shown in one study of obese nondiabetic men *(85)*. A recent study, however, reported

Table 3
Testosterone Therapy Effects on Bone in Older Men

Treatment (mo)	Study N	Parameters of bone turnover		Bone density		Ref.
		Formation	Degradation	Spine	Other	
3	13	NC	↓	—	—	76
3	8	↑	—	—	—	77
7–14	6	↓	↓	—	—	78
12	34	NC	NC	NC	↑[a]	79
18	29	↓	↓	↑	—	80
36	54	NC	NC	↑	NC	81

Note: ↓, decrease; ↑, increase; NC, no change.
[a]Compared to placebo treated.

Table 4
Testosterone-Replacement Effects on Body Composition
and Strength in Older Men

Months of treatment	No. of men treated	Body fat	Lean mass	Strength[a]
		(Trend and mean percent change)		
1	6	—	—	↑ (LE)
2	9	—	—	↑ (grip)
3	7	—	↔	↑ (LE, grip)
3	13	↔	↑ (3.2%)	↔ (grip)
3	8	↔	—	↑ (grip)
9	31	↓ (6.4%)	↔	—
12	17	↔	—	↑ (grip)
18	29	↓ (14%)	↑ (5%)	—
36	54	↓ (14%)	↑ (3.8%)	↔

Note: ↔, no change; ↑, increase; ↓, decrease.
[a]Grip, strength by handheld dynamometry; LE, lower extremity strength, usually by isokinetic testing.

in abstract form only, did not demonstrate that overtly diabetic men improved their insulin sensitivity with T treatment. When comparing the increase in LBM in older men with ART and that seen with T treatment in young adult hypogonadal men or with supraphysiological treatment in eugonadal young men, the magnitude of the changes are roughly similar to those seen in treated hypogonadal young men.

The strength changes reported thus far with ART are variable (see Table 4). When strength was shown to improve with treatment, the magnitude of the change seen was not large. More recent studies, as yet unpublished, which have evaluated muscle power rather than isokinetic strength, have shown somewhat more robust effects from ART. For the average older man, however, the overall clinical relevance of the changes in strength seen with ART is uncertain. Only two studies have evaluated the effect of ART on some aspect of physical function (83,88), and only one of these showed any effect (83). Some of the difficulty with ascertaining from the data available whether ART might have a positive impact on function has been the study of relatively healthy men using function measures that are insensitive or have "ceiling effects." The increases in muscle strength that occur with ART may have more of a clinical impact on function when evaluated with different measures or when used in men who are more frail at baseline. In this regard, it should be noted that the one study to date that has demonstrated an improvement in function with ART used the treatment in men who were not robust *(83)*.

ART and CVD Risk

Studies on the cardiovascular effects of ART in older men have been done by evaluating the response of various CVD risk factors to treatment. As has been shown with female HRT, this may not be the most clinically accurate way to assess true CV benefits and/or risks. Nonetheless, until there are long-term large multicenter trials of ART in which clinical CV end points, such as myocardial infarction or stroke, are assessed, this is the best method and these are the best data available.

In terms of changes in cholesterol profiles with ART, the effects generally appear to be beneficial (*see* Table 5). Blood pressure has not been reported to increase in any of the ART studies, even though there is transient increase in body weight that is assumed to be the result of fluid retention. None of the ART trials to date has measured the effects of treatment on vasoactive factors.

ART and Libido and Mood

Studies in older men with low libido have generally reported an improvement in libido and sexual arousal with therapy *(52,89)*. There have been a few blinded placebo-controlled studies involving ART that have included evaluation of mood using self-report questionnaires with graded scales for items such as energy or general well-being *(76,85)*. In these studies, men on androgen therapy reported increased energy levels and sense of well-being compared to that reported on placebo therapy.

ART and Cognition

There have been only a few small clinical trials of ART and its effects on cognitive function in older men. Several studies reported an effect on visual spatial memory *(59,90)*; another study showed no effects on tested memory *(87)*. Several other studies, which have been reported in abstract form only, have reported improvement in trail-making ability and spatial and verbal memory with T.

ART and Polycythemia

Most studies of ART have reported a significant increase in hemoglobin and hematocrit levels with therapy (*see* Table 6) *(76,77,79,81,84,87,89,91,92)*. The increases reported are much larger than those usually seen with T treatment in younger hypogonadal adult men. Because older men tend to have slightly lower hematocrits than do young adult men, the increase in hemoglobin and hematocrit may be beneficial in some men. It is possible that it is this increase in oxygen-carrying capacity that contributes, in part, to the decrease in fatigue and improved energy levels reported by some men on ART. In some cases, however, the increases in hematocrit have necessitated termination in therapy, phlebotomy, or a decrease in the T dose. Although the coexistence of sleep apnea and elevated body mass index may contribute to the development of polycythemia, these have not been contributing factors in most cases. The method of T replacement may

Table 5
ART in Older Men and Serum Cholesterol (15 studies; n = 325)

Reported cholesterol change	No. of studies reporting	Mean percent change (if applicable)
Total cholesterol		
Increase	0	—
Decrease	6	−11%
No change	9	—
LDL cholesterol		
Increase	0	—
Decrease	4	−12%
No change	7	—
HDL cholesterol		
Increase	0	—
Decrease	3	−18%
No change	9	—

Table 6
Hemoglobin/Hematocrit Changes in Older Men on Testosterone

Treatment regimen	Duration (mo)	Hemoglobin mean % change	% of men getting Hct >52%	Study ref.
TE 300 mg/3 wk	3	+20	60	91
TE 200 mg/2 wk	3	+17	ND	77
TE 200 mg/2 wk	3	+9	ND	84
TE 200 mg/2 wk	12	+7	24	87
TE 200 mg/2 wk	24	+5	24	89
TE 150 mg/2 wk	6	+[a]	25	92
TE 100 mg/wk	3	+5	15	76
Scrotal patch	36	+6	6	81
Nonscrotal patch	12	+2	0	79

Note: TE, testosterone enanthate intramuscular injections; ND, no data.
[a]No data given to calculate percentage.

affect the magnitude of the change in hemoglobin levels, with those methods that provide a more uniform level of T within physiological range throughout the dosing period resulting in a smaller increase in the hematocrit (see Table 6).

ART and the Prostate

There have been no large long-term trials of ART to evaluate the effect of therapy on the incidence of prostate cancer or symptomatic BPH, and most studies that have been done are a year or less in duration. Therefore, although men in ART studies are monitored for the development of prostate cancer and lower urinary tracts symptoms (LUTS), it has it been necessary to utilize surrogate markers, such as serum PSA measurements, to evaluate the prostatic effects of therapy. Based on data from studies where hypogonadal younger adult men were given testosterone replacement and the effects on the prostate followed for years (74), some small increase in PSA or prostate size might be expected with ART, especially if the recipient has been testosterone deficient for years. On the other hand, there have been data to suggest that older men who have T deficiency may have lower PSA values, even when prostate cancer is present *(75)*. Therefore, given the lack of data to interpret PSA changes over time in older men on ART, PSA changes with therapy should be interpreted in the same age-appropriate manner as for men not on ART, and the presence or history of prostate cancer is an absolute contraindication to the use of ART.

To date, there have been at least 32 studies in which men between the ages of 40 and 89 yr have been given T and the serum levels of PSA measured. Of these studies, 22 (69%) reported no change in PSA with T treatment, and the other 10 reported a small, but statistically significant, change in PSA. The average change in PSA for the men on T in those 10 studies was 0.61 ng/mL. In 7 of those 10 studies, where the men were followed for a least 1 yr, a PSA velocity can be calculated; the average PSA velocity was 0.39 ng/mL/yr, well within the normal range of change resulting from benign disease (<0.75 ng/mL).

There was no reported increase in the incidence of prostate cancer in men in the ART trials, but neither the number of men studied nor the length of time monitored has been long enough to make any conclusions about the long-term effects of ART and clinically significant prostate cancer. The total experience thus far with ART is limited to about 1500 man-years of experience.

As far as ART and the development or worsening of LUTS in older men with BPH, there have been 12 studies in which older men have been evaluated for parameters of prostate size, LUTS, or urinary function parameters, such as urine flow rates or postvoid urine residual volumes (PVR). None of the studies reported any changes in these measures with T therapy. Selection criteria for these studies, however, required exclusion on the basis of significant baseline LUTS, slow urine flow rates, or high PVR. In addition, these studies were all relatively short in duration (the longest was 3 yr). Therefore, because BPH has a very long natural history, it should not be concluded that the lack of effects of ART on LUTS from the experience to date implies that long-term use, or use in men who have significant LUTS pretreatment, would be expected to have little effect. Without more data, symptomatic BPH is currently considered a relative contraindication to ART, and the use of T therapy in men with symptomatic BPH should be done with caution and monitoring.

ART and Other Possible Risk Factors

It has been reported that T therapy can worsen pre-existing obtructive sleep apnea (OSA) *(93)*. Conversely, some men with OSA and low serum T levels have been shown to normalized their T levels with OSA treatment alone *(94)*. The relationship between T and OSA is not understood, and the incidence of the coexistence of androgen deficiency and OSA is not known. A recent study in 54 men given ART for 3 yr reported no increase in apneic or hypoapneic episodes during sleep while on T *(81)*, suggesting that ART-induced OSA may not be a common occurrence. Physicians, however, should be sensitized to this potential problem and evaluate for sleep apnea by history prior to and throughout the course of ART.

Occasionally, men on ART develop tender breasts or gynecomastia. Many older men, when given ART, demonstrate a relatively greater percentage increase in serum estradiol levels than in serum T levels, and this may contribute to the breast changes. Often the increase in estradiol is larger when the serum T levels are high, so this adverse effect may be overcome with either a downward adjustment in the T dose or a switch to a form of therapy that gives lower but more uniform levels of T.

ANDROGEN REPLACEMENT METHODS

To date, almost all of the ART trials have utilized T as the replacement androgen, although the method of T replacement has varied. There is little experience with nonaromatizable androgens, such as DHT, and this hormone is not commercially available for clinical use in North America. Because it is not yet known how much of the effect of ART on target organs such as bone are the result of the conversion of the T to estrogens, at this time it is recommended that some form of T be the replacement androgen for therapy.

The androgen dose–response of the various target organs in older men is not known, but it has been shown that replacement of endogenous T with equivalent levels of exogenous T has no measurable effect. Therefore, it should be the treatment goal to have some significant increase in T over that at pretreatment while maintaining levels within the physiological normal range for young adult men.

All methods for T replacement are probably efficacious if adequate serum T levels are achieved. Selecting the form of therapy largely depends on recipient preference, but in a few instances, selection on the basis of the possible relative side effects unique to the T delivery form may be appropriate.

Listed in Table 7 are the major T delivery forms available in the United States that are considered safe for use in older men. Because of the potential for liver toxicity, the oral methylated testosterones are not considered in this category (95). Also in Table 7 are the recommended starting doses for older men and the possible side effects unique to the particular delivery form.

The injectable esters, T enanthate and T cypionate, have similar pharmacokinetics and the recommended administration is every 1–2 wk. This form of T administration has been around for over 50 yr, and if the man can learn to give himself the intramuscular (im) injections or it can be administered by a family member, the cost of the therapy is quite low. Although most men complain of little or no pain from T injections, some men do not accept the idea of im injections, or because they are on warfarin, it is not appropriate for them to receive the injections. In addition, the serum T levels obtained with this method of therapy are far from physiologic. Especially with the every 2-wk dosing regimen, T levels can be supraphysiologic within the first few days after injection and fall to levels below the normal physiologic range just prior to the next dose. This form of therapy often leads to a larger increase in hemoglobin and estradiol levels than seen with other forms of T replacement, and in some men, the changes in T levels during the dosing interval can be paralleled by changes in their libido and/or mood. As noted earlier, however, the mood and libido changes with ART in older occur much less frequently than with younger men. Because T metabolism slows with age, the recommended initial doses of T for older men are lower than those usually used in younger adults.

The pellet form of T requires implantation with a trocar. Local extrusion of the pellets and infection at the site of placement are possible problems. The pellets may be active up to 6 mo, tend to give unpredictable plasma T levels, and require pellet removal if dosage adjustment is necessary or adverse events occur. Therefore, it is a form of therapy not generally recommended for use in most older men.

Table 7
Testosterone Delivery Forms for Use in ART

Preparation	Recommended initial dose regimen	Potential specific adverse effects
Injectable Esters		
Testosterone enanthate	75 mg im/wk	Pain at injection site
or cypionate	or 150 mg im/2 wk	Mood swings
		Large increase in hemoglobin/hematocrit
		Elevated serum estradiol
Pellets	224 mg/4–6 mo	Local-site infection
		Extravasations of pellet
		Large increase in hemoglobin/hematocrit
Patches		
Scrotal	40 cm^2 patch/d	Shaving of scrotum necessary
		Adhesion problems
		Elevated DHT levels
Nonscrotal	5 mg/d	Adhesion problems
		Dermatitis at application site
Gel	5-g packet/d	Mildly elevated DHT levels

The patch delivery forms of T provide physiologic levels of T throughout most of the 24-h dosing period and, if needed, allow for rapid discontinuation of therapy. The transdermal patch also provides physiologic levels of estradiol and DHT, whereas the scrotal patch yields supraphysiologic levels of serum DHT. If applied in the evening, patch therapy can mirror the diurnal variation in blood levels of T, although the importance of this has not been demonstrated. Hemoglobin and hematocrit changes with the patch forms of therapy are usually quite small. Limitations of patch therapy include the following: lack of flexibility in the dosing because only whole-patch adjustments can be made; strong dependence of T levels obtained on patient compliance with skin preparation and application instructions; lack of acceptance by some men because of cosmetic reasons; and the incidence of skin reactions to the patch, which seems to occur more often in older men than in younger men and more often with the first-generation transdermal patch (Androderm) than with the other patch forms. Coapplication of 0.1% triamcinolone cream may lessen or negate the skin reaction.

The gel form of T provides about 24 h of midrange physiologic levels of T and estradiol while producing serum DHT levels that are mildly supraphysiologic. The application of the gel requires a moderate amount of skin area, but the gel is colorless and the skin surface area utilized has only a small influence on T levels achieved. The gel comes in two different dose packets, and application of less than a full packet is possible, allowing for some dosing flexibility. Skin reactions to the gel have not proven to be a problem to date. At this time, the major drawback to the gel form of therapy is its cost.

Monitoring for appropriateness of serum level of T obtained, for efficacy of therapy, and for possible adverse effects is an ongoing process. The initial monitoring should be within about 3 mo after initiating therapy and should include an evaluation for weight gain, peripheral edema, gynecomastia or breast tenderness, LUTS, problems with sleep, bothersome changes in mood or libido, and a digital rectal examination of the prostate.

Laboratory tests should include a serum T level, hemoglobin and hematocrit, and a PSA. In the absence of obvious problems, a trial of ART should last for at least 6 mo, because it often takes that amount of time to differentiate true benefits of therapy from placebo effects. This necessitates a second follow-up visit for monitoring at about mo 6 of treatment. If the treatment is felt to have been efficacious and no significant adverse events have arisen, the therapy can be continued, but it should be reassessed at least on a yearly basis.

CONCLUSION

The potential rejuvenation of certain functions in aging men through treatment with a testicular "invigorating agent" is not a new concept. Studies involving ART date back to the late 19th century with Brown-Séquard's self-experimentation using animal testicular extracts *(96)*. Since the 1930s, when T was synthesized, a great deal has been learned about its physiology and clinical effects. Yet, there remains a lack of both solid clinical data to define which older men are good candidates to receive ART and consensus guidelines on how to diagnose and treatment PADAM. The data that are available give support to the hypothesis that ART should have a number of beneficial effects for some older men and that its adverse effects may not be so severe as to overwhelm efficacy. Until such time as more clinical data on ART are forthcoming, especially data as relates to effects on the development of fractures, cardiovascular events, LUTS caused by BPH, and prostate cancer, it is important to continually reassess the benefits and risks of ART therapy for each man.

REFERENCES

1. Vermeulen A. Clinical Review 24: Androgens in the aging male. J Clin Endocrinol Metab 1991;73:221–224.
2. Gray A, Berlin JA, McKinlay JB, Longcope C. An examination of research design effects on the association of testosterone and male aging: results of a meta-analysis. J Clin Epidemiol 1991;44:671–684.
3. Deslypere JP, Vermeulen A. Leydig cell function in normal men: effect of age, life-style, residence, diet and activity. J Clin Endocrinol Metab 1984;59:955–962.
4. Ferrini RL, Barrett-Connor E. Sex hormones and age: a cross-sectional study of testosterone and estradiol and their bioavailable fractions in community-dwelling men. Am J Epidemiol 1998;147:750–754.
5. Gray A, Feldman HA, McKinlay JB, Longcope C. Age, disease, and changing sex hormone levels in middle-aged men: results of the Massachusetts Male Aging Study. J Clin Endocrinol Metab 1991;73: 1016–1025.
6. Morley JE, Kaiser FE, Perry HM, et al. Longitudinal changes in testosterone, luteinizing hormone, and follicle stimulating hormone in healthy older men. Metabolism 1997;46:410–413.
7. Znuda JM, Cauley JA, Kriska A, et al. Longitudinal relation between endogenous testosterone and cardiovascular disease risk factors in middle-aged men: a 13-year follow-up of former Multiple Risk Factor Intervention Trial participants. Am J Epidemiol 1997;146:609–617.
8. Harman SM, Metter EJ, Tobin JD, Pearson J, Blackman MR. Longitudinal effects of aging on serum total and free testosterone levels in healthy men. J Clin Endocrinol Metab 2001;86:724–731.
9. Perry HM, Miller DK, Patrick P, Morley JE. Testosterone and leptin in older African-American men: relationship to age, strength, function, and season. Metabolism 2000;49:1085–1091.
10. Usanachitt C, Leepipatpaiboon AAS, Numchaisrika P. Relationship of male hormonal levels and aging in Thai males. Aging Male 2000;3(Suppl 1):47.
11. Geller J, Albert J, Lopez D, et al. Comparison of androgen metabolites in benign prostatic hypertrophy (BPH) and normal prostate. J Clin Endocrinol Metab 1976;43:686–690.
12. Harman SM, Tsitouras PD. Reproductive hormones in aging men. I. Measurement of sex steroids, basal luteinizing hormone, and leydig cell response to human chorionic gonadotropin. J Clin Endocrinol Metab 1980;51:35–40.

13. Baker HWG, Burger HG, deKretser DM, et al. Changes in the pituitary–testicular system with age. Clin Endocrinol (Oxf) 1976;5:349–372.
14. Nieschlag E, Lammers U, Freischem CW, et al. Reproductive functions in young fathers and grandfathers. J Clin Endocrinol Metab 1982;55:676–681.
15. Mulligan T, Iranmanesh A, Hohnson ML, et al. Aging alters feed-forward and feedback linkings between LH and testosterone in healthy men. Am J Physiol 1997;273:R1407–R1413.
16. Marrama P, Montanini V, Celani MR, et al. Decrease in luteinizing hormone biological activity/immunoactivity ratio in elderly men. Maturitas 1984;5:223–231.
17. Tenover JS, Matsumoto AM, Plymate SR, Bremner WJ. The effects of aging in normal men on bioavailable testosterone and luteinizing hormone secretion: response to clomiphene citrate. J Clin Endocrinol Metab 1987;5:1118–1126.
18. Bannister P, Oakes J, Sheridan P, Mosowsky MS. Sex hormone changes in chronic liver disease: a matched study of alcoholic versus non-alcoholic liver disease. Q J Med 1987;240:305–313.
19. Kley HK, Niederau C, Stremmel W, et al. Conversion of androgens to estrogens in idiopathic hemochromatosis: comparison with alcoholic liver disease. J Clin Endocrinol Metab 1985;61:1–6.
20. Turner HE, Wass JAH. Gonadal function in men with chronic illness. Clin Endocrinol (Oxf) 1997;47:379–403.
21. Pont A, Graybill JR, Craven PC, et al. High-dose ketoconazole therapy and adrenal and testicular function in humans. Arch Intern Med 1984;144:2150–2153.
22. Lardinois CK, Mazzaferri EL. Cimetidine blocks testosterone synthesis. Arch Intern Med 1985;145:920–922.
23. MacAdams, MR, White RH, Chipps BE. Reduction of serum testosterone levels during chronic glucocorticoid therapy. Ann Intern Med 1986;104:648–651.
24. Gaigulli VA, Kauman JM, Vermeulen A. Pathogenesis of the decreased androgen levels in obese men. J Clin Endocrinol Metab 1994;79:997–1000.
25. van den Beld AW, deJong FH, Grobbee DE, et al. Measures of bio-available serum testosterone and estradiol and their relationship with muscle strength, bone density, and body composition in elderly men. J Clin Endocrinol Metab 2000;85:3276–3282.
26. Nilsson P, Moller L, Solkad K. Adverse effects of psychosocial stress on gonadal function and insulin levels in middle aged males. J Intern Med 1995;237:479–486.
27. Khosla S, Melton LJ, Atkinson EJ, et al. Relationship of serum sex steroid levels and bone turnover markers with bone mineral density in men: a key role for bio-available estrogen. J Clin Endocrinol Metab 1998;83:2266–2275.
28. Nankin HR, Calkins JH. Decreased bioavailable testosterone in aging normal and impotent men. J Clin Endocrinol Metab 1986;63:418–420.
29. Tenover JS, Matsumoto AM, Clifton DK, Bremner WJ. Age-related alterations in the circadian rhythms of pulsatile luteinizing hormone and testosterone secretion in healthy elderly men. J Gerontol Med Sci 1988;43:M163–M169.
30. Morley JE, Charlton E, Patrick P, et al. Validation of a screening questionnaire for androgen deficiency in aging males. Metabolism 2000;49:1239–1242.
31. Vermeulen A, Verdonck L, Kaufman JM. A critical evaluation of simple methods for the estimation of free testosterone in serum. J Clin Endocrinol Metab 1999;84:3666–3672.
32. Haren M, Nordin BEC, Pearce CEM, et al. The calculation of bioavailable testosterone. In: Robaire R, Chemes H, Morales CA, eds. Andrology in the 21st Century. Medimond Medical Publishing, Englewood, NJ, 2001, pp. 209–215.
33. Forbes GB, Reina JC. Adult lean body mass declines with age: some longitudinal observations. Metabolism 1970;19:653–663.
34. Melton LJ, Khosla S, Riggs BL. Epidemiology of sarcopenia. Mayo Clin Proc 2000;75(Suppl):S10–S13.
35. Lexell J, Henriksson-Larsen K, Wimblod B, Sjostrom M. Distribution of different fiber types in human skeletal muscles: effects of aging studied in whole muscle cross section. Muscle Nerve 1983;6:588–595.
36. Larsson LG, Grimby G, Karlsson J. Muscle strength and speed of movement in relation to age and muscle morphology. J Appl Physiol 1979;46:451–456.
37. Wolfson L. Judge J, Whipple R, King M. Strength is a major factor in balance, gait, and the occurrence of falls. J Gerontol 1995;50:A64–A67.
38. Bhasin S, Storer TW, Berman N, et al. Testosterone replacement increases fat-free mass and muscle size in hypogonadal men. J Clin Endocrinol Metab 1997;82:407–413.
39. Bhasin S, Storer TW, Berman N, et al. The effects of supraphysiologic doses of testosterone on muscle size and strength in normal men. N Engl J Med 1996;335:1–7

40. Kohrt WM, Malley MT, Dalsky GP, Holloszy JO. Body composition of healthy sedentary and trained, young and older men and women. Med Sci Sports Exerc 1992;24:832–837.
41. Bjorntorp P. Visceral obesity: a civilisation syndrome. Obes Res 1993;1:206–222.
42. Vermeulen A, Goemaere S, Kaufman J. Sex hormones, body composition and aging. Aging Male 1999;2:8–15.
43. Seidell JC, Bjorntorp P, Sjostrom L, et al. Visceral fat accumulation in men is positively associated with insulin, glucose and C-peptide levels, but negatively with testosterone levels. Metabolism 1990;39:897–901.
44. Orwoll ES, Klein RF. Osteoporosis in men. Endocr Rev 1995;16:87–116.
45. Gallagher JC, Melton LJ, Riggs BL, et al. Epidemiology of fractures of the proximal femur in Rochester, Minnesota. Clin Orthoped 1980;150:163–168.
46. Magaziner J, Simonsick EM, Kashner TM, et al. Survival experience of aged hip fracture patients. Am J Public Health 1989;79:274–235.
47. Stanley HL, Schmitt BP, Poses RM, Deiss WP. Does hypogonadism contribute to the occurrence of minimal trauma hip fracture in elderly men? J Am Geriatr Soc 1991;39:766–771.
48. Stephan JJ, Lachman M, Zverina J, et al. Castrated men exhibit bone loss: effect of calcitonin treatment on biochemical indices of bone remodeling. J Clin Endocrinol Metab 1989;69:523–527.
49. Goldray D, Weisman Y, Jaccard N, et al. Decreased bone density in elderly men treated with the gonadotropin-releasing hormone agonist decapeptyl (D-Tryp⁶-GnRH). J Clin Endocrinol Metab 1993;76:288–290.
50. Finkelstein JS, Klibanski A, Neer RM, et al. Osteoporosis in men with idiopathic hypogonadaotropic hypogonadism. Ann Intern Med 1987;106:354–361.
51. Behre HM, Kliesch S. Leifke E, et al. Long-term effects of testosterone therapy on bone mineral density in hypogonadal men. J Clin Endocrinol Metab 1997;82:2386–2390.
52. Schiavi RC. Androgens and sexual function in men. In: Oddens BJ, Vermeulen A, eds. Androgens and the Aging Male. Parthenon, New York, 1996, pp. 111–128.
53. Korenman SG, Morley JE, Mooradian AD, et al. Secondary hypogonadism in older men: its relation to impotence. J Clin Endocrinol Metab 1990;71:963–969.
54. Kwan M, Greenleaf WJ, Mann J, et al. The nature of androgen action on male sexuality: a combined laboratory-self-report study on hypogonadal men. J Clin Endocrinol Metab 1983;57:557–562.
55. Carani C, Zini D, Baldini A, et al. Effects of androgen treatment in impotent men with normal and low levels of free testosterone. Arch Sex Behav 1990:19:223–234.
56. Wang C, Alexander G, Berman N, et al. Testosterone replacement therapy improves mood in hypogonadal men—a clinical research center study. J Clin Endocrinol Metab 1996;81:3578–3583.
57. Margolese HC. The male menopause and mood: testosterone decline and depression in the aging male—is there a link? J Geriatr Psychiatry Neurol 2000;13:93–101.
58. Barrett-Connor E, Von Muhlen DG, Kritz-Silverstein D. Bioavailable testosterone and depressed mood in older men: the Rancho Bernardo Study. J Clin Endocrinol Metab 1999;84:573–577.
59. Janowsky JS, Oviatt SK, Orwoll ES. Testosterone influences spatial cognition in older men. Behav Neurosci 1994;108:325–332.
60. Barrett-Connor E, Goodman-Gruen D, Patay B. Endogenous sex hormones and cognitive function in older men. J Clin Endocrinol Metab 1999;84:3681–3685.
61. Shahidi NT. Androgens and erythropoiesis. N Engl J Med 1971;289:72–80.
62. Claustres M, Sultan C. Androgen and erythropoiesis: evidence for an androgen receptor in erythroblasts from human bone marrow cultures. Horm Res 1988;29:17–22.
63. Vahlquist B. The cause of the sexual differences in erythrocyte, hemoglobin and serum iron levels in human adults. Blood 1950;5:874–875.
64. McCullagh EP, Jones R. Effect of androgens on the blood count of men. J Clin Endocrinol 1942;2: 243–247.
65. Matsumoto AM. Effects of chronic testosterone administration in normal men: safety and efficacy of high dosage testosterone and parallel dose-dependent suppression of luteinizing hormone, follicle stimulating hormone, and sperm production. J Clin Endocrinol Metab 1990;70:282–287.
66. Garry PJ, Goodwin JS, Hunt WC. Iron status and anemia in the elderly. J Am Geriatr Soc 1983;31: 389–394.
67. Kirkland RT, Keenan BS, Probstfield JL, et al. Decrease in plasma high density lipoprotein cholesterol at puberty in boys with delayed adolescence. Correlation with plasma testosterone levels. JAMA 1987;27:502–507.

68. Friedl KE, Hannan CJ, Jones RE, Plymate SR. High-density lipoprotein cholesterol is not decreased if an aromatizable androgen is administered. Metabolism 1990;39:69–74.

69. Goldberg RB, Rabin AN, Alexander AN, et al. Suppression of plasma testosterone leads to an increase in serum total and high density lipoprotein cholesterol and Apo A and B. J Clin Endocrinol Metab 1985;60:203–207.

70. Barrett-Connor E, Khaw RT, Yen SS. Testosterone and risk factors for cardiovascular disease in men. Diabetes Metab 1995;21:156–161.

71. Caron P, Bennet A, Camare L, et al. Plasminogen activator inhibitor in plasma is related to testosterone in man. Metabolism 1989;38:1010–1013.

72. Webb CM, McNeill JG, Hayward CS, et al. Effects of testosterone on coronary vasomotor regulation in men with coronary heart disease. Circulation 1999;100:1690–1696.

73. Webb CM, Adamson DL, deZeigler D, Collins P. Effect of acute testosterone on myocardial ischemia in men with coronary artery disease. Am J Cardiol 1999;83:437–439.

74. Behre HM, Bohmeyer J. Nieschlag E. Prostate volume in testosterone-treated and untreated hypogonadal men in comparison to age-matched normal controls. Clin Endocrinol (Oxf) 1994;40:341–349.

75. Morgenthaler A, Bruning CO, DeWolf WC. Occult prostate cancer in men with low serum testosterone levels. JAMA 1996;276:1904–1906.

76. Tenover JS. Effects of testosterone supplementation in the aging male. J Clin Endocrinol Metab 1992;75:1092–1098.

77. Morley JE, Perry HM, Kaiser FE, et al. Effects of testosterone replacement therapy in hypogonadal males: a preliminary study. J Am Geriatr Soc 1993;41:149–152.

78. Jackson JA, Kleerekoper M, Parfitt AM, et al. Bone histomorphometry in hypogonadal and eugonadal men with spinal osteoporosis, J Clin Endocrinol Metab 1987;65:53–58.

79. Kenny AM, Prestwood KM, Gruman CA, et al. Effects of transdermal testosterone on bone and muscle in older men with low bioavailable testosterone levels. J Gerontol Med Sci 2001;56A:M266–M272.

80. Katznelson L, Finkelstein JS, Schoenfeld DA, et al. Increase in bone density and lean body mass during testosterone administration in men with acquired hypogonadism. J Clin Endocrinol Metab 1996;81:4358–4365.

81. Snyder PJ, Peachey H, Hannoush P, et al. Effect of testosterone treatment on bone mineral density in men over 65 years of age. J Clin Endocrinol Metab 1999;84:1966–1972.

82. Reid IR, Wattie DJ, Evans MC, Stapleton JC. Testosterone therapy in gluco-corticoid treated men. Arch Intern Med 1996;156:1173–117.

83. Bakhshi V, Elliott M, Gentili A, et al. Testosterone improves rehabilitation outcomes in ill older men. J Am Geriatr Soc 2000;48:550–553.

84. Clague JE, Wu FCW, Horan MA. Difficulties in measuring the effect of testosterone replacement therapy on muscle function in older men. Int J Androl 1999;22:261–265.

85. Marin P, Holmang S, Gustafsson C, et al. Androgen treatment of abdominally obese men. Obes Res 1993;1:245–251.

86. Urban RJ, Bodenburg YH, Gilkison C, et al. Testosterone administration to elderly men increases skeletal muscle strength and protein synthesis. Am J Physiol 1995;269:E820–E826.

87. Sih R, Morley JE, Kaiser FE, et al. Testosterone replacement in older hypogonadal men: a 12-month randomized controlled trial. J Clin Endocrinol Metab 1997;82:1661–1667.

88. Snyder PJ, Peachey H, Hannoush P, et al. Effect of testosterone treatment on body composition and muscle strength in men over 65 years of age. J Clin Endocrinol Metab 1999;84:2647–2653.

89. Hajjar RR, Kaiser RE, Morley JE. Outcomes of long-term testosterone replacement in older hypogonadal males: a retrospective analysis. J Clin Endocrinol Metab 1997;82:3793–3796.

90. Cherrier MM, Asthana S, Plymate S, et al. Testosterone supplementation improves spatial and verbal memory in healthy older men. Neurology 2001;57:80–88.

91. Krauss DJ, Taub HA, Lantiga LJ. Risks of blood volume changes in hypogonadal men treated with testosterone enanthate for erectile impotence. J Urol 1991;146:1566–1570.

92. Drinka PJ, Jochen AL, Cuisinier M, et al. Polycythemia as a complication of testosterone replacement therapy in nursing home men with low testosterone levels. J Am Geriatr Soc 1995;43:899–901.

93. Matsumoto AM, Sandblom RE, Schoene RB, et al. Testosterone replacement in hypogonadal men: effects on obstructive sleep apnoea, respiratory drives, and sleep. Clin Endocrinol (Oxf) 1985; 22:713–721.

94. Santamaria JD, Prior JC, Fleetham JA. Reversible reproductive dysfunction in men with obstructive sleep apnea. Clin Endocrinol (Oxf) 1988;28:461–470.

95. Mooradian AD, Morley JE, Korenman SG. Biological action of androgens. Endocr Rev 1987;8:1–28.
96. Brown-Séquard, CE. Experience demontrant la puissance dynamogenique chez l'homme d'un liquide extrait de testicules d'animaux. Arch Phys Norm Pathol 1889;21:651–656.

19 Rationale for Treating Hypoandrogenism in Women

Susan R. Davis, *PhD, MBBS, FRACP*

CONTENTS

INTRODUCTION
PHYSIOLOGY
ANDROGENS AND MOOD
LOW TESTOSTERONE IS ASSOCIATED WITH DIMINISHED
   LIBIDO IN WOMEN
INFLUENCE ON BONE
CARDIOVASCULAR DISEASE RISK
EFFECTS ON BODY COMPOSITION
ANDROGENS AND BREAST CANCER
SUMMARY OF THE POTENTIAL RISKS OF TESTOSTERONE REPLACEMENT
DIAGNOSING HYPOANDROGENISM
TESTOSTERONE ADMINISTRATION
CONCLUSIONS
REFERENCES

INTRODUCTION

Traditionally, androgenic disorders in women have been limited to androgen excess. There is now growing awareness that not only are androgens physiologically important for women, but that insufficient levels result in adverse clinical sequelae (*see* Table 1). The focus of most research and discussion in this field to date has been on the use of testosterone to restore libido in postmenopausal women. The fundamental flaw in this approach is that androgen levels change little, if not at all, across menopause, whereas circulating levels of total testosterone and its precursor hormones androstenedione (A) and dehydroepiandrosterone (DHEA) begin to decline in the middle to late reproductive years. Thus, many women insidiously develop symptoms of androgen deficiency prior to menopause. Furthermore, the effects of androgens in women are more far reaching than sexual interest. Areas that need to be explored further include the role of androgens in premenopausal women, effects on mood and well-being, as well as effects on bone, muscle, breast, and the cardiovascular system.

Although the therapeutic window is small, the increasing availability of preparations designed specifically for use in women is opening the door for clinical research and treatment of women.

From: *Contemporary Endocrinology: Androgens in Health and Disease*
Edited by: C. Bagatell and W. J. Bremner © Humana Press Inc., Totowa, NJ

Table 1
Proposed Androgen Deficiency
Symptoms and Signs

Low libido
Persistent fatigue
Blunted motivation
Depression
Inadequate vaginal lubrication with intercourse
Bone loss
Loss of lean mass

PHYSIOLOGY

Circulating androgens are of either ovarian or adrenal origin. DHEA, DHEA-sulfate and A are pro-hormones from which circulating testosterone and dihydrotestosterone (DHT) are derived. They have little biological activity or specific target tissue activity. DHEA and A are produced by both the adrenals and ovaries, whereas the adrenals are the main source of DHEAS. Approximately half of the circulating testosterone is produced by peripheral conversion from these pre-androgens, with A being the main precursor (1). Testosterone is secreted directly by the ovaries. Whether there is direct secretion of testosterone by the adrenals is controversial. In the ovaries, DHEA-S serves as the main precursor for intrafollicular synthesis of testosterone and DHT. Testosterone itself is also further metabolized in target tissues to the DHT.

There is significant cyclicity in plasma levels of A and testosterone in regularly ovulating women, with increases in the mean circulating levels of both of these hormones in the middle third of the menstrual cycle (2,3). This is followed by a second rise in A production by the corpus luteum during the late luteal phase (2). Ovarian androgens are produced by the thecal cells under the control of luteinizing hormone (LH).

The blood level of DHEA in adulthood is higher than any other circulating steroid except cholesterol. DHEA secretion is acutely stimulated by adrenocorticotropic hormone (ACTH) (4,5); however DHEA-S, which has a long plasma half-life, does not acutely increase following ACTH administration (1). DHEA and DHEA-S are converted peripherally into A and then into the potent androgens testosterone and DHT as well as to estrogens.

Under normal physiological conditions, only 1–2% of total circulating testosterone is free or biologically available. The rest is bound by sex hormone-binding globulin (SHBG) and albumin, with SHBG binding 66% of total circulating testosterone (6). The binding affinity for steroids bound by SHBG is DHT> testosterone > androstenediol > estradiol > estrone (7). SHBG also weakly binds DHEA, but not DHEA-S (7). Therefore, variations in the plasma levels of SHBG impact significantly on the amount of free or bioavailable testosterone (7). Elevations in estradiol and thyroxine increase SHBG, where as increases in testosterone, glucocorticosteroids, growth hormone, and insulin suppress SHBG production.

In women, androgens may act directly via the androgen receptor, or indirectly after conversion to estrogen. Androgens are the precursor hormones for estrogen production not only in the ovaries but also in extragonadal tissues, including bone, adipose, and brain. Therefore, maintenance of physiological circulating androgen levels in women ensures adequate supply of substrate for estrogen biosynthesis in extragonadal sites, such as bone, in which high tissue estrogen concentrations may be required physiologically. The preovulatory phase of the menstrual cycle is associated with a rise in intrafollicular and circulating androgen levels, such that peripheral A and testosterone increase 15–20% at midcycle, followed by a secondary rise in A in the late luteal phase (2). The mean daily production rate of testosterone in young healthy women is 0.04–0.144 mg/d when measured in the follicular phase, with a diurnal variation, the highest rate of production occurring between 4 AM and midday (8). The mean circulating level of testosterone declines gradually with increasing age rather than a precipitous fall at the menopause transition (9) such that the levels in women aged 40 are approximately half that of women in their early twenties (10). Because the percent of free testosterone does not vary with age, there is an absolute decline in free testosterone with age. Longcope et al. noted the mean concentration of testosterone in women transiting the menopause to be significantly less than that of premenopausal women sampled between d 5 and 7 of their regular cycles (9). Women approaching the menopause have loss of the midcycle surge of free testosterone and A despite apparently regular menstrual cycle (3). Acutely following bilateral oophorectomy, levels of both testosterone and A decrease by about 50% (11) with a lesser reduction following unilateral oophorectomy (12). Following menopause, peripheral conversion of A becomes the major source of circulating testosterone, although there are varying degrees of ongoing ovarian production (13).

Dehydroepiandrosterone and DHEA-S levels fall linearly with age, and this further contributes to the decline in testosterone (14). Little is known of absolute testosterone levels beyond menopause, as published studies have either included few women or have been extensively statistically manipulated (12). Other iatrogenic causes of low testosterone include nonsurgical oophorectomy—for example, the use of gonadotropin-releasing hormone (GnRH) antagonists, chemotherapy or radiotherapy, and the use of exogenous oral estrogens or glucocorticosteroids (15). The oral contraceptive pill or oral estrogen-replacement therapy (ERT) significantly lowers circulating free-testosterone levels (16) by increasing SHBG and suppressing pituitary LH secretion and, thus, may render a woman hypoandrogenic.

Miller et al. have elegantly demonstrated profound androgen deficiency in women with hypopituitism (17). Similarly, women with premature ovarian failure have reduced circulating androgens (18).

ANDROGENS AND MOOD

Following surgical menopause, the addition of intramuscular testosterone therapy to estrogen replacement results in women feeling more composed, elated, and energetic than with estrogen alone (19). Other studies have demonstrated positive effects of testosterone in perimenopausal and naturally postmenopausal women (20,21).

Transdermal testosterone replacement in surgically menopausal women significantly improves the Psychological General Well-being Index score over placebo, with the greatest change being in improved general well-being and less depressed mood (22). We have recently demonstrated improvements in all the parameters of the Psychological Well-being Index in premenopausal women presenting with low libido treated with transdermal testosterone compared with placebo (author's unpublished data) in a 12-wk double-blind crossover trial.

Dedydroepiandrosterone given orally (50 mg/d) *(23)* or transdermally (by a 10% DHEA cream) *(24)* is associated with a marked improvement in well-being over placebo. Oral DHEA improves well-being and depression and anxiety scores in women with adrenal insufficiency *(25)*. However, not all DHEA trials have been positive *(26,27)*. Larger prospective trials with this steroid are required before definitive guidelines can be developed for its clinical use.

LOW TESTOSTERONE IS ASSOCIATED WITH DIMINISHED LIBIDO IN WOMEN

Androgens also play a major role, particularly in stimulating sexual motivation behaviors, maintaining optimal levels of sexual desire, and possibly contributing to sexual gratification *(28–30)*. Acute decline in sexual interest at the time of natural menopause appears unrelated to testosterone levels *(31)*, consistent with testosterone levels not falling acutely at this time. Sexual dysfunction, primarily low libido, tends to be more prevalent in women as they age or following oophorectomy *(32)*. There is an age-related reduction in sexual frequency among women and lessening of coital frequency associated with the menopausal transition independent of age *(33)*. Testosterone is inversely correlated with reduced coital frequency and loss of sexual desire *(34,35)*. Antiandrogens have adverse effects on female sexual function *(36)*, and among lactating women, testosterone and A levels are lowest in those reporting the greatest reduction in sexual interest *(37)*.

It is generally accepted that estrogen replacement improves vasomotor symptoms, vaginal atrophy, and general well-being, but may not restore libido *(32,33,38)*. Postmenopausal women treated with intramuscular estradiol and testosterone have improvements in sexual motivational behaviors (desire, fantasy, and arousal) and increased frequencies of coitus and orgasm *(29)*, with the improvements in these sexual parameters covarying with plasma testosterone, not estradiol *(29)*. The effects of esterified estrogens (EE) alone vs EE plus methyltestosterone (ET) in postmenopausal women described as being "dissatisfied" with their hormone-replacement therapy (HRT) regimens have been reported. SHBG increased in the EE group and decreased in the ET group. Those taking ET had significant improvements in sexual desire, satisfaction, and coital frequency, whereas those treated with EE alone had no improvement *(39)*. Subcutaneous testosterone implants significantly improve sexual activity, satisfaction, pleasure, and orgasm over and above the effect achieved with estrogen alone *(40–43)*. Moreover, there are no adverse effects on blood lipids with parenteral therapy and no virilization effects.

Acute sublingual testosterone therapy results in an increase in vaginal pulse amplitude peaking at about 4 h post-administration in association with increased subjective sexual excitement and lust scores in young women *(44)*. The findings of Laan and Van Luunsen *(45)* indicate that complaints of vaginal dryness and dyspareunia should not be attributed to vaginal atrophy because of estrogen deficiency but rather reflect inadequate sexual arousal. Leiblum et al. have shown that women with a lower vaginal atrophy index have higher androgen levels *(46)*. Taken together with the favorable effects of testosterone on vascular function *(47)*, testosterone appears to be important for both central sexual arousal and the vaginal responses of vasocongestion and lubrication.

INFLUENCE ON BONE

Androgenic steroids have an important physiologic role in the development and maintenance of bone mineralization in women and men, although the mechanisms of androgen action on bone is still a matter of debate. The skeletal effects of androgens appear to be mediated in part via the estrogen receptor after local aromatization of androgens to estrogen, and mutations in either the estrogen receptor gene or the aromatase gene are associated with osteoporosis (48,49). Abundant aromatase activity has been reported in fetal osteoblasts and cell lines of osteoblastic origin (50). Androgen receptors have been demonstrated in human osteoblast-like cell lines, and androgens directly stimulate bone cell proliferation and differentiation (51,52). DHT increases alkaline phosphatase activity, type 1 procollagen synthesis and insulin-like growth factor-II messenger RNA in the SAOS2 cell line (53). Androgen receptor mRNA is expressed in human osteoblasts, osteocytes, hypertrophic chondrocytes, marrow mononuclear cells and vascular endothelial cells within bone, but not in osteoclasts (54). The pattern and number of cells expressing the androgen receptor is similar in female and male tissues (54). In addition, androgen receptors are upregulated in osteoblastic cells by both testosterone and DHT in vitro (55).

Total and bioavailable testosterone and DHEA-S, not estradiol, are the greatest predictors of bone mineral density (BMD) and bone loss in premenopausal women (56–59). Women who experience bone loss from the hip prior to menopause have lower total- and free-testosterone concentrations by 14% and 22% respectively, than those who do not significantly lose bone (58). Consistent with these findings, hyperandrogenic women have higher BMD, after correction for body mass index, than their normal female counterparts (60). In the premenopausal years, BMD is also strongly positively correlated with body weight (57). In obesity, SHBG is suppressed, with a resultant increase in free testosterone (61), and this may partially explain the relationships among obesity, free testosterone, and increased BMD, with the greater endogenous levels of biologically active free testosterone in more corpulent women directly enhancing bone mass.

Androgen insufficiency may also be a factor underlying bone loss in young women with premature ovarian failure. Despite adequate standard estrogen–progestin therapy, two-thirds of such women have significantly reduced BMD to levels associated with increased hip fracture risk. Of these, 47% have reductions in BMD within 18 mo of their diagnosis (62).

In postmenopausal women, low circulating free testosterone is predictive of subsequent height loss (a surrogate measure of vertebral compression fractures) and hip fracture (7,63,64). Circulating DHEA and DHEA-S are positively correlated with BMD in aging women (65–67), and the progressive decline in DHEA with increasing age is believed to contribute to senile osteoporosis. Suppression of adrenal production of DHEA and DHEA-S with chronic glucocorticosteroid therapy may also contribute to the pathogenesis of osteoporosis and osteopenia, which are known complications of this therapy in women and men. DHEA or testosterone administration may be effective in preventing and or treating this common and serious side effect of glucocorticosteroid therapy. Postmenopausal women treated with oral DHEA have restoration of circulating A, DHT, and testosterone to premenopausal levels, as well as increases in DHEA and DHEA-S, with no changes in circulating levels of estrone or estradiol from baseline (68). Similarly, the daily percutaneous administration of 10 mL of a 20% DHEA solution results in an increase in circulating total testosterone of approx 50%, with no consistent effect on estradiol or estrone *(59)*. Circulating DHEA-S, but not estradiol, in postmenopausal women is positively correlated with BMD *(65)*, and daily application of a 10% DHEA cream has been reported to increase hip BMD in older women *(24)*. Thus, DHEA therapy may prove, in time, to be an alternative to administering testosterone replacement to androgen-deficient women.

Studies of both oral and parenteral estrogen and estrogen-plus-testosterone therapy in postmenopausal women have shown beneficial effects of testosterone replacement on BMD *(40,63,64)*. Oral EE–ET treatment has been shown to increase spinal BMD over a 2-yr period. In contrast estrogen-only therapy prevented bone loss but did not increase bone mass *(69)*. The ET combination not only suppresses biochemical markers of bone reabsorption (as seen with estrogen alone) but is also associated with increases in markers of bone formation *(70)*. Treatment of postmenopausal women with nandrolone decanoate increases vertebral BMD and has been used successfully for many years to treat osteoporosis *(71)*. Combined estradiol and testosterone replacement with subcutaneous implant pellets increases bone mass in postmenopausal women *(72,73)*, with the effects in the hip and spine being greater than with estradiol implants alone *(40)*. Thus, it appears that estradiol alone has an anti-reabsorptive effect on bone in postmenopausal women, whereas the addition of testosterone, either orally or parentally, enhances bone formation.

Increasing BMD is only clinically important if it is associated with enhanced mechanical strength and a reduced fracture rate. As yet, no studies have addressed the impact of androgens on fracture incidence. However, the effects of androgens on the mechanical properties of bone have been studied in feral female cynomolgus monkeys *(74)*. In this primate model, increases in intrinsic bone strength and resistance to mechanical stress were associated with increased BMD following testosterone therapy. Treatment also resulted in increased bone torsional rigidity and bending stiffness.

In summary, current data indicates androgen replacement, in the form of testosterone, and, possibly, DHEA, is potentially an effective alternative to the prevention of bone loss and the treatment of osteopenia and osteoporosis. The use of testosterone to prevent bone loss in individuals on long-term glucocorticosteroids has not been studied but warrants further research.

CARDIOVASCULAR DISEASE RISK

Menopause, both natural and surgically induced, is associated with the development of a more adverse lipoprotein profile, which is unrelated to endogenous testosterone levels *(75)*. The incidence of coronary heart disease in postmenopausal women is not associated with levels of testosterone or DHEA-S *(76,77)*. Postmenopausal ERT lowers total and low-density lipoprotein (LDL) cholesterol, and these favorable effects are not diminished with either oral or parenteral testosterone replacement *(40,69,70)*. Parenteral testosterone replacement does not affect high-density lipoprotein (HDL) cholesterol *(40)*; however, HDL cholesterol and apolipoprotein A1 decrease significantly when oral methyltestosterone is administered with oral estrogen *(78,79)*. The addition of oral methyltestosterone also results in a reduction in triglycerides *(70)*.

Combined oral EE and methyltestosterone therapy reduces arterial LDL degradation and cholesterol ester content in cynomolgus monkeys; this effect does not differ from the effects of estrogen if given alone *(80)*. Combined estrogen and methyltestosterone therapy is also associated with reduced plasma concentrations of apolipoprotein B, reduced LDL particle size and increased total-body LDL catabolism *(80)*. Small LDL particles are more susceptible to oxidation and are, hence, considered to be more athero-genic. Because estrogens appear to increase oxidative modification of LDL in the arterial wall *(80)*, the reduction in LDL particle size observed with both oral estrogen and combined therapy may not be deleterious, but may merely reflect selective removal of large LDL particles from the circulation.

Intracoronary testosterone administration to anesthetized male and female dogs induces increases in coronary artery cross-sectional area peak flow velocity and calcu-lated volumetric blood flow, which is blocked by pretreatment with an inhibitor of nitric oxide synthesis *(81)*. The beneficial effects of ERT on coronary artery reactivity in cynomolgus monkeys is not lost with the addition of oral methyltestosterone *(82)*. Exogenous testosterone implants improve both endothelial-dependent (flow mediated) and endothelium-independent (glyceryl trinitrate [GTN] mediated) brachial artery vasodilation in postmenopausal women using long-term ERT *(47)*.

Cardiac myocytes and fibroblasts contain functional estrogen receptors and express cyp450 aromatase *(83)*. Incubation of cardiac myocytes with A or testosterone results in transactivation of an estrogen-receptor (ER)-specific reporter, and both A and testoster-one upregulate inducible nitric oxide synthase in cardiac myocytes *(83)*.

In summary, exogenous testosterone does not appear to adversely influence the car-diovascular system, but may have favorable effects as a consequence of local aromati-zation to estradiol.

EFFECTS ON BODY COMPOSITION

In postmenopausal women, neither measured nor estimated free testosterone is asso-ciated with waist-to-hip ratio measurements, and there does not appear to be a direct relationship between androgens and visceral adiposity in this population *(84)*. Neither oral nor parenteral ERT significantly increase body weight *(40,85,86)* and there is also no evidence that the addition of testosterone replacement causes weight gain *(40)*. We have reported an increase in fat-free mass (reflecting muscle mass) and a reduced fat mass–to–fat-free mass ratio in postmenopausal women treated with concurrent estro-gen–testosterone therapy *(87)*. As aging is associated with loss of muscle mass, this is a beneficial effect of testosterone therapy in the older woman and may contribute to preservation of muscle strength and skeletal stability.

Testosterone levels are frequently lower in human immunodeficiency virus (HIV)-positive premenopausal women and augmentation of testosterone levels in HIV-positive premenopausal women using a transdermal patch is associated with overall increased mean body weight and body mass index as well as improved quality of life *(88)*.

ANDROGENS AND BREAST CANCER

Early studies have indicated both positive *(78,89)* and negative *(90)* relationships between androgens and breast cancer. Androgen receptors are found in over 50% of breast tumors *(91)* and are associated with longer survival in women with operable breast cancer and a favorable response to hormone treatment in advanced disease *(92)*. There is also evidence that the mechanism by which high-dose medroxyprogesterone acetate exerts a negative effect on breast cancer growth is mediated via the androgen receptor

(93). Most recently, Zhou et al. have shown a reduction in ER mRNA expression and epithelial proliferation when testosterone is coadministered with estrogen *(94)*.

SUMMARY OF THE POTENTIAL RISKS OF TESTOSTERONE REPLACEMENT

The potential masculinizing effects of androgen therapy include development of acne, hirsutism, deepening of the voice, and excessive libido. These cosmetic side effects are rare if supraphysiological hormone levels are avoided *(41–43,72,73,95,96)*. Fluid retention is uncommon and appears to be more idiosyncratic than dose related. Hirsutism, androgenic alopecia, and/or acne are relatively strong contradictions to androgen replacement. Enhancement of libido is currently the most common indication for testosterone therapy; however, circumstances in which this would be an undesirable effect is a relative contraindication to therapy. Syndromes of endogenous androgen excess are clearly associated with increased cardiovascular risk, perturbations in lipid and carbohydrate metabolism, a more android weight distribution, and virilization. In contrast, data at hand does not indicate that exogenous testosterone therapy in postmenopausal women concomittantly treated with estrogen and with testosterone maintained close to, or within, the normal female reproductive range has any adverse metabolic consequences. Absolute contraindications are listed in Table 2.

DIAGNOSING HYPOANDROGENISM

There is no clinical or biochemical definition of female androgen deficiency. However, we have proposed a clinical cluster of symptoms that we believe characterizes female hypoandrogenism *(97)*. This includes low sexual desire in the setting of lowered mood, blunted motivation, and persistent fatigue in a woman who is adequately estrogenized. Women who have undergone surgical-, chemical-, or radiation-induced menopause and women with premature ovarian failure are likely to be symptomatic. However, clinical suspicion should also be raised for otherwise healthy women presenting with lowered mood and low libido irrespective of their menopausal status (*see* Table 3). Most importantly, women with hypopituitism or adrenal insufficiency may have persistent subtle low well-being without androgen replacement.

Most published studies report normal ranges of total and free testosterone for women from samples taken early in the menstrual cycle, when levels are at their nadir.

When investigating women for possible testosterone depletion, blood should be drawn before midday, because of the diurnal variation, and after the early follicular phase in menstruating women. Otherwise, falsely low levels may be determined.

Biochemical measurements that should be performed include total testosterone and SHBG, as well as any other clinically indicated investigations such as thyroid function and iron studies. Free testosterone alone is not particularly useful, as it does not indicate total-testosterone production and how much is unavailable because of high binding to SHBG.

For example, a woman on postmenopausal oral estrogen with a normal testosterone level but high SHBG (therefore low bioavailable testosterone) should be initially changed to nonoral therapy and the profile repeated and clinical reassessment conducted after 6–8 wk. This may obviate the need for testosterone therapy. Similarly taking young women off the oral contraceptive pill may be effective. In general, total

Table 2
Contraindications to Testosterone Treatment

Relative
Severe acne
Moderate–severe hirsutism
Androgenic alopecia
Circumstances in which enhanced libido would be undesirable
Absolute
Pregnancy or lactation
Known or suspected androgen-dependent neoplasia

Table 3
Clinical and Potential Indications for Androgen Replacement and Use in Women

---

Clinical Indications for Androgen Replacement

Symptomatic testosterone deficiency following natural menopause
Symptomatic testosterone deficiency because of surgical menopause, chemotherapy,
 or irradiation
Premature ovarian failure
Premenopausal loss of libido with diminished serum non-SHBG-bound testosterone

Potential Indications for Androgen Use

Management of premenstrual syndrome
Glucocorticosteroid-induced bone loss
Premenopausal/postmenopausal bone loss
Management of wasting syndromes secondary to HIV and malignancy
Premenopausal iatrogenic androgen deficiency states including GnRH-analog treatment
 of endometriosis
Adjunctive therapy for rheumatoid arthritis or systemic lupus erythematosis (SLE)

---

testosterone is measured with assays that do not discriminate low testosterone from the mid-to-low normal range.

Because most laboratories do not use highly sensitive total testosterone assays, a woman with a very low testosterone level may have a level reported within the normal range. We have verified this recently by comparing values between a standard and a very sensitive assay. Hence, until highly sensitive assays become routine, women manifesting characteristic symptoms who have a total testosterone within the lower quartile for the specific assay and an SHBG level that is normal or elevated should be offered treatment based on clinical assessment *(98)*.

TESTOSTERONE ADMINISTRATION

Various testosterone preparations are currently used for androgen replacement (*see* Table 4). Although widely available for men with hypogonadism, such is not the case for women. Availability currently remains limited with varying approval in different states and countries. Despite this, specialist menopause clinics have had a range of experience with the use of testosterone in women.

Table 4
Androgen Replacement Therapy Formulations Used for Women

	Dose range	Frequency	Route
Methyltestosterone[a] (in combination with esterified estrogen)	1.25–2.5 mg	Daily	Oral
Mixed testosterone esters	50–100 mg	4–6 weekly	Intramuscular
Testosterone implants	50 mg	3–6 monthly	Subcutaneous
Transdermal testosterone Patch[b]	150-300 µg	Every 3.5 d	Topical
Testosterone cream 1%[b]	5–10 mg	Daily	Topical
Testosterone undecanoate	40 mg	Daily	Oral
Nandrolone decanoate	50 mg	8–12 weekly	Intramuscular

[a]Currently available in the United States.
[b]Undergoing clinical trial.

Oral estrogen/androgen therapy is available in the United States in two strengths: EE 0.625 mg plus methyltestosterone 1.25 mg, or EE 1.25 mg plus methyltestosterone 2.5 mg. Methyltestosterone is not available in some countries because liver damage has been reported with long-term high-dose therapy (99); however, recent data do not support any detrimental effects of the above doses on hepatic enzymes or blood pressure over 24 mo (99,100). Women should be regularly reviewed for clinical manifestation of androgen excess, but no specific biochemical monitoring should be undertaken routinely.

Testosterone implants were approved for postmenopausal women in the United Kingdom in the early 1990s. A 50-mg dose is effective in improving BMD without causing virilizing side effects (40). Testosterone levels increase acutely after each implant to well above the normal female range with considerable inter-individual variation. Despite this, side effects (i.e., virilization) are virtually never seen with this dose implant, but are not infrequent when 100 mg is inserted. It is suggested that testosterone levels be measured before each implant and a subsequent implant should not be inserted until total-testosterone levels are within the low normal range for young women.

Tibolone is a unique compound that, along with its metabolites, exerts tissue-specific estrogenic, progestogenic, and weak androgenic effects. It reduces postmenopausal vasomotor symptoms without stimulating the endometrium or breast tissue (101). Furthermore, tibolone lowers SHBG (102) and, therefore, increases the bioavailability of endogenous testosterone. Tibolone appears to enhance libido in postmenopausal women (103) and should be considered as a therapeutic option in terms of androgen replacement. It is taken as a total hormonal regimen and should not be co-prescribed with estrogens. Tibolone 2.5 mg is now available in most countries, but has not yet been approved in the United States. It is well tolerated with very low rates of mastalgia or vaginal bleeding (104).

Nandrolone decanoate is a weakly aromatizable androgen used for the treatment of osteoporosis and is administered intramuscularly. The dose of 50 mg should not be exceeded, and frequency of administration should be titrated according to the patient's build. In general, it is given every 6 wk, but at longer intervals for a body mass index less than 20.

Testosterone and its esters are available as an intramuscular injection. A dose of 50–100 mg may be administered 4–6 weekly. Although the pharmacokinetics have not been extensively studied in women, it appears to have a more rapid onset of effects, with women reporting enhanced libido 2–3 d after treatment. There is a high incidence of acne and virilizing side effects, possibly because of rapid high peak levels after administration, and, thus, should not be used routinely or long term.

Testosterone undecanoate is an oral preparation that is widely used for treatment of hypogonadal men. In women, however, pharmacokinetic studies have demonstrated that even very low doses result in supraphysiological peak levels *(105)*.

A transdermal matrix patch has been developed specifically for use in women. Studies thus far are encouraging because it appears well tolerated and produces stable levels, with little variation between individuals. The exact dosing and frequency is still being determined, but it is designed to deliver 150 or 300 µg/d with twice-weekly application. Testosterone creams and gels are currently being used in clinical trials.

CONCLUSIONS

Controversy continues to surround the issue of testosterone therapy for women. This review summarizes most of the pertinent data available, but, clearly, there are vast gaps that need to be filled.

As more women enjoy longer and healthier lives, the demand to optimize quality of life will increase. Testosterone therapy is an important quality-of-life issue. No woman will die from testosterone deficiency, but if the link between testosterone depletion and depression and well-being is established, in addition to the effects on libido, testosterone therapy will be a therapy to be considered by all women.

The emphasis must be made that no specific testosterone product is approved for use in women in most countries; yet, historically, its use has been and continues to be widespread.

In the near future, specific formulations for women are likely to revolutionize this aspect of women's health, but in the interim, all women treated with testosterone should be reviewed carefully and blood testosterone levels should be monitored regularly.

REFERENCES

1. Haning RV Jr, Cabot M, Flood CA, et al. Metabolic clearance rate (MCR) of dehydroepiandrosterone sulfats (DS) its metabolism to dehydroepiandrosterone, androstenedione testosterone and dihydrotestosterone, and the effects of increased plasm DS concentration on DS MCR in normal women. J Clin Endocrinol Metab 1989;69:1047–1052.
2. Judd HL, Yen SSC. Serum androstenedione and testosterone levels during the menstrual cycle. J Clin Endocrinol Metab 1973;36:475–481.
3. Mushayandebvu T, Castracane DV, Gimpel T, et al. Evidence for diminished midcycle ovarian androgen production in older reproductive aged women. Fertil Steril 1996;65:721–723.
4. Vaitukaitis JL, Dale SL, Melby JC. Role of ACTH in the secretion of free DHA and its sulphate ester in man. J Clin Endocrinol Metab 1969;29:1443–1447.
5. Vermeulen A, Ando S. Prolactin and adrenal androgen secretion. Clin Endocrinol (Oxf) 1978;8:295–303.
6. Rannevik G, Jeppsson S, Johnell O. A longitudinal study of the perimenopausal transition: altered profiles of steroid and pituitary hormones, SHBG and bone mineral density. Matuitas 1986;8:189–196.
7. Dunn JF, Nisula BC, Rodboard D. Transport of steroid hormones. Binding of 21 endogenous steroids to both testosterone-binding globulin and cortico-steroid-binding globulin in human plasma. J Clin Endocrinol Metab 1981;53:58–68.

8. Vierhapper H, Nowotny P, Waldhausl W. Determination of testosterone production rates in men and women using stable isotope'dilution and mass spectromety. J Clin Endocrinol Metab 1997;82: 1492–1496.

9. Longcope C, Franz C, Morello C, et al. Steroid and gonadotropin levels in women during the peri-menopausal years. Maturitas 1986;8:189–196.

10. Zumoff B, Strain GW, Miller LK, Rosner W . Twenty-four hour mean plasma testosterone concentration declines with age in normal premenopausal women. J Clin Endocrinol Metab 1995;80: 1429–1430.

11. Judd HL. Hormonal dynamics associated with the menopause. Clin Obstet Gynecol 1976;19: 775–788.

12. Laughlin G.A, Barrett-Connor E, Kritz-Silverstein D, Von Muhlen D. Hysterectomy, oophorectomy, and endogenous sex hormone levels in older women: the Rancho Bernardo Study. J Clin Endocrinol Metab 2000;85(2):645–651.

13. Procope BJ. Studies on the urinary excretion, biological effects and origina of estrogens in postmenopausal women. Acta Endocrinol (Copenh) 1969;135:1–86.

14. Labrie F, Belanger A, Cusan L, et al. Marked decline in serum concentrations of adrenal C19 sex steroid precursors and conjugated andrgoen metaboliltes during aging. J Clin Endocrinol Metab 1997;82(8):2396–2402.

15. Abraham GE. Ovarian and adrenal contribution to peripheral androgens during the menstrual cycle. J Clin Endocrinol Metab 1974;39:340–346.

16. Mathur RS, Landgreve SC, Moody LO, et al. The effect of estrogen treatment on plasma concentrations of steroid hormones, gonadotropins, prolactin and sex hormone-binding globulin in postmenopausal women. Maturitas 1985;7:129–133.

17. Miller K, Sesmilo G, Schiller A, et al. Androgen deficiency in women with hypopituitarism. J Clin Endocrinol Metab 2001;86(2):561–567.

18. Doldi N, Belvisi L, Bassan M, et al. Premature ovarian failure:steroid synthesis and autoimmunity. Gynecol Endocrinol 1998;12(1):23–28.

19. Sherwin BB. Affective changes with estrogen and androgen replacement therapy in surgically menopausal women. J Affect Disord 1988;14(2):177–187.

20. Montgomery J, Brincat M, Appleby L, et al. Effect of oestrogen and testosterone implants on psychological disorders in the climacteric. Lancet 1987;1:297–299 (abstract).

21. Brincat M, Studd JWW, O'Dowd T, et al. Subcutaneous hormone implants for the control of climacteric symptoms. Lancet 1984;1:16–18 (abstract).

22. Shifren JL, Braunstein G, Simon J, et al. Transdermal testosterone treatment in women with impaired sexual function after oophorectomy. N Engl J Med 2000;343(10):682–688.

23. Morales AJ, Nolan JJ, Nelson JC, Yen SSC. Effects of replacement dose of dehydroepiandrosterone in men and women of advancing age. J Clin Endocrinol Metab 1997;78:1360–1367.

24. Labrie F, Diamond P, Cusan L, et al. Effect of 12-month dehydroepiandrosterone replacement therapy on bone, vagina and endometrium in postmenopausal women. J Clin Endocrinol Metab 1997;82(10):3498–3505.

25. Wiebke A, Callies F, Van Vlijmen JC, et al. Dehydroepiandrosterone replacement in women with adrenal insufficiency. N Engl J Med 1999;341(14):1013–1020.

26. Barnhart KT, Freeman E, Grisso JA, et al. The Effect of dehydroepiandrosterone supplementation to symptomatic perimenopausal women on serum endocrine profiles, lipid parameters and health-related quality of life. J Clin Endocrinol Metab 1999;84:(11)3896–3902 (abstract).

27. Flynn M, Weaver-Osterholtz D, Sharpe-Timms K, et al. Dehydroepiandrosterone replacement in aging humans. J.Clin Endocrinol Metab 1999;84:(5)1527–1533 (abstract).

28. Steiner M, Steinberg S, Stewart D, et al. Fluoxetine in the treatment of premenstrual dysphoria. N Engl J Med 1995;332:1529–1534.

29. Sherwin BB, Gelfand MM. The role of androgen in the maintenance of sexual functioning in oophorectomized women. Psychosom Med 1987;49(4):397–409.

30. Persky H, Dreisbach L, Miller WR, et al. The relation of plasma androgen levels to sexual behaviours and attitudes of women. Psychosom Med 1982;44(4):305–319.

31. Dennerstein L, Smith A, Morse, Burger H. Sexuality and the menopause. J Psychsom Obstet Gynecol 1994;15:56–59.

32. Nathorst-Boos J, von Schoultz H. Psychological reactions and sexual life after hysterectomy with and without oophorectomy. Gynecol Obstet Invest 1992;34:97–101.

33. Frock J, Money J. Sexuality and the menopause. Psychother Psychosom 1992;57:29–33.
34. Bachmann GA, Leiblum SR. Sexuality in sexagenarian women. Maturitas 1991;13:45–50.
35. McCoy NL, Davidson JM. A longitudinal study of the effects of menopause on sexuality. Maturitas 1985;7:203–210.
36. Appelt H, Strauss SB. The psychoendocrinology of female sexuality. A research project. German J Psychol 1986;10:143–156.
37. Alder EM, Cook A, Davidson D, et al. Hormones, mood and sexuality in lactaing women. Br J Psychiatry 1986;148:74–79.
38. Utian WH. The true clinical features of postmenopausal oophorectomy and their response to estrogen replacement therapy. S Afr Med J 1972;46:732–737.
39. Sarrel P, Dobay B, Wiita B. Estrogen and estrogen-androgen replacement in postmenopausal women dissatisfied with estrogen-only therapy. sexual behaviour and neuroendocrine response. J Reprod Med 1998;43:847–856.
40. Davis SR, McCloud PI, Strauss BJG, Burger HG. Testosterone enhances estradiol's effects on postmenopausal bone density and sexuality. Maturitas 1995;21:227–236.
41. Studd JWW, Chakravarti S, Oram D. The climacteric. Clin Obstet Gynecol 1977;4:3–29.
42. Studd JWW, Colins WP, Chakravarti S. Estradiol and testosterone implants in the treatment of psychosexual problems in postmenopausal women. Br J Obstet Gynaecol 1977;84:314–315.
43. Burger HG, Hailes J, Nelson J, Menelaus M. Effect of combined implants of estradiol and testosterone on libido in postmenopausal women. Br Med J 1987;294:936–937.
44. Tuiten A, Von Honk J, Koppeschaar H, et al. Time course of effects of testosterone administration on sexual arousal in women. Arch Gen Psychiatry 2000;57:149–153.
45. Laan E, Van Lunsen RH. Hormones and sexuality in postmenopausal women: a psychophysiological study. J Psychosom Obset Gynaecol 1997;18(2):126–133.
46. Leiblum S, Bachmann GA, Kemmann E, et al. The importance of sexual activity and hormones. JAMA 1983;249:2195–2198.
47. Worboys S, Kotsopoulos D, Teede H, et al. Parental testosterone improves endothelium-dependent and independent vasodilation in postmenopausal women already receiving estrogen. J Clin Endocrinol Metab 2001;86(1):158–161.
48. Smith EP, Boyd J, Frank GR, et al. Estrogen resistance caused by a mutation in the oestrogen-receptor gene in a man. N Engl J Med 1994;331:1056–1061.
49. Morishima A, Grumbach MM, Simpson ER. Aromatase deficiency in male and female siblings caused by a novel mutuation and the physiological role of estrogens. J Clin Endocrinol Metab 1995;80:3689–3698.
50. Shozu M, Simpson ER. Aromatase expression of human osteoblast-like cells. Mol Cell Endocrinol 1998;139:117–129.
51. Colvard DS, Eriksen EF, Keeting PE. Identification of androgen receptors in normal human osteoblast-like cells. Proc Natl Acad Sci USA 1989;86:854–857.
52. Kasperk CH, Wergedal JE, Farley JR, et al. Androgens directly stimulate proliferation of bone cells in vitro. Endocrinology 1989;124:1576–1578.
53. Kasperk CH, Fitzsimmons R, Strong D, et al. Studies of the mechanism by which androgens enhance mitogenesis and differentiation in bone cells. J Clin Endocrinol Metab 1990;71:1322–1329.
54. Abu EO, Horner V, Kusec V, et al. The localization of androgen receptors in human bone. J Clin Endocrinol Metab 1997;82(10):3493–3497.
55. Wiren KM, Keenan EJ, Orwoll ES, et al. Transcriptional U-regulation of the human androgen receptor by androgen in bone cells. Endocrinology 1997;138(6):2291–2300.
56. Carlson LA, Rosehamer G. Reduction of mortality in The Stockholm Ishcaemic Heart Disease Secondary Prevention Study by combined treatment with clofibrate and nicotinic acid. Acta Med Scand 1988;(223):405–418.
57. Nilas L, Christiansen C. Bone mass and its relationship to age and the menopause. J Clin Endocrinol Metab 1987;65:697–699.
58. Slemenda C, Longcope C, Peacock M, et al. Sex steroids, bone mass, and bone loss. A propspective study of pre-, peri-, and postmenopausal women. J Clin Invest 1996;97:14–21.
59. Labrie F, Belanger A, Cusan L, Candas B. Physiological changes in dehydroepiandrosterone are not reflected by serum levels of active androgens and estrogens but of their metabolites: intracrinology. J Clin Endocrinol Metab 1997;82(8):2403–2409.

60. Simberg N, Titinen A, Silfrast A, et al. High bone density in hyperandrogenic women: effect of gonadotropin-releasing hormone agonist alone or in conjunction with estrogen–progestin replacement. J Clin Endocrinol Metab 1995;81:646–651.

61. Heiss CJ, Sanborn CF, Nichols DL. Associations of body fat distribution, circulating sex hormones and bone density in postmenopausal women. J Clin Endocrinol Metab 1995;80:1591–1596.

62. Anasti JN, Kalantaridou SN, Kimzey LM, et al. Bone loss in young women with karyotypically normal spontaneous premature ovarian failure. Obstet Gynecol 1998;91(1):12–15.

63. Jassal SK, Barrett-Connor E, Edelstein S. Low bioavailable testosterone levels predict future height loss in postmenopausal women. J Bone Miner Res 1995;10(4):650–653.

64. Davidson BJ, Ross RK, Paganni Hill A, et al. Total free estrogens and androgens in post menopausal women with hip fractures. J Clin Endocrinol Metab 1982;54:115–120.

65. Nawata H, Tariaka S. Aromatase in bone cell: association with osteoporosis in post menopausal women. J Steroid Biochem Molec Biol 1995;53:165–174.

66. Taelman P, Kayman JM, Janssens X, Vermeulen A. Persistence of increased bone resorption and possible role of dehydroepiandrosterone as a bone metabolism determinant in osteoporotic women in late menopause. Maturitas 1989;11:65–73.

67. Nordin BEC, Robertson A, Seamark RF, et al. The relation between calcium absorption serum DHEA and vertebral mineral density in postmenopausal women. J Clin Endocrinol Metab 1985;60:651–657.

68. Morales AJ, Nolan JJ, Nelson JC, Yen SSC. Effects of replacement dose of dehydroepiandrosterone in men and women of advancing age. J Clin Endocrinol Metab 1994;78:1360–1367.

69. Watts NB, Notelovitz M, Timmons MC. Comparison of oral estrogens and estrogens plus androgen on bone mineral density, menopausal symptoms and lipid–lipoprotein profiles in surgical menopause. Obstet Gynecol 1995;85:529–537.

70. Raisz LG, Wiita B, Artis A, et al. Comparison of the effects of estrogen alone and estrogen plus androgen on biochemical markers of bone formation and resoprtion in postmenopausal women. J Clin Endocrinol Metab 1995;81:37–43.

71. Need GA, Horowitz M, Bridges A, et al. Effects of nandrolone decanoate and antiresorptive therapy on vertebral density in osteoporotic women. Arch Intern Med 1989;149:57–60.

72. Savvas M, Studd JWW, Fogelman I, et al. Skeletal effects of oral estrogen compared with subcutaneous oestrogen and testosterone in postmenopausal women. Br Med J 1988;297:331–333.

73. Savvas M, Studd JWW, Norman S, et al. Increase in bone mass after one year of percutaneous oestradiol and testosterone implants in post menopausal women who have previously received long-term oral oestrogens. Br J Obstet Gynaecol 1992;99:757–760.

74. Kasra M, Grynpas MD. The effects of androgens on the mechanical properties of primate bone. Bone 1995;17:265–270.

75. Wakatsuki A, Sagara Y. Lipoprotein metabolism in postmenopausal and oophorestomized women. Obstet Gynecol 1995;85:523–528.

76. Barrett-Connor E, Goodman-Gruen D. Prospective study of endogenous sex hormones and fatal cardiovascular disease in postmenopausal women. Br Med J 1995;311:1193–1196.

77. Barrett-Connor E, Goodman-Gruen D. Dehydroepiandrosterone sulfate does not predict cardiovascular death in postmenopausal women. The Rancho Bernardo Study. Circulation 1995;91: 1757–1760.

78. Secreto G, Toniolo P, Pisani P, et al. Androgens and breast cancer in premenopausal women. Cancer Res 1989;49:471–476.

79. Hickok LR, Toomey C, Speroff L. A comparison of esterified estrogens with and without methyltestosterone: effects on endometrial histology and serum lipoproteins in postmenopausal women. Obstet Gynecol 1993;82:919–924.

80. Wagner JD, Zhang L, Williams JK, et al. Esterified estrogens with and without methyltesterone decrease arterial LDL metabolism in Cynomolgus monkeys. Arteriosclerosis Thromb Vasc Biol 1996;16:1473–1479.

81. Chou TM, Sudhir K, Hutchison SJ, et al. Testosterone induces dilation of canine coronary conductance and resistsance arteries in vivo. Circulation 1996;94:2614–2619.

82. Honore EK, Williams JK, Adams MR, et al. Methyltestosterone does not diminish the beneficial effects of estrogen replacement therapy on coronary arter reactivity in cynomolgus monkeys. Menopause 1996;3:20–26.

83. Grohe C, Kahlert S, Lobbert K, Vetter H. Expression of oestrogen receptor alpha and beta in rat heart: role of local oestrogen synthesis. J Endocrinology 1998;156:R1–R7.

84. Goodman-Gruen D, Barrett-Connor E. Total but not bioavailable testosterone is a predictor of central adiposity in postmenopausal women. Int J Obes 1995;19:293–298.
85. Darling GM, Johns JA, McCloud PI, Davis SR. Estrogen and progestin compared with simvastatin for hypercholesterolemia postmenopausal women. N Engl J Med 1997;337(9):595–601.
86. The Writing Group for the PEPI Trial. Effects of estrogen or estrogen/progestin regimens on heart disease risk factors in postmenopausal women. JAMA 1995;273:199–208.
87. Davis SR, Walker KZ, Strauss BJ. Effects of estradiol with and without testosterone on body composition and relationships with lipids in post-menopausal women. Menopause 2000;7:395–401.
88. Miller K, Corcoran C, Armstrong C, et al. Transdermal testosterone administration in women with acquired immunodeficiency syndrome wasting: A pilot study. J Clin Endocrinol Metab 1998;83: 2717–2725.
89. Secreto G, Toniolo P, Berrino E, et al. Serum and urinary androgens and risk of breast cancer in postmenopausal women. Cancer Res 1991;51:2572–2576.
90. Bulbrook RD, Thomas BS. Hormones are ambiguous risk factors for breast cancer. Acta Oncol 1989;28:841–847.
91. Recchione C, Venturelli E, Manzari A, et al. Testosterone, dihydrotestosterone and oestradiol levels in postmenopausal breast cancer tissues. J Steroid Biochem Mol Biol 1995;52:541–546.
92. Bryan RM, Mercer RJ, Rennie GC, et al. Androgen receptors in breast cancer. Cancer 1984;54: 2436–2440.
93. Birrell SN, Roder DM, Horsfall DJ, et al. Medroxyprogesterone acetate therapy in advanced breast cancer: the predictive value of androgen receptor expression. J Clin Oncol 1995;13(7):1572–1577.
94. Zhou J, Ng S, Adesanya-Famuiya O, et al. Testosterone inhibits estrogen-induced mammary epithelial proliferation and suppresses estrogen receptor expression. FASEB J 2000;14(12):1725–1730.
95. Sherwin BN, Gelfand MM, Brender W. Androgen enhances sexual motivation in females: a prespective, crossover study of sex steroid administration in surgical menopause. Psychosom Med 1997;47:339–351.
96. Burger HG, Hailes J, Menelaus M. The management of persistent symptoms with estradiol–testosterone implants: clinical, lipid and hormonal results. Maturitas 1984;6:351–358.
97. Davis SR. Androgen replacement in women: a commentary. J Clin Endocrinol Metab 1999;84(6): 1886–1891.
98. Bachmann GA, Bancroft J, Braunstein G, et al. Female androgen insufficiency: the Princeton Consensus Statement on definition, classification and assessment. Fertil Steril 2002;77(4):660–665.
99. Barrett-Connor E, Timmons MC, Young R, Wiita B, Estratest Working Group. Interim safety analysis of a two-year study comparing oral estrogen-androgen and conjugated estrogens in surgically menopausal women. J Women's Health 1996;5:593–602.
100. Barrett-Connor E, Young R, Notelovitz M, et al. A two-year, double-blind comparison of estrogen-androgen and conjugated estrogens in surgically menopausal women. Effects on bone mineral density, symptoms and lipid profiles. J Reprod Med 1999;44:(12)1012–1020.
101. Tax L, Goorssen E, Kicovic P. Clinical profile of Org OD 14. Maturitas 1987;(Suppl 1):3–13.
102. Doren M, Rubig A, Coelingh Bennink H, and Holzgreve W. Differential effects of the androgen status of postmenopausal women treated with tibolone and continuous combined estradiol and norethindrone acetate replacement therapy. Fertil Steril 2001;75(3):554–549.
103. Nathorst-Boos J, Hammar M. Effect on sexual life—a comparison between tibolone and a continous estradiol–norethisterone acetate regimen. Maturitas 1997;26:15–20.
104. Kloosterboer H. Tibolone: a steroid with tissue-specific mode of action. J Steroid Biochem Mol Biol 2001;76:231–238.
105. Buckler HM, Robertson WR, Wu FCW. Which androgen replacement therapy for women? J Clin Endocrinol Metab 1998;83(11):3920–3924.

20 Androgens as Anabolic Agents

Shalender Bhasin, MD, Linda J. Woodhouse, PhD, and Thomas W. Storer, PhD

CONTENTS

HISTORICAL PERSPECTIVE
EFFECTS OF SPONTANEOUS AND EXPERIMENTALLY
    INDUCED ANDROGEN DEFICIENCY ON BODY COMPOSITION IN MEN
TESTOSTERONE REPLACEMENT INCREASES MUSCLE MASS AND MAXIMAL
    VOLUNTARY STRENGTH IN HEALTHY YOUNG HYPOGONADAL MEN
EFFECT OF SUPRAPHYSIOLOGICAL DOSES OF TESTOSTERONE
    ON BODY COMPOSITION AND MUSCLE STRENGTH
TESTOSTERONE DOSE–RESPONSE RELATIONSHIPS
    IN HEALTHY YOUNG MEN
MECHANISMS OF TESTOSTERONES'S ANABOLIC EFFECTS ON THE MUSCLE
USE OF TESTOSTERONE AS AN ANABOLIC THERAPY IN SARCOPENIA
    ASSOCIATED WITH CHRONIC ILLNESS AND AGING
HETEROGENEITY IN RESPONSE AND PREDICTORS
    OF ANABOLIC RESPONSE TO ANDROGEN ADMINISTRATION
TESTOSTERONE EFFECTS ON FAT METABOLISM
THE ABUSE OF ANDROGENIC STEROIDS BY ATHLETES
    AND RECREATIONAL BODYBUILDERS
SUMMARY
REFERENCES

HISTORICAL PERSPECTIVE

The idea that secretions of the testis might regulate body composition is as old as humanity itself. Humans have known since antiquity that "...you can take away the vigor of men by removing their testes." Many cannibal tribes practiced castration on their victims several weeks prior to the sacrificial ritual. Ancient Hindus, Romans, and Egyptians advocated the use of the testicles of wild animals as treatment of impotence. The testicular transplantation experiments of Hunter and Berthold established that the secretions of the testis could regulate the growth of capon and male behavior, remote from the site of production. Brown-Sequard claimed to have rejuvenated himself by injecting himself with the extracts of guinea pig testis; these claims invited ridicule at the time, but

From: *Contemporary Endocrinology: Androgens in Health and Disease*
Edited by: C. Bagatell and W. J. Bremner © Humana Press Inc., Totowa, NJ

his prescient prediction that secretions of the testis would reverse age-related changes in body composition and muscle strength has once again gained currency. In the 1920s, several surgeons in Europe and the United States amassed substantial wealth by practicing transplantation of testis from young, male prisoners, or those dying on the battlefield, to older men to reverse changes associated with aging.

The modern era of androgen biology and pharmacology began in 1937 with the chemical synthesis of testosterone by Ruzicka and Butenandt, for which they shared a Nobel Prize. With the availability of pure testosterone for animal experiments, it was soon discovered that testosterone promoted nitrogen retention in castrated males of many species, in boys before puberty, and in women, indicating that testosterone had anabolic properties in addition to its masculinizing effects. These observations led to considerable efforts to develop derivatives of testosterone that had preferential anabolic effects. These congeners of testosterone, with presumably greater anabolic than androgenic activity, became known as anabolic steroids (1,2). In the early 1950s, members of the Russian weight-lifting team were the first to use anabolic steroids in sports. As word of the assumed potency of these compounds in enhancing athletic prowess became known, the abuse of androgenic steroids in sports spread rapidly. This abuse has continued in spite of concerted efforts of many national and international sports agencies to discourage the use of anabolic steroids by instituting screening programs and penalties for their use.

The decades of the 1970s and 1980s witnessed considerable polarization of views on the anabolic effects of androgens (3). Although athletes and many sports medicine physicians believed that androgenic steroids increased muscle size and strength, the academic community decried their use citing the absence of verifiable data (see Table 1). The controversy about the anabolic effects of androgens on the muscle was a consequence of the shortcomings of previous studies; several reviews have discussed these study design issues (3,4). Many previous studies that examined the effects of androgenic steroids were neither blinded nor randomized. Some studies included competitive athletes whose desire to win at any cost might prevent them from complying with a standardized regimen of diet and exercise. Nutritional intake was not controlled in many of the studies; changes in energy and protein intake might have had independent effects on nitrogen balance. Exercise stimulus was not standardized and, in some studies, the participants were allowed to exercise ad libitum. Consequently, the effects of androgen administration could not be separated from the effects of resistance exercise training. Most of the studies used relatively small doses of androgenic steroids. In contrast, athletes not only use much larger doses of androgenic steroids than those used in controlled clinical trials, but they often stack multiple androgenic steroids simultaneously. Not surprisingly, the results of these studies that used relatively low doses of androgens in eugonadal men were inconclusive. However, studies published in the last 6 yr by a number of groups have now established that testosterone is an important regulator of body composition and that testosterone supplementation increases muscle mass and strength (5–14).

EFFECTS OF SPONTANEOUS AND EXPERIMENTALLY INDUCED ANDROGEN DEFICIENCY ON BODY COMPOSITION IN MEN

Healthy young hypogonadal men have higher fat mass and lower fat-free mass compared to age-matched eugonadal controls (15). Epidemiological studies have revealed

Table 1
Beliefs Held by the Athletic and the Academic Communities
About the Effects of Androgenic Steroids in the 1970s and 1980s

Beliefs held by recreational body-builders and athletic community about androgenic steroids	The academic view in the 1980s and early 1990s	What have recent studies revealed?
Androgenic steroids increase muscle mass, strength, and athletic performance.	Only replacement doses of testosterone when given to hypogonadal men and prepubertal boys have anabolic effects. Supra-physiological doses of testosterone do not further increase muscle mass.	Replacement doses of testosterone when administered to hypogonadal men and supraphysiological doses when administered to eugonadal men increase fat-free mass, muscle size, and strength.
Higher doses of androgenic steroids promote greater increases in muscle mass and strength than lower doses; administering more than one androgenic steroid simultaneously (stacking) produces greater increases in muscle mass and strength than any single agent alone.	Beyond the physiologic range, further increases in the dose of androgenic steroid would produce no further gains in fat-free mass and muscle strength.	A linear dose–response relationship exists between testosterone dose and its anabolic effects over a wide range of concentrations extending from subphysiologic to supraphysiologic range.
The anabolic and androgenic activities of androgens can be dissociated, so that some derivatives of testosterone have preferentially greater anabolic activity than androgenic activity.	The anabolic and androgenic activity cannot be dissociated; they are described by the same dose–response relationship.	Different androgen-dependent processes have different dose–response relationships.
The anabolic and androgenic effects are mediated through separate mechanisms and thus can be dissociated.	The anabolic effects are mediated through an androgen-receptor-mediated mechanism.	The anabolic effects are likely mediated through an androgen-receptor-mediated mechanism that involves recruitment of tissue-specific coactivators and corepressors.

an inverse relationship between serum-free testosterone concentrations and intra-abdominal fat, measured by computed tomography (CT) scan *(16,17)*. Similarly, in a series of elegant studies, Mauras et al. *(18)* have demonstrated that lowering of serum testosterone concentrations in healthy, young men is associated with loss of fat-free mass (FFM), gain of fat mass, and a reduction in fractional muscle protein synthesis rates.

Table 2
Effects of Testosterone Replacement on Body Composition in Hypogonadal Men

Study	Age (yr)	Testosterone regimen	Change in fat-free mass	Change in fat mass	Change in muscle strength
Bhasin et al. (1997)	19–47	Testosterone enanthate 100 mg weekly for 10 wk	5.0 ± 0.7 kg (9.9 ± 1.4%) increase by underwater weight and D_2O	No change in fat mass by underwater weight and D_2O	+22 ± 3%
Katznelson et al. (1996)	22–69	Testosterone enanthate or testosterone-cypionate 100 mg weekly for 18 mo	7 ± 2% increase by bioelectrical impedance	14 ± 4% decrease in percent body fat, 13 ± 4% decrease in sc fat	Not measured
Brodsky et al. (1996)	33–57	Testosterone cypionate 3 mg/kg/2 wk for 6 mo	15% increase by DEXAscan	11% decrease in fat mass	Not measured
Wang et al. (1996)	19–60	Sublingual testosterone 5 mg three times a day for 6 mo	0.9 kg (2%) increase by DXA scan	No change in fat mass	No change in arm press, 8.7-kg increase in leg press
Snyder et al. (2000)	22–78	Transdermal testosterone patch for 12–36 mo	3.1 ± 3.3 kg increase by DXA scan	No change in fat mass	No change in isokinetic strength of knee extension
Wang et al. (2000)	19–68	Testosterone gel (50–100 mg/d) × 180 d	2.7 ± 0.3 kg increase by DXA scan	1-kg decrease in fat mass	Leg press strength increased by 11–13 kg

TESTOSTERONE REPLACEMENT INCREASES MUSCLE MASS AND MAXIMAL VOLUNTARY STRENGTH IN HEALTHY YOUNG HYPOGONADAL MEN

Over 50 yr ago, it was shown that testosterone replacement increases nitrogen retention in castrated males of several mammalian species (19), eunuchoidal men, boys before puberty, and women (20). Several more recent studies have re-examined the effects of testosterone on body composition and muscle mass in hypogonadal men in more detail (see Table 2). For instance, we administered 100 mg of testosterone enanthate weekly for 10 wk to seven hypogonadal men after a 10–12-wk washout period (6). Testosterone replacement was associated with a 4.5- to 0.6-kg ($p = 0.005$) increase in body weight caused predominately by an increase in fat-free mass, estimated from underwater weight while body fat did not change. Similar increases in fat-free mass were observed using the deuterium water dilution method. More importantly, the ratio of fat-free mass to total-body water did not change after testosterone administration, indicating that the testosterone-induced increase in apparent fat-free mass was not simply the result of water retention in excess of that associated with protein accretion. Arm and leg muscle cross-sectional areas, assessed by magnetic resonance imaging (MRI) increased significantly. Substantial increases in maximal voluntary muscle strength were also noted following treatment.

A number of other studies are in agreement that testosterone replacement, regardless of the testosterone formulation used, increases fat-free mass, although the effects of testosterone supplementation on fat mass and muscle performance remain less well established. Brodsky et al. (8) reported a 15% increase in fat-free mass and an 11% decrease in fat mass in hypogonadal men. The muscle mass of testosterone-treated, hypogonadal men, increased by 20% and accounted for 65% of the increase in fat-free mass. The muscle accretion during testosterone treatment was associated with a 56% increase in fractional muscle protein synthesis. A cyclodextrin-complexed, testosterone formulation produced a modest increase in fat-free mass (+0.9 kg) and muscle strength (+8.7 kg) in hypogonadal men (13); however, the testosterone dose used in this study was lower than the doses used in previous studies. Snyder et al. (12) recorded the changes in body composition in healthy hypogonadal men over a 3-yr period of testosterone replacement. These studies demonstrate that maximal gains in fat-free mass are achieved within 3 mo of testosterone administration and that these gains are sustained when testosterone administration is continued for up to 3 yr.

EFFECT OF SUPRAPHYSIOLOGIC DOSES OF TESTOSTERONE ON BODY COMPOSITION AND MUSCLE STRENGTH

Intense controversy persisted, until recently, with respect to the effects of supraphysiologic doses of androgenic steroids on body composition and muscle strength (3,4,21). We conducted a placebo-controlled, double-blind, randomized clinical trial to separately assess the effects of supraphysiologic doses of testosterone and resistance exercise on fat-free mass, muscle size, and strength (5). Healthy men, 19–40 yr of age, who were within 15% of their ideal body weight, were randomly assigned to one of four groups: placebo but no exercise; testosterone but no exercise; placebo plus exercise; and testosterone plus exercise. The men received 600 mg testosterone enanthate or placebo weekly for 10 wk. Serum total- and free-testosterone levels, measured 7 d after each injection, increased fivefold; these were nadir levels and serum testosterone levels at other times must have been higher. Serum LH levels were markedly suppressed in the two testosterone-treated but not the placebo-treated men, providing additional evidence of compliance. Men in the exercise groups underwent weight-lifting exercises thrice weekly; the training stimulus was standardized based on the subjects' initial 1-repetition maximum (1-RM) and the sessions were well supervised. Fat-free mass by underwater weighing, muscle size by MRI, and maximal muscle strength of the arms and legs using bench press and squat exercises were measured before and after 10 wk of treatment.

The men randomized to receive testosterone alone had greater gains in muscle size of the arm (mean ± SEM change in triceps area 13.2 ± 3.3 vs $-2.1 \pm 2.9\%$, $p < 0.05$) and leg (change in quadriceps area 6.5 ± 1.3 vs $-1.0 \pm 1.1\%$, $p < 0.05$), than those who received placebo injections. Testosterone treatment was also associated with greater gains in strength in the bench press (increase 10 ± 4 vs $-1 \pm 2\%$, $p < 0.05$) and squat exercise capacity (increase 19 ± 6 vs $3 \pm 1\%$, $p < 0.05$) compared to placebo injections. The effects of testosterone and exercise were additive, resulting in greater increase in fat-free mass ($+9.5 \pm 1.0\%$), and muscle size ($+14.7 \pm 3.1\%$ in triceps area and $+14.1 \pm 1.3\%$ in quadriceps area) compared to either placebo or exercise alone, and greater gains in muscle strength ($+24 \pm 3\%$ in bench press strength, and $+39 \pm 4\%$ in squat exercise capacity) than either nonexercising group. Serum prostate-specific antigen (PSA) levels did not change during treatment and no abnormalities in the prostate were detected on digital rectal examination during the 10-wk treatment period. These results demonstrate that supraphysiologic doses of testosterone, especially when combined with strength training, increase fat-free mass, muscle size, and strength in healthy men.

Griggs et al. (22) administered testosterone enanthate at a dose of 3 mg/kg/wk to healthy men, 19–40 yr of age. This was an open-label study that was not placebo controlled. Muscle mass, estimated from creatinine excretion, increased by 20% and potassium-40 (^{40}K) mass increased 12% after 12 wk of testosterone treatment. In a separate study, a similar dose of testosterone enanthate was given to men with muscular dystrophy for a period of 12 mo. There was an associated 4.9-kg increase in lean body mass (approx 10%) at 3 mo that was maintained for 12 mo (23).

Young et al. (24) examined fat-free mass by dual-energy X-ray absorptiometry (DEXA) scan in 13 nonathletic men treated with 200 mg testosterone enanthate weekly for 6 mo during the course of a male contraceptive study. This was an open-label study that included untreated men as controls. Testosterone treatment increased serum testosterone levels by 90% and was associated with a 9.6% increase in fat-free mass and 16.2% decrease in fat mass.

Collectively, these data demonstrate that when dietary intake and exercise stimulus are controlled, supraphysiologic doses of testosterone produce further increases in fat-free mass and strength in eugonadal men. It is likely that strength training may augment androgen effects on the muscle.

TESTOSTERONE DOSE–RESPONSE RELATIONSHIPS IN HEALTHY YOUNG MEN

Testosterone increases muscle mass and strength and regulates other physiologic processes, but we do not know whether testosterone effects are dose dependent and whether dose requirements for maintaining various androgen-dependent processes are similar *(25–27)*. Androgen receptors in most tissues are either saturated or downregulated at physiologic testosterone concentrations *(3,25–27)*. This has led to speculation that there might be two separate dose–response curves: one in the hypogonadal range, with maximal response at low normal testosterone concentrations, and a second in supraphysiologic range, representing a separate mechanism of action *(3,28–30)*. However, testosterone dose–response relationships for a range of androgen-dependent functions in humans have not been studied.

To determine the effects of graded doses of testosterone on body composition, muscle size, strength, power, sexual and cognitive functions, PSA, plasma lipids, hemoglobin, and insulin-like growth factor 1 (IGF-1) levels, 61 eugonadal men, 18–35 yr, were randomized to one of 5 groups. Each group received monthly injections of a long-acting gonadopropin-releasing hormone (GnRH) agonist to suppress endogenous testosterone secretion, plus weekly injections of either 25, 50, 125, 300, or 600 mg testosterone enanthate for 20 wk *(29,30)*. Energy and protein intake were standardized. The administration of GnRH agonist plus graded doses of testosterone resulted in mean nadir testosterone concentrations of 253, 306, 542, 1345, and 2370 ng/dL at the 25-, 50-, 125-, 300-, and 600-mg doses, respectively. Fat-free mass increased dose-dependently in men receiving 125, 300 or 600 mg of testosterone weekly (change: +3.4, 5.2, and 7.9 kg, respectively). The changes in fat-free mass were highly dependent on testosterone dose (Figs. 1 and 2, $p = 0.0001$) and linearly correlated with both testosterone ($R = 0.69$, $p < 0.0001$) and log testosterone concentrations ($R = 0.73$, $p < 0.0001$). Changes in leg press strength, leg power, thigh and quadriceps muscle volumes, hemoglobin, and IGF-I were positively correlated with testosterone concentrations, while changes in fat mass and plasma high-density lipoprotein (HDL) cholesterol were negatively correlated (*see* Figs. 1 and 2). Sexual function, visual–spatial cognition and mood, and PSA levels did not change significantly at any dose (*see* Figs. 1 and 2). These data demonstrate that changes in circulating testosterone concentrations, induced by GnRH agonist and testosterone administration, are associated with testosterone dose- and concentration-dependent changes in fat-free mass, muscle size, strength and power, fat mass, hemoglobin, HDL cholesterol, and IGF-I levels, in conformity with a single, linear dose–response relationship. However, different androgen-dependent processes have different testosterone dose–response relationships.

MECHANISMS OF TESTOSTERONE'S ANABOLIC EFFECTS ON THE MUSCLE

The prevalent view that testosterone produces muscle hypertrophy by increasing fractional muscle protein synthesis *(8,31)* is supported by a number of studies. However, as discussed in this section, recent observations suggest that increase in muscle protein synthesis probably occurs as a secondary event and may not be the sole or the primary mechanism by which testosterone induces muscle hypertrophy *(32)*.

Testosterone Supplementation Increases Satellite Cells in the Muscle of Healthy Young Men

In order to determine whether the testosterone-induced increase in muscle size is the result of muscle fiber hypertrophy or hyperplasia, muscle biopsies were obtained from

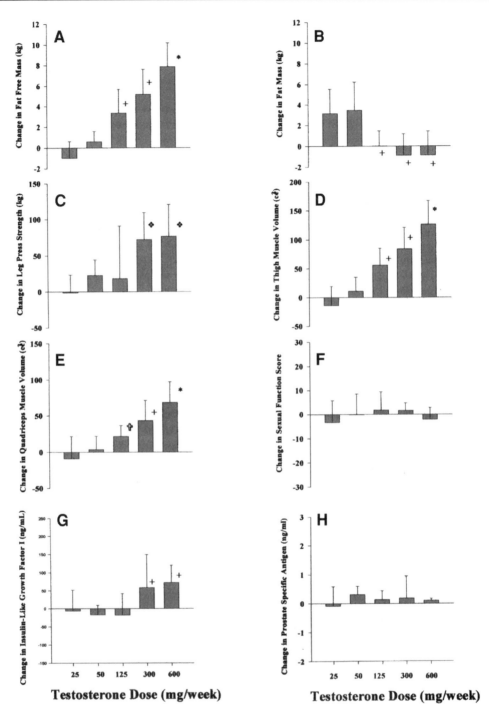

Fig. 1. Change in fat-free mass (**A**), fat mass (**B**), leg press strength (**C**), thigh muscle volume (**D**), quadriceps muscle volume (**E**), sexual function (**F**), IGF-I (**G**), and PSA (**H**). Data are mean ± SEM. The asterisk denotes significant differences from all other groups ($p < 0.05$); ❖ denotes significant difference from 25-, 50-, and 125-mg doses ($p < 0.05$); + denotes significant difference from 25- and 50-mg doses ($p < 0.05$); and ✝ denotes significant difference from the 25-mg dose ($p < 0.05$). (From ref. *29*; reproduced with permission.)

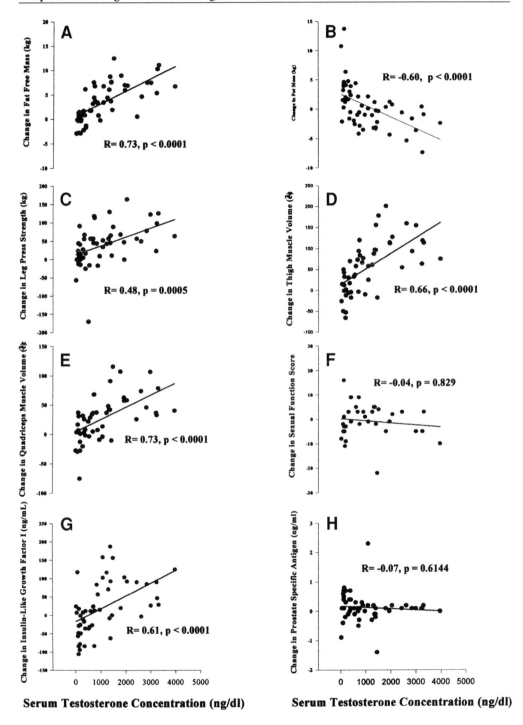

Fig. 2. Relationship between serum testosterone concentrations (*T*) during treatment (wk 16) and change in fat-free mass (**A**), fat mass (**B**), leg press strength (**C**), thigh muscle volume (**D**), quadriceps muscle volume (**E**), sexual function (**F**), IGF-I (**G**), and PSA (**H**). The correlation coefficient, *R*, was calculated using the logarithmic model, $Y = a + b\,X$, where $X = \log(T)$ and *a* and *b* represent the intercept and slope, respectively. (From ref. *29*, reproduced with permission.)

the vastus lateralis in 39 men before and after 20 wk of combined treatment with GnRH agonist and weekly injections of either 25, 50, 125, 300, or 600 mg testosterone enanthate *(32)*. Graded doses of testosterone administration were associated with testosterone dose and concentration-dependent increase in muscle fiber cross-sectional area. Changes in cross-sectional areas of both type I and II fibers were dependent on testosterone dose and significantly correlated with total-testosterone ($R = 0.35$ and 0.44, $p < 0.0001$ for type I and II fibers, respectively) and ($R = 0.34$ and 0.35, $p < 0.005$) free-testosterone concentrations during treatment. The men receiving 300 and 600 mg of testosterone enanthate (TE) weekly experienced significant increases from baseline in type I fiber area (baseline vs 20 wk, 3176 ± 163 vs 4201 ± 163 μm^2, $p < 0.05$ at a 300-mg dose, and 3347 ± 253 vs 4984 ± 374 μm^2, $p = 0.006$ at a 600-mg dose); the men in the 600-mg group also had significant increments in cross-sectional area of their type II fibers (4060 ± 401 vs 5526 ± 544 μm^2, $p = 0.03$). The relative proportions of type I and type II fibers did not change significantly after treatment in any group. The myonuclear number per fiber increased significantly in men receiving the 300- and 600-mg doses of TE and was significantly correlated with testosterone concentration and muscle fiber cross-sectional area *(32)*. These data demonstrate that increases in muscle volume in healthy eugonadal men treated with graded doses of testosterone are associated with concentration-dependent increases in muscle fiber cross-sectional area and myonulcear number, but not muscle fiber number. We conclude that the testosterone-induced increase in muscle volume is the result of muscle fiber hypertrophy. In our study, the myonuclear number increased in direct relation to the increase in muscle fiber diameter *(32)*. Because myonuclei in muscle fibers are derived from fusion of satellite cells, it is likely that the increase in myonuclear number was preceded by testosterone-induced increase in satellite cell number and their fusion with muscle fibers. There is substantial evidence supporting a role for the modulation of myonuclear number during muscle remodeling in response to injury or disease *(33–35)*. Satellite cells are cells of the myogenic lineage that are located inside the basilar lamina but outside the sarcolemma and retain the potential for cell replication in response to muscle injury or other appropriate stimuli. The hypertrophy of the levator ani muscle in the female rat, induced by exogenous testosterone administration, is indeed associated with satellite cell proliferation *(35)*. Muscle remodeling and repair following injury often involve satellite cell replication and recruitment of new stem cells into the myogenic cell lineage *(34–36)*. The mechanisms by which testosterone might increase satellite cell number are not known. An increase in satellite cell number could occur by an increase in satellite cell replication, inhibition of satellite cell apoptosis, and/or increased differentiation of stem cells into the myogenic lineage. We do not know which of these processes is the site of regulation by testosterone. The hypothesis that testosterone promotes muscle fiber hypertrophy by increasing the number of satellite cells should be further tested. Because of the constraints inherent in obtaining multiple biopsy specimens in humans, the effects of testosterone on satellite cell replication and stem cell recruitment would be more conveniently studied in an animal model.

The molecular mechanisms that mediate androgen-induced muscle hypertrophy are not well understood. Urban et al. *(31)* have proposed that testosterone stimulates the expression of IGF-1 and downregulates insulin-like growth factor binding protein-4 (IGFBP-4) in the muscle. Reciprocal changes in IGF-1 and its binding protein thus provide a potential mechanism for amplifying the anabolic signal.

It is not clear whether the anabolic effects of supraphysiologic doses of testosterone are mediated through an androgen-receptor-mediated mechanism. In vitro binding studies *(37)* suggest that the maximum effects of testosterone should be manifest at about 300 ng/dL (i.e., serum testosterone levels that are at the lower end of the normal male range). Therefore, it is possible that the supraphysiologic doses of androgen produce muscle hypertrophy through androgen-receptor-independent mechanisms, such as through an antiglucocorticoid effect *(38)*. We cannot exclude the possibility that some androgen effects may be mediated through nonclassical binding sites. Testosterone effects on the muscle are modulated by a number of other factors such as the genetic background, growth hormone secretory status *(39)*, nutrition, exercise, cytokines, thyroid hormones, and glucocorticoids. Testosterone may also affect muscle function through its effects on neuromuscular transmission *(40–41)*.

The Role of 5-α-Reduction of Testosterone in the Muscle

Although the enzyme 5-α-reductase is expressed at low concentrations within the muscle *(42)*, we do not know whether conversion of testosterone to dihydrotestosterone is required for mediating the androgen effects on the muscle. Men with benign prostatic hypertrophy who are treated with the 5-α-reductase inhibitor do not experience muscle loss. Similarly, individuals with congenital 5-α-reductase deficiency have normal muscle development at puberty. These data suggest that 5-α-reduction of testosterone is not obligatory for mediating its anabolic effects on the muscle. Because testosterone effects on the prostate require its obligatory conversion to dihydrotestosterone (DHT), selective androgen-receptor modulators that bind the androgen receptor, but are not 5-α-reduced would be very attractive. Such agents could achieve the desired anabolic effects on the muscle without the undesirable effects on the prostate.

Sattler et al. *(43)* have reported that serum DHT levels are lower and testosterone to DHT levels are higher in human immunodeficiency virus (HIV)-infected men compared to healthy men. These investigators have proposed that a defect in testosterone to DHT conversion may contribute to wasting in a subset of HIV-infected men. If this hypothesis were true, then it would be rational to treat such patients with DHT rather than testosterone. A DHT gel is currently under clinical investigation. However, unlike testosterone, DHT is not aromatized to estradiol. Therefore, there is concern that suppression of endogenous testosterone and estradiol production by exogenous DHT may produce osteoporosis.

USE OF TESTOSTERONE AS AN ANABOLIC THERAPY IN SARCOPENIA ASSOCIATED WITH CHRONIC ILLNESS AND AGING

In many chronic illnesses, including HIV, end-stage renal disease, chronic obstructive lung disease, and some types of cancer, we can now achieve disease stability but not cure. In these chronic disorders, muscle wasting occurs frequently and is associated with debility, impaired quality of life, and poor disease outcome. Similarly, as men grow older, their muscle mass decreases and fat mass increases in association with a decline in testosterone levels. Therefore, strategies that can reverse muscle wasting and augment muscle function may reduce the burden of disease, improve quality of life, and reduce utilization of health care resources.

A number of placebo-controlled randomized clinical trials have demonstrated that testosterone replacement in older men with low or low normal testosterone levels

Table 3
Effects of Testosterone Supplementation in Older Men

Study	Subjects	Treatment regimen	Changes in body composition	Changes in muscle function	Comments
Tenover (1992)	60–75 yr, serum testosterone <400 ng/dL	Testosterone enanthate 100 mg weekly for 3 mo	1.8-kg increase in fat-free mass; no change in fat mass	No change in grip strength	Mild increases in PSA and hematocrit
Morley et al. (1993)	69–89 yr, bioavailable testosterone <75 ng/dL	Testosterone enanthate 200 mg every 2 wk for 3 mo	No change in fat mass or body weight	Increase in grip strength	
Sih et al. (1997)	Healthy men, 51–79 yr, serum bioavailable testosterone <60 ng/dL	Testosterone cypionate 200 mg every 2 wk for 12 mo	0.9-cm (3%) increase in mid-arm circumference, no change in fat mass	4- to 5-kg increase in grip strength	No change in PSA, increase in
Urban et al. (1995)	Healthy elderly, 67 ± 2 yr, testosterone <480 ng/dL	Testosterone enanthate weekly for 4 wk to increase testosterone to 500–1000 ng/dL	Body composition not reported	Increase in hamstring and quadriceps work per repetition; no change in endurance rate	Approximately twofold increase in fractional muscle protein synthesis
Snyder et al. (1999)	Healthy older men, >65 yr of age	Scrotal testosterone patch, 6 mg/d for 3 yr	Lean body mass increased by 1.9 kg; fat mass decreased by 3 kg	No change in strength of knee extension and flexion	Improved perception of physical function
Tenover (2000)	Healthy, older men	Testosterone enanthate, ~150 mg/2 wk for 3 yr	Fat-free mass increased and fat mass decreased	Improvements in some measures of muscle strength	
Kenny et al. (2001)	Healthy older men >65 yr, bioavailable testosterone <4.4 nmol/L	Testosterone patch 5 mg daily vs placebo × 1 yr	1-kg gain in FFM; a reduction in fat mass; no change in body mass	Improved strength in association with testosterone replacement, but not significantly greater in comparison to placebo	

increases fat-free mass and grip strength and decreases fat mass (Table 3). However, testosterone effects on objective measures of physical function and health-related outcomes have not been studied.

Of the various anabolic interventions being considered for promoting restitution of body cell mass in HIV-infected men, testosterone is particularly attractive because it is safe and relatively inexpensive. Although testosterone can increase fat-free mass and muscle strength under specific experimental paradigms, we do not know whether replacement doses of testosterone can produce clinically meaningful changes in body composition and muscle function in chronic illnesses associated with muscle wasting.

There is a high frequency of low testosterone levels in chronic illnesses associated with muscle wasting. Approximately, 20–30% of HIV-infected men have serum total- and free-testosterone levels in the hypogonadal range *(44–53)*. Twenty percent of HIV-infected men with low testosterone levels have elevated luteinizing hormone (LH) and follicle-stimulating hormone (FSH) levels and thus have hypergonadotropic hypogonadism *(44)*. The remaining 80% have either normal or low LH and FSH levels; these men with hypogonadotropic hypogonadism either have a central defect at the hypothalamic or pituitary site or a dual defect involving both the testis and the hypothalamic–pituitary centers. Similarly, there is a high frequency of hypogonadism in patients with cancer, chronic obstructive lung disease, end-stage renal disease, and liver disease.

Low testosterone levels correlate with adverse disease outcome in HIV-infected men. Serum testosterone levels are lower in HIV-infected men who have lost weight than in those who have not *(51)*. A longitudinal follow-up of HIV infected homosexual men revealed a progressive decrease in serum testosterone levels *(48)*; this decrease is much greater in HIV-infected men who progress to acquired immunodeficiency syndrome (AIDS) than in those who do not *(48)*. Serum testosterone levels decline early in the course of events that culminate in wasting *(49)*. Testosterone levels correlate with muscle mass and exercise capacity in HIV-infected men *(50)*, leading to speculation that hypogonadism may contribute to muscle wasting and debility. There is a high prevalence of sexual dysfunction in HIV-infected men *(54)*. With the increasing life expectancy of HIV-infected men, frailty and sexual dysfunction have emerged as important quality-of-life issues.

Several studies on the effects of androgen supplementation in HIV-infected men have been reported *(55–64)*; placebo-controlled studies of testosterone replacement are shown in Table 4. Most of the studies were of short duration, ranging from 12 to 24 wk. Several androgenic steroids have been studied in a limited fashion, including nandrolone decanoate, oxandrolone, oxymetholone, stanozolol, testosterone cypionate, and testosterone enanthate.

In a placebo-controlled, double-blind clinical trial, we examined the effects of physiological testosterone replacement by means of the nongenital patch *(56)*. Forty-one HIV positive men with serum testosterone level less than 400 ng/dL were randomly assigned to receive either two placebo patches nightly or two testosterone patches, designed to release 5 mg testosterone over a 24-h period. Results indicate that physiological testosterone replacement of HIV-infected men with low testosterone levels was associated with a 1.34-kg increase in lean body mass ($p = 0.02$) as well as a significantly greater reduction in fat mass than that achieved with placebo treatment alone. There were no significant changes in liver enzymes, plasma HIV–RNA copy number, and CD4 and CD8+ T-cell counts. There were no significant differences in the change in muscle strength between the two treatment groups over the 12-wk treatment duration. The

Table 4

Effects of Testosterone Supplementation in HIV-Infected Men

Study	Subjects	Treatment regimen	Changes in body composition	Changes in muscle function	Comments
Bhasin et al. (1998)	HIV-infected men with serum T <400 ng/dL	Testosterone patch (5 mg daily) vs placebo patch × 10 wk	1.3-kg gain in FFM after testosterone replacement	Strength gains in placebo and testosterone-treated men not significantly different effect	Strength measurements confounded by learning
Grinspoon et al. (1998)	HIV-infected men with AIDS wasting syndrome and free-testosterone levels <42 pmol/L	300 mg every 3 wk × 6 mo	2-kg increase in FFM; no change in fat mass	Muscle strength not measured; no change in exercise functional capacity	Testosterone-treated patients reported feeling better, improved quality of life, and appearance
Bhasin et al. (2000)	HIV-infected men with >5% weight loss and serum testosterone less than 350 ng/dL	100 mg testosterone enanthate weekly × 16 wk with or without resistance training; placebo controlled	2.9-kg gain in testosterone-treated men	Significantly greater gains in muscle strength with testosterone treatment than with placebo	
Grinspoon et al. (2001)	HIV-infected men with AIDS wasting syndrome	200 mg testosterone enanthate weekly with or without strength training; placebo controlled × 12 wk	Greater increments in muscle mass and volume in response to testosterone and resistance exercise training as compared to placebo	Strength gains not significantly greater in testosterone or resistance training groups in comparison to placebo group	
Dobs et al. (2000)	HIV-infected men with AIDS and 5–10% weight loss, and baseline testosterone <400 ng/dL or free testosterone <16 pg/mL	Testoderm 6-mg scrotal patch vs placebo patch × 12 wk	Changes in body weight or body cell mass by bioelectrical impedance not significantly different between testosterone and placebo groups	Not measured	Quality of life measure not changed
Coodley et al. (1995)	HIV-infected men with > 5% weight loss, and CD4 counts <200/cmm	Testosterone cypionate 200 mg every 2 wk × 12 wk vs placebo in a crossover design	No significant differences in change in body weight between testosterone and placebo periods	Not measured	Testosterone treatment associated with improved well-being

placebo-treated men also experienced a significant increase in muscle strength, presumably because of the learning effect. The patients in this study were recruited based on low testosterone levels and weight loss was not an entry criterion. Therefore, in a second study (57), we examined the effects of testosterone replacement with or without a program of resistance exercise in HIV-infected men who had lost at least 5% body weight. To minimize confounding because of training effect, the participants underwent several training sessions with the equipment until stability of measurement was achieved. This study demonstrated that both resistance exercise and testosterone replacement significantly increased lean body mass and effort-dependent muscle strength in HIV-infected men with weight loss (57).

Although these preliminary data in HIV-positive men (55–59) are encouraging and suggested that anabolic factors such as testosterone promote weight gain and an increase in lean body mass, most of these studies were of short duration and it remains to be seen whether physiological androgen replacement can produce sustained and meaningful reduction in the burden of disease with improvements in quality of life, utilization of health care resources, and muscle function in HIV-infected men. Testosterone treatment probably does not affect HIV titers, but its effects on virus shedding in the genital tract are not known.

Patients with autoimmune disorders, particularly those receiving glucocorticoids, often experience muscle wasting and bone loss (65–66). In a placebo-controlled study, Reid et al. (65) administered a replacement dose of testosterone to men receiving glucocorticoids. Testosterone replacement was associated with a greater increase in fat-free mass and bone density than placebo.

There is a high frequency of low total- and free-testosterone levels, sexual dysfunction, infertility, delayed puberty, and growth failure in patients with end-stage renal disease (67,68). Androgen administration does not consistently improve sexual dysfunction in these patients. Similarly, the effects of androgen treatment on growth and pubertal development in children with end-stage renal disease remain unclear (69,70). Controlled clinical trials of nandrolone decanoate (71–74) have reported increased hemoglobin levels with androgen treatment of men with end-stage renal disease who are on hemodialysis. Testosterone increases red cell production by stimulating erythropoieitin and by augmenting erythropoieitin action. Further studies are needed to determine whether testosterone administration can reduce blood transfusion and erythropoieitin requirements in patients with end-stage renal disease on hemodialysis. A recent placebo-controlled study (73) demonstrated that nandrolone administration in men on hemodialysis is associated with greater grains in fat-free mass, muscle strength, and hemoglobin levels in patients on hemodialysis than those associated with placebo administration.

HETEROGENEITY IN RESPONSE AND PREDICTORS OF ANABOLIC RESPONSE TO ANDROGEN ADMINISTRATION

Although testosterone supplementation increases fat-free mass and muscle size in healthy, hypogonadal men (6–10), HIV-infected men with low testosterone levels (55–61), and older men with low testosterone levels (11,31,75–79), there are striking qualitative and quantitative differences in the anabolic response to testosterone administration among different reports. Of the six, placebo-controlled clinical trials of testosterone administration in HIV-infected men (56–61), two found no significant differences in the change in fat-free mass between the placebo- and testosterone-treated men. The magnitude of gains in fat-free mass also varied considerably among the studies that did show significant gains in lean body mass during androgen administration (56,57,60,61). In one study (56) in which HIV-infected men with low testosterone levels were treated with placebo or testosterone patches, the mean gain in fat-free mass in testosterone-treated men was 1.3 kg, whereas in another study (57), administration of 100 mg testosterone enanthate weekly was associated with a mean 2.9-kg gain in fat-free mass.

Studies of testosterone supplementation in older men have demonstrated similar variability in results (11,31,75–79). Although Sih et al. (75) reported no significant gains in fat-free mass during testosterone administration, others (11,76,77) found greater gains in older men treated with testosterone than in those treated with placebo. These data are similar to anecdotal reports that athletes using androgenic steroids differ significantly in their anabolic response to these agents. We do not know whether the differences in the results of these studies in HIV-infected men and older men are the result of differences in testosterone dose, the baseline characteristics of the subjects, or the methods of body composition assessment.

The magnitude of gain in fat-free mass in healthy hypogonadal men after testosterone replacement has also varied considerably in different reports (6–10,12); these reports differ from one another in testosterone dose, patient's age and pretreatment body composition, duration of washout prior to initiation of testosterone replacement, pubertal status, and methods of body composition assessment. For instance, the studies that included relatively young, lean hypogonadal men (6) have demonstrated greater increments in fat-free mass than those that included older men (12–14). Empiric experience indicates that prepubertal or peripubertal boys experience greater increments in fat-free mass when given testosterone replacement than postpubertal men. Similarly, in hypogonadal men who have been on stable testosterone-replacement therapy, the gains in muscle mass after reinitiation of testosterone therapy may be modest if the washout period is insufficient to restore the body composition to its androgen-deficient status.

We sought to determine whether testosterone dose, steady-state testosterone concentrations, and/or subject characteristics could be used to predict anabolic response, defined as the change in FFM (by DEXA) during testosterone (T) treatment. In our testosterone dose–response study (29), increasing doses of TE were associated with dose-dependent changes in serum total- and free-T concentrations, FFM, and muscle size. Of the models tested, a linear model best described the relationship between T dose and steady-state concentrations. However, despite the high degree of overall correlation between T dose and changes in FFM and muscle size, there was considerable heterogeneity in individual responses to a given T dose. Multiple regression analysis was used to identify the subset of baseline measures that best predicted change in total-body lean body mass (by DEXA) and thigh muscle volume (by MRI), age, testosterone dose administered, measures of body composition (including weight, height, body mass index, total-body fat and lean body mass, measures of leg muscle performance (leg press strength, power, and local muscular endurance), measures of skeletal muscle morphometry (mean fiber area and fiber type from biopsies of the vastus lateralis musculature), serum hormone concentrations (total and free testosterone, sex hormone-binding globulin [SHBG], LH, LH/T and log[LH/T] ratios, and FSH), concentrations of IGF-1 and its binding protein IGFBP-3, lipid profile including triglycerides, high-density (HDL) and low-density (LDL) lipoprotein levels, blood counts (hematocrit [Hct] and hemoglobin [HGB]), PSA levels, and genetic factors, including polymorphisms in exon 1 of the androgen-receptor gene (i.e., lengths of the polyglutamine : CAG and polyglycine : GGC trinucleotide tracts). The same two-variable model of TE dose and age explained 77% and 70% of the variance in change in lean body mass (by DEXA) and thigh muscle volume (MRI), respectively, during testosterone administration. The length of CAG and GGC tracts were only weak predictors of change in LBM and muscle volume in this small sample. These analyses indicate that the anabolic response of healthy young men to exogenous testosterone administration is largely predicted by the testosterone dose. Further studies are needed in a larger sample of men to elucidate the genetic basis of natural variation in androgen responsiveness.

TESTOSTERONE EFFECTS ON FAT METABOLISM

Percent body fat is higher in hypogonadal men *(15)*. Induction of androgen deficiency in healthy men by administration of a GnRH agonist leads to an increase in fat mass *(18)*. Some studies of young hypogonadal men have reported a decrease in fat mass with testosterone-replacement therapy *(8,10)* whereas others *(6,13)* found no change. In contrast, long-term studies of testosterone supplementation of older men have consistently demonstrated a decrease in fat mass *(11)*. Epidemiologic studies *(16,17)* have shown that serum testosterone levels are lower in middle-aged men with visceral obesity than age-matched controls. Serum testosterone levels correlate inversely with visceral fat mass and directly with plasma HDL levels. Testosterone replacement in middle-aged men with visceral obesity improves insulin sensitivity and decreases blood glucose and blood pressure *(80,81)*. Testosterone is an important determinant of regional fat distribution and metabolism in men *(80,82)*. Therefore, it has been hypothesized that testosterone supplementation might be beneficial in HIV-infected men with fat-redistribution syndromes; this hypothesis is being tested in ongoing studies in HIV-infected men with HIV-associated visceral obesity.

THE ABUSE OF ANDROGENIC STEROIDS
BY ATHLETES AND RECREATIONAL BODYBUILDERS

Use of Andogenic Steroids by Athletes and Recreational Bodybuilders Is Widespread

The historical aspects of the use of androgenic/anabolic steroids have been extensively reviewed *(1–4)*. Although their use is most common among weight lifters and heavy throwers, almost all types of athlete whose event requires explosive strength or power, including football players, swimmers, and track and field athletes, have been known to use steroids *(1–4)*. Their use has spread to high school athletes and to amateur bodybuilders. Disqualification of highly celebrated athletes like Ben Johnson and some members of the Chinese swim team has focused considerable media attention on this issue. The recreational bodybuilders and occupational users, including policemen and prison wardens, are the other groups with high prevalence of androgenic steroid use *(1–4,83–85)*. Pope et al. *(86)* have pointed out that because of the pressures exerted by extraordinary dimensions assumed by our superheroes and figures, body dysmorphia has become a significant clinical problem for young men. In his recent book, *Adonis*

Complex, Pope et al. *(86)* point out that superheroes of the current times are far more hypermuscular than those of 50 yr ago. The chiseled and rippled hypermuscularity associated with superheroes and male models creates unrealistic expectations of a body image that is unlikely to be achieved by most healthy men. Therefore, it is not surprising that many healthy young men, in their desire to attain improbable body composition and proportions, feel an enormous pressure to use bodybuilding drugs. Since 1986, anabolic steroids have been the most frequently detected substance found in screening tests of competitive athletes *(1)*. A survey of school children in England revealed that anabolic steroids were the third most commonly offered drug to school children, behind marijuana and amphetamines *(2,83,84)*. In another survey, 6.6% of 12th-grade male students had used and were using anabolic steroids *(85)*. Korkia and Stimson *(84)* found 5% of gym users in the United Kingdom to be using anabolic steroids.

Effects of Androgens on Athletic Performance

There is agreement that testosterone supplementation increases maximal voluntary strength but that it does not improve specific tension (force produced per unit of muscle mass). Therefore, testosterone would be expected to improve performance in weight-lifting events because performance in these events is critically dependent on absolute maximal voluntary strength. It is not surprising that the abuse of androgenic steroids is most prevalent among power lifters. The effects of testosterone on other measures of muscle performance such as fatigability and power (the rate of force generation) are unknown. Previous studies have failed to demonstrate any improvements in performance in endurance events *(78)*. The abuse of androgenic steroids by sprint runners or swimmers is therefore surprising. It is possible that testosterone might improve athletic performance in sprint events by decreasing reaction time, as testosterone has been shown to regulate neuromuscular transmission *(40,41)*. Others have proposed that testosterone use might enhance recovery from exercise, thus allowing the athletes to train harder. This speculation has not been tested, and unequivocal improvements in measures of athletic performance have not been demonstrated in any study.

Detection of Androgenic Steroid Use

Many sports organizations, including the International Olympic Committee, the US Olympic Committee, and the National Collegiate Athletic Association, have implemented screening programs based on urine testing *(87)*. The analysis of urinary steroids by gas chromatography–mass spectrometry has been an effective but not foolproof method for majority of anabolic steroids. However, the detection of exogenous testosterone abuse has been a particularly difficult problem. Several methods have been explored for the screening of exogenous testosterone abuse, including the measurement of testosterone-to-epitestosterone (T : E) ratio, LH-to-testosterone ratio and, more recently, the use of the carbon isotope ratio method *(87–89)*. In healthy men, the ratio of testosterone to epitestosterone is typically 1; less than 0.8% of healthy men not using exogenous androgen will have a ratio of greater than 6 *(87,90)*. Therefore, the Medical Commission of the International Olympic Committee in 1982 adapted a T : E ratio of greater than 6 as evidence of exogenous testosterone use *(87,90)*. There are several problems associated with the use of this screening criterion. There are ethnic differences in testosterone-to-epitestosterone ratio, and some individuals have high T : E ratio even without exogenous testosterone use. Furthermore, the athletes have started

spiking urine with epitestosterone to evade detection. Therefore, a urinary epitestosterone concentration greater than 150 µg/L should be viewed suspiciously *(91,92)*.
The T : E ratio should decline to 1 on repeated testing of urine if the athlete discon-
tinues steroid use; in contrast, the high T : E ratio persists in individuals who have a
naturally increased T : E ratio. Because exogenous testosterone suppresses LH excretion more than it suppresses testosterone and epitestosterone excretion, the measurement of T-to-LH ratios in the urine has been suggested as an additional, confirmatory
test. Perry et al. *(92)* reported that a urinary T-to-LH ratio of greater than 30 is a more
sensitive marker of anabolic steroid use than the T : E ratio, and it remains positive for
a longer period than the urinary T : E ratio.

Most recently, Aguilera et al. *(89)* have validated the use of carbon isotope ratio method
to determine whether the urinary steroids are of endogenous or pharmaceutical origin. The
androgenic steroids synthesized for pharmaceutical use are obtained from starting materials such as diosgenin and stigmasterol, which are derived from plants. These plant-
derived compounds have less carbon-13 (^{13}C) than their endogenous homologs in humans;
therefore, the ^{13}C-to-^{12}C ratio in steroids of pharmaceutical origin is less than that in
endogenous human steroids. The ^{13}C value of steroids extracted from urine can be determined by gas chromatography–combustion–isotope mass spectrometry (GC-C-IRMS).
Aguilera et al. *(89)* have demonstrated that a GC-C-IRMS assay of urinary diols has
acceptable within-assay and between-assay coefficients of variation and is an accurate
method for detecting doping. It can be particularly effective in individuals who have high
T : E ratios in determining whether high T : E ratio is the result of natural variations in
steroid metabolism or the administration of exogenous steroid *(89)*.

In recent years, a variety of xenobiotic steroids such as androstenedione and
dehydroepiandrosterone (DHEA) have become widely available through nutrition and
health food stores. Their urinary metabolites can confound the results of the tests in
unexpected ways. Several reports have suggested that the use of these dietary supple-
ments can cause positive urine tests for metabolites of nandrolone *(88)*.

In spite of the implementation of screening programs, the use of performance-
enhancing drugs in competitive sports has not decreased. The failure of these efforts to
stem the growing use of these illicit compounds is the result of a confluence of several
factors: the extraordinary motivation of the competitive athlete to go to extreme lengths
to maximize the chances of winning, the covert involvement of the national Olympic
organizations, the ambivalent attitudes of the academic community and society at large
toward the use of these compounds, and the enormous cultural pressures to attain an
unrealistic body image.

SUMMARY

It is ironic that many dogmas about the effects of androgenic steroids on the muscle,
held sacred by the academic community for over three decades, have not held up in the
face of rigorous investigation. In contrast, many of the empiric beliefs and observations
of the sports medicine community have turned out to be true. Undoubtedly, testosterone
supplementation is associated with increase in muscle mass, size, and maximal voluntary strength in healthy hypogonadal men, older men with low testosterone levels, and
in men with chronic illness. However, we do not know whether testosterone-induced
increase in muscle mass will translate into clinically meaningful improvements in physical function, balance, quality of life, or other disease outcomes, or whether these changes

will reduce the risk of disability or falls. The mechanisms of testosterone's anabolic action on the muscle are not well understood, but likely involve muscle fiber hypertrophy and increases in myonuclear number and satellite cell number. The molecular basis of androgen effects on satellite cells requires further investigation.

REFERENCES

1. Verroken M. Ethical aspects and the prevalence of hormone abuse in sport. J Endocrinol 2001;170: 49–54.
2. Dawson RT. Drugs in sport - the role of the physician. J Endocrinol 2001;170:55–61.
3. Wilson JD. Androgen abuse by athletes. Endocr Rev 1988;9:181–199.
4. Bardin CW. The anabolic action of testosterone. N Engl J Med 1996;335:52–53.
5. Bhasin S, Storer TW, Berman N, et al. The effects of supraphysiologic doses of testosterone on muscle size and strength in men. N Engl J Med 1996;335:1–7.
6. Bhasin S, Storer TW, Berman N, et al. A replacement dose of testosterone increases fat-free mass and muscle size in hypogonadal men. J Clin Endocrinol Metab 1997;82:407–413.
7. Bhasin S, Woodhouse L, Storer TW. The proof of androgen action on the muscle. J Endocrinol 2001; 170:71–76.
8. Brodsky IG, Balagopal P, Nair KS. Effects of testosterone replacement on muscle mass and muscle protein synthesis in hypogonadal men-a Clinical Research Center Study. J Clin Endocrinol Metab 1996;81:3469–3475.
9. Bross R, Casaburi R, Storer TW, Bhasin S. Androgen effects on body composition and muscle function: implications for the use of androgens as anabolic agents in sarcopenic states. Baillieres Clin Endocrinol Metab 1998;12:365–378.
10. Katznelson L, Finkelstein JS, Schoenfeld DA, et al. Increase in bone density and lean body mass during testosterone administration in men with acquired hypogonadism. J Clin Endocrinol Metab 1996;81: 4358–4365.
11. Snyder PJ, Peachey H, Hannoush P, et al. Effect of testosterone treatment on body composition and muscle strength in men over 65. J Clin Endocrinol Metab 1999;84:2647–2653.
12. Snyder PJ, Peachey H, Berlin JA, et al. Effects of testosterone replacement in hypogonadal men. J Clin Endocrinol Metab 2000;85:2670–2677.
13. Wang C, Eyre DR, Clark R, et al. Sublingual testosterone replacement improves muscle mass and strength, decreases bone resorption, and increases bone resorption markers in hypogonadal men—a Clinical Research Center Study. J Clin Endocrinol Metab 1996;81:3654–3662.
14. Wang C, Swerdloff RS, Iranmanesh A, et al. Transdermal testosterone gel improves sexual function, mood, muscle strength, and body composition parameters in hypogonadal men. Testosterone Gel Study Group. J Clin Endocrinol Metab 2000;85:2839–2853.
15. Katznelson L, Rosenthal DI, Rosol MS, et al. Using quantitative CT to assess adipose distribution in adult men with acquired hypogonadism. Am J Roentgenol 1998;170:423–427.
16. Seidell J, Bjorntorp P, Sjostrom L, et al. Visceral fat accumulation in men is positively associated with insulin, glucose and C-peptide levels, but negatively with testosterone levels. Metabolism 1990;39: 897–901.
17. Barrett-Connors E, Khaw K-T. Endogenous sex-hormones and cardiovascular disease in men. A prospective population-based study Circulation 1988;78:539–545.
18. Mauras N, Hayes V, Welch S, et al. Testosterone deficiency in young men: marked alterations in whole body protein kinetics, strength and adiposity. J Clin Endocrinol Metab 1998;83:1886–1892.
19. Kochakian CD. Comparison of protein anabolic properties of various androgens in the castrated rat. Am J Physiol 1950;60:553–558.
20. Kenyon AT, Knowlton K, Sandiford I, et al. A comparative study of the metabolic effects of testosterone propionate in normal men and women and in eunuchoidism. Endocrinology 1940;26: 26–45.
21. Casaburi R, Storer T, Bhasin S. Androgen effects on body composition and muscle performance. In: Bhasin S, Gabelnick H, Spieler JM, et al., eds. Pharmacology, Biology, and Clinical Applications of Androgens: Current Status and Future Prospects. Wiley-Liss, New York, 1996, pp. 283–288.
22. Griggs RC, Kingston W, Josefowicz RF, et al. Effect of testosterone on muscle mass and muscle protein synthesis. J Appl Physiol 1989;66:498–503.

23. Griggs RC, Pandya S, Florence JM, et al. Randomized controlled trial of testosterone in myotonic dystrophy. Neurology 1989;39:219–222.
24. Young NR, Baker HWG, Liu G, Seeman E. Body composition and muscle strength in healthy men receiving testosterone enanthate for contraception. J Clin Endocrinol Metab 1993;77:1028–1032.
25. Antonio J, Wilson JD, George FW. Effects of castration and androgen treatment on androgen-receptor levels in rat skeletal muscles. J App Physiol 1999;87:2016–2019.
26. Dahlberg E, Snochowski M, Gustafsson JA. Regulation of the androgen and glucocorticoid receptors in rat and mouse skeletal muscle cytosol. Endocrinology 1981;108:1431–1440.
27. Rance NE, Max SR. Modulation of the cytosolic androgen receptor in striated muscle by sex steroids. Endocrinology 1984;115:862–866.
28. Bhasin S. The dose-dependent effects of testosterone on sexual function and on muscle mass and function. Mayo Clin Proc 2000;75(Suppl):S70–S75.
29. Bhasin S., Woodhouse L, Casaburi R, et al. Testosterone dose response relationships in healthy young men. Am J Physiol (Endo Metab) 2001;281:E1172–R1181.
30. Singh AB, Hsia S, Alaupovic P, et al. The effects of varying doses of T on insulin sensitivity, plasma lipids, apolipoproteins, and C-reactive protein in healthy young men. J Clin Endocrinol Metab 2002;87(1):136–143.
31. Urban RJ, Bodenburg YH, Gilkison C, et al.Testosterone administration to elderly men increases skeletal muscle strength and protein synthesis. Am J Physiol 1995;269:E820–E826.
32. Sinha-Hikim I, Artaza J, Woodhouse L, et al. Testosterone-induced increase in muscle size in healthy, young men is associated with muscle fiber hypertrophy. Am J Physiol (Endo Metab) 2002; 283:E154–E164.
33. Allen DL, Roy RR, Edgerton VR. Myonuclear domains in muscle adaptation and disease Muscle Nerve 1999;22:1350–1360.
34. Kadi F, Thornell LE. Concomitant increases in myonuclear and satellite cell content in female trapezius muscle following strength training. Histochem Cell Biol 2000;113:99–103.
35. Nnodim J. Testosterone mediates satellite cell activation in denervated rat levator ani muscle. Anat Rec 2001;263:19–24.
36. Reimann J, Irintchev A, Wering A. (2000) Regenerative capacity and the number of satellite cells in soleus muscles of normal and mdx mice. Neuromusc Disord 2000;10:276–282.
37. Saartok T, Dahlberg E, Gustaffsson JA. Relative binding affinity of anabolic-androgenic steroids, comparison of the binding to the androgen receptors in skeletal muscle and in prostate as well as sex hormone binding globulin. Endocrinology 1984;114:2100–2107.
38. Konagaya M, Max SR. A possible role for endogenous glucocorticoid in orchiectomy-induced atrophy of the rat levator ani muscle: studies with RU38486, a potent glucocorticoid antagonist. J Steroid Biochem 1986;25:305–311.
39. Fryburg DA, Weltman A, Jahn LA, et al. Short-term modulation of the androgen milieu alters pulsatile, but not exercise- or growth hormone (GH)-releasing hormone-stimulated GH secretion in healthy men: impact of gonadal steroid and GH secretory changes on metabolic outcomes. J Clin Endocrinol Metab 1997;82:3710–3719.
40. Leslie M, Forger NG & Breedlove SM. Sexual dimorphism and androgen effects on spinal motoneurons innervating the rat flexor digitorum brevis. Brain Res 1991;561:269–273.
41. Blanco CE, Popper P, Micevych P. Anabolic-androgenic steroid induced alterations in choline acetyltransferase messenger RNA levels of spinal cord motoneurons in the male rat. Neuroscience 1997;78:973–882.
42. Bartsch W, Krieg M, Voigt KD. Quantitation of endogenous testosterone, 5-alpha-dihydrotest-osterone and 5-alpha-androstane-3-alpha, 17-beta-diol in subcellular fractions of the prostate, bulbocavernosus/levator ani muscle, skeletal muscle, and heart muscle of the rat. J Steroid Biochem 1980;13:259–267.
43. Sattler FR, Antonipillai I, Allen J, Horton R. Wasting and sex hormones: evidence for the role of dihydrotestosterone in AIDS patients with weight loss. XI International Conference on AIDS, 1996, abstract Tu.B.2376.
44. Arver S, Sinha-Hikim I, Beall G, et al. Serum dihydrotestosterone and testosterone concentrations in human immunodeficiency virus-infected men with and without weight loss. J Androl 1999;20:611–618.
45. Rietschel P, Corcoran C, Stanley T, et al. Prevalence of hypogonadism among men with weight loss related to human immunodeficiency virus infection who were receiving highly active antiretroviral therapy. Clin Infect Dis 2000;31:1240–1244.

46. Salehian B, Jacobson D, Grafe M, et al. Pituitary-testicular axis during HIV infection: a prospective study. 18th Annual Meeting of the American Society of Andrology, 1993.
47. Laudat A, Blum L, Guechot J, et al. Changes in systemic gonadal and adrenal steroids in asymptomatic human immunodeficiency virus-infected men: relationship with the CD4 cell counts. Eur J Endocrinol 1995;133:418–424.
48. Dobs AS, Few WL 3rd, Blackman MR, et al. Serum hormones in men with human immunodeficiency virus-associated wasting. J Clin Endocrinol Metab 1996;81:4108–4112.
49. Dobs AS, Dempsey MA, Ladenson PW, Polk BF. Endocrine disorders in men infected with human immunodeficiency virus. Am J Med 1988;84:611–616.
50. Grinspoon S, Corcoran C, Lee K, et al. Loss of lean body and muscle mass correlates with androgen levels in hypogonadal men with acquired immunodeficiency syndrome and wasting. J Clin Endocrinol Metab 1996;81:4051–4058.
51. Coodley GO, Loveless MO, Nelson HD, Coodley MK. Endocrine function in the HIV wasting syndrome. [see comments]. J Acquired Immune Defic Syndrome 1994;7:46–51.
52. Raffi F, Brisseau JM, Planchon B, et al. Endocrine function in 98 HIV-infected patients: a prospective study. AIDS 1991;5:729–733.
53. Sellmeyer DE, Grunfeld C. Endocrine and metabolic disturbances in human immunodeficiency virus infection and the acquired immune deficiency syndrome. Endocr Rev 1996;17:518–532
54. Newshan G, Taylor B, Gold R. Sexual functioning in ambulatory men with HIV/AIDS. Int J STD AIDS 1998;9:672–676.
55. Bhasin S, Javanbakht M. Can androgen therapy replete lean body mass and improve muscle function in wasting associated with human immunodeficiency virus infection? J Parenteral Enteral Nutr 1999;23:S195–S201.
56. Bhasin S, Storer TW, Asbel-Sethi N, et al. Effects of testosterone replacement with a non-genital, transdermal system, Androderm, in human immunodeficiency virus-infected men with low testosterone levels. J Clin Endocrinol Metab 1998;83:3155–3162.
57. Bhasin S, Storer TW, Javanbakht M, et al. Effects of testosterone replacement and resistance exercise on muscle strength, and body composition in human immunodeficiency virus-infected men with weight loss and low testosterone levels. JAMA 2000;283:763–770.
58. Dobs AS, Cofrancesco J, Nolten WE, et al. The use of a transscrotal testosterone delivery system in the treatment of patients with weight loss related to human immunodeficiency virus infection. Am J Med 1999;107:126–132.
59. Coodley GO, Coodley MK. A trial of testosterone therapy for HIV-associated weight loss. AIDS 1997;11:1347–1352.
60. Grinspoon S, Corcoran C, Askari H, et al. Effects of androgen administration in men with the AIDS wasting syndrome: a randomized, double-blind, placebo-controlled trial. Ann Intern Med 1998; 129:18–26.
61. Grinspoon S, Corcoran C, Parlman K, et al. Effects of testosterone and progressive resistance training in eugonadal men with AIDS wasting. A randomized, controlled trial. Ann Intern Med 2000;133(5): 348–355.
62. Sattler FR, Jaque SV, Schroeder ET, et al. Effect of pharmacological doses of nandrolone decanoate and progressive resistance training in immunodeficient patients infected with the human immunodeficiency virus. J Clin Endocrinol Metab 1999;84:1268–1276.
63. Strawford A, Barbieri T, Neese R, et al. Effects of nandrolone decanoate therapy in borderline hypogonadal men with HIV-associated weight loss. J Acquired Immune Defic Syndromes Hum Retrovirol 1999;20:137–146.
64. Strawford A, Barbieri T, Van Loan M, et al. Resistance exercise and supraphysiologic androgen therapy in eugonadal men with HIV-related weight loss. JAMA 1999;281:1282–1290.
65. Reid IR, Wattie DJ, Evans MC, Stapleton JP. Testosterone therapy in glucocorticoid-treated men. Arch Intern Med 1996;156:1173–1177.
66. Reid IR, Ibbertson HK, France JT, Pybus J. Plasma testosterone concentrations in asthmatic men treated with glucocorticoids. Br Med J 1985;291:574–577.
67. Handelsman DJ, Dong Q. Hypothalamic-pituitary gonadal axis in chronic renal failure. Endocrinol Metab Clin North Am 1993;22:145–161.
68. Handelsman DJ, Liu PY. Androgen therapy in chronic renal failure. Baillieres Clin Endocrinol Metab 1998;12:485–500.

69. Jones RW, El Bishti MM, Bloom SR, et al. The effects of anabolic steroids on growth, body composition, and metabolism in boys with chronic renal failure on regular hemodialysis. J Pediatr
1980;97:559–566.

70. Kassmann K M, Rappaport R, Broyer M. The short term effect of testosterone on growth in boys on
hemodialysis. Clin Nephrol 1992;37:148–154.

71. Berns JS, Rudnick MR, Cohen RM. A controlled trial of recombinant erythropoieitin and nandrolone
decanoate in the treatment of anemia in patients on chronic hemodialysis. Clin Nephrol 1992;37:
264–267.

72. Buchwald D, Argyres S, Easterling RE, et al. Effect of nandrolone decanoate on the anemia of chronic
hemodialysis patients. Nephron 1977;18:232–238.

73. Johansen KL, Mulligan K, Schambelan M. Anabolic effects of nandrolone decanoate in patients
receiving dialysis: a randomized controlled trial. [see comments]. JAMA 1999;281:1275–1281.

74. Williams JL, Stein JH, Ferris TF. Nandrolone decanoate therapy for patients receiving hemodialysis.
A controlled study. Arch Intern Med 1974;134:289–292.

75. Sih R, Morley JE, Kaiser FE, et al. Testosterone replacement in older hypogonadal men: a 12-month
randomized controlled trial. [see comments]. J Clin Endocrinol Metab 1997;82:1661–1667.

76. Tenover JS. Effects of testosterone supplementation in the aging male. J Clin Endocrinol Metab
1992;75(4):1092–1098.

77. Tenover JL. Experience with testosterone replacement in the elderly. Mayo Clin Proc 2000;75(Suppl):
S77–S81, discussion S82.

78. Kenny AM, Prestwood KM, Gruman CA, et al. Effects of transdermal testosterone on bone and muscle
in older men with low bioavailable testosterone levels. J Gerontol A: Biol Sci Med Sci 2001;56(5):
M266–M272.

79. Morley JE, Perry HMD, Kaiser FE, et al. Effects of testosterone replacement therapy in old hypogonadal
males: a preliminary study. J Am Geriatr Soc 1993;41:149–152.

80. Marin P, Krotkiewski M, Bjorntorp P. Androgen treatment of middle-aged, obese men: effects on
metabolism, muscle, and adipose tissues. Eur J Med 1992;1:329–336.

81. Marin P, Oden B, Bjorntorp P. Assimilation and mobilization of triglycerides in subcutaneous abdominal and femoral adipose tissue in vivo in men: effects of androgens. J Clin Endocrinol Metab
1995;80:239–243.

82. Munzer T, Harman SM, Hees P, et al. Effects of GH and/or sex steroid administration on abdominal
subcutaneous and visceral fat in healthy aged women and men. J Clin Endocrinol Metab 2001;86(8):
3604–3610.

83. Dawson RT. Hormones and sport: Drugs in sport—the role of the physician. J Endocrinol 2001;170:
55–61.

84. Korkia P, Stimson GV. Anabolic steroid use in Great Britain. An exploratory investigation. A Summary of a Report for the Department of Health, England, Scotland, and Wales. The Centers for
Research on Drugs and Health Behavior, London, 1993.

85. Buckley WE, Yesalis CE, Friedl KE, et al. Estimated prevalence of anabolic steroid use among male
high school seniors. JAMA 1988;260:3441–3445.

86. Pope H, Phillips K, Olivardia R. The Adonis Complex—The Secret Crisis of the Male Body Obses-
sion. The Free Press, New York, 2000.

87. Catlin DH, Hatton CK, Starcevic SH. Issues in detecting abuse of xenobiotic anabolic steroids and
testosterone by analysis of athletes' urine. Clin Chem 1997;43:1280–1288.

88. Catlin DH, Leder BZ, Ahrens B, et al. Trace contamination of over-the-counter androstenedione and
positive urine test for a nandrolone metabolite. JAMA 2000;284:2618–2621.

89. Aguilera R, Chapman TE, Starcevic B, et al. Performance characteristics of a carbon isotope ratio
method for detecting doping with testosterone based on urine diols: controls and athletes with elevated
testosterone/epitestosterone ratios. Clin Chem 2001;47:292–300.

90. Dehennin L. Detection of simultaneous self-administration of testosterone and epitestosterone in
healthy men. Clin Chem 1994;40:106–109.

91. Dehennin L, Matsumoto AM. Long-term administration of testosterone enanthate to normal men:
alterations of the urinary profile of androgen metabolites potentially useful for the detection of testosterone misuse in sport. J Steroid Biochem Mol Biol 1993;44:179–189.

92. Perry PJ, MacIndoe JH, Yates WR, et al. Detection of anabolic steroid administration: ratio of urinary
testosterone to epitestosterone vs the ratio of urinary testosterone to luteinizing hormone. Clin Chem
1997;43: 731–735.

21 Androgens and Male Contraception

John K. Amory, MD

CONTENTS

INTRODUCTION
TESTOSTERONE ALONE AS A CONTRACEPTIVE
NEWER ANDROGENS FOR MALE CONTRACEPTION
GNRH ANALOGS AND TESTOSTERONE COMBINATIONS
PROGESTINS/TESTOSTERONE COMBINATIONS
FUTURE DIRECTIONS
CONCLUSIONS
REFERENCES

INTRODUCTION

Exogenously administered testosterone suppresses the release of pituitary gonadotropins and, hence, spermatogenesis, and it is central to efforts to create a hormonal contraceptive for men. When given alone, however, currently used forms of testosterone are not completely effective at reducing sperm counts to zero in all men. Therefore, newer androgens and agents such as progestins and gonadotropin-releasing hormone (GnRH) analogs that synergistically suppress gonadotropin release are being studied in efforts to develop a safe, effective, and commercially viable hormonal contraceptive for men.

Despite currently available contraceptives, the world's population continues to increase exponentially. In many parts of the world, overpopulation is a leading cause of human suffering, poverty, and environmental degradation. Inadequate contraception leads to high rates of undesired pregnancy and resultant high rates of abortion (often lethal in countries where it is not legal and/or available from trained providers) and infanticide, or it results in unwanted children who suffer disproportionately from poverty and neglect. Therefore, there is a pressing need for better contraceptives, and male-directed ones in particular. The two contraceptive options currently available to men, condoms and vasectomy, although accounting for roughly one-third of all current contraceptive use, have substantial drawbacks. A hormonal contraceptive for men analogous to the estrogen/progesterone hormonal contraceptive used by women has the potential to be safe, effective, and easy to use. When surveyed, the majority of men indicated a willingness to use such a contraceptive if available *(1)*. Importantly, 98% of women surveyed were willing to trust their partner to use a hormonal method of contraception *(2)*. Clearly, the time is ripe for the widespread

From: *Contemporary Endocrinology: Androgens in Health and Disease*
Edited by: C. Bagatell and W. J. Bremner © Humana Press Inc., Totowa, NJ

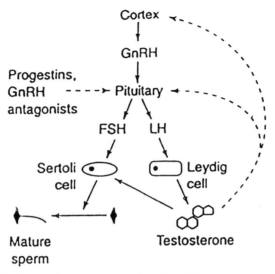

Fig. 1. The endocrinology of spermatogenesis and male hormonal contraception. Solid arrows: promotes spermatogenesis; dashed arrows: inhibits spermatogenesis.

introduction of hormonal male contraceptives to help diminish population pressures, prevent unintended pregnancy, and improve reproductive freedom for men, "the forgotten 50% of contraception."

When administered to a normal male, testosterone (T) functions as a contraceptive by suppressing secretion of the pituitary gonadotropins luteinizing hormone (LH) and follicle-stimulating hormone (FSH) (*see* Fig. 1). Low levels of LH and FSH deprive the testis of the signals required for normal spermatogenesis, leading to markedly decreased sperm counts and reversible infertility in most, but not all, men. Because of the failure of T alone to completely suppress sperm production in some men, compounds such as GnRH analogs and progestins that further suppress pituitary gonadotropins are being studied in combination with T to optimize its contraceptive efficacy.

In normal men, sperm counts vary from 20 million to 200 million sperm per milliliter of ejaculate. The absence of spermatozoa in the ejaculate (azoospermia) renders fertilization impossible and is the ultimate goal of hormonal male contraceptives. Most studies to date, however, demonstrate that some men sustain partial but incomplete reduction of their sperm counts (oligozoospermia) *(3)*. There is good evidence from efficacy trials of T alone as a contraceptive that sperm counts below 3 million sperm per milliliter of ejaculate are associated with decreased rates of pregnancy *(4)*. "Severe oligozoospermia" (counts less than 1 million sperm/mL) decreases the chances of conception even further and is, therefore, considered a reasonable short-term goal for male contraceptive research.

Most hormonal contraceptives do not incapacitate existing sperm; they hinder sperm production. Because sperm take an average of 72 d to reach maturity, it is likely that any contraceptive based on manipulation of the hormonal axis will be associated with some delay in the onset of the full contraceptive effect.

In addition, it is important to consider ethnic differences in interpreting results of contraceptive trials. Study volunteers in Asia are more susceptible to T-induced suppression of spermatogenesis, with rates of azoospermia in the 90–100% range. Men studied

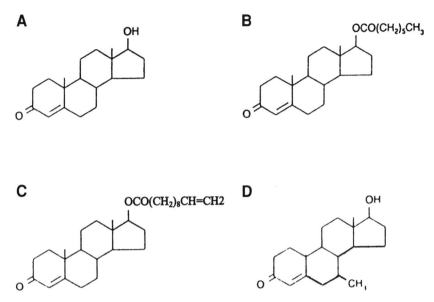

Fig. 2. Androgens used in contraceptive research: (**A**) Testosterone; (**B**) testosterone enanthate; (**C**) testosterone undecanoate; (**D**) 5α-methyl-19-nortestosterone.

in Europe, North America, and Australia, however, have rates of azoospermia closer to 60% on the same regimens *(4,5)*. Although the explanation for this difference is unclear, it is important in the interpretation of trial results and complicates extrapolation of data to different populations.

TESTOSTERONE ALONE AS A CONTRACEPTIVE

Administration of T (*see* Fig. 2A) itself is impractical because when given orally or by injection, the liver promptly degrades it. Most orally active androgens can cause liver damage and are, therefore, not considered safe for long-term use in oral contraceptives *(6)*. Therefore, most current regimens use T esters such as T enanthate (TE; *see* Fig. 2B) given by intramuscular injection on a weekly to fortnightly basis. The onset of azoospermia is around 2–3 mo, and recovery of normal sperm counts occurs 3–4 mo after T is discontinued.

The World Health Organization (WHO) has conducted two large, multicenter trials of TE as a male contraceptive. The first study enrolled 271 subjects who were administered 200 mg TE im weekly for a 6-mo induction phase *(7)*. Sixty percent of these men achieved azoospermia, and an additional 30% were rendered severely oligozoospermic. The fertility of the azoospermic men was then tested in a 12-mo efficacy phase. Of the 119 couples in which the man became azoospermic, continued the injections, and used no other form of birth control, only 1 pregnancy occurred. This pregnancy rate of 0.8 pregnancies per 100 person-years compares favorably with that of the estrogen/progestin birth control pill for women.

The second WHO study examined the fertility of both the men who became azoospermic and the men who achieved severe oligozoospermia on the TE regimen *(4)*. A total of 399 mostly Asian men were enrolled in this study. Of these, all but eight (2%) became severely oligozoospermic or azoospermic. In terms of fertility, there were no pregnancies fathered by the men who became azoospermic. In men whose sperm counts were suppressed to below 3 million/mL, fertility was reduced to 8.1 pregnancies per 100 person-years. The combined fertility rate for oligozoospermic and azoospermic men was 1.4 per 100 person-years. Therefore, the overall failure rate (including the eight men who failed to suppress to oligozoospermia) was 3.4%, for an overall contraceptive efficacy of 96.6%.

These studies demonstrated that TE is safe, fully reversible, and effective as a contraceptive in the majority of men. However, some men fail to suppress below 3 million sperm/mL and, therefore, remain fertile. In addition, the necessity of weekly intramuscular injections is a deterrent. It is important to note that 12% of patients in the second WHO study discontinued involvement for personal or medical reasons or the result of a dislike of the injection schedule. Finally, high-dose TE has been shown to decrease serum high-density lipoprotein (HDL) cholesterol, which could contribute to accelerating atherosclerosis (8,9).

NEWER ANDROGENS FOR MALE CONTRACEPTION

Newer methods of more sustained delivery for T suitable for use in a contraceptive regimen are being pursued. Testosterone buciclate, a synthetic ester given by depot injection, maintains physiologic androgen levels for up to 3 mo in hypogonadal men (10). Recently, this agent has been successfully combined for an experimental contraceptive regimen with the progestin cyproterone acetate in bonnet monkeys, but human testing has not yet been undertaken (11).

Testosterone undecanoate (TU; see Fig. 2C) is a long-chain ester that is absorbed via lymphatics. When given orally, TU therefore escapes first-pass hepatic metabolism (12). It can be given orally two to four times a day or by injection, where it maintains serum T levels for at least 6 wk in hypogonadal men (13,14).

Recently, trials of TU injections for male contraception have been conducted in China (15) and Germany (16,17). In the Chinese study, volunteers received monthly doses of 500 mg or 1000 mg TU. Eleven of 12 in the 500-mg group and 12/12 in the 1000-mg group became azoospermic, with the 1000-mg group achieving azoospermia more quickly. Serum T was elevated but remained within the normal range. Importantly, no significant changes in HDL or serious side effects were found, proving this to be a promising androgen for future studies, especially in Asian populations.

In the German study, TU was studied with and without the addition of a progestin (discussed in a later section). In the TU-only arm of the study, 8/14 men given 1000 mg TU every 6 wk achieved azoospermia, with 4 of the remaining 6 suppressing their sperm counts below 3 million sperm/mL. Therefore, as anticipated, it is proving more difficult to suppress sperm counts in non-Asian populations even with long-acting androgens such as TU. In addition, significant reductions in HDL cholesterol were seen in this predominately Caucasian group of subjects.

Other esters such as 19-nortestosterone (19-NT) have been evaluated as a potential substitute for TE. In addition to its potent androgenic effects, 19-NT has 10 times the progestational activity of testosterone and, therefore, inhibits FSH and LH production to a greater degree than TE (18). 19-NT has been used in contraceptive trials in conjunction with both progestins and the GnRH antagonist cetrorelix and been shown to be as effective in suppressing sperm counts as TE (19) but was unable to maintain suppression of gonadotropins well when cetrorelix was discontinued *(20)*. A derivative of 19-NT, 7α-methyl-19-nortestosterone (MENT; *see* Fig. 2D) is of considerable interest. The 7-methylation of this compound prevents 5α-reduction, effectively preventing the compound from exhibiting any dihydrotestosterone (DHT)-like effects *(21)*. DHT is thought to stimulate prostate enlargement and blocking DHT production by the exogenous administration of MENT could reduce the long-term risk of symptomatic prostate disease and possibly prostate cancer. In addition, DHT is the T metabolite most closely associated with acne and male-pattern baldness, so a contraceptive containing MENT might have appeal to men for reasons other than contraception. Such noncontraceptive health benefits have been well established with the estrogen/progesterone combined oral contraceptive for women (a reduction in the risk of endometrial and ovarian cancer, acne, and dysmennorhea) *(22)* and could significantly approve the appeal of a male hormonal contraceptive to men.

In one recent study in castrated monkeys, MENT showed a 10-fold greater potency (vs T) in terms of LH inhibition, but only a twofold greater potency at stimulating prostate growth *(23)*. Preliminary work on the pharmacokinetics of MENT has been undertaken. Single injections of 2, 4, and 8 mg of micronized MENT injected intramuscularly in healthy men have a short half-life, probably because that MENT does not appear to bind to sex hormone-binding globulin (SHBG) *(24)*. Subsequent studies with MENT implants seem to have overcome this hurdle. In healthy men, MENT-acetate implants suppressed serum T, DHT, and gonadotropins by 80–90% throughout a 1-mo test period *(25)*. A contraceptive study using MENT implants has been published in abstract form and demonstrates that MENT is as effective as T in inducing azoospermia *(26)*. Combinations of MENT with a progestin may be promising.

Transdermal T patches for the treatment of male hypogonadism have been in use for the last several years, but they have only recently been tested for male contraception. A study combining 5.4 mg of T daily delivered via transdermal patch with the progestin levonorgestrel was recently described *(27)*. This combination, however, resulted in azoospermia in only 2 of 11 men, and counts below 3 million sperm/mL in three others. This low success rate was probably the result of the insufficient doses of T delivered by the patch. Transdermal delivery of T is also hampered by the skin irritation caused by the patches. In another study combining T patches with the progestin desogestrel *(28)*, 24% of participants withdrew from the study because of skin irritation. The only reported use of an androgen gel combined a DHT gel with the progestin levonorgestrel *(29)*. Contraceptive efficacy was poor with no individuals reaching azoospermia. In addition, the DHT gel was found to be uncomfortable by the majority of subjects.

Recently, nonsteroidal androgenic compounds have been described *(30,31)*. These compounds can safely be administered orally to rats, and if safe in humans, they could easily be incorporated into a contraceptive regimen. Further animal testing, however, will be required before these compounds can be studied in humans.

GNRH ANALOGS AND TESTOSTERONE COMBINATIONS

The failure to achieve uniform azoospermia with T alone has led to the study of T combined with second agents, such as GnRH analogs or progestins, to improve contraceptive efficacy. The combination of T with the widely available GnRH agonists has proven disappointing, but the use of GnRH antagonists remains promising. These GnRH antagonists can suppress FSH and LH production within hours of administration, and their inhibition of gonadotrophin secretion is more complete than can be produced by agonists. Three human trials have been conducted using the GnRH antagonist "Nal-Glu" with testosterone. The first two trials showed promise, with seven of eight subjects in one study achieving azoospermia by 6–10 wk of treatment *(32,33)*. A third trial, however, demonstrated no difference in azoospermia when compared to TE alone *(34)*. The time required to reach azoospermia was roughly 7–10 wk. Normal sperm counts returned in roughly the same amount of time, demonstrating the reversibility of this approach. GnRH antagonists may be useful in the initiation of spermatogenic arrest. It has recently been demonstrated that administration of Nal-Glu in conjunction with T for 12 wk can be used to induce azoospermia that can then be maintained by TE alone for a subsequent period of 20 wk *(35)*.

A newer GnRH antagonist, Cetrorelix, has recently been licensed for use in Europe. Administration of this agent to cynomolgus monkeys safely reduces serum gonadotropins and androgens by 80% within 16 d *(36)*. Similar results were obtained in trials of healthy male volunteers *(37)*, and Cetrorelix was successful in inducing azoospermia in six of six volunteers in a recent small clinical trial *(20)*.

Newer and even more potent GnRH antagonists have been recently developed. Acyline, a novel GnRH antagonist, has been shown to almost completely suppress gonadotropins and androgens after administration *(38)*. Furthermore, this suppression lasts for up to 3 wk. Given the improvements in gonadotropin suppression and duration of action, these newer GnRH antagonists are obvious choices for testing in male contraceptive trials.

The GnRH antagonists have some drawbacks. Because they are peptides, they are expensive to make and must by injected subcutaneously to avoid degradation in the intestine; also, most older antagonists have very short half-lives and must be injected daily. Side effects noted by trial volunteers included mild burning sensations at the injection site and occasional nontender, subcutaneous nodules at the injection site that resolve within weeks. Happily, the newer compounds seem to have fewer side effects, and because they are very effective, additional work is being undertaken with these agents. Orally active nonpeptide antagonists have recently been described *(39)*. These compounds will require further testing, but they are exciting prospects for future contraceptive trials.

PROGESTINS/TESTOSTERONE COMBINATIONS

The idea of using a progestin synergistically with T to block sperm production has been extensively tested. This work showed that progestins possessed the ability to inhibit LH and FSH secretion in men and suggested that progestins may also have a direct suppressive effect on spermatogenesis *(40–42)*. Combinations of T and depot medroxyprogesterone acetate (DMPA; *see* Fig. 3A) were shown to induce azoospermia in half of the subjects, and some degree of oligozoospermia in most others. The contraceptive efficacy of these combinations, however, was poor, with nine couples conceiving while on therapy despite simultaneous use of other contraceptives *(43)*. In addition, drawbacks to this class of 17-hydroxyl progestational agents were significant—patients experienced weight gain and decreases in HDL cholesterol.

Recent studies of progestins have focused on compounds with fewer side effects, such as the potent oral progestin levonorgestrel (LNG; *see* Fig. 3B). A randomized, controlled

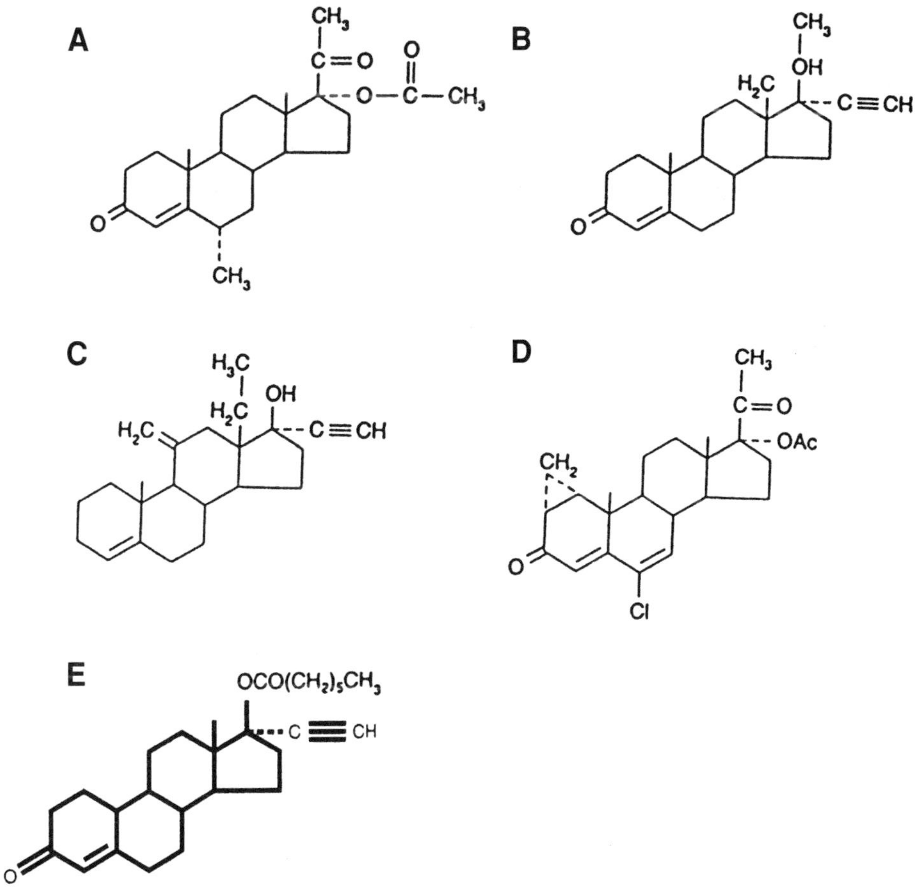

Fig. 3. Progestins used in male contraceptive research: (**A**) Medroxyprogesterone acetate; (**B**) levonorgestrel; (**C**) cyproterone acetate; (**D**) desogestrel; (**E**) norethisterone enanthate.

trial of LNG (500 μg orally daily) with TE (100 mg im/wk) showed the LNG–TE combination was superior to TE alone in terms of azoospermia (67% vs 33%) by 6 mo *(44)*. In addition, the total achieving either severe oligozoospermia or azoospermia was 94% in the LNG–TE group compared to 61% of the TE-alone group. Drawbacks to the LNG–TE regimen included greater weight gain and decreases in HDL cholesterol when compared to the TE-alone group. Recently, the same research group demonstrated that lower doses of LNG were as effective at achieving azoospermia, but weight gain and reductions of HDL cholesterol were minimized with the decreased dose of LNG *(45)*. LNG has recently been tested in combination with 1000 mg of TU injected every 6 wk; however, there was no additive benefit of LNG in terms of suppression of spermatogenesis when compared to TU alone in this study *(16)*.

Another new progestin, desogestrel (DSG; *see* Fig. 3C), has been recently tested in male contraceptive regimens *(46,47)*. DSG differs from LNG only by a methylene group in the 11 position, however, it is thought to possess less inherent androgenicity than LNG. In both studies, 150 or 300 μg of DSG daily was combined with 50- and

100-mg doses of weekly TE. In the first study, after 24 wk, 18 of 23 patients became azoospermic and all but 1 suppressed to less than 3 million sperm/mL. This DSG–TE regimen is notable for larger drops in HDL cholesterol (around 20–25%) than have been seen with LNG–TE.

In the second study, azoospermia was attained in 8/8 men in receiving 150 mg of daily DSG plus 100 mg of weekly TE and 7/8 men in the 300-mg DSG/100-mg TE group. Similar reductions in HDL cholesterol were noted. These studies have demonstrated that DSG is a potent progestin for the suppression of spermatogenesis in normal men, however, significant HDL suppression may limit its clinical utility.

Progestins with antiandrogenic effects such as cyproterone acetate (CPA; *see* Fig. 3D) have also been tested as potential male contraceptives. CPA functions as an antiandrogen by blocking the binding of T and DHT to androgen receptors *(48)*. Therefore, it may interfere with androgen-dependent spermatogenesis in the testis. In addition, CPA suppresses FSH and LH production at the pituitary level.

In a promising trial, two groups of men received CPA at either 50 or 100 mg orally daily, and 100 mg TE im weekly; a third group received weekly TE only *(49)*. All men receiving CPA became azoospermic, whereas only three out of five in the TE alone group attained azoospermia *(see* Fig. 4). In addition, the time required to achieve azoospermia in the CPA groups was half of that needed in the T-alone group (49 vs 98 d). This result is encouraging given the 72-d maturation time of sperm, and it implies that this regimen both blocks the generation of new spermatids and prevents the maturation of already developing sperm. No major adverse side effects, such as changes in HDL cholesterol, liver function, libido, or sexual potency, were noted in this small sample of men. The sole drawbacks noted were slight decreases in body weight and serum hemoglobin level that were dependent on the dose of CPA. Recently, the same group published a study using a lower doses of CPA (12.5 mg and 25 mg daily) with the same dose of TE *(50)*. All men in the 25-mg group attained azoospermia, although one later demonstrated some sperm in his ejaculate. Azoospermia was achieved in only 3/5 men in the 12.5 mg group, demonstrating the need for higher doses of CPA to achieve full contraceptive efficacy. In addition, this group has reported on the first combination of CPA with oral testosterone undecanoate—the first "all-oral" male contraceptive regimen *(51)*. In this study, CPA was combined with oral T undecanoate twice daily. Of eight subjects, one became azoospermic, five were suppressed below 3 million sperm/mL, and the two remaining subjects were suppressed to 4 million and 6 million sperm/mL. It is hoped that alterations in the regimen will lead to more complete and reliable spermatogenic suppression and the eventual availability of a true oral male contraceptive.

Recently, the long-acting progestin norethisterone enanthate (NETE; *see* Fig. 3E; also known as norethindrone enanthate) has been tested in contraceptive trials. A single 200-mg im injection of this agent has been shown to suppress serum gonadotropins and sperm counts for up to 1 mo after injection *(52)*. NETE and TU were recently tested in a combined regimen for male contraception. Thirteen of 14 men who received the combination of 1000 mg TU and 200 mg TE every 6 wk achieved azoospermia after 32 wk of treatment, with HDL suppression and mild weight gain in line with prior studies of progestin/testosterone combinations *(16)*. Because both TU and NETE can be given at 6-wk intervals, however, this approach is a vast improvement over the requirement for weekly injections of TE in most prior studies. NETE can also be administered orally with injectable TU and rates of azoospermia in excess of 90% *(53)*.

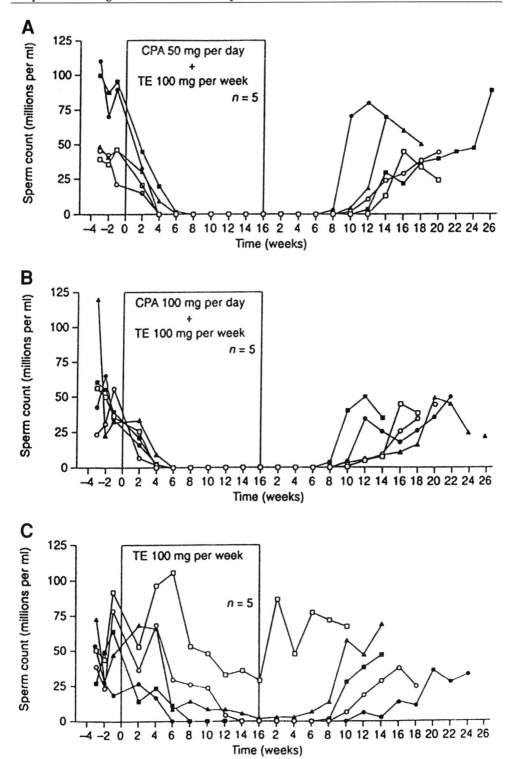

Fig. 4. Sperm concentrations in individual subjects during the control period, throughout 16 wk of hormone administration with testosterone and cyproterone acetate and during 26 wk of recovery phase. (From ref. *46*, reproduced with permission of The Endocrine Society.)

FUTURE DIRECTIONS

Given the encouraging results from recent combinations of T and progestins, many researchers now feel that this combination is the most likely to result in a viable contraceptive method for use in non-Asian populations, whereas long-acting injections of T (e.g., T undecanoate) alone may prove effective in Asian men. Current research is focused on both improving the method of androgen administration and finding combinations that optimize sperm count suppression in all populations while minimizing side effects.

One mystery in the field of male contraceptive research is why some men fail to suppress their sperm counts to zero despite the extremely low levels of serum gonadotropins. It is clear from recent contraceptive trials using testosterone/progestin combinations that the additional suppression of serum gonadotropins mediated by the addition of a progestin improves rates of azoospermia to 70–90% compared with 50–60% with TE alone. In these studies, the levels of circulating gonadotropins in subjects receiving TE in combination with a progestin are significantly lower than control groups receiving TE alone. However, there are no apparent differences in the gonadotropin levels among men who suppress to azoospermia and those who do not *(54,55)*. One must conclude, therefore, that whereas further lowering of serum gonadotropin levels improves the percentage of subjects who achieve azoospermia, it is also suggests that serum gonadotropin levels within a given hormonal regimen may not distinguish between men who will achieve azoospermia and those who will not.

Explanations for differences between subjects who attain azoospermia and those who do not on contraceptive regimens have been proposed. For example, it has been suggested that this difference may be the result of greater 5α-reductase (type II) activity in the testes resulting in higher DHT levels in the serum and seminal plasma of patients who failed to suppress to azoospermia on 200 mg weekly TE *(56)*. However, two recent studies have demonstrated that the coadministration of testosterone and a type II 5α-reductase inhibitor (finasteride) does not enhance suppression of spermatogenesis any more than T alone *(57)* or T plus DSG *(58)*.

Recent research in cynomolgus monkeys implies that FSH suppression may be more important than low levels of intratesticular T in the maintenance of spermatogenesis on contraceptive dose T *(59)*. Moreover, a recent highly sensitive gonadotropin assay has detected FSH immunoreactivity in men on hormonal contraceptive regimens *(60)*. Because it has recently been demonstrated that estrogen and not T is the major source of feedback inhibition of FSH in men at the pituitary *(61)*, and the addition of estrogen has been shown to enhance T-induced suppression of spermatogenesis *(62)*, enhancing estrogen feedback to limit FSH activity may be crucial in future male contraceptive trials. Further investigation directed toward understanding the innate differences in the intratesticular environment that allow some men to continue to produce sperm in an extremely low gonadotropin environment will be instrumental in efforts to develop safe, reversible, and effective hormonal contraception for men.

CONCLUSIONS

Research has demonstrated the feasibility of the hormonal approach to male contraception. Androgen-based combinations are able to reversibly suppress human spermatogenesis without severe side effects in most men; however, a regimen with 100% effectiveness has remained elusive. GnRH antagonists improve the efficacy of T, but are, at present, impractical for widespread use. T combinations with progestins appear promising. Ongoing trials with T plus LNG, DSG, CPA, or NETE may offer a usable option for men, but difficulties in T delivery continue to hinder commercial use. Newer androgens such as injectable TU and MENT may help improve T delivery, avoid undesirable effects on the prostate, and aid in the development of a marketable contraceptive regimen.

REFERENCES

1. Martin CW, Anderson RA, Cheng L, et al. Potential impact of hormonal meal contraception: cross-cultural implications for development of novel male preparations. Hum Reprod 2000;15:637–645.
2. Glasier AF, Anakwe R, Everington D, et al. Would women trust their partners to use a male pill? Hum Reprod 2000;15:646–649.
3. Amory JK, Bremner WJ. The use of testosterone as a male contraceptive. Balliere's Clin Endocrinol Metab 1998;12:471–484.
4. World Health Organization Task Force on Methods for the Regulation of Male Fertility. Contraceptive efficacy of testosterone-induced azoospermia and oligozoospermia in normal men. Fertil Steril 1996;65:821–829.
5. Handelsman DJ, Farley TM, Peregoudov A,Waites GM. Factors in nonuniform induction of azoospermia by testosterone enanthate in normal men. Fertil Steril 1995;63:125–133.
6. Bagatell CJ, Bremner WJ. Androgens in men-uses and abuses. N Engl J Med 1996;334:707–714
7. World Health Organization. Contraceptive efficacy of testosterone-induced azoospermia in normal men. Lancet 1990;336:995–999.
8. Bagatell CJ, Heiman JR, Matsumoto AM, et al. Metabolic and behavioral effects of high-dose, exogenous testosterone in healthy men. J Clin Endocrinol Metab 1994;79:561–567.
9. Meriggiola MC, Marcovina S, Paulsen CA, Bremner WJ. Testosterone enanthate at the dose 200 mg/week decreases HDL-cholesterol levels in healthy men. Int J Androl 1995;18:237–242.
10. Behre HM, Nieschlag E. Testosterone buciclate (20 Aet-1) in hypogonadal men: pharmacokinetics and pharmacodynamics of the new long-acting androgen ester. J Clin Endocrinol Metab 1992;75:1204–1210.
11. Sharma RS, Rajalakshmi M, Pal PC, et al. Evaluation of efficacy, safety, and reversibility of combination regimen of cyproterone acetate and testosterone buciclate in bonnet monkeys. Contraception 2000;62:195–201.
12. Coert A, Geelen J, de Visser J, VanderVies J. The pharmacology and metabolism of testosterone undecanoate (TU), an new orally active androgen. Acta Endocrinol (Copenh) 1975;79:789–800.
13. Zhang GY, Gu YQ, Wang XH, et al. A pharmacokinetic study of injectable testosterone undecanoate in hypogonadal men. J Androl 1998;19:761–768.
14. Behre AM, Abshagen K, Oettel M, et al. Intramuscular injection of testosterone undecanoate for the treatment of male hypogonadism: phase I studies. Eur J Endrocrinol 1999;140:414–419.
15. Zhang GY, Gu YQ, Wang XH, et al. Injectable testosterone undecanoate for contraception in Chinese men. J Clin Endocrinol Metab 1999;84:3642–3647
16. Kamischke A, Ploger D, Venherm S, et al. Intramuscular testosterone undecanoate with or without oral levonorgestrel: a randomized placebo-controlled feasibility study for male contraception. Clin Endocrinol 2000;53:43–52.
17. Kamischke A, Venherm S, Ploger D, et al. Intramuscular testosterone undecanoate and norethisterone enanthate in a clinical trial for male contraception. J Clin Endocrinol Metab 2001;86:303–309.
18. Schurmeyer T, Knuth UA, Belkien L, Nieschlag E. Reversible azoospermia induced by the anabolic steroid 19-nortestosterone. Lancet 1984;1:417–420.
19. World Health Organization. Comparison of two androgens plus depot-medroxyprogesterone acetate for suppression to azoospermia in Indonesian men. Fertil Steril 1993;60:1062–1068.
20. Behre HM, Kliesch S, Lemcke B, et al. Suppression of spermatogenesis to azoospermia by combined administration of GnRH antagonist and 19-nortestosterone cannot be maintained by this non-aromatizable androgen alone. Hum Reprod 2001;16:2570–2577.
21. Sundaram K, Kumar N, Bardin CW. 7-Alpha-methyl-19-nortestosterone: an ideal androgen for replacement therapy. Recent Prog Horm Res 1994;49:373–376.

22. Oral contraception. In: Speroff L, Glass RH, Kase NG, eds. Clinical Gynecologic Endocrinology and Infertility, 6th Edition. Williams and Wilkins, Baltimore, MD, 1999, pp. 867–945.

23. Cummings DE, Kumar N, Bardin CW, et al. Prostate-sparing tissue specific effects of the potent androgen 7α-methyl-19-nortestosterone (MENT) in primates. J Clin Endocrinol Metab 1998;83: 4212–4219.

24. Suvissari J, Sundaram K, Noe G, et al. Pharmacokinetics and pharmacodynamics of 7α-methyl-19-nortestosterone and intramuscular administration in healthy men. Hum Reprod 1997;12:967–973.

25. Noe G, Suvisaari J, Martin C, et al. Gonadotropin and testosterone suppression by 7α-methyl-19-nortestosterone acetate administered by subdermal implant to healthy men. Hum Reprod 1999;14: 2200–2206.

26. Von Eckardstein, Nieschlag E, Croxatto H, et al. 7α-Methyl-19-nortestosterone (MENT) implants for male contraception: a dose-finding study. VIIth International Congress for Andrology, 2001, abstract 140.

27. Buchter D, Von Eckardstein S, Von Eckardstein A, et al. Clinical trial of transdermal testosterone and oral levonorgestrel for male contraception. J Clin Endocrinol Metab 1999;84:1244–1249.

28. Hair WM, Kitteridge K, O'Conner DB, Wu FC. A novel male contraceptive pill-patch combination: oral desogestrel and transdermal testosterone in the suppression of spermatogenesis in normal men. J Clin Endocrinol Metab 2001;86:5201–5209.

29. Pollanen P, Nikkanen V, Huhtaniemi I. Combination of subcutaneous levonorgestrel implants and transdermal dihydrotestosterone gel for male hormonal contraception. Int J Androl 2001;24:369–380.

30. Hamann LG, Mani NS, Davis RL, et al. Discovery of a potent, orally active, nonsteroidal androgen receptor agonist: 4-ethyl-1,2,3,4-tetrahydro-6-(trifluoromethyl)-8-pyridono[5,6-g]-quinoline (LG121071). J Med Chem 1999;42:210–212.

31. Van Dort ME, Robins DM, Wayburn F. Design, synthesis, and pharmacological characterization of 4-[4,4-dimethyl-3-(4-hydroxybutyl)-5-oxo-2-thioxo-1-imidazolidinyl]-2-iodobenzonitrile as a high-affinity nonsteroidal androgen receptor ligand. J Med Chem 2000;43:3344–3347.

32. Pavlou SN, Brewer K, Farley MG et al. Combined administration of a gonadotropin-releasing hormone antagonist and testosterone in men induces reversible azoospermia without loss of libido. J Clin Endocrinol Metab 1991;73:1360–1369.

33. Tom L, Bhasin S, Salameh W et al. Induction of azoospermia in normal men with combined Nal-Glu gonadotropin-releasing hormone and testosterone enanthate. J Clin Endocrinol Metab 1992;75: 476–483.

34. Bagatell CJ, Matsumoto AM, Christensen RB, et al. Comparison of a gonadotropin releasing-hormone antagonist plus testosterone (T) versus T alone as potential male contraceptive regimens. J Clin Endocrinol Metab 1993;77:427–432.

35. Swerdloff RS, Bagatell CJ, Wang C, et al. Suppression of spermatogenesis in man induced by Nal-Glu gonadotropin releasing hormone antagonist and testosterone enanthate (TE) is maintained by TE alone. J Clin Endocrinol Metab 1998;83:3527–3533.

36. Yeung CH, Weinbauer GF, Cooper TG. Effect of acute androgen withdrawal by GnRH antagonist on epididymal sperm motility and morphology in the cynomolgus monkey. J Androl 1999;20:72–79.

37. Rolf C, Gottschalk I, Behre HM, et al. Pharmacokinetics of new testosterone transdermal therapeutic systems in gonadotropin-releasing hormone antagonist-supressed normal men. Exp Clin Endocrinol Diabetes 1999;107:63–69.

38. Herbst KL, Anawalt BD, Amory JK, et al. Acyline: a novel GnRH antagonist in men. J Clin Endocrinol Metab 2002;87:3215–3220.

39. Cho N, Harada M, Imaeda T, et al. Discovery of a novel, potent and orally active nonpeptide antagonist of the human luteinizing hormone-releasing hormone (LHRH) receptor. J Med Chem 1998;41: 4190–4195.

40. Schearer SB, Alvarez-Sanchez F, Anselmo J et al. Hormonal contraception for men. Int J Androl 1978;2:680–695.

41. Fotherby K, Davies JE, Richards DJ, Bodin M. Effect of low doses of synthetic progestagens on testicular function. Int J Fertil 1972;17:113–119.

42. Meriggiola MC, Bremner WJ. Progestin-androgen combination regimens for male contraception. J Androl 1997;18:240–244.

43. Barfield A, Melo J, Coutinho E, et al. Pregnancies associated with sperm concentrations below 10 million/ml in clinical studies of a potential male contraceptive method, monthly depot medroxyprogesterone acetate and testosterone esters. Contraception 1977;20:121–127.

44. Bebb RA, Anawalt BD, Christensen RB, et al. Combined administration of levonorgestrel and testosterone induces more rapid and effective suppression of spermatogenesis than testosterone alone: a promising male contraceptive approach. J Clin Endocrinol Metab 1996;81:757–762.

45. Anawalt BD, Bebb RA, Bremner WJ, Matsumoto AM. A lower dosage levonorgestrel and testosterone combination effectively suppresses spermatogenesis and circulating gonadotropin levels with fewer metabolic effects than higher dosage combinations. J Androl 1999;20:407–414.

46. Wu FC, Balasubramanian R, Mulders TIM, et al. Oral progestogen combined with testosterone as a potential male contraceptive: additive effects between desogestrel and testosterone enanthate in suppression of spermatogenesis, pituitary-testicular axis, and lipid metabolism. J Clin Endocrinol Metab 1999;84:112–122.

47. Anawalt BD, Herbst KL, Matsumoto AM, et al. Desogestrel plus testosterone effectively suppresses spermatogenesis but also causes modest weight gain and high-density lipoprotein suppression. Fertil Steril 2000;74:707–714.

48. Neumann F, Topert M. Pharmacology of antiandrogens. J Steroid Biochem 1986;25:885–895.

49. Meriggiola MC, Bremner WJ, Paulsen CA, et al. A combined regimen of cyproterone acetate and testosterone enanthate as a potentially highly effective male contraceptive. J Clin Endocrinol Metab 1996;81:3018–3023.

50. Meriggiola MC, Bremner WJ, Constantino A, et al. Low dose of cyproterone acetate and testosterone enanthate for contraception in men. Hum Reprod 1998;13:1225–1229.

51. Meriggiola MC, Bremner WJ, Constantino A, et al. An oral regimen of cyproterone acetate and testosterone for spermatogenic suppression in men. Fertil Steril 1997;68:844–850.

52. Kamischke A, Diebacker J, Nieschlag E. Potential of norethisterone enanthate for male contraception: pharmacokinetics and suppression of pituitary and gonadal function. Clin Endocrinol (Oxf) 2000;53:351–358.

53. Kamischke A, Heuermann T, Kruger K, et al. An effective hormonal male contraceptive using testosterone undecanoate with oral or injectable norethisterone preparations. J Clin Endocrinol Metab 2002;87:530–539.

54. Wallace EM, Gow SM, Wu FCW. Comparison between testosterone enanthate-induced azoospermia and oligoazoospermia in a male contraceptive study I: plasma luteinizing hormone, follicle stimulating hormone, testosterone, estradiol and inhibin concentrations. J Clin Endocriol Metab 1993;777:290–293.

55. Amory JK, Anawalt BD, Bremner WJ, Matsumoto AM. Daily testosterone and gonadotropin levels are similar in azoospermic and nonazoospermic normal men administered weekly testosterone: implications for male contraceptive development. J Androl 2001;22:1053–1060.

56. Anderson RA, Wallace AM, Wu FC. Comparison between testosterone enanthate-induced azoospermia and oligozoospermia in a male contraceptive study. III. Higher 5α-reductase activity in oligozoospermic men administered supraphysiological doses of testosterone. J Clin Endocrinol Metab 1996;81:902–908

57. McLachlan RI, McDonald J, Rushford D, et al. Efficacy and acceptability of testosterone implants, alone or in combination with a 5α-reductase inhibitor, for male hormonal contraception. Contraception 2000;62:73–78.

58. Kinniburgh D, Anderson RA, Baird DT. Suppression of spermatogenesis with desogestrel and testosterone pellets with not enhanced by addition of finasteride. J Androl 2001;22:88–95.

59. Weinbauer GF, Schlatt S, Walter V, Nieschlag E. Testosterone-induced inhibition of spermatogenesis is more closely related to suppression of FSH than to testicular androgen levels in the cynomolgus monkey model (*Macaca fascicularis*). J Endocrinol 2001;168:25–38.

60. Robertson DM, Pruysers E, Stephenson T, et al. Sensitive LH and FSH assays for monitoring low serum levels in men undergoing steroidal contraception. Clin Endocrinol (Oxf) 2001;55:331–339.

61. Hayes FJ, Decrz S, Seminara SB, et al. Differential regulation of gonadotropin secretion by testosterone in the human male: absence of a negative feedback effect of testosterone on follicle-stimulating hormone secretion. J Clin Endocrinol Metab 2001;86:53–58.

62. Handelsman DJ, Wishart S, Conway AJ. Oestradiol enhances testosterone-induced suppression of human spermatogenesis. Hum Reprod 2000;15:672–679.

22 Androgens in Primary Care

Bradley D. Anawalt, MD

CONTENTS

INTRODUCTION
DEFINITION OF THE SYNDROME OF MALE HYPOGONADISM
EPIDEMIOLOGY
CLINICAL MANIFESTATIONS OF HYPOGONADISM
DIAGNOSIS OF HYPOGONADISM
COMMON CLINICAL SYNDROMES ASSOCIATED WITH LOW SERUM
    TESTOSTERONE LEVELS
TREATMENT
SIDE EFFECTS OF ANDROGEN THERAPY IN HYPOGONADAL MEN
CONCLUSION
REFERENCES

INTRODUCTION

Disturbances in the male gonadal axis are common and often create vexing dilemmas for primary care clinicians. The principal clinical questions are the following: Does my patient have hypogonadism or does he have a transient disturbance as a result of an acute illness? What is the underlying etiology for his hypogonadism? What is the appropriate evaluation? Will my patient benefit from treatment? If androgen supplementation or replacement therapy is used, what mode of therapy should be selected?

Although we do not have all of the data yet to answer the above questions with complete certainty, we can attempt to make rational decisions for each of our individual patients. In this chapter, I describe an approach to the diagnosis and treatment of male hypogonadism in common clinical scenarios in the primary care setting.

DEFINITION OF THE SYNDROME OF MALE HYPOGONADISM

Male hypogonadism is defined by decreased androgen effect (usually by impaired secretion of testosterone) and/or sperm production. In this chapter I will focus on androgen deficiency, and I will not discuss defects in spermatogenesis in this chapter. Normal serum androgen (testosterone and dihydrotestosterone) levels are important for bone and muscle mass, strength, erythropoiesis, cognition, sexual function, and sense of well-being. However, it is essential to acknowledge that male hypogonadism is not defined exclusively by serum androgen levels. Hypogonadism is a syndrome associated with

From: *Contemporary Endocrinology: Androgens in Health and Disease*
Edited by: C. Bagatell and W. J. Bremner © Humana Press Inc., Totowa, NJ

inadequate androgen effect. This syndrome may be associated with osteoporosis, weakness and frailty, hypoproliferative anemia, decreased libido and sexual dysfunction or inanition, and malaise. As clinicians, we treat our patients for hypogonadism to either ameliorate or prevent the effects of this syndrome. Thus, we must integrate our clinical assessment (history and physical examination) with our biochemical measurements of a man's gonadal status in determining whether a man is hypogonadal and would benefit from exogenous androgen therapy.

EPIDEMIOLOGY

Male hypogonadism is very common. For example, Klinefelter's syndrome, a congenital cause of hypogonadism, occurs in about 1 : 400 live male births *(1)*. As men age, the prevalence of hypogonadism increases. The prevalence of hypogonadism (based on low serum total- or free-testosterone levels) increases from approx 5% of men in the 20- to 29-yr-old group to 20%, 30%, and 50% in the 60–69, 70–79, and 80+ groups, respectively *(2)*.

CLINICAL MANIFESTATIONS OF HYPOGONADISM

The clinical manifestations of hypogonadism depend on whether the onset of hypogonadism occurred before or after puberty (*see* Tables 1 and 2). Androgen deficiency that occurs before puberty is associated with absent or decreased secondary sexual characteristics, including little or no terminal facial hair, a high-pitched voice (vocal cords do not develop usual male thickness), and small testes. In addition, prepubertal androgen deficiency results in abnormal skeletal proportions with very long limbs ("eunuchoidal") because the absence of normal androgen activity during puberty results in delayed closure of the epiphyses of the long bones. Men who become hypogonadal before puberty might not notice a low libido because they have never experienced a normal androgen-driven libido. The physical manifestations of postpubertal hypogonadism (soft testes, slowly growing terminal facial hair) are subtle because most men with postpubertal hypogonadism have developed normal secondary sexual characteristics. The symptoms of postpubertal hypogonadism such as decreased libido, weakness, decreased assertiveness, and decreased sense of well-being are nonspecific, and these manifestations are often dismissed as the effects of aging or depression.

DIAGNOSIS OF HYPOGONADISM

The diagnosis of hypogonadism can be straightforward when men present with overt symptoms of testosterone deficiency such as osteoporosis, weakness, and decreased libido plus profoundly low serum testosterone levels. However, many cases of hypogonadism are much subtler and require careful evaluation. Hypogonadism should be considered in men who complain of decreased libido or sexual dysfunction, decreased energy, weakness, or depressed mood. When clinicians evaluate for male hypogonadism, they should determine serum testosterone and gonadotropin levels.

Measurement of Serum Testosterone

There is a great controversy about the best method of determining androgen levels. Ideally, clinicians would like to measure a patient's serum bioactive androgen level.

Table 1
Manifestations of Hypogonadism
Acquired Prepubertally

Scant body hair and terminal facial hair
High-pitched voice
Female escutcheon
Small testes: volume < 6 cm^3; length < 2.5 cm
Small penis: length < 5 cm
Little or no scrotal rugae or hyperpigmentation
Small prostate
Eunuchoidal proportions

Table 2
Manifestations of Hypogonadism
Acquired Postpubertally

Loss of libido
Facial terminal hair present but slow growth
Body hair present but decreased
Normal male pitch
Testes > 10 cm^3; sometimes soft
Normal penile length
Scrotal rugae and hyperpigmentation
Adult prostate size
Decreased bone and muscle mass
Normal skeletal proportions

However, we do not have a precise method of measuring serum androgen bioactivity. The majority of testosterone that circulates in the blood is bound to plasma proteins. In men, about 40% of serum testosterone is avidly bound to sex hormone-binding globulin (SHBG) and about 58% is weakly bound to albumin; only about 1–2% of testosterone is "free" or unbound *(3)*. Testosterone that is unbound or "free" is unequivocally bioactive, but testosterone that is weakly bound to albumin is supposedly bioavailable (because of rapid disassociation from albumin) as a source of androgen for tissues *(4–6)*. Thus, we can measure total-testosterone, bioavailable ("weakly bound") testosterone, and free-testosterone levels.

Although it would be ideal to measure the bioactive testosterone levels, the most appropriate assay for the clinical use in men is the total-testosterone assay. The total-testosterone assay is inexpensive, widely available and reliable. In addition, we have considerable normative data for the total-testosterone assay, and most of the clinical studies of the effects of androgen supplementation or replacement in men have used total-testosterone levels to determine the subjects' gonadal status. Therefore, when primary care clinicians are using the literature to determine the benefit of androgen therapy for their patients, the serum total-testosterone level is the most clinically germane.

Serum free-testosterone levels may be measured accurately and reliably by equilibrium dialysis, but this is an expensive, time-consuming assay that is only available in a few specialty commercial laboratories. Serum free-testosterone levels can be determined with many commercial kits, but the results are often inaccurate, particularly when SHBG levels are abnormally high or low such as in obesity, diabetes mellitus 2, or hypothyroidism *(7,8)*. Serum bioavailable testosterone levels classically are determined by precipitating the SHBG-bound testosterone with cold 50% ammonium sulfate *(9)*. However, this is a time-consuming procedure that is infeasible for most clinical laboratories. Serum free and bioavailable testosterone levels also can be calculated if the total testosterone, SHBG, and albumin levels are known *(10,11)*. The calculated serum free and bioavailable testosterone measurements might become the most useful means of assessing the gonadal status of men when this method has been used widely and normative ranges have been validated in clinical laboratories.

Measurement of Serum Gonadotropins (FSH and LH)

Male hypogonadism is categorized into primary and secondary hypogonadism based on the site of dysfunction in the gonadal axis (*see* Fig. 1). In primary hypogonadism, the testes are dysfunctional and fail to produce adequate amounts of testosterone despite supranormal serum levels of FSH and LH that are high because of the absence of negative feedback on the hypothalamus and pituitary. In secondary and tertiary hypogonadism, the defect is in the pituitary and hypothalamus, respectively, and serum testosterone levels are low while serum FSH and LH levels are low or *inappropriately normal*. For clinical purposes, pituitary and hypothalamic causes are often lumped into a single category of secondary hypogonadism because GnRH cannot be measured in peripheral blood. Thus, pituitary and hypothalamic hypogonadism are biochemically indistinguishable.

It is essential to measure serum gonadotropin levels in addition to serum testosterone levels when evaluating for male hypogonadism. It is not adequate to determine only serum testosterone levels. In a pattern analogous to primary hypothyroidism, patients with primary hypogonadism may have low-normal serum testosterone levels but unequivocally elevated serum gonadotropins; testing for serum testosterone alone would lead to the incorrect assessment of eugonadism. Furthermore, determination of primary vs secondary hypogonadism dictates the extent of the remainder of the evaluation. Patients with primary hypogonadism do not require any further workup, although some clinicians will order a serum karyotyping for the definitive diagnosis or exclusion of Klinefelter's (*see* Table 3). Finally, the distinction between primary hypogonadism vs secondary hypogonadism has clinical implications for subsequent fertility. In general, patients with primary hypogonadism are infertile. Occasionally, patients with primary hypogonadism are fertile after the use of assisted reproductive techniques that include harvesting sperm directly from the testes and the use of intracytoplasmic sperm injection *(12)*. Patients with secondary hypogonadism may be fertile when treated with gonadotropin therapy or gonadotropin-releasing hormone.

It is useful to measure both serum FSH and LH levels in the evaluation of the male gonadal axis. Serum FSH levels may be elevated in men with an isolated defect in spermatogenesis and decreased inhibin B production from Sertoli cells in the testes. These men have normal serum testosterone and LH levels (*see* Fig. 1E). Serum LH levels may vary considerably in normal men because LH is secreted in a pulsatile pattern and it has a very short serum half-life. Thus, a normal eugonadal man may have slightly low or high LH levels, intermittently reflecting nadirs and peaks in secretion.

A   Normal

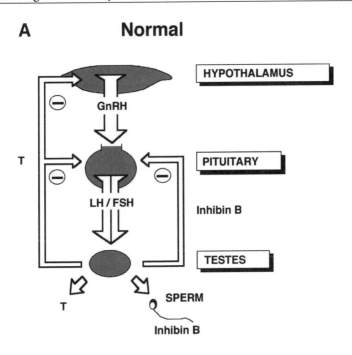

B   Primary Hypogonadism

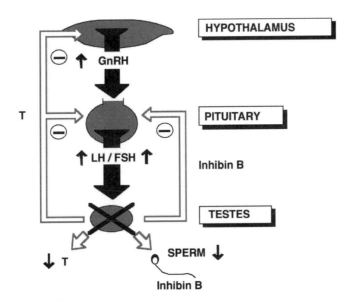

Fig. 1. The gonadal axis in health and disease: **(A)** normal gonadal axis; **(B)** primary hypogonadism. *(Figure continues.)*

C   Secondary Hypogonadism

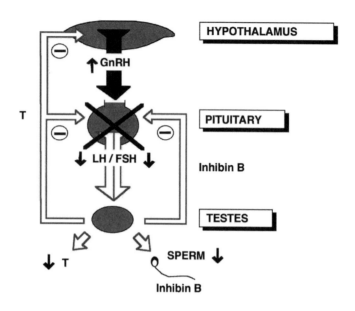

D   Tertiary Hypogonadism

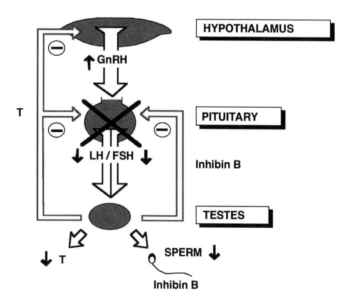

Fig. 1. (C) Secondary hypogonadism caused by pituitary disease (note that GnRH is not measurable in peripheral blood); **(D)** tertiary hypogonadism caused by hypothalamic disease. *(Figure continues.)*

E   Sertoli cell dysfunction and decreased inhibin B secretion

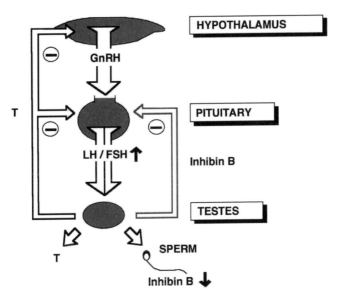

Fig. 1. (E) Dysfunction of Sertoli cells leads to abnormal spermatogenesis, decreased inhibin B secretion, and isolated elevation of circulating FSH and LH levels.

Table 3
Common Causes of Primary Hypogonadism

Prepubertal onset (small testes)
    Klinefelter's syndrome (XXY males)

Postpubertal onset (normal testes)
    Mumps orchitis (usually does not cause hypogonadism if prepubertal)
    Autoimmune orchitis
    Trauma
    Testicular irradiation or surgery

Summary of the Evaluation of Gonadal Axis

When male hypogonadism is being considered, clinicians should order a serum total testosterone (or calculated free and bioavailable testosterone when this assay has been validated in the primary care setting) plus serum LH and FSH levels (Fig. 2). If the patient has primary hypogonadism with low serum testosterone plus elevated gonadotropins, no further work-up is necessary. If the patient has a pattern suggesting secondary hypogonadism (low serum testosterone plus low or normal gonadotropins), the laboratory assessment should be repeated. Any acute systemic illness may suppress the gonadal axis and cause a biochemical profile identical to secondary hypogonadism. Thus, it would be best to repeat the gonadal assessment when the man has been healthy for some period of time.

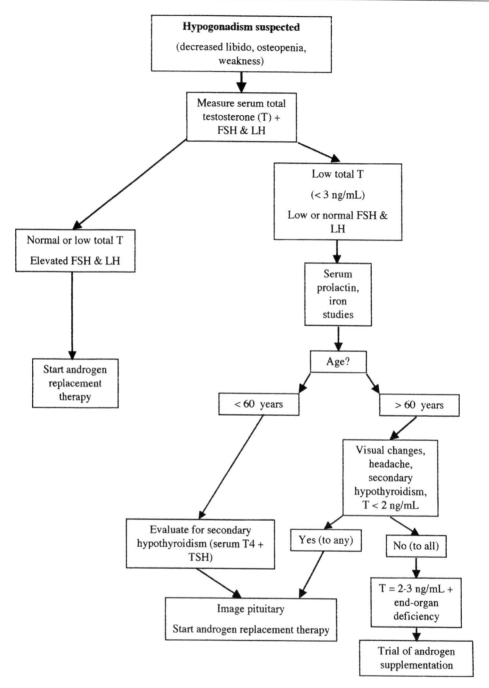

Fig. 2. Evaluation and treatment of male hypogonadism in the primary care clinic.

In younger men (< 60 yr), the repeat laboratory assessment should be done before 10 AM because the normal range of testosterone is based on peak testosterone levels that occur in the morning. In older men, the timing of the phlebotomy for hormone levels is less important because older men lose the normal circadian rhythm of gonadal secretion and have fairly constant gonadal steroid levels throughout the day (13).

Table 4
Common Causes of Secondary Hypogonadism

Prepubertal onset (small testes)
    Kallmann's syndrome
    Idiopathic hypogonadotropic hypogonadism
    Pituitary tumor (craniopharyngioma)
    Uremia
    Severe systemic illness
    Cranial irradiation
    Hyperprolactinemia
Postpubertal onset (normal testes)
    Acquired idiopathic hypogonadotropic hypogonadism
    Pituitary macroadenomas
    Uremia
    Severe systemic illness
    Cranial irradiation
    Hyperprolactinemia
    Hemochromatosis
    Cushing's syndrome
    Cirrhosis
    Morbid obesity

Table 5
Drugs Commonly Associated with Male Hypogonadism

Primary hypogonadism
  Decreased Leydig cell production of testosterone
    Corticosteroids
    Ethanol
    Ketoconazole (high dosages)
  Decreased conversion of testosterone to dihydrotestosterone
    Finasteride (rarely cause decreased libido and erectile dysfunction)
  Androgen-receptor blockade
    Spironolactone
    Flutamide
    Cimetidine
    Cyproterone
Secondary hypogonadism
  Decreased pituitary secretion of gonadotropins
    Corticosteroids
    Ethanol
    GnRH analogs (e.g., Lupron)
    Estrogens
    Medications that raise prolactin levels (psychotropic drugs, metoclopramide, opiates)

After secondary hypogonadism has been confirmed with repeat biochemical testing, common causes of gonadotropin deficiency should be excluded. Common causes include idiopathic hypogonadotropic hypogonadism, hyperprolactinemia, Cushing's syndrome, pituitary macroadenomas (>1 cm^2), hemochromatosis, and drugs (*see* Tables 4 and 5).

All men with secondary hypogonadism should be evaluated with a serum prolactin level and iron studies to exclude hyperprolactinemia and hemochromatosis. The recommended screening test for hemochromatosis is serum transferrin saturation (serum iron concentration divided by total iron-binding capacity, multiplied by 100). Iron saturation less than 45% excludes hemochromatosis as a cause of male hypogonadism, and virtually all men who are homozygotic for hemochromatosis will have an iron saturation greater than 62% *(14,15)*. Because serum iron concentration and transferrin saturation are increased by meals, the specificity of transferrin saturation for hemochromatosis is better when the patient is fasting. The possibility of Cushing's syndrome should be evaluated by history and physical examination (careful examination of the skin for decreased thickness, easy bruisability, violaceous striae, and evaluation of the musculoskeletal system for weakness and osteoporosis). If indicated, Cushing's syndrome may be screened for with a 24-h collection for urinary free cortisol or an overnight low-dose dexamethasone suppression test.

Men with secondary hypogonadism who are younger than age 50 and who do not have hemochromatosis should have an imaging study of the pituitary to exclude a large, compressive pituitary macroadenoma. Either a computed tomography (CT) or magnetic resonance imaging (MRI) scan would suffice, but CT is less expensive. MRI is clearly superior when smaller pituitary lesions need to be evaluated. Because men older than age 65 yr often have low or low-normal serum testosterone and gonadotropin levels without any pituitary disease, it would not be cost-effective to do imaging studies on all of them. If prolactin levels are normal and thyroid function tests do not suggest a pituitary source of hypothyroidism (low serum T4 plus low or inappropriately normal thyroid-stimulating hormone [TSH]), an imaging study may be waived unless the patient complains of frequent headaches or visual disturbances that might suggest a sellar mass. Men with secondary hypogonadism with very low serum testosterone levels (<200 ng/dL) should have a pituitary imaging study regardless of the age of the patient.

COMMON CLINICAL SYNDROMES ASSOCIATED WITH LOW SERUM TESTOSTERONE LEVELS

Men who are hypogonadal as a result of specific defects in the hypothalamus (e.g., Kallmann's syndrome), the pituitary (e.g., pituitary macroadenoma), or testes (e.g., Klinefelter's syndrome) clearly benefit from androgen-replacement therapy. For hypogonadal men, adequate androgen-replacement therapy will cause significant increases in bone mass, lean body mass (and decreased fat mass), strength, and hematocrit *(16–24)*. In addition, hypogonadal men who are adequately treated report improved sexual function and mood *(23,25)*.

Older Men (> 65 yr) with Low-Normal Serum Testosterone Levels

Serum testosterone levels decline in aging men because of a dual defect in the hypothalamus and in the testes. Aging is associated with the aberrant secretion of gonadotropin-releasing hormone (GnRH) and a blunted response of the Leydig cell to gonadotropin stimulation *(26–28)*. Pituitary gonadotropin function is spared in older men as the gonadotropes continue to produce LH normally when stimulated by GnRH *(27,29,30)*. More than 20% of all men ≥ 60 yr have serum total- and free-testosterone levels below the threshold of hypogonadism for healthy young men *(2)*. Most of these men will have normal serum gonadotropin levels and thus have a biochemical profile similar to young men with secondary hypogonadism. The age-related decline in male serum testosterone levels has been cited as a potential cause for the age-related sarcopenia, osteopenia, decreased sexual function, and depression *(31,32)*.

Three longer-term (≥ 1 yr) studies have shown positive effects on body composition and bone mineral density in older men with low to low-normal serum testosterone levels. In Sih's study of 32 men older than 50 yr with low bioavailable testosterone levels, 1 yr of treatment with intramuscular testosterone (200 mg every 2 wk) resulted in significant increases in grip strength in the testosterone group only *(33)*. In a 3-yr study of older men, Tenover demonstrated that intramuscular testosterone (150–200 mg every 2 wk) produced significant increases in lean body mass and hand-grip strength in older men with pretreatment low to low-normal total-testosterone levels (<3.5 ng/mL) *(34,35)*. In the largest published study, Snyder et al. randomized 108 men over age 65 yr with total-testosterone levels < 4.75 ng/mL to 3 yr of transdermal testosterone or a placebo patch *(36)*. In Snyder et al.'s study, which included men with normal serum testosterone levels, exogenous transdermal testosterone increased lean body mass and improved self-reported physical functioning, but did not increase lower extremity strength.

Tenover's and Snyder et al.'s studies also showed that exogenous testosterone increased bone mineral density in older men *(35,37)*. In Tenover's study of the effects of intramuscular testosterone, there was a significant increase in bone mineral density in the testosterone-treated group compared to placebo group. In Snyder et al.'s study of the effects of transdermal testosterone, both the testosterone-treated and placebo groups had significant increases (approx 4% and 2%, respectively) in bone mineral density compared to baseline. Both groups were treated with calcium + vitamin D, and there were no significant differences in bone mineral density between the groups after 3 yr of treatment. However, men with the lowest baseline total-testosterone levels (<2 ng/mL) had a larger (approx 6%) increase in bone mineral density, and this increase was significantly greater than that of the placebo group.

Overall, these small long-term studies suggest that older men with low-normal testosterone levels might benefit from exogenous supplemental testosterone. However, we need data about safety plus clinically relevant outcomes such as the effects on physical function (e.g., ability to live independently and fractures) before making recommendations about screening and treating a large percentage of the older male population. Older men with very low serum total-testosterone levels (<2 ng/mL) are most likely to benefit from exogenous androgen therapy. Selected older men with total-testosterone levels between 2 and 3.5 ng/mL plus clinical evidence of androgen deficiency (osteopenia, decreased libido, unexplained hypoproliferative anemia) might benefit with androgen supplementation. A 6- to 12-mo trial of exogenous androgen therapy would be reasonable in this setting because most of the anabolic effects of testosterone are achieved by 12 mo (although bone mineral density will continue to increase for an additional 12–24 mo). Older men with testicular disease and elevated serum gonadotropins or older men with documented pituitary disease (e.g., hemochromatosis or a pituitary macroadenoma) should be considered for exogenous androgen therapy regardless of their age.

Men with Renal Failure

There are some data supporting the use of androgen administration to men with renal failure. Men with any severe systemic illness including uremia may develop hypotestosteronemia. In men with uremia, androgen therapy was historically used to treat anemia *(38)*. With the advent of human recombinant erythropoietin, androgen therapy fell out of favor. There has been renewed interest in the use of androgens in patients with end-stage renal disease because androgen therapy is less expensive than erythropoietin, and, unlike erythropoietin, androgens increase serum albumin, lean body mass, and bone mass but do not cause hypertension *(39,40)*. Until we have results from large clinical trials of the use of androgens in patients with renal disease, it would be reasonable and prudent for primary care clinicians to restrict the use of androgens to those men with renal disease with established hypogonadism or the occasional patient with low-normal testosterone levels and who is intolerant or refractory to the effects of erythropoeitin.

Men with HIV Disease

Gonadal dysfunction is very common in human-immunodeficiency virus (HIV)-infected men, and 20–50% of men with progressive HIV disease develop hypogonadism *(41–43)*. Primary hypogonadism may occur with acquired immunodeficiency syndrome (AIDS) because HIV directly damages the testes, but men with HIV disease often have secondary hypogonadism because of the effects of malnutrition, severe systemic illness, or medications used in the treatment of the patients with AIDS (e.g., megesterol acetate) *(42,43)*. Exogenous androgens have been shown to increase lean body mass and result in significantly increased strength or improved sense of well-being and quality of life in men with low testosterone levels and symptomatic HIV infection *(44–47)*. Supra-physiological dosages of androgen increase lean body mass and strength in men with HIV infection and also normal testosterone levels *(48–50)*. The effects of androgens on body composition and strength appear to be dose dependent, and the results from trials using transdermal therapy are much less impressive than the trials using intramuscular testosterone or synthetic androgens *(50,51)*. In summary, men with symptomatic HIV infection and low or low-normal testosterone levels may benefit with exogenous testosterone administration.

TREATMENT

When treating male hypogonadism, it is important to recall that the testes have two important functions: steroid hormone synthesis and spermatogenesis. In primary care, the focus of therapy of male hypogonadism is directed toward androgen replacement. If a hypogonadal man desires fertility, he should be referred to a specialist. There are several treatment options available for androgen replacement or supplementation therapy. In men with hypogonadism, the goal of androgen therapy generally is to provide physiological levels of testosterone safely, inexpensively, and conveniently. Although there are now many different formulations of testosterone available for androgen replacement, none of these options are optimal (*see* Table 6).

Intramuscular Testosterone Esters

Testosterone that is administered orally or parenterally is rapidly metabolized by the liver (approx 10 min). Therefore, testosterone that is esterified to enanthate or cypionate to give it a longer half-life. Testosterone enanthate and testosterone cypionate have similar pharmacokinetics and may be administered at a dosage of 100–200 mg every 7–14 d. An intramuscular injection of 200 mg of testosterone enanthate or testosterone cypionate raises serum testosterone levels to a peak slightly

Table 6
Commercially Formulations of Testosterone Therapy

	Dosage	Treatment serum testosterone	Adverse drug effects	Cost per mo
Androderm® patch (Watson)	5-mg patch on torso, arms, or legs daily	Low- to mid-normal range	~35–70% develop skin rash	~$110
Testoderm® scrotal patch (Alza)	5-mg patch on shaved scrotal skin daily	Low- to mid-normal range	Poor adherence to scrotal skin	~$95
Testoderm TTS® patch (Alza)	4- or 6-mg patch on torso, arms, or buttocks daily	Low- to mid-normal range	~10% develop skin rash	~$100
Androgel® (Unimed)	5–10 g on upper arm or abdomen daily	Mid- to upper-normal range	Possible transfer to female partners	~$150
Testosterone cypionate or testosterone enanthate	100–250 mg im every 7–14 d	Mid- to slightly supraphysio-logical range	Pain with injections	$2–4 ± office visit

Source: Data from refs. *52–54*.

above the normal male range 24–48 h after administration, and then serum levels gradually decline and remain in the normal eugonadal range over the next 2 wk *(55,56)*. Serum gonadotropins are often suppressed by exogenous intramuscular testosterone therapy, and serum gonadotropins cannot be used as reliable markers to adjust the dosage of androgen replacement (unlike TSH in hypothyroidism). Therefore, adjustment of the dosage of intramuscular testosterone is generally based on a patient's symptomatology and not on serum hormone levels. Some experts recommend checking a serum total-testosterone on the day halfway between injections to verify that levels are in the midnormal range, but this is not essential *(57)*. In general, the starting dosage of intramuscular testosterone is 150–200 mg every 2 wk. For older men or younger men with very low serum testosterone levels, rapid normalization of serum androgen levels may be unpleasant (analogous to the abrupt onset of a second puberty). In these clinical situations, it is prudent to start with lower dosages of intramuscular testosterone ester (50–100 mg every 2 wk) or to use transdermal androgen-replacement therapy. Because older men are more likely to develop erythrocytosis while being administered intramuscular testosterone, 150 mg biweekly is often the maximum tolerable dosage *(58)*. Some men who are receiving intramuscular testosterone 150–200 mg every 14 d will notice disturbing fluctuations in mood, energy, and sexual function associated with rapidly fluctuating testosterone levels. Reducing the interval between injections to 75–100 mg every 7 d or switching to a transdermal therapy that gives more physiologic variations in testosterone levels might be useful.

Intramuscular testosterone injections are generally well tolerated *(59)*. In fact, anecdotal reports suggest that many hypogonadal men seem to prefer the higher peak testosterone levels achieved within 1–2 d after the injection. Intramuscular testosterone is also the least expensive form of androgen therapy and can be safely administered to virtually all hypogonadal men, even those patients with bleeding diatheses. Most men can be taught how to self-administer the intramuscular injections although some men are too fearful and require either a friend or a health professional to administer the injection. Although many men tolerate intramuscular testosterone therapy, this regimen does not provide physiological testosterone replacement, and many hypogonadal men would strongly prefer a less invasive route of delivery.

Transdermal Testosterone Patch Systems

There are three testosterone patch systems available for hypogonadal men. All of the patch systems are applied daily in the evening and produce a physiological circadian rhythm of testosterone levels with peak levels in the early-morning hour and a gradual decline in serum testosterone levels throughout the day (52). The first patch developed was Testoderm (Alza, Palo Alto, CA), which is applied to shaved scrotal skin. Scrotal skin is very thin and vascular and readily absorbs steroid hormones. However, the scrotal patch has not proven to be a very popular therapy because men object to shaving their scrota and because Testoderm does not adhere very well. Two nonscrotal systems have been developed for application to the torso, arms and buttocks (Androderm from Watson, Corona, CA, USA; Testoderm TTS from Alza, Palo Alto, CA). Both of these patches may commonly cause a rash although Testoderm TTS might cause a rash less frequently than Androderm (60).

Transdermal patch systems developed in the 1990s were a major advance for the treatment of male hypogonadism because they provided a safe, noninvasive mode of providing physiological androgen replacement. However, transdermal patch systems do not always provide adequate serum testosterone levels for many hypogonadal men, and it is very difficult to adjust the dosage. In contradistinction to intramuscular androgen replacement, testosterone levels must be monitored in men using transdermal patches to verify that adequate serum testosterone levels have been achieved.

Transdermal Testosterone Gel

A testosterone gel (Androgel; Unimed, Buffalo Grove) has recently been approved for use in hypogonadal men (53). Its pharmacokinetics are similar to the nonscrotal patches, but it causes significant skin irritation much less frequently (23,54). The chief advantages of Androgel are that the dosage may be adjusted more easily than patches and the gel raises serum testosterone levels formulation more reliably into the upper half of the normal range. The major drawback of Androgel is the possibility of vicariously transferring testosterone to female sexual partners and household contacts. This vicarious transfer of exogenous testosterone to sexual partners and household contacts might be avoided by showering shortly after applying the testosterone gel. In addition, the current price of Androgel is exorbitant. As with transdermal testosterone patches, serum testosterone levels must be monitored in hypogonadal men treated with Androgel.

Oral Androgen Therapy

Unmodified testosterone has a short half-life when ingested orally. Aklylated (at the 17α position), testosterone has a longer half-life. These alkylated androgens may cause serious hepatoxicity and should not be used in the treatment of hypogonadal men.

Novel Therapies

There are several novel therapies being tested that are likely to become available in the United States in the next decade. These therapies include oral testosterone undecanoate, long-acting testosterone esters that permit longer intervals between intramuscular injections (every 6–10 wk), and buccal testosterone formulations (61–63).

Treatment of Male Infertility Due to Secondary or Tertiary Hypogonadism

Men with primary hypogonadism have infertility that is untreatable with hormonal intervention. These men occasionally might have a few intratesticular sperm that can be harvested by a variety of microsurgical techniques; these sperm may then be used to fertilize an egg by one of the available assisted reproductive techniques such as intracytoplasmic injection (64,65).

Most men with infertility as a result of secondary hypogonadism may have spermatogenesis and fertility restored with appropriate hormonal therapy. In general, men with infertility due to pituitary disease will respond to gonadotropin replacement therapy. Gonadotropin replacement therapy generally requires both LH and FSH activity. LH replacement therapy is initiated after all exogenous androgens are discontinued, and LH replacement is generally administered as hCG (1000–2000 U subcutaneously 2–3 times weekly). These dosages might be excessive, and it is possible that 375–750 IU would be as effective as the conventional higher dosages (66). The dosage of hCG is adjusted after 3 mo if the serum testosterone has not normalized. Because some men produce sperm and become fertile with hCG treatment alone, and because FSH therapy is quite expensive, treatment with hCG alone is continued for 6–12 mo while sperm counts are performed monthly. Spermatogenesis takes a little over 10 wk, and sperm counts should not be expected to rise until at least 4–6 mo of treatment and may take 2–3 yr. FSH replacement may be accomplished with hMG (extracted and purified from urine of postmenopausal women) or human recombinant FSH. The usual starting dosage of FSH or hMG is 75 IU subcutaneously every other day. The dosage of FSH or hMG may be doubled if conception has not occurred within 6 mo of combination therapy with hCG. It should be noted that many gonadotropin-deficient men become fertile after appropriate treatment despite sperm counts (e.g., <5 million/mL) that are much lower than levels usually associated with fertility.

Most (80–90%) men with hypogonadotropism due to a hypothalamic defect (e.g., Kallmann's syndrome) can be successfully treated with either gonadotropin replacement therapy (as described above) or GnRH replacement therapy (subcutaneously every 2 h by a programmable mini-pump) with improvement in spermatogenesis and subsequent fertility (67–69). Although anecdotal reports suggest that GnRH replacement therapy might be slightly more effective than gonadotropin replacement therapy for men with hypothalamic infertility, gonadotropin therapy is more readily available.

Although appropriate exogenous gonadotropin or GnRH therapy normalize serum androgen levels in men with secondary hypogonadism, these therapies are much more expensive and complicated than testosterone administration. Thus, all men with primary hypogonadism and men with secondary hypogonadism who do not wish to be fertile should be treated with exogenous testosterone.

SIDE EFFECTS OF ANDROGEN THERAPY IN HYPOGONADAL MEN

Androgen-replacement therapy is well tolerated, and serious side effects are very rare. The most common side effect of androgen therapy is erythrocytosis, a side effect more common in older men (>65 yr). Other side effects that occur very infrequently include acne (usually in younger men), worsening fluid retention in patients with underlying edematous states, and precipitation or worsening of sleep apnea *(70,71)*. Hepatotoxicity is seen only with oral alkylated androgens. Some men will develop gynecomastia or transient breast tenderness initially with testosterone therapy (particularly with intramuscular testosterone); this effect is presumably the result of increased estrogen levels because of conversion by enzymatic aromatization of testosterone. Some men with very low serum testosterone levels are disturbed by the rapid increase in libido or altered mood when testosterone replacement is begun at full dose. These effects may be avoided by a gradual titration of the dosage or by using transdermal testosterone therapy that causes less dramatic shifts in sex steroid levels.

There is no evidence that exogenous testosterone stimulates the development of severe symptomatic prostatic hyperplasia or prostate cancer. When hypogonadal men are administered testosterone-replacement therapy, their prostate volumes and prostate-specific antigen levels rise to the level of age-matched controls *(72,73)*. It seems unlikely that exogenous testosterone therapy for hypogonadal men will raise the risk of prostatic disease above that of eugonadal men.

Although cardiovascular disease is more common in men than women, epidemiological studies of physiological levels of testosterone suggest that testosterone has a neutral or favorable effect on cardiovascular disease *(74)*. Testosterone has multiple effects on cardiovascular risk factors. Exogenous testosterone administration tends to suppress serum high-density cholesterol levels, but it also tends to suppress serum levels of atherogenic lipoprotein(a) *(75–77)*. In addition, exogenous testosterone acts as a coronary vasodilator in men with cardiovascular disease *(78)*. Thus, based on limited data, it appears that exogenous testosterone administration does not have hazardous cardiovascular effects and might even be beneficial for hypogonadal men.

CONCLUSION

Male hypogonadism is common and causes considerable morbidity. When a man presents with an atraumatic fracture or complaints of decreased libido or sexual dysfunction, unexplained weakness, decreased energy, or depressed mood, hypogonadism should be considered. When symptoms or physical examination findings (small testes, gynecomastia) suggest the possibility of hypogonadism, serum testosterone and gonadotropin levels should be determined. The total-testosterone assay is the most reliable clinical assay at this time, but a calculated bioavailable testosterone level might become the best indicator of circulating androgens when this method has been validated by more extensive use in primary care settings. It is essential to measure serum gonadotropins to distinguish between primary and secondary hypogonadism. Primary hypogonadism does not require any additional laboratory evaluation although some clinicians will order serum karyotyping for the definitive diagnosis of Klinefelter's syndrome. Secondary hypogonadism requires an evaluation to exclude hemochromatosis, hyperprolactinemia, Cushing's syndrome, and pituitary disease. Older men (>65 yr) with serum total-testosterone levels ≥ 2 ng/mL, normal serum transferrin, prolactin, T4, and TSH levels, no evidence of corticosteroid excess, and no complaints of headache or visual disturbances do not need to pituitary imaging. All other men with secondary hypogonadism should have a pituitary CT or MRI to exclude a macroadenoma. Men who are seeking fertility should be referred to an endocrinologist or reproductive specialist.

The benefits of androgen-replacement therapy outweigh the hazards for most hypogonadal men. Men with very low total testosterone levels (<2 ng/mL) unequivocally benefit from exogenous treatment. Those men with serum testosterone levels < 3.5 ng/mL and primary hypogonadism (elevated gonadotropins) should also be treated with exogenous testosterone. Men with secondary hypogonadism and levels between 2.0 and 3.5 ng/mL should be treated if they have clinical manifestations of hypogonadism.

Many men with low or low-normal serum testosterone levels such as older men, men with symptomatic HIV disease, men with end-stage renal disease and anemia, and men with other serious systemic illnesses might also benefit from androgen supplementation, but it is not clear what the marginal benefit is in these settings. When a clinician elects to treat such men with androgen therapy, it would be prudent to advise the patient that long-term consequences are unknown. Some experts advocate that the patient sign an informed consent form prior to beginning treatment. Six months of androgen therapy is adequate for most of the effects of androgen therapy except the trophic effects on bone that may take >24 mo for maximal benefit. Therefore, if a patient and physician elect to embark on a trial of testosterone therapy, 6 mo is generally an adequate trial. Most patients who do not experience a benefit will discontinue androgen therapy on their own after 6 mo.

The choice of androgen replacement depends on cost, convenience, and amount of androgen administration clinically necessary. Intramuscular testosterone is the least expensive therapy, but it requires biweekly intramuscular injections. Transdermal patches and gel offer a less invasive route of administration, but they must be applied daily and are much more costly than intramuscular testosterone therapy. Testosterone gel is more likely to restore serum testosterone levels than any of the patch systems, and the gel formulation is less likely to cause skin irritation. However, testosterone gel is very expensive and carries a risk of vicarious transfer of testosterone to household contacts and sexual partners.

There is a great deal of research and development occurring in the area of androgen effects in men. As we learn more about the effects and develop new therapies, we shall be better prepared to identify which men will benefit from exogenous androgen administration, and we will have the ability to tailor the androgen therapy for their individual needs.

REFERENCES

1. Amory JK, Anawalt BD, Paulsen CA, Bremner WJ. Klinefelter's syndrome. Lancet 2000;356:333–335.
2. Harman SM, Metter EJ, Tobin JD, et al. Longitudinal effects of aging on serum total and free testosterone levels in healthy men. J Clin Endocrinol Metab 2001;86:724–731.
3. Hammond G, Nisker J, Jones L, Siiteri P. Estimation of the percentage of free steroid in undiluted serum by centrifugal ultrafiltration dialysis. J Biol Chem 1980;255:5023–5026.
4. Pardridge W. Selective delivery of sex steroid hormones to tissues *in vivo* by albumin and by sex hormone-binding globulin. Ann NY Acad Sci 1988;538:173–192.
5. Plymate SR. Which testosterone assay should be used in older men? J Clin Endocrinol Metab 1998;83:3436–3438.
6. Cumming DC, Wall SR. Non-sex hormone-binding globulin-bound testosterone as a marker for hyperandrogenism. J Clin Endocrinol Metab 1985;61:873–876.

7. Rosner W. Errors in the measurement of plasma free testosterone. J Clin Endocrinol Metab 1997;82:2014–2015.

8. Winters SJ, Kelley DE, Goodpaster B. The analog free testosterone assay: are the results in men clinically useful? Clin Chem 1998;44:1278–1282.

9. Wheeler MJ. The determination of bio-available testosterone. Ann Clin Biochem 1995;32:345–357.

10. Sodergard R, Backstrom T, Shanbhag V, Carstensen H. Calculation of free and bound fractions of testosterone and estradiol 17β to human plasma protein at body temperature. J Steroid Biochem 1982;16:801–810.

11. Vermeulen A, Verdonck L, Kaufman JM. A critical evaluation of simple methods for the estimation of free testosterone in serum. J Clin Endocrinol Metab 1999;84:3666–3672.

12. Palermo GP, Schlegel PN, Sills ES, et al. Births after intracytoplasmic injection of sperm obtained by testicular extraction from men with nonmosaic Klinefelter's syndrome. N Engl J Med 1998;338:588–590.

13. Bremner WJ, Prinz PN. A loss of circadian rhythmicity in blood testosterone levels with aging in normal adult males. J Clin Endocrinol Metab 1983;56:1278–1281.

14. McDonnell SM, Pradyumna DP, Felitti V, et al. Screening for hemochromatosis in primary care settings. Ann Intern Med 1998;129:962–970.

15. Powell LW, George DK, McDonnell SM, Kowdley KV. Diagnosis of hemochromatosis. Ann Intern Med 1998;129:925–931.

16. Bhasin S, Storer TW, Berman N, et al. Testosterone replacement increases fat-free mass and muscle size in hypogonadal men. J Clin Endocrinol Metab 1997;82:407–413.

17. Finkelstein JS, Klibanski A, Neer RM, et al. Increases in bone density during treatment of men with idiopathic hypogonadotropic hypogonadism. J Clin Endocrinol Metab 1989;69:776–782.

18. Greenspan SL, Oppenheim DS, Klibanski A. Importance of gonadal steroids to bone mass in men with hyperprolactinemic hypogonadism. Ann Intern Med 1989;110:526–531.

19. Katznelson L, Finkelstein JS, Schoenfeld DA, et al. Increase in bone density and lean body mass during testosterone administration in men with acquired hypogonadism. J Clin Endocrinol Metab 1996;81:4358–4365.

20. Kubler A, Schulz G, Cordes U, et al. The influence of testosterone substitution on bone mineral density in patients with Klinefelter's syndrome. Exp Clin Endocrinol 1992;100:129–132.

21. Leifke E, Korner H-C, Link TM, et al. Effects of testosterone replacement therapy on cortical and trabecular bone mineral density, vertebral body area and paraspinal muscle area in hypogonadal men. Eur J Endocrinol 1998;138:51–58.

22. Wang C, Eyre DR, Clark R, et al. Sublingual testosterone replacement improves muscle mass and strength, decreases bone resorption, and increases bone formation markers in hypogonadal men—a clinical research center study. J Clin Endocrinol Metab 1996;81:3654–3662.

23. Wang C, Swerdloff RS, Iranmanesh A, et al. Transdermal testosterone gel improves sexual function, mood, muscle strength, and body composition parameters in hypogonadal men. J Clin Endocrinol Metab 2000;85:2839–2853.

24. Snyder PJ, Peachey H, Berlin JA, et al. Effects of testosterone replacement in hypogonadal men. J Clin Endocrinol Metab 2000;85:2670–2677.

25. Burris AS, Banks SM, Carter CS, et al. A long-term prospective study of the physiologic and behavioral effects of hormone replacement in untreated hypogonadal men. J Androl 1992;13:297–304.

26. Harman SM, Tsitouras PD, Costa PT, Blackman MR. Reproductive hormones in aging men. I. Measurement of sex steroids, basal luteinizing hormone and Leydig cell response to human chorionic gonadotropin. J Clin Endocrinol Metab 1980;51:35–41.

27. Veldhuis JD. Recent insights into neuroendocrine mechanisms of aging of the human male hypothalamo–pituitary–gonadal axis. J Androl 1999;20:1–17.

28. Veldhuis JD, Zwart A, Mulligan T, Iranmanesh A. Muting of androgen negative feedback unveils impoverished gonadotropin-releasing hormone/luteinizing hormone secretory reactivity in healthy older men. J Clin Endocrinol Metab 2001;86:529–535.

29. Harman SM, Tsitouras PD, Costa PT, Blackman MR. Reproductive hormones in aging men. II. Basal pituitary gonadotropins and gonadotropin responses to luteinizing hormone-releasing hormone. J Clin Endocrinol Metab 1982;54:547–551.

30. Snyder PJ, Reitano JF, Utiger RD. Serum LH and FSH responses to synthetic gonadotropin releasing hormone in normal men. J Clin Endocrinol Metab 1975;41:938–945.

31. Morley JE. Andropause, testosterone therapy and quality of life in aging men. Cleveland Clin J Med 2000;67:880–882.
32. Tenover JL. Male hormone replacement therapy including "Andropause." Endocrinol Metab Clin North Am 1998;27:969–987.
33. Sih R, Morley JE, Kaiser FE, et al. Testosterone replacement in older men: a 12-month randomized controlled trial. J Clin Endocrinol Metab 1997;82:1661–1667.
34. Bross R, Javanbakht M, Bhasin S. Anabolic interventions for aging-associated sarcopenia. J Clin Endocrinol Metab 1999;84:3420–3430.
35. Tenover JL. Testosterone for all? Proceedings of the 80th Meeting of the Endocrine Society, 1998.
36. Snyder PJ, Peachey H, Hannoush P, et al. Effect of testosterone treatment on body composition and muscle strength in men over 65 years of age. J Clin Endocrinol Metab 1999;84:2647–2653.
37. Snyder PJ, Peachey H, Hannoush P, et al. Effect of testosterone treatment on bone mineral density in men over 65 years of age. J Clin Endocrinol Metab 1999;84:1966–1972, 1999.
38. Johnson CA. Use of androgens in patients with renal failure. Sem Dial 2000;13:36–39.
39. Gaughan WJ, Liss KA, Dunn SR, et al. A 6-month study of low-dose recombinant human erythropoietin alone and in combination with androgens for the treatment of anemia in chronic hemodialysis patients. Am J Kidney Dis 1997;1997:495–500.
40. Teruel JL, Marcen R, Navarro-Antolin J, et al. Androgen *versus* erythropoietin for the treatment of anemia in hemodialyzed patients: a prospective study. J Am Soc Nephrol 1996;7:140–144.
41. Corcoran C, Grinspoon S. Treatments for wasting in patients with the acquired immunodeficiency syndrome. N Engl J Med 1999;340:1740–1750.
42. Grinspoon S, Corcoran C, Lee K. Loss of lean body and muscle mass correlates with androgen levels in hypogonadal men with acquired immunodeficiency and wasting. J Clin Endocrinol Metab 1996;81:4051–4058.
43. Salehian B, Jacobson D, Swerdloff RS, et al. Testicular pathologic changes and the pituitary-testicular axis during human immunodeficiency virus infection. Endocr Pract 1999;5:1–9.
44. Bhasin S, Storer TW, Javanbakht M, et al. Testosterone replacement and resistance exercise in HIV-infected men with weight loss and low testosterone levels. JAMA 2000;283:763–770.
45. Grinspoon S, Corcoran C, Askari H, et al. Effects of androgen administration in men with AIDS wasting syndrome. Ann Intern Med 1998;129:18–26.
46. Grinspoon S, Corcoran C, Stanley T, et al. Effects of hypogonadism and testosterone administration on depression indices in HIV-infected men. J Clin Endocrinol Metab 2000;85:60–65.
47. Rabkin JG, Wagner GJ, Rabkin R. A double-blind, placebo-controlled trial of testosterone therapy for HIV-positive men with hypogonadal symptoms. Arch Gen Psychiatry 2000;57:141–147.
48. Grinspoon S, Corcoran C, Parlman K, et al. Effects of testosterone and progressive resistance training in eugonadal men with AIDS wasting: a randomized, controlled trial. Ann Intern Med 2000; 133:348–355.
49. Sattler FR, Jaque SV, Schroeder ET, et al. Effects of pharmacological doses of nandrolone decanoate and progressive resistance training in immunodeficient patients infected with human immunodeficiency virus. J Clin Endocrinol Metab 1999;84:1268–1276.
50. Strawford A, Barbieri T, Van Loan M, et al. Resistance exercise and supraphysiologic androgen therapy in eugonadal men with HIV-related weight loss. JAMA 1999;281:1282–1290.
51. Bhasin S, Storer TW, Asbel-Sethi N, et al. Effects of testosterone replacement with a nongenital transdermal system, Androderm, in human immunodeficiency virus-infected men with low testosterone levels. J Clin Endocrinol Metab 1998;83:3155–3162.
52. Amory JK, Matsumoto AM. The therapeutic potential of testosterone patches. Exp Opin Invest Drugs 1998;7:1977–1985.
53. Letter TM. Androgel. Med Lett 2000;42:49-51.
54. Swerdloff RS, Wang C, Cunningham G, et al. Long-term pharmacokinetics of transdermal testosterone gel in hypogonadal men. J Clin Endocrinol Metab 2000;85:4500–4510.
55. Nankin HR. Hormone kinetics after intramuscular testosterone cypionate. Fertil Steril 1987;47:1004–1009.
56. Snyder PJ, Lawrence DA. Treatment of male hypogonadism with testosterone enanthate. J Clin Endocrinol Metab 1980;51:1335–1339.
57. Matsumoto AM. Hormonal therapy of male hypogonadism. Endocrinol Metab Clin North Am 1994;23:857–875.
58. Hajjar RR, Kaiser FE, Morley JE. Outcomes of long-term testosterone replacement in older hypogonadal males: a retrospective analysis. J Clin Endocrinol Metab 1997;82:3793–3796.

59. Mackey MA, Conway AJ, Handelsman DJ. Tolerability of intramuscular injections of testosterone ester in oil vehicle. Human Reprod 1995;10:862–865.

60. Jordan WP, Atkinson LE, Lai C. Comparison of the skin irritation potential of two testosterone transdermal systems: an investigational system and a marketed product. Clin Ther 1998;20:80–87.

61. Gooren LJG. A ten-year safety study of oral androgen testosterone undecanoate. J Androl 1994;15:212–215.

62. Dobs AS, Hoover DR, Chen M-C, Allen R. Pharmacokinetic characteristics, efficacy, and safety of buccal testosterone in hypogonadal males: a pilot study. J Clin Endocrinol Metab 1998;83:33–39.

63. Nieschlag E, Buchter D, von Eckardstein S, et al. Repeated intramuscular injections of testosterone undecanoate for substitution therapy in hypogonadal men. Clin Endocrinol 1999;51:757–763.

64. Khorram O, Patrizio P, Wang C, Swerdloff R. Reproductive technologies for male infertility. J Clin Endocrinol Metab 2001;86:2373–2379.

65. Kolettis PN. The evaluation and management of the azoospermic patient. J Androl 2002;23:293–305.

66. Bhasin S, Salehian B. Gonadotropin Therapy of Men with Hypogonadotropic Hypogonadism. Mosby-Year, St Louis, MO, 1997.

67. Nachtigall L, Boepple P, Pralong F, Crowley WFJ. Adult-onset idiopathic hypogonadotropic hypogonadism—a treatable form of male infertility. N Engl J Med 1997;336:410–415.

68. Christensen RB, Matsumoto AM, Bremner WJ. Idiopathic hypogonadotropic hypogonadism with anosmia (Kallmann's syndrome). Endocrinologist 1992;2:332–340.

69. Kliesch S, Behre HM, Nieschlag E. High efficacy of gonadotropin or pulsatile gonadotropin-releasing hormone treatment in hypogonadotropic hypogonadal men. Eur J Endocrinol 1994;131:347–354.

70. Matsumoto AM, Sandblom RE, Schoene RB, et al. Testosterone replacement in hypogonadal men: effects of obstructive sleep apnoea, respiratory drives, and sleep. Clin Endocrinol (Oxf) 1985;22:713–721.

71. Sandblom RE, Matsumoto AM, Schoene RB, et al. Obstructive sleep apnea syndrome induced by testosterone administration. N Engl J Med 1983;308:508–510.

72. Meikle AW, Arver S, Dobs AS. Prostate size in hypogonadal men treated with a nonscrotal permeation-enhanced testosterone transdermal system. Urology 1997;49:191–196.

73. Behre HM, Bohmeyer J, Nieschlag E. Prostate volume in testosterone-treated and untreated hypogonadal men in comparison to age-matched normal controls. Clin Endocrinol (Oxf) 1994;40:341–349.

74. Alexandersen P, Haarbo J, Christiansen C. The relationship of natural androgens to coronary disease in males: a review. Atherosclerosis 1996;125:1–13.

75. Bagatell CJ, Bremner WJ. Androgen and progestagen effects on plasma lipids. Prog Cardiovasc Dis 1995;38:255–271.

76. Bagatell CJ, Bremner WJ. The effects of aging and testosterone on lipids and cardiovascular risk. J Clin Endocrinol Metab 1998;83:3440–3441.

77. von Eckardstein A, Kliesch S, Nieschlag E, et al. Suppression of endogenous testosterone in young men increases serum levels of high density lipoprotein subclass lipoprotein A-I and lipoprotein(a). J Clin Endocrinol Metab 1997;82:3367–3372.

78. Webb CM, McNeill JG, Hayward CS, et al. Effects of testosterone on coronary vasomotor regulation in men with coronary heart disease. Circulation 1999;100:1690–1696.

INDEX

A

Acne,
  androgen replacement therapy induction,
    326, 327
  dutasteride studies, 83
  steroid 5α-reductase inhibitor therapy, 83
  virilization, 126
Aging,
  androgen replacement therapy,
    benefits and risks, 353, 429
    benign prostatic hyperplasia, 356, 357
    body composition effects,
      men, 249, 250, 353–355, 392, 429
      women, 253, 254
    bone response, 353, 429
    cardiovascular disease risks, 355
    clinical trial limitations, 352
    cognition effects, 297, 299, 355
    delivery system, 358–360
    gynectomastia, 357, 358
    polycythemia, 355, 356
    prostate cancer, 356, 357
    response heterogeneity and predictors, 396
    sexual function effects in men, 261, 262, 355
    sleep apnea, 357
  body composition changes, 249, 350
  bone loss, 350, 351
  cardiovascular disease, 352
  cognition effects of androgens, see Cognition,
    androgen effects
  demographics, 347
  erythropoiesis effects, 351, 352
  hypogonadism, 68, 69
  mood and cognitive function changes, 351
  prostate changes, 352
  sex hormone-binding globulin changes, 349
  sexual function changes, 351
  testosterone level changes,
    men, 178, 249, 297, 347–349, 428, 429*
    women, 271
AIDS wasting syndrome, see Human
    immunodeficiency virus
AIS, see Androgen insensitivity syndrome
Albumin, testosterone binding, 23
Alcoholism, hypogonadism, 69
Alopecia,
  androgen replacement therapy induction, 327
  male pattern baldness and steroid 5α-reductase
    inhibitor therapy, 82, 83
Anabolic steroids, see also Body composition,
    androgen effects,
  athletic performance effects, 398
  beliefs by athletic and academic communities,
    382, 383
  coronary artery disease risks, 194, 195
  detection of use, 398, 399
  dose–response in healthy young men, 386, 387
  history of use, 382
  incidence of use in athletes and bodybuilders,
    397, 398
  response heterogeneity and predictors, 395–397
  testosterone supraphysiologic dose effect on
    body composition and strength, 385, 386
Androgen ablation therapy, see also specific
    drugs,
  adjunctive therapy for prostate cancer, 177
  apoptosis induction,
    mitochondrial pathway, 174
    prostate cancer cell line studies, 175, 176
    rat ventral prostate studies, 174, 175
    receptor-mediated apoptosis, 172, 173
  benign prostatic hyperplasia, 178
  metastatic prostate cancer, 176–178
  side effects, 177
Androgen deficiency, female,
  bone effects, 369, 370
  diagnosis, 372, 373
  menopause, hormonal changes, 365
  risks and contraindications to testosterone
    treatment, 370–373
  signs and symptoms, 365, 366
  testosterone preparations and delivery, 373–375
Androgen excess, female, see also Hirsutism;
    Polycystic ovarian syndrome;
    Virilization,
  androgen sources, 123, 124
  Cushing's syndrome, 131
  differential diagnosis, 125
  nonclassical congenital adrenal hyperplasia, 130
  pathophysiology, 123–125
  phenotypic spectrum, 123

From: *Contemporary Endocrinology: Androgens in Health and Disease*
Edited by: C. Bagatell and W. J. Bremner © Humana Press, Totowa, NJ

polycystic ovaries, 131
Androgen insensitivity syndrome (AIS),
    androgen receptor mutations,
        DNA-binding domain mutations, 111, 112
        ligand binding absence,
            large-scale deletions, 105, 107
            point mutations, 109
            premature termination codons, 108
            small deletions and insertions, 107, 108
            splice variants, 108, 109
        ligand binding decreased levels, 112, 113
        ligand binding qualitative abnormalities,
            109–111
        minimal defects of virilization, 113, 114
        phenotype-genotype correlations, 114
    bone mineral density, 225
    infertility, 60
    phenotypic spectrum, 37, 38, 104, 105,
        114, 115
    Reifenstein syndrome, 59, 105
    testicular feminization, 58, 59, 104
Androgen receptor (AR),
    antiandrogens, 25
    coactivators, 35, 36, 159–161
    corepressors, 35, 36
    gene,
        locus, 158
        polymorphisms, 115
        structure, 27, 158
    ligand-independent activation, 36, 37
    mutations, see also Androgen insensitivity
        syndrome; Prostate cancer,
        distribution of mutations, 116, 117
        male infertility, 39
        spinal bulbar muscular atrophy, 38, 39,
            115–117
    phosphorylation, 27, 37
    steroid response elements, 33, 34
    structure,
        DNA-binding domain, 29-31
        hinge region, 32
        ligand-binding domain, 32, 33
        nuclear localization signal, 31, 32
        overview, 28, 105
        transactivation domain, 28, 29
    transcriptional activation mechanism, 23, 24,
        34, 35, 158
Androgen replacement therapy (ART),
    body composition effects, see Body composition,
        androgen effects
    bone response,
        men, 226
        women, 226, 227

cognition effects, see Cognition, androgen
    effects,
coronary artery disease effects,
    eugonadal men and lipid profiles, 201, 202
    hemostatic system effects, 204
    high-density lipoprotein, 199, 203
    hypogonadal men and lipid profiles, 200, 201
    lipoprotein(a), 203
    men, 195
    overview, 209
    women, 195, 196
delivery systems
    selection, 150, 151
    types, 141, 358, 359, 373–375
dosing and frequency of administration, 146,
    358, 359
female androgen deficiency, see Androgen
    deficiency, female
formulations under development, 324-326, 433
history of study, 360, 381, 382
hypogonadism treatment, see Hypogonadism,
    male
implants, 147, 148, 324
injectables, 144, 146
intramuscular testosterone esters, 430-432
local side effects, 329, 330
monitoring, 359, 360
older men supplementation, see Aging
oral preparations, 142–144, 432
parenteral testosterone esters for hypogonadism
    treatment, 317, 320–322
prostate cancer risks, 178, 328
puberty,
    constitutional delay of growth and puberty,
        341, 342
    permanent hypogonadism, 342–344
response heterogeneity and predictors, 395–397
selective androgen receptor modulators, 150, 326
sexual function effects, see Sexual function
testosterone derivatives, 142, 317–319
transdermal preparations, 148–150,
    322–324, 432
women, 373–375
Andropause, see Aging
Anorexia nervosa, sexual function response to
    testosterone, 281, 282
Aplastic anemia, androgen therapy, 237, 238
AR, see Androgen receptor
Aromatase,
    estrogen synthesis from testosterone, 16
    knockout mouse studies,
        clinical relevance, 98, 99
        follicle-stimulating hormone levels, 93
        luteinizing hormone levels, 92, 93

prostate differentiation and function, 97
seminal vesicle development, 98
sexual behavior, 91, 92
spermatogenesis, 94, 96, 97
mutation effects in males, 16, 17, 98
ART, *see* Androgen replacement therapy
Autoimmune testicular failure, types, 63

B

Benign prostatic hyperplasia (BPH),
α_1-blocker studies, 80, 81
androgen replacement therapy risks, 178, 328,
356, 357
antihormonal treatment, 178
definition, 170
epidemiology, 157, 170, 171
estrogen role, 171, 172
growth factors, 172
histopathology, 171
race differences, 170, 171
steroid 5α-reductase inhibitor therapy, 79–81
testosterone role, 171
Body composition, androgen effects,
aging,
androgen replacement therapy, *see* Aging
changes with aging, 249, 250, 350, 353–355
eugonadal men, testosterone response, 247–249
fat metabolism, 397
human immunodeficiency virus,
AIDS wasting syndrome and androgen
replacement therapy, 250, 252–254
testosterone deficiency, 250
hypogonadal men,
body composition, 382, 383
testosterone response, 243–247, 384, 385
muscle satellite cell response to testosterone,
387, 390, 391, 400
overview, 243, 255
puberty changes, 336
testosterone supraphysiologic dose effect on
body composition and strength, 385, 386
women studies,
AIDS wasting syndrome, 254, 371
menopause, 253, 254, 371
transsexuals, 253
Bone,
aging effects, 350, 351
androgens,
androgen replacement therapy response,
men, 226, 353
women, 226, 227, 369, 370
animal model studies, 224
bioavailability, 223
deficiency and osteoporosis, 225, 226

direct effects on bone cells, 223
human studies, 224, 225
metabolism, 224
prospects for study, 227
estrogen roles, 224
marrow, *see* Erythropoiesis
modeling, 222
puberty maturation and sex steroids,
336–341
remodeling and regulation, 222, 223
BPH, *see* Benign prostatic hyperplasia
Breast cancer,
androgen inhibition, 371, 372
androgen receptor,
distribution, 371
mutations, 112

C

CAD, *see* Coronary artery disease
CAH, *see* Congenital adrenal hyperplasia
Chemotherapy, hypogonadism induction, 63
Cholesterol,
mitochondrial transport, 7, 8
sources for steroidogenesis, 6
uptake, 6
Cirrhosis, hypogonadism, 69
Clitoromegaly, features, 126
Cognition, androgen effects,
aging effects, 351
androgen replacement therapy effects in aging,
297, 299, 355
animal studies,
activational effects, 293
organizational effects, 292, 293
central nervous system effects of testosterone,
291, 292
congenital adrenal hyperplasia studies,
299–301
endogenous androgen levels and cognitive
performance, 293, 294
exogenous androgen effects, 296
functional magnetic resonance imaging studies,
295, 296
history of study, 291
hypogonadism studies,
isolated hypogonadotropic hypogonadism,
301, 302
Kallmann's syndrome, 301, 302
Klinefelter's syndrome, 302–304
prospects for study, 304
sex differences, 294
spatial task considerations, 294, 295
Congenital adrenal hyperplasia (CAH),
cognition studies, 299–301

lipoid congenital adrenal hyperplasia,
  steroidogenic acute regulatory protein
  mutations, 7
nonclassical form and androgen excess in
  women, 130
Contraception, *see* Male contraception; Oral
  contraceptives
Coronary artery disease (CAD),
  dehydroepiandrosterone effects, 208
  epidemiology, 191, 192
  estrogen effects in men, 208, 209
  hematocrit levels and cardiovascular disease
    risks, 239, 240
  macrophage effects of testosterone, 206–208
  platelet effects of testosterone, 208
  serum testosterone levels and risks,
    animal studies, 196, 197
    men,
      anabolic steroid users, 194, 195
      androgen replacement therapy effects,
        195, 355
      cross-sectional clinical studies, 192
      endogenous androgen deprivation
        effects, 194
      prospective cohort studies, 192
    women,
      androgen replacement therapy effects,
        195, 196, 370, 371
      overview, 192, 193
      polycystic ovarian syndrome, 193, 194
  testosterone effects on risk factors,
    adipose tissue and insulin resistance effects
      of endogenous testosterone,
      men, 198
      polycystic ovarian syndrome, 198, 199
      women, 198
    androgen replacement therapy effects,
      eugonadal men and lipid profiles,
        201, 202
      hemostatic system effects, 204
      high-density lipoprotein, 199, 203
      hypogonadal men and lipid profiles, 200,
        201, 329
      lipoprotein(a), 203
      overview, 209
    vasoreactivity effects of androgens, 204–206
CPA, *see* Cyproterone acetate
Cryptorchidism, features, 61
Cushing's syndrome, androgen excess in
  women, 131
CYP11A,
  luteinizing hormone induction, 8
  testosterone synthesis, 4
CYP19, *see* Aromatase

Cyproterone acetate (CPA),
  deviant sexual behavior control, 266
  male contraception, 412
  sexual function effects on females, 281

D

Dehydroepiandrosterone (DHEA),
  aging effects on levels, 367
  bone effects in women, 369, 370
  coronary artery disease effects, 208
  metabolism, 366
  puberty levels, 338
  regulation of secretion, 366
  replacement effects on female sexual function,
    278, 279, 367, 368
Desogestrel (DSG), male contraception, 411, 412
DHEA, *see* Dehydroepiandrosterone
DHT, *see* Dihydrotestosterone
Dihydrotestosterone (DHT), *see also* Steroid 5α-
    reductase,
  cognition effects, 293
  deficiency in human immunodeficiency
    virus, 391
  functions, 78, 79, 142
  gels for androgen replacement therapy, 149,
    150, 325
  inactivation, 16
  metabolism, 26, 77, 78
  protein binding, 78
  synthesis from testosterone, 15, 16, 26, 77
DSG, *see* Desogestrel
Dutasteride, acne studies, 83

E

End-stage renal disease, *see* Uremia
ER, *see* Estrogen receptor
Erectile dysfunction, testosterone levels, 267, 268
Erythropoiesis, androgen stimulation,
  aging effects, 351, 352
  clinical applications,
    anemia of renal failure,
      androgen plus erythropoietin trial, 237
      androgen vs erythropoietin comparison
        trial, 236
      anephric vs intact kidney patients, 236
      erythropoietin response, 236
      overview, 235, 236
    aplastic anemia, 237, 238
    hemolytic anemia, 238
    myelodysplastic syndrome, 238
    polycythemia risks, 238, 239
    side effects, 238
  hematocrit levels and cardiovascular disease
    risks, 239, 240

history of study, 233, 234
mechanism of action,
    bone marrow response, 234
    erythropoietin induction, 234
    glucose uptake and red cell glycolysis, 235
    iron incorporation into red blood cells, 235
response in normal men, 235
Estrogen, *see also* Hormone replacement therapy,
    benign prostatic hyperplasia role, 171, 172
    bone effects, 224
    cognition effects, 293
    coronary artery disease effects in men, 208, 209
    puberty levels, 338
    replacement, *see* Hormone replacement therapy
    synthesis from androgens, 16, 366, 367
    testosterone synthesis regulation, 10, 11
Estrogen receptor (ER),
    deficiency effects in males, 16, 17, 98
    knockout mouse studies,
        clinical relevance, 98, 99
        follicle-stimulating hormone levels, 93
        luteinizing hormone levels, 92, 93
        prostate differentiation and function, 97
        seminal vesicle development, 98
        sexual behavior, 91, 92
        spermatogenesis, 94, 96, 97
        types, 90
Eugonadal men, androgen replacement therapy,
    body composition response, 247–249
    lipid profiles, 201, 202

F

Fat mass, *see* Body composition, androgen effects
Finasteride,
    benign prostatic hyperplasia studies, 79–81
    hirsutism studies, 83
    inhibition, 79
    male pattern baldness studies, 82, 83
    polycystic ovary syndrome management, 135
    prostate cancer studies, 81, 82
    safety, 84
    steroid 5α-reductase,
Flutamide, puberty effects, 340
Follicle-stimulating hormone (FSH),
    deficiency and hypogonadism, 66
    hypogonadism evaluation in males, 422, 425, 426
    knockout mouse studies, effects on levels,
        aromatase, 93
        estrogen receptor, 93
    male contraception targeting, 409, 410, 414
    puberty secretion, 336, 337
    testosterone synthesis regulation studies, 8
    therapy for infertility in hypogonadism, 433

FSH, *see* Follicle-stimulating hormone
Functional prepubertal castrate syndrome, hypogonadism, 54, 55

G

GH, *see* Growth hormone
Glucocorticoids, testosterone replacement in chronic users, 395
GnRH, *see* Gonadotropin-releasing hormone
Gonadotropin-releasing hormone (GnRH),
    antagonists for male contraception, 409, 410, 414
    pulsatile secretion, 9, 10
    receptor signaling, 10
    therapy for infertility in hypogonadism, 433
Growth hormone (GH),
    sex steroid interactions in puberty, 338, 339
    testosterone synthesis regulation studies, 8, 9
Gynecomastia, androgen replacement therapy induction, 327, 328, 357, 358

H

hCG, *see* Human choroinic gonadotropin
HDL, *see* High-density lipoprotein
Hematocrit, levels and cardiovascular disease risks, 239, 240, 327
Hemochromatosis, hypogonadism, 68, 428
Hemolytic anemia, androgen therapy, 238
High-density lipoprotein (HDL), androgen replacement therapy effects, 199, 203, 329
Hirsutism, *see also* Polycystic ovarian syndrome,
    definition, 127
    differential diagnosis, 127, 128
    mechanisms, 127
    steroid 5α-reductase inhibitor therapy, 83
    treatment, 131, 132, 135
    virilization, 126
HIV, *see* Human immunodeficiency virus
Hormone replacement therapy (HRT), sexual function effects,
    natural menopause, 274, 275
    overview of considerations, 273, 274, 368
    summary of studies, 278
    surgical menopause, 275–278
HRT, *see* Hormone replacement therapy
Human choroinic gonadotropin (hCG), testosterone synthesis regulation studies, 10
Human immunodeficiency virus (HIV),
    AIDS wasting syndrome and androgen replacement therapy,
        men, 250, 252, 253, 393–395, 430
        rationale, 393
        response heterogeneity and predictors, 395, 396

women, 254
dihydrotestosterone deficiency, 391
testosterone deficiency, 250, 393, 430
Hyperandrogenism, *see* Androgen excess, female
Hypoandrogenism, *see* Androgen deficiency,
        female; Hypogonadism, male
Hypogonadism, male,
    aging, 68, 69
    androgen receptor defects,
        infertility, 60
        Reifenstein syndrome, 59
        testicular feminization, 58, 59
    androgen replacement therapy,
        body composition response, 243–247,
            384, 385
        contraindications, 326, 330
        formulations,
            development, 324–326, 433
            intramuscular testosterone esters,
                430–432
            parenteral testosterone esters, 317,
                320–322, 432
            subcutaneous pellets, 324
            table, 318, 319
            transdermal formulations, 322–324, 432
        illness, *see* Human immunodeficiency virus
        initiation, 315, 316, 435
        lipid profile response, 200, 201
        older men, *see* Aging
        renal failure, *see* Uremia
        response heterogeneity and predictors, 396
        risks and monitoring, 326–330, 434
        sexual function response, 260, 261
        therapeutic goals and benefits, 316, 330
    autoimmune testicular failure, 63
    body composition, 382, 383
    chemotherapy induction, 63
    cirrhosis, 69
    classification, 46, 48, 422–424
    clinical presentation, 45–48, 420
    cognition studies of androgen effects,
        isolated hypogonadotropic hypogonadism,
            301, 302
        Kallmann's syndrome, 301, 302
        Klinefelter's syndrome, 302–304
    cryptorchidism, 61
    definition, 45, 419, 420
    diagnosis and work-up,
        gonadotropin serum assay, 422, 425, 426
        overview, 314–316, 330, 434, 435
        testosterone serum assay, 420–422, 425, 426
    enzyme deficiencies,
        steroid 5α-reductase, 56, 57
        testosterone biosynthesis enzymes, 55, 56

follicle-stimulating hormone deficiency, 66
functional prepubertal castrate syndrome, 54, 55
gonadotropin-resistant testis, 57
hemochromatosis, 68, 428
hypogonadotropic hypogonadism, 64–66
illness induction, 67, 68, 313
infertility treatment, 433, 434
irradiation of testes, 62, 63
Kallmann syndrome, 64, 65
Klinefelter syndrome,
    etiology, 51
    incidence, 49
    laboratory findings, 50
    phenotype, 49
    psychopathology, 50, 51
leprosy, 61
luteinizing hormone deficiency, 66
mumps orchitis, 60
myotonic dystrophy, 53, 54
Noonan syndrome, 53
persistent Müllerian duct syndrome, 58
pituitary adenoma, 428
prevalence, 420
primary hypogonadism features, 46, 48, 49
prolactinoma, 66, 67
secondary hypogonadism differential diagnosis,
    427, 428, 434
Sertoli-cell-only syndrome, 54
sickle cell disease, 69, 70
testicular trauma, 61, 62
uremia, 68, 429, 430
XX males, 51, 52
XY/XO mixed gonadal genesis, 52
XYY syndrome, 53

I

IGF-1, *see* Insulin-like growth factor-1
IL-1, *see* Interleukin-1
Illness, *see also* Human immunodeficiency virus;
        Uremia,
    hypogonadism induction, 67, 68, 313
    muscle wasting, 391
Insulin-like growth factor-1 (IGF-1), muscle
        anabolism role, 390
Insulin resistance,
    coronary artery disease, endogenous
            testosterone effects,
        men, 198
        polycystic ovarian syndrome, 198, 199
        women, 198
    polycystic ovary syndrome and management,
        129, 134
Interleukin-1 (IL-1), testosterone synthesis
        regulation studies, 9

K

Kallmann syndrome,
cognition studies of androgen effects, 301, 302
features, 64, 65
Klinefelter syndrome,
cognition studies of androgen effects, 302-304
etiology, 51
incidence, 49
laboratory findings, 50
phenotype, 49
psychopathology, 50, 51

L

Lean mass, *see* Body composition, androgen effects
Leprosy, hypogonadism, 61
Levonorgestrel (LNG), male contraception, 410, 411
Leydig cell,
features, 3
steroid receptors, 9
testosterone synthesis, 3, 4
LH, *see* Luteinizing hormone
Libido, *see* Sexual function
Lipoid congenital adrenal hyperplasia (LCAH),
steroidogenic acute regulatory protein mutations, 7
Lipoprotein(a), androgen replacement therapy effects, 203
LNG, *see* Levonorgestrel
Luteinizing hormone (LH),
deficiency and hypogonadism, 66
estrogen regulation, 10, 11
gonadotropin-resistant testis, 57
hypogonadism evaluation in males, 422, 425, 426
knockout mouse studies, effects on levels,
aromatase, 92, 93
estrogen receptor, 92, 93
puberty secretion, 336, 337
receptor signaling, 6
testosterone suppression, 10
testosterone synthesis regulation,
acute regulation, 6–8
long-term regulation, 8
therapy for infertility in hypogonadism, 433

M

Macrophage, effects of testosterone, 206–208
Male contraception,
19-nortestosterone, 408, 409
gonadotropin-releasing hormone antagonists
and testosterone combinations, 409, 410
MENT, 409
progestin and testosterone combinations, 410–412
prospects, 414
rationale, 405, 406
testosterone suppression of spermatogenesis,
ethnic differences, 406, 407
sperm count, 406
testosterone enanthate contraception trials, 407, 408
testosterone undecanoate, 408
Male pattern baldness, steroid 5α-reductase
inhibitor therapy, 82, 83
Medroxyprogesterone acetate, deviant sexual
behavior control, 266
Menopause, *see* Aging; Androgen deficiency, female
MENT,
male contraception, 409
potency, 326
Metformin, polycystic ovary syndrome
management, 134
Mumps orchitis, features, 60
Muscle, *see* Body composition
Myelodysplastic syndrome, androgen therapy, 238
Myotonic dystrophy, hypogonadism, 53, 54

N

NETE, *see* Norethisterone enanthate
Noonan syndrome, hypogonadism, 53
Norethisterone enanthate (NETE), male
contraception, 412

O

Obesity, control in polycystic ovary syndrome, 132, 133
OC, *see* Oral contraceptives
Oral contraceptives (OC),
effects on sexual function, 280, 281
testosterone suppression, 367
Ornithine decarboxylase inhibitors, polycystic
ovary syndrome management, 133
Osteoporosis, androgen deficiency, 225, 226
Oxandrolone, role in pubertal growth, 339, 340

P

P450c17,
luteinizing hormone induction, 8
testosterone synthesis, 5, 6
P450scc, *see* CYP11A
PACAP, *see* Pituitary adenylate cyclase-activating
polypeptide
PCOS, *see* Polycystic ovarian syndrome
Persistent Müllerian duct syndrome,
hypogonadism, 58

Pituitary adenoma, male hypogonadism, 428
Pituitary adenylate cyclase-activating polypeptide
        (PACAP), fetal testosterone
        biosynthesis regulation, 8
Platelet, effects of testosterone, 208
Polycystic ovarian syndrome (PCOS),
    cardiovascular disease, 129, 130
    coronary artery disease, 193, 194, 198, 199
    diagnostic criteria, 125
    gynecological cancer association, 129
    infertility, 128, 129
    insulin resistance, 129
    natural history, 128
    treatment,
        antiandrogens, 134, 135
        finasteride, 135
        hirsutism, 131, 132, 135
        insulin sensitizers,
            metformin, 134
            thiazolidinediones, 134
        lifestyle modification, 132, 133
        ornithine decarboxylase inhibitors, 133
        ovarian suppressive therapies, 133
        overview, 131, 132
        spironolactone, 134, 135
        surgery, 136
Polycythemia, androgen therapy association, 238,
        239, 355, 356
Precocious puberty, definition, 335
Pregnenolone, testosterone conversion pathways, 4–6
Progestins, male contraception, 410–412
Prolactin, testosterone synthesis regulation studies, 8
Prolactinoma, hypogonadism, 66, 67
Prostate,
    aging effects, 352
    androgen receptor expression, 157, 158
    development, 157
    knockout mouse studies, effects on differentiation
        and function,
        aromatase, 97
        estrogen receptor, 97
Prostate cancer,
    androgen ablation therapy,
        adjunctive therapy, 177
        apoptosis induction,
            mitochondrial pathway, 174
            prostate cancer cell line studies, 175, 176
            rat ventral prostate studies, 174, 175
            receptor-mediated apoptosis, 172, 173
        metastatic prostate cancer, 176–178
        side effects, 177
    androgen dependence, 164
    androgen receptor,
        activation,

        ligand-independent activation, 169, 170
        nongenomic effects, 170
    mutations,
        androgen-independent cancer, 164
        CAG repeats, 168, 169
        detection, 165
        gain-of-function mutations, 165, 167, 168
        latent prostate cancer mutations, 167
        loss-of-function mutations, 168
        overview, 38, 116, 117, 166, 167
    androgen replacement therapy risks, 178, 328,
        356, 357
    epidemiology, 157, 161
    steroid 5α-reductase inhibitor therapy, 81, 82
    testosterone levels and cancer risks,
        fetal development, 161, 162
        nested case control studies, 163
        racial differences, 163
Prostate serum antigen (PSA), androgen replacement
        therapy monitoring, 328, 329
PSA, see Prostate serum antigen
Puberty,
    androgen replacement therapy,
        constitutional delay of growth and puberty,
            341, 342
        permanent hypogonadism, 342–344
    body composition changes, 336
    bone maturation and sex steroids, 336–341
    definition, 335
    dehydroepiandrosterone levels, 338
    estrogen levels, 338
    flutamide effects, 340
    gonadotropin secretion, 336, 337
    growth hormone-sex steroid interactions,
        338, 339
    growth spurt, 336
    oxandrolone role in growth, 339, 340
    precocious puberty, 335
    secondary sexual characteristics, 336
    sexual function and androgens,
        females, 269, 270
        males, 264–266
    tamoxifen effects, 340
    testosterone levels, 337

R

Radiation therapy, hypogonadism induction, 62, 63
Red blood cell, see Erythropoiesis
Reifenstein syndrome, features, 59
Renal failure, see Uremia

S

SARMs, see Selective androgen receptor modulators
SBMA, see Spinal bulbar muscular atrophy

Selective androgen receptor modulators (SARMs),
        clinical use, 150, 326
Seminal vesicle, knockout mouse studies of
        development,
    aromatase, 98
    estrogen receptor, 98
Sertoli-cell-only syndrome, hypogonadism, 54
Sex hormone-binding globulin (SHBG),
    aging changes, 349
    androgen-binding protein variant, 13, 26
    female production in aging, 272
    functions, 13, 23
    insulin resistance role, 13, 14
    levels across lifespan, 13
    ligands, 25, 366
    receptors, 25
    regulation of levels, 14
    structure, 13, 25
    testosterone level correlation, 14, 15
Sexual differentiation, overview, 103, 104
Sexual function, men,
    aging,
        androgen replacement therapy response, 355
        effects, 261, 262, 351
    developmental aspects in puberty, 264–266
    deviant sexual behavior control,
        cyproterone acetate, 266
        medroxyprogesterone acetate, 266
    erectile dysfunction and testosterone levels,
        267, 268
    experimental manipulation of testosterone and
        effects,
        increasing testosterone, 263, 264
        lowering testosterone, 263
        varying levels within normal range, 264
    hypogonadism and androgen replacement
        therapy response, 260, 261
    medication side effects, 267
    sex differences in testosterone effects,
        desensitization hypothesis, 284, 285
        findings, 282–284
    variations in testosterone levels, 263
Sexual function, women,
    anorexia nervosa response to testosterone,
        281, 282
    clinical studies of low sexual desire, 279
    cyproterone acetate effects, 281
    dehydroepiandrosterone replacement effects,
        278, 279, 367, 368
    endocrine abnormalities, 280
    hormone replacement therapy effects,
        natural menopause, 274, 275
        overview of considerations, 273, 274, 368
        summary of studies, 278

surgical menopause, 275–278
    masturbation onset, 269, 270
    oral contraceptive effects, 280, 281
    overview of testosterone effect findings, 282
    postmenopausal function, 271–273
    sex differences in testosterone effects,
        desensitization hypothesis, 284, 285
        findings, 282–284
    testosterone production,
        development, 269
        lactation, 271
        menstruation, 270, 271, 367
        pregnancy, 271
SHBG, see Sex hormone-binding globulin
Sickle cell disease, hypogonadism, 69, 70
Sleep apnea, androgen replacement therapy
        induction, 327, 357
Spermatogenesis,
    androgen replacement therapy effects, 329
    gonadotropin therapy for infertility in
        hypogonadism, 433
    knockout mouse studies,
        aromatase, 94, 96, 97
        estrogen receptor, 94, 96, 97
    maturation of sperm, 406
    testosterone suppression,
        ethnic differences, 406, 407
        sperm count, 406
        testosterone enanthate contraception trials,
            407, 408
Spinal bulbar muscular atrophy (SBMA), androgen
        receptor mutations, 38, 39, 115–117
Spironolactone,
    polycystic ovary syndrome management,
        134, 135
    sexual side effects, 267
Steroid 5α-reductase,
    deficiency, 26, 27, 56, 57
    dihydrotestosterone synthesis from testosterone,
        15, 16, 26, 77
    inhibitors and applications,
        acne, 83
        benign prostatic hyperplasia studies, 79–81
        dutasteride, 83
        finasteride, 79
        hirsutism, 83
        male pattern baldness, 82, 83
        polycystic ovary syndrome, 135
        prostate cancer, 81, 82
        safety, 84
    isoforms, 26, 27, 78, 79, 83, 84
    ligands, 26, 27
    muscle, 391
Steroidogenic acute regulatory protein (StAR),

lipoid congenital adrenal hyperplasia
    mutations, 7
luteinizing hormone induction, 7, 8
Stroke, hematocrit levels and cardiovascular dis-
    ease risks, 239, 240

T

Tamoxifen, puberty effects, 340
Testicular trauma, hypogonadism, 61, 62
Testosterone,
    aging changes,
        men, 178, 249, 297, 347–349, 428, 429
        women, 271
    assays, 349, 420–422, 425, 426
    benign prostatic hyperplasia role, 171
    bioavailability in serum, 348, 349
    circulating levels, 11, 13, 23
    contraception, *see* Male contraception
    coronary artery disease role, *see* Coronary
        artery disease
    dose-response in healthy young men, 386, 387
    female production,
        development, 269
        lactation, 271
        menstruation, 270, 271, 367
        pregnancy, 271
    female production,
        aging, 271
        development, 269
        lactation, 271
        menstruation, 270, 271
        pregnancy, 271
    functional overview, 89
    metabolism, 15–17, 26, 292
    prostate cancer risks, *see* Prostate cancer
    protein binding, *see* Albumin; Sex hormone-
        binding globulin
    puberty levels, 337
    replacement therapy, *see* Androgen
        replacement therapy

suppression by medications, 348
supraphysiologic dose effect on body
    composition and strength, 385, 386
synthesis,
    biosynthetic pathway, 4–6
    enzyme defects and male hypogonadism,
        55, 56
    hormone interactions, 8–10
    Leydig cells, 3, 4
    luteinizing hormone regulation,
        acute regulation, 6–8
        long-term regulation, 8
    negative feedback, 10
    prospects for study, 17
    sites, 3
    target tissues, 142
Thiazolidinediones, polycystic ovary syndrome
    management, 134

U

Uremia,
    anemia of renal failure, androgen therapy,
        androgen plus erythropoietin trial, 237
        androgen vs erythropoietin comparison
            trial, 236
        anephric vs intact kidney patients, 236
        erythropoietin response, 236, 395
        overview, 235, 236
    hypogonadism, 68, 429, 430

V

Virilization,
    clinical presentation, 125, 126
    differential diagnosis, 126, 127

X

XX males, hypogonadism, 51, 52
XXY males, *see* Klinefelter syndrome
XY/XO mixed gonadal genesis, features, 52
XYY syndrome, hypogonadism, 53